MW01115625

Herbal Therapeutics
For Women, Pregnancy, & Children

Jesse Wolf Hardin & Kiva Rose Hardin – Editors

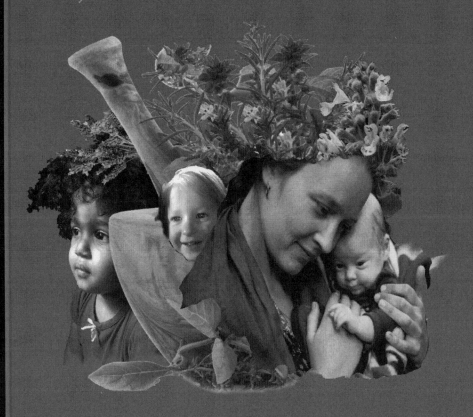

From The Pages of Plant Healer Quarterly

(c) MMXX Plant Healer LLC

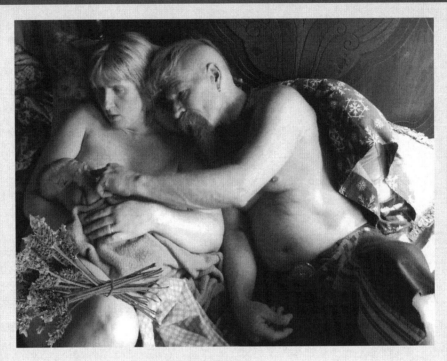

PREFACE

Giving birth miles from pavement, and a hundred miles from the nearest medical assistance, is not something I would be comfortable recommending. And yet, it was exactly those circumstances that my wife Kiva and I found ourselves in. A midwife who had promised to attend, cancelled a couple weeks before the delivery. Kiva is uncommonly sensitive and suffers anxiety around strangers and crowds, so we chose to read up on potential difficulties and stock up on herbal remedies… and to take the risk of delivering at home in our wilderness sanctuary.

The emergency birthing manuals and scary online case studies did nothing to ease our trepidation, but we were greatly comforted by what our friend Dr. Kenneth Proefrock said:

"With some rare exceptions, we need to understand that giving birth is not a medical procedure."

Labor was lengthy and painful, with Kiva eventually needing to break the amniotic sac digitally in oder to make our son Aelfyn's entry into the world possible. It was medicinal plants that staunched her bleeding after the birth, and Ashwaghanda that helped most to regulate the moods and hormonal system the birth had disrupted.

I had the honor of pressing my thumbs into the small of her back for literally hours in order to ease the pain, and to be the first to hold what has become a most wondrous addition to our already meaningful existence. I almost daily recall handing him to his mother, and the wondrous look on her face.

It is to her, and to our child, that this book is dedicated.

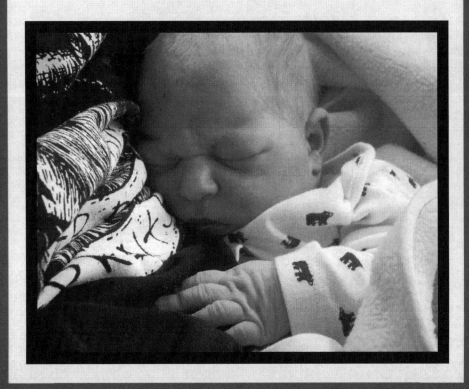

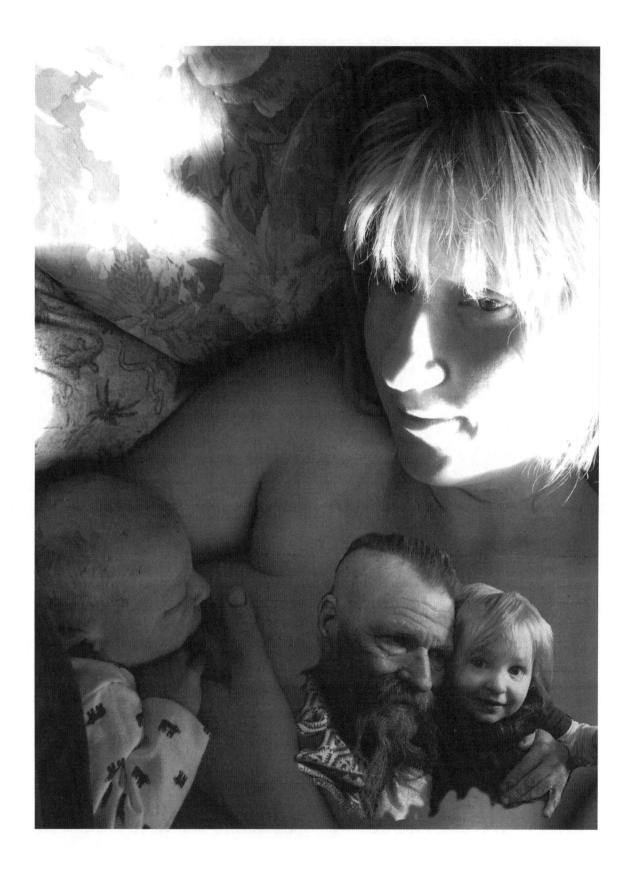

Herbal Therapeutics For Women, Pregnancy & Children is a compilation with chapters drawn directly from past issues of the esteemed Plant Healer Quarterly, appearing in the exact form they appeared in the Quarterly's pages. While other PHQ compilations cover treatments and materia medica, this is the first time we have devoted an entire book to the wellbeing of women and offspring.

As always, we are thankful to the experience, skills, perspectives and insights of our often incredible Plant Healer authors and plant practitioners:

Juliette Abigail Carr • Dr. Kenneth Proefrock • Dr. Aviva Romm
Juanita Nelson • Sabrina Lutes • Juliet Blankespoor
Julie James • Alanna Whitney • Katja Swift • Briana Wiles
Jennie Isbell Shinn • Elaine Sheff • Debra Swanson
Wendy Hounsel • Anja Robinson • Erin Piorier
Angela Justis • Adrie Lester • Astrid Grove • Rosalee de la Foret

Not every course of action described here may prove efficacious over time, applicable to you personally, or be the best course of action for women's and children's varying constitutions. As with all assessment and treatment, be cautions with your suggestions and amend them according to effects. Observance, caution, study, critical thinking, and your personal experiences are your best tools and guides as you seek to foster health in yourself and others. And this book can start you on the way to safely tend and bolster your self, your family, clients and community.

–Jesse Wolf Hardin
Anima Botanical Sanctuary, NM

Jesse Wolf Hardin & Kiva Rose Hardin, Editors
(C) MMXX by Plant Healer
All other rights remain exclusively with the contributing authors
PlantHealer.org – PlantHealerMagazine.com

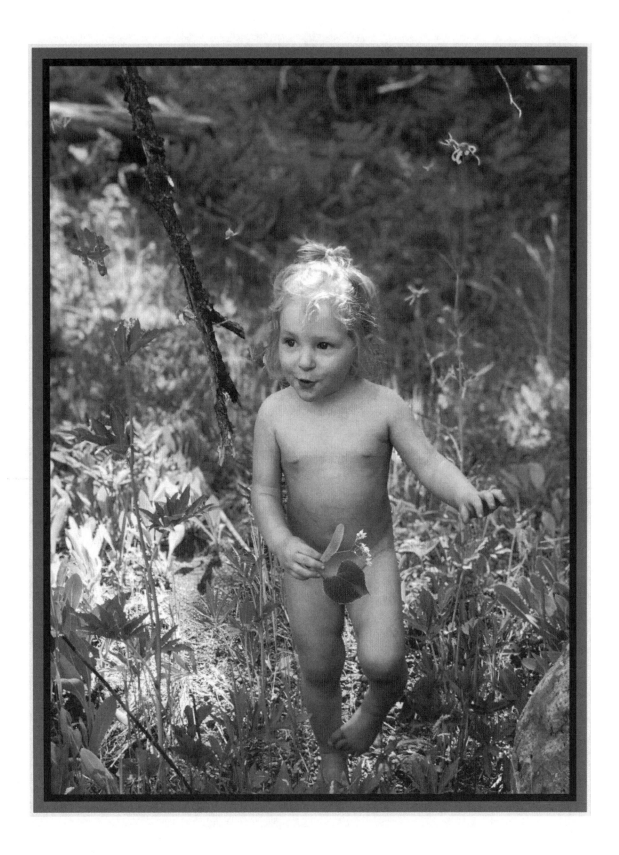

CONTENTS

PART II

HERBAL THERAPEUTICS & PREGNANCY

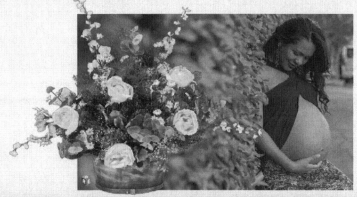

Part III

Herbal Therapeutics For Children

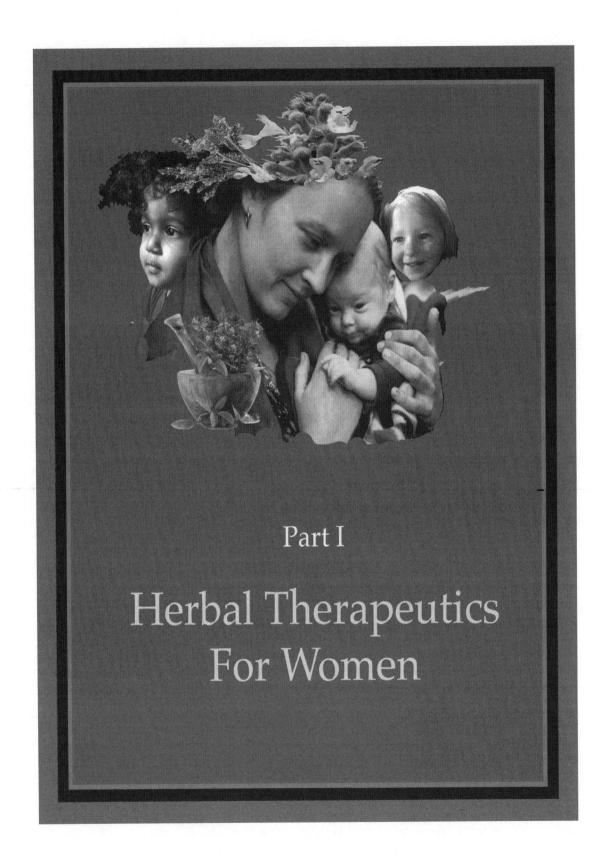

Part I

Herbal Therapeutics
For Women

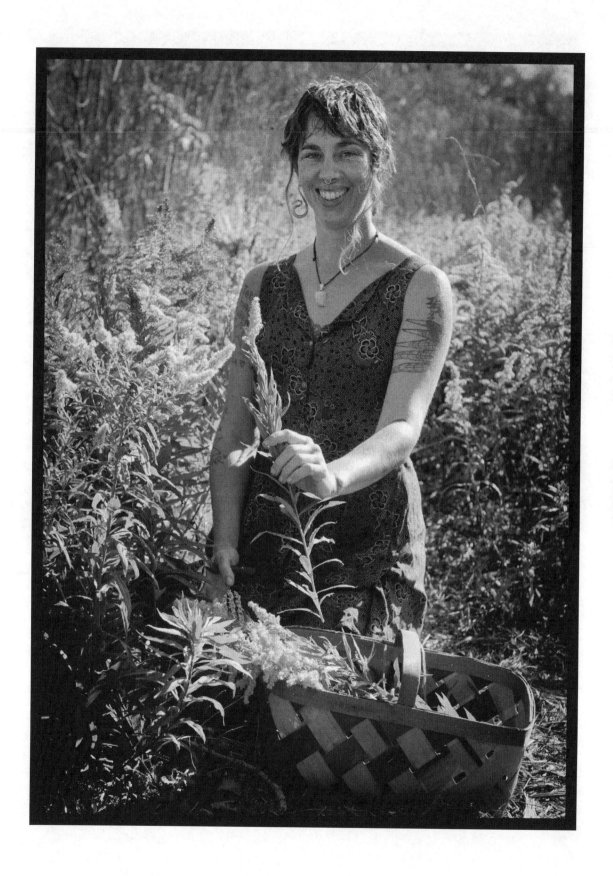

TAKING CARE OF OUR PINK PARTS

by Jen Stovall

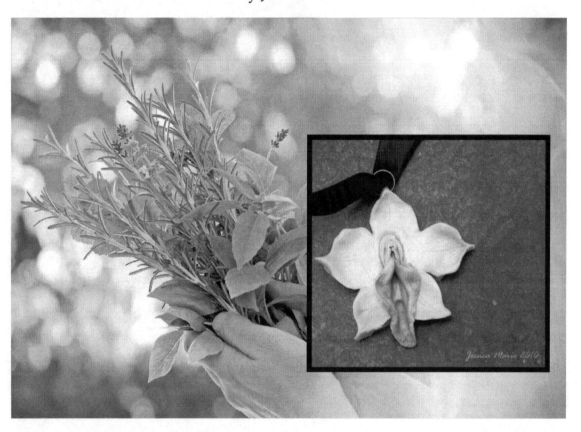

Talking about those areas where the sun don't shine can prove to be difficult in a society where our main associations with these parts of us are shame and/or sex. However, not having body positive conversations about how we can care for our bits can leave our clients stuck in the dark struggling with no one to turn to for these sensitive matters. We herbalists all too often spend our time developing wonderful herb formulas for internal use or recommending a topical treatment when there is skin irritation or muscle and joint pain. Yet when dealing with imbalances in the pelvic region, our approach to topical treatments frequently lacks creativity. This is often a detriment to our treatment plans where these applications can be extremely helpful. It can also be healing to address the importance of care and attention for these oft-neglected parts.

One of the major tenets of herbal medicine is direct contact with affected tissues for as long of a time as possible in order to have the best effect, which is simple when we are trying to use herbs on our skin and some of our more accessible mucous membranes. But, what about when someone has an issue that revolves around their generative organs that needs attention? Caring for these tender tissues can be a delicate issue to address with a client and many of us steer clear of these discussions.

Yet, it is important that we as herbalists have as many tools in our back pockets as possible and being able to educate our clients on ways to care for their genitals is one of these useful tools. This is true when we want to support folks dealing with more obvious issues like STIs, bacterial and/or yeast infections, UTIs, and hemorrhoids. But it is equally useful in situations of sexual trauma, pelvic stagnation, abortion/miscarriage, and discomfort due to long term tucking for some trans women. To be clear, I don't advise these applications as the only treatment necessary for many of these situations but I find that they are invaluable additions to our treatment plans and often make the difference of bringing the system back into balance much quicker. Unfortunately, I find them to be extremely underused.

Many times, these parts of our body are left unnamed, addressed as slang or taboo hush words, called private, or not referred to at all. They may be tucked into clothes and constricting underwear that don't breathe or are too tight and are not allowed to see the light of day or feel the wind drift across their delicate tissues often enough. These parts of us are often kept in the dark; hold feelings of shame, or memories of trauma. These parts are often only talked about being cared for when we focus on ways to make them look appealing to others or fit a mainstream idea of what beauty looks like. These parts are often taught that they are shameful and a source of embarrassment...or pride, based on other's assessment of their inherent value and worth. It is vitally important to remember all of these feelings, connotations, and possibilities when we discuss ways to ask people to open up, contact, look at, care for, and address these parts of ourselves. This is not an issue for everyone we work with, but for those that it is, it is important to be aware of and not something to dismiss lightly. I would also argue that these associations are the reason that many herbalists struggle to discuss these treatments and applications. And that this is why we need to try even harder to be comfortable discussing them. Overcoming these stigmas and having healing conversations about these parts of our body can be empowering for both our clients and us.

There are many different types of genital care that can be used and some applications definitely seem to work better than others for certain issues. I will address how each of the applications can affect different types of genitalia, which application is best for certain issues, and some herbs that work best for each type. I am not going to go into each herb and how it might be used because I find that just as with internal treatments, genital treatments should also be individualized. Not everyone experiences the same response to an infection or the same reason why the infection settled in and took up residence in those tissues as everyone else. So, I will give a brief overview of herbs that are commonly used but encourage everyone to research the herbs that might be best for each person's constitution and the particular energetics of their imbalance/experience. I also want to acknowledge that many of these treatments are often discussed as being only for people with vaginas, but I don't find that to be true. There can be cautions for those folks with more dangly parts that I will discuss in those sections, but all of these applications can work for everyone. I encourage everyone to experiment with each of these applications before recommending any of them to others.

A quick note on pelvic stagnation: so many people I work with have some amount of pelvic stagnation. This can be due to wearing constrictive clothes, too much time spent sitting, a stagnant/ liver/colon/insert other organ here, or stemming from emotions. Therefore, I find that knowing ways we can address this condition from many angles is extremely important. The first two applications below are external ways we can get some lymph and blood flow to the area in order to break up some of that stagnant energy.

Pelvic Steams

One of the ones that I see a lot of media about these days is pelvic steams. You might have heard these referred to as bajos, chai-yok, V- steam, or a Yoni Steam…some of these are names that refer to it's use for people with vaginas but I've also seen it used to good effect for people with penises too. These have been used traditionally in many different cultures and have been co-opted by folks in this country as of late. Thanks to all the traditional cultures who have lent (whether willing or not) their healing traditions to benefit the generative organs of ours. So, lets give a collective nod of thanks to those traditions and also think of healing our relationship with those communities who we have benefited from but who have often not benefited from that same relationship as we acknowledge where this wisdom flows from. On with the essay…

Pelvic steams warm and relax the pelvic floor, stimulating blood and lymph flow to those areas, cleansing and nourishing the pelvic region. The warmth of the steam and the increased blood and lymph flow all help to cleanse the area, shedding excess energy and menses while stimulating healthy tissue growth. Steams are really helpful for people with stagnant blood and lymph that settles in the pelvic region. This can look like dark, thick menses blood, painful periods/dysmenorrhea, irregular periods, PMS symptoms, fibroids, cysts, hemorrhoids, chronic prostatitis (post inflammatory state), chronic bacterial and fungal infections, and uterine prolapse. They are also used to increase fertility, during menopause to slough off old tissue, post-partum or post-abortion, post prostate surgery, for chronic vulvar pain, pelvic muscle spasms and tension, endometriosis, constipation, urinary incontinence (stress and urgency), and overall circulation and lymph support. They can also be helpful to symbolically cleanse the area after sexual trauma, abortion, or miscarriage. By bringing warmth and attention to the area along with the use of cleansing herbs, people can incorporate ritual to cleanse and let go of past trespasses or pain that may be held in this region.

Pelvic steams are commonly done tonically 1 – 4 times a year or more often for acute situations or chronic imbalances, up to 4 times a week. For people with uteruses, it is recommended to do the steam as close to the onset of menses (but not while menstruating) as possible. The timing is not as important for folks with penises. When steaming post-abortion or miscarriage be sure to wait about two weeks and at least six weeks post-birth in order for the tissues to heal before introducing heat and volatile oils. Sometimes when first beginning steams, people will notice that their menses looks quite different and that they pass gritty, thick tissue. Usually this will shift to bright red blood by the third month of regular steams. Other changes that people might notice are both vaginal and penile discharges, which are normal cleansing reactions. It is important to note that there are times when you should not use pelvic steams. Such as when you are menstruating (though it is commonly done the day before menses onset), when you are pregnant or think you might be pregnant (unless directed by your midwife), if you have an IUD, if you have an infection including a current herpes outbreak or an active yeast or bacterial infection, or if you use any hormonal creams. If you notice any unusual reactions or discharge, stop using pelvic steams and talk to a knowledgeable practitioner about what you are experiencing. There is a list of a few I know of at the bottom of this essay if you want further information.

There is lots of information in books and on the internet as to how to actually give yourself a pelvic steam and it can be helpful to do one on yourself before you try to teach clients how to do them. The basic recipe for pelvic steams is to make a strong tea (1 cup of herbs to 2 quarts of water) using your chosen plants. Allow the tea to steep for 5 – 15 minutes before beginning your steam. For those who don't want to invest in a lot of equipment, pelvic steams can be done in a toilet. This involves scrubbing out the toilet, draining the water, and placing the hot tea/steam inside the toilet bowl and then draping a blanket or towel around yourself and the toilet to hold the steam in while sitting on the toilet seat. This is the most simple way, though it does tend to skeeve some people out since we use the toilet for waste products and therefore, it doesn't always feel as cleansing as some might like. Other ways to do pelvic steams that require a bit more investment involve purchasing a shower chair with a hole in it, drilling a hole out of an old chair, or building/purchasing a steaming box built specifically for this purpose. The basic idea is to find any way that you can allow steam to contact your generative organs while sitting comfortably and keeping the steam in for as long as possible. Having a box for steaming can help to insulate the steam and keep the heat in but a blanket wrapped around the lower body and the steaming pot can work just as well. I also know some people who steam by digging a hole in the ground outside and putting the pot in it and then squatting above it with a blanket wrapped around them.

This is a great way to do a steam if you are able bodied to squat for long enough to receive the benefits. The earth is a natural insulator to keep your tea hot for the necessary amount of time to receive benefits and for some people, the very idea of being outside for this process is cleansing in itself. No matter which method you choose, be sure to test that the steam is not too hot before settling your delicate tissues over it. It should be warm and pleasant to the point of tingly, but not too hot to the point of stinging. Be aware that for those of us who have more protruding anatomy, we will need to be sure that there is enough space between the source of the steam and our bodies so that we are not burnt/injured by the steam or hot water. When it is a comfortable temperature, sit over the steam and find a way to place your feet on a support that will bring your knees slightly higher than your hips. Sit over your herbal steam for at least 20 minutes and then rest quietly for at least an hour after your steam. Make sure that you are warm during the time that you are steaming and afterwards as you rest and absorb the benefits of the herbs.

Aromatic herbs are often chosen as their volatile oils are released in steam and act on the uterus and prostate to stimulate and cleanse the tissues. Some herbs that have been traditionally used include a lot of our mint family plants, such as Basil, Rosemary, Oregano, Motherwort, Lemon Balm, Lavender, and Sage. Other powerful herbs that are often used include Calendula, Rose Petals, Marshmallow, Mugwort, Gotu Kola, Chamomile, Yarrow, Marigold, Raspberry leaf, Cedar, Comfrey leaf, and Plantain. You can combine any number of these to address the imbalance that you are currently working with. A few ideas are using herbs such as Marshmallow, Comfrey, and Plantain which are moistening and cooling to soothe inflamed tissues or herbs such as Yarrow, Plantain, Rose, Cedar, and Raspberry leaf to tonify and strengthen boggy tissues or herbs such as Calendula, Basil, Oregano, Sage, Lavender, and Mugwort to support and balance bacterial and fungal populations. There are many other amazing herbs that you can use that are too numerous to list in this publication and I encourage you to research and find the ones that are right for your situation. Please do not use essential oils in your steam…I have seen them cause some serious injuries and they are just too strong for these gentle places.

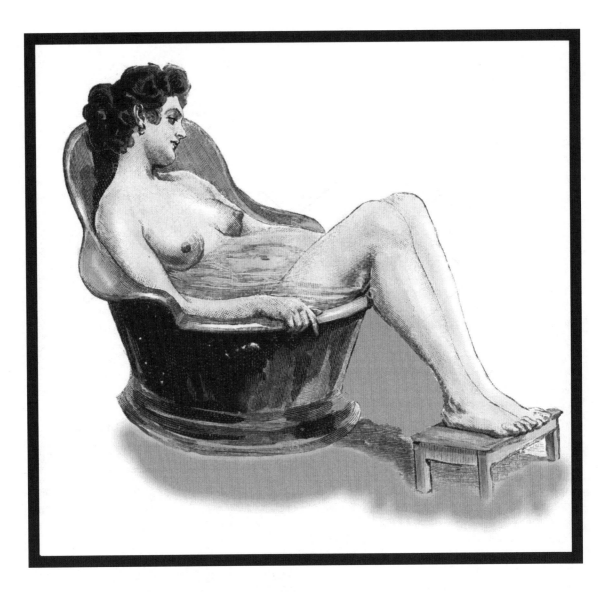

Sitz Baths/Hip Baths

Another option to focus healing on the pelvic region is a sitz bath or hip bath, in which you soak only your pelvic region in a tub of water or tea. This concentrated soak stimulates blood flow to the area, which encourages tissue healing and also increases the ability of the body to carry waste products away from the area. These are a more tonifying and less cleansing choice than a pelvic steam and are great for drawing fresh energy and circulation to the pelvic area. I find them especially useful for folks who are trying to heal a wound or tear in the pelvic region. They are also beneficial for hemorrhoids, cysts, fibroids, cervical dysplasia, infertility, yeast and bacterial infections, and overall boggy tissues with a tendency to chronic discharge, urinary incontinence, and chronic UTIs. You can use just hot water or both hot and cold water to alternately dilate and constrict the blood vessels in this region. This alternating action is similar to a pump that removes stuck energy and stagnant blood and lymph and helps to tonify the tissues.

16

You can use sitz baths monthly as a tonic treatment or more frequently when addressing acute issues. I've known some people to use them up to four times a day when they are dealing with painful hemorrhoids or tears in the perineal area, as they can be quite pain relieving. For post-birth or post-abortion situations, sitz baths should be done at least 6 weeks afterwards. They can be used at any time in the menstrual cycle. It can be important for folks who are doing lots of sitz baths to be sure to dry the area well afterwards and allow it to air out before putting on underwear or pants.

I also find that sitz baths are great for people who are struggling with painful sex due to scar tissue from past trauma. Sitz baths can bring a lot of warmth to the area and soften tissues so that people can more easily break up the scar tissue. This can be done with a wooden gua-sha or a nice polished stone with round edges that are warmed up before beginning to use it. I encourage folks to choose a rock that feels good to them, perhaps Rose Quartz to invite in loving energy or Black Tourmaline to absorb negative energy, and then to warm it in the sitz bath or a cup of tea. The edge of it can be gently rubbed in areas with lots of scar tissue in order to begin waking up the tissues and slowly breaking down the ones that cause constriction when stretched and stimulated. This process is obviously really difficult for many people and it is really important that they feel safe and held while doing it…nourishing heart herbs, nervines, and embodying herbs taken internally can be really helpful here. The point is not to do this so much that you feel pain while undertaking this process, but to do it often enough that it slowly makes a difference. For some people it can take many months to get to a point where they are no longer in pain during sex. I generally encourage people to work on the tissues once a week or so as doing it more often than that can be draining physically and mentally.

You can use similar herbs for a sitz bath as you would for a pelvic steam. There are many different herbs to choose from and again, I encourage anyone interested to further research those herbs that seem specific to the case that you are working with. For folks with bacterial and yeast infections, Calendula, Lavender, and Yarrow can make a nice soak in combination with other herbs specific to your situation. For folks struggling with hemorrhoids, using the alternating hot/cold method with astringing and drawing herbs such as Rose, Plantain, and Raspberry leaf can be really helpful. To prevent infection and support tissue healing for perineal tears, sitz baths can make a big difference.

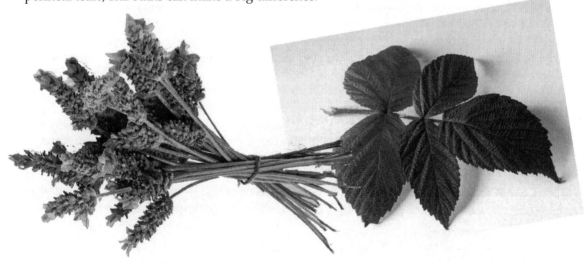

Suppositories

Using suppositories, both anally and vaginally, is another great way to apply herbs topically to the pelvic region. These can be really useful for herpes, chronic bacterial and fungal infections, cysts, fibroids, prostate inflammation, BPH, genital warts, hemorrhoids, anal fissures, and tumors located in any of the pelvic tissues. All of these are situations where it is helpful to allow the herbs to be in contact with the tissues for as long as possible in order to have their maximum healing effect. Using suppositories while also working on bringing the gut flora and other protective immunity back into balance is key; these are not a stand-alone. On the other hand, attempting to balance gut flora and struggling with long-term chronic gut dysbiosis and infection that can contribute to chronic bacterial and fungal infections can often benefit greatly from the addition of suppository use. These can be used both anally and vaginally depending on where the infection is and what parts you are working with.

Suppositories are not something that I encourage people to use tonically, unlike pelvic steams and sitz baths. I use them for both chronic and acute situations and find that the more often they are used, the better they work. Again, that herbal principle that the longer the herbs are in direct contact with affected tissues the better applies here. If you are planning to use suppositories long term, I encourage people to take a five – seven daylong break every 10 days. This means that folks can do 2 rounds of treatments over a month.

There are a few different ways to make suppositories but all involve the addition of herbs to a base of a more solid oil/substance. This can be gelatin or cocoa butter or coconut oil. The simplest method is to mix approximately 3 parts melted cocoa butter to 1 part finely powdered herbs. This should be the consistency of a thick paste, if it's not add more powdered herbs to thicken it or oils to make it more pliable. Be sure that your herbs are finely powdered…if they aren't you will notice as soon as you try to insert them into these sensitive areas. You then pour this into a suppository or pessary mold (make your own with aluminum foil!) and let it cool. After wrapping them, they can then be stored in the fridge for up to two weeks or in the freezer for up to 6 months. Making suppositories with gelatin can be more complicated, but there is a link with detailed directions at the end of this essay. The herbs will stay in contact with the tissues until the base oil melts and it begins to leak out. I usually encourage people to use a cloth or pad in their underwear while using suppositories for this reason. It is important to use the suppositories at night when the body is horizontal and the medicine will remain inside for as long as possible but for people who are dealing with more serious and chronic issues, I encourage them to use suppositories around the clock. You can add herbs that are specific for your situation to the base. For instance, many people use Echinacea, Calendula, and strong essential oils for cervical dysplasia suppositories or Black Walnut, Calendula, Usnea, Yarrow, Oregon Grape Root, and probiotic powders for yeast and bacterial infections. For folks who already have inflamed tissues, the addition of a demulcent herb can really soothe the tissues, which can improve pain levels and allow the tissues to heal. Making suppositories that are primarily demulcent herbs can also be helpful when there are chronically dry vaginal tissues, as often seen in menopause. You can use all of the herbs mentioned in the applications above and others specific to your situation.

When choosing herbs for suppositories, there is a tendency to choose strong heroic herbs and essential oils to match the virulence of some of the infections that folks have often struggled with long term before reaching for herbal support. Remember that these tissues are very delicate and strongly absorb anything you put into them. They are also often inflamed and irritated from long term infection once people choose to use suppositories. I have seen people have allergic reactions to many herbs that other people have no issue with so I caution people to test a small amount of herb on these tender spots before investing lots of time and money into a whole batch of suppositories only to swell up ferociously and not be able to sit/stand/walk. Some plant medicines that I have seen people react to are Chaparral, Tea Tree essential oil, and Thuja essential oil. Since essential oils are such strong medicines, you can choose whether you want to use them or not. In cases of intractable infection they can be helpful but they can also contribute to an inflammatory state and dry tissues out. I generally urge people to begin with a less intense method and use them more often and for longer rather than to use strong herbs for a short time. For some people who are dealing with high-grade cervical dysplasia and other serious conditions, this is not an option but I still urge everyone to move forward with caution.

Sunshine

Hang it out there! Find the time and way to put your head down/ass up in the sunshine as often as possible! Finding ways to air out our pelvic region and get some sunshine directly on these areas can feel really great as well as help to warm up those tissues and dry out an area that can be a moist breeding ground for bacteria and yeast. Finding a way to do this for a few minutes every month can be really helpful in ensuring long-term health of our pelvic region. Get some sunshine where the sun don't shine!

Using these applications with our clients can be vitally important in finding ways to shift imbalances in the pelvic region. I encourage us all to find sex and body positive ways to talk about generative organs with each other and our clients. Having these tools in our pocket can be extremely healing to our work, our clients, and our own bodies.

Suppository Recipes

Suppository for Vaginal Infections:

2 parts powdered Goldenseal

2 parts powdered Plantain

1 part powdered Lavender

1 part powdered Calendula

Blend herbs together with enough cocoa butter to form pellets the size of the last joint of the little finger. Refrigerate to harden before using.

Suppository for Abnormal Pap Smear:

Echinacea angustifolia root

Vegetable glycerin

Flour

Usnea tincture

Calendula tincture

Powder the Echinacea as finely as you can, then mix it with enough vegetable glycerin to bring it to the consistency of cookie dough. At this point it will be a bit sticky, so mix it with enough flour (any kind – chlorella or spirulina can be used) to bring it to the consistency of bread dough. Once you have, take a bit of the mix and press it into the shape of a suppository, about the size of your thumb. Repeat until you've used up all the mixture. Place the suppositories on a tray and put them in the freezer. They won't freeze; they will remain pliable but manageable.

Each evening, after you are in bed, place one suppository up against the cervix. The next morning, use a douche made from a mix of equal parts Calendula and Usnea tincture, ½ ounce in 1 pint of water (otherwise, the remains of the suppository will drip out throughout the day). Repeat every day for 14 days.

Resources

(Michael Moore – SWSBM: HPV and Cervical Dysplasia
Recipe: http://www.swsbm.com/ManualsMM/Formulary2.txt)

Thomas Easley & Steven Horne: The Modern Herbal Dispensatory, p167

Stephen Harold Buhner – Herbal Antibiotics, p355–356

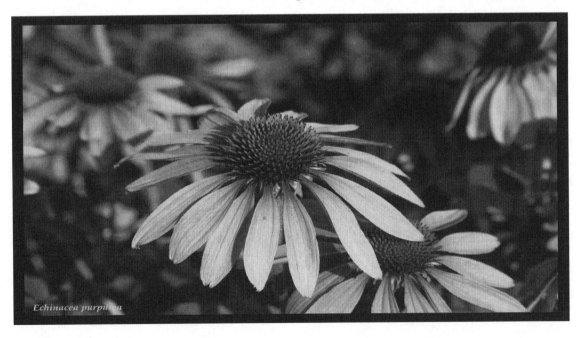

Echinacea purpurea

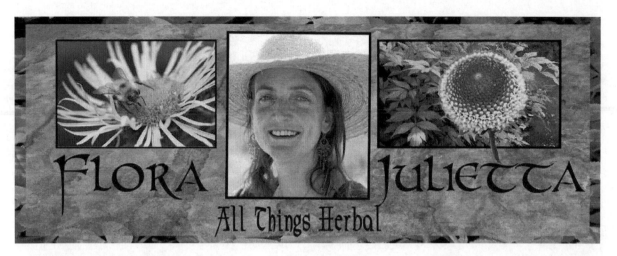

Women today live in a very different world than our foremothers. We have benefited immensely from cultural advances around gender equality, but our bodies are suffering the consequences of modern life. Our pre-industrial predecessors began menstruating later in life, had more children, breastfed longer, underwent menopause earlier, ate whole food, and lived in a cleaner environment. Women today have approximately ten times the menstrual cycles as earlier women. Our bodies did not evolve with the hormonal inputs of perpetual ovulation and menstruation.

In this article, we will explore various factors affecting the hormonal ecology, or hormonal environment, of contemporary women. Most women are aware of the hormonal complexities of the menstrual cycles, even if they don't fully grasp all the intricate details. I will start by outlining the three major sources of estrogens, each of which is described in detail later in the article. The term endogenous is used to describe any substance

The Ecology of Estrogen In The Female Body

Text & Photos by
Juliet Blankespoor

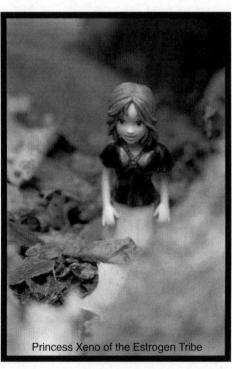
Princess Xeno of the Estrogen Tribe

generated from within an organism. Thus, endogenous estrogens are estrogens produced by the human body. Phytoestrogens are compounds, produced by plants, with an ability to bind to estrogen receptor sites. In contrast, xenoestrogens are human-made chemicals, which are also capable of binding to estrogen receptor sites. Xenoestrogens are a subclass of endocrine disruptors, which are described below.

It is important to understand that a variety of compounds have the ability to fit into estrogen receptor sites— natural and human-made molecules will alter a woman's overall estrogen pool. A woman's ovaries may be producing healthy levels of estrogen and progesterone, but her cells may be bombarded with strong estrogenic inputs from unnatural substances in her diet, water and air. Humans are exposed to environmental chemicals beginning at conception, absorbing novel compounds through the placenta, and then through breast milk. These endocrine disruptors (chemicals which

21

disrupt hormonal physiology) have the potential to alter the reproductive ecology of the body, often with drastic effects, such as reproductive cancers and chronic female reproductive disorders, such as uterine fibroids and endometriosis.

Phytoestrogens have the ability to bind to hormonal receptor sites; they exert a beneficial effect on the female physiology. Our bodies' hormonal systems have evolved with phytoestrogens, which are helpful in treating estrogen dominance (relative imbalance of estrogen to progesterone), as well as reducing menopausal symptoms. Most modern peoples in wealthy industrialized nations consume very little phytoestrogens and are regularly exposed to endocrine disruptors. I believe that these two factors play a large role in the increasing rates of reproductive pathologies.

Our diets are different than those of our great great grandmothers - with easy access to processed "foods", as well as chemically grown and genetically modified foods. We are often not as active as our foremothers, and many women are overweight and obese. The world is a different place; in many ways the decisions about how we live, eat and reproduce are not as simple. Some health care professionals believe the increase in modern women's estrogen pools should be mediated with oral contraceptives. I do not agree with that strategy, and instead propose the judicious intake of dietary and herbal phytoestrogens, along with specific lifestyle changes aimed at lessening the stress of excess estrogen.

Males are also exposed to novel chemicals in the environment, which present equal challenges to their hormonal systems. Much of the following information will be relevant to both sexes, especially the info on phytoestrogens and xenoestrogens.

Phytoestrogens are a diverse group of compounds, found in plants, which have the ability to bind to estrogen receptor sites and elicit an estrogenic effect (*phyto* = plant, *estrogen* = estrus [period of fertility for female mammals] + *gen* = to generate). These "plant estrogens" are fairly abundant in a whole foods diet, and are found in many commonly eaten seeds, grains, and beans. In addition, many medicinal herbs used to treat female reproductive disorders contain phytoestrogenic compounds.

To understand how phytoestrogens work, it is important to grasp the following: varying substances can bind to the same receptor site and elicit differing effects, depending on the exact molecular fit. Phytoestrogens exert a weaker estrogenic effect on cells than endogenous estrogens and xenoestrogens. Phytoestrogens have an anti-estrogenic effect premenopausally by competitive inhibition of hormone receptor sites. When receptor sites are occupied with the less estrogenic phytoestrogens, there are fewer sites available for the more potent endogenous estrogens or xenoestrogens. Imagine a lock on a doorknob (estrogen receptor site), now picture a key (phytoestrogen) fitting into the lock and turning the key. Now imagine a second key coming along (endogenous estrogen); it can't fit into the lock because there's already a key there, blocking its way (phytoestrogen). The phytoestrogen key opens the door gently, while the endogenous estrogen would cause the door to fling open with wild abandon. Why do we want to gently open the door? Because most modern women have estrogen dominance, or a relative imbalance of estrogen to progesterone— turning down the estrogen dial by slowly opening the door is a good thing.

In menopausal and post-menopausal women, estrogen production from the ovaries slows, and then stops. As menstruation ceases, phytoestrogens have a positive effect by increasing the estrogenic effect on the body. Although phytoestrogens are less estrogenic than endogenous estrogens, they still increase the net estrogenic effect. This is evidenced by epidemiological studies demonstrating fewer menopausal symptoms, greater bone density, and lower breast cancer in populations of women who regularly consume phytoestrogens as part of their diet. [1]

Isoflavones (genistein, daidzein, formononetin, and biochanin A) are primarily found in the bean family (Fabaceae) and are some of the most potent and researched phytoestrogens. Soybeans (*Glycine max*,

Fabaceae) appear to be the most concentrated dietary source of isoflavones. Soy foods, listed in order of isoflavone concentration, include miso, tempeh, soymilk, tofu, and edamame. Soy is one of the most controversial foods today, either vilified as a harmful substance or praised for its nutritional superiority. There are some possible negative aspects to soy: it is a common allergen, difficult for many to digest, and typically grown as a genetically modified monoculture. However, it is a traditional food, consumed by Asians for millennia, and can be grown organically, without any chromosomal foul play. It is crucial to understand the difference between its traditional whole foods forms (tempeh, miso, tamari, edamame, and tofu) and the industrially produced processed "food"—soy protein isolate. Much of American soy consumption is from the latter form in processed meats from fast foods.

Traditional Asian cultures ingest about one ounce of soy daily on average, often in fermented forms such as tempeh, miso, and tamari. These fermented foods are easier to digest than other forms of soy. When eaten in moderation, they are beneficial as a high protein phytoestrogen, with the following benefits: increased bone density; fewer menopausal symptoms; and lowered incidence of breast, uterine, and prostate cancers. It appears that soy consumption via breastfeeding (with mothers who consume soy foods) and in youth, reduces breast and prostate cancer later in life.[2] Population studies

show that early consumption of soy is also linked to a reduced amount of menopausal symptoms.

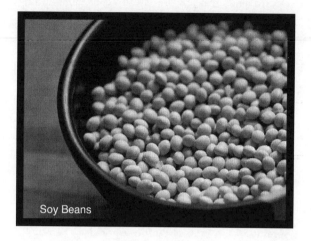
Soy Beans

Lignans are the most widely consumed phytoestrogen precursors found in the western diet and are found in high concentrations in flax and sesame seeds and to a lesser extent in other seeds, whole grains, fruits, vegetables, and beans.[3] Flax has about ten times the lignan levels as sesame. Intestinal flora metabolize the lignans, converting them to their active forms: enterodiol and enterolactone. These phytoestrogen metabolites produce a weaker estrogenic effect compared to the isoflavones. Lignans are not present in the oil portion of the seed, so sesame and flax oil are not good sources. Both flax and sesame seeds, in their

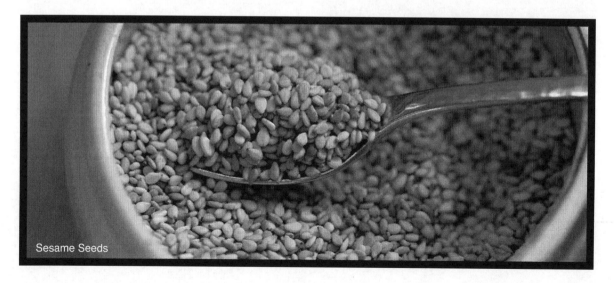
Sesame Seeds

whole form, pass through the gastro-intestinal system intact, and thus are not assimilated. I recommend grinding the fresh seeds and adding them to food after the food has been cooked. Grind flax with a hand grinder, coffee grinder, or blender and store it refrigerated for a week. Add the flax meal to oatmeal, or other breakfast gruels, salads, stir-fries, and baked goods. Gomasio is a traditional Japanese condiment made from toasted sesame seeds; try it sprinkled on salads, soup, and stir-fries. Prepare gomasio by toasting the seeds in a dry cast iron skillet and then grinding them after they have cooled, with the addition of salt or seaweed. Tahini, or sesame butter, is another excellent source of lignans.

Clinical Significance: Encourage the ample intake of sesame in the form of tahini or gomasio. Sesame is traditionally used in Ayurvedic medicine as an aphrodisiac and to strengthen the bones, hair and teeth. The seeds are considered to be a rejuvenative for Vata constitutions. In Chinese medicine, the black sesame seeds are used medicinally as a galactagogue (stimulate breast milk production) and to tonify the yin and blood. Sesame seeds are rich in calcium and protein. Two tablespoons of ground flax seed daily is a good dosage of lignans, with the additional benefit of flax's soluble fiber (which is protective against cardio-vascular disease and helps to promote healthy intestinal flora).

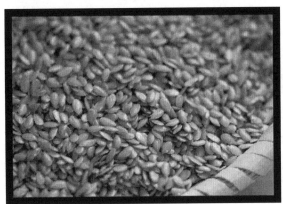
Flax Seeds

For women who are able to effectively digest soy: I recommend tamari and/or miso daily. Both miso and tamari are naturally eaten in moderation, as they are so salty tasting. Tempeh or tofu can be eaten two to three times a week. Counsel women to avoid soy protein and soy protein isolate. I am not a fan of isolated isoflavone supplements, such as genistein, and believe that dietary sources from whole foods and herbs are a better choice. Herbal sources of isoflavones include Red clover (*Trifolium pratense*, *Fabaceae*) and Alfalfa (*Medicago sativa*, *Fabaceae*).

Endocrine disruptors, or hormone disruptors, are human-made chemicals in the environment that interfere with the development and function of all body systems in animals, including humans. Endocrine disruptors can bind to hormone receptor sites, triggering a body-wide hormonal influence. They may also inhibit our natural hormones, such as androgens (male hormones), thyroid hormones, and progesterone. In addition, these chemicals can affect the production, elimination and metabolism of our endogenous hormones.

Most of the chemicals used in modern conventional (*euphemism for chemical*) agriculture are known endocrine disruptors. These same chemicals are also used in home gardens and lawns. Home use of garden herbicides and insecticides are typically devoid of the same regulation and education inherent in agricultural settings. Many of the ingredients in cleaning and body care products have also demonstrated binding to hormone receptor sites. Additional exposure may come from absorbing compounds found in electronic devices and shopping receipts.

Clinical Significance: Educate your clients about endocrine disruptors without overwhelming them to the point of feeling powerless. It is a common response to feel disheartened and concerned for the future generations of all life when first hearing about endocrine disruptors. That's a good sign of humanness! However, it is beneficial to balance the facts with hope, by offering concrete suggestions around reducing personal and planetary exposure to endocrine disruptors.

Avoid any type of plastic coming into contact with food and beverages. Use glass and stainless steel containers instead. Buy or make natural cleaning and body care products. Buy or grow food organically. If finances are an issue, focus on organic

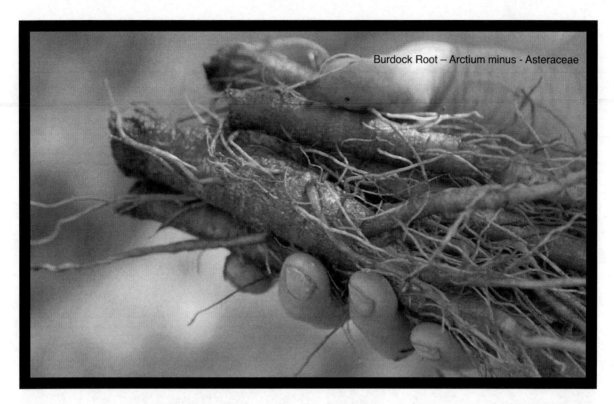
Burdock Root – Arctium minus - Asteraceae

meat and dairy, as the bulk of our exposure to agricultural chemicals comes from these animal foods. Many forms of packaging contain endocrine disruptors: the inside lining of canned foods, aseptic containers, and plastic wrap to name a few. Filter water unless it is absolutely pure spring or well water (lucky few). Avoid chemicals in clothing (fire-retardant children's pajamas) and freshly manufactured synthetic fabrics. Try to avoid the chemicals found in conventional building materials. It can be maddening to think about all the ways we absorb environmental chemicals! Living simply is a good start, along with breathing deeply and laughing through the madness.

For many women, fasting and cleansing can be extremely beneficial if undertaken slowly and carefully. This is especially important for a woman considering motherhood, as most of her lifetime stores of fat-soluble chemicals are passed on to her infant via breast-milk. It is beyond the scope of this article to thoroughly discuss fasting and cleansing, but I will say that it is imperative to tailor the cleanse to the woman's constitution and lifestyle. For someone who eats mainly processed foods and lives a fairly typical western lifestyle, a good start would be to eat a mono diet like kicheree (a traditional Indian dish, made from mung beans, rice and spices) for four days. During this time, offer herbal support in the form of alteratives, diuretics, and liver and kidney tonics. Examples would be dandelion leaf and root (*Taraxacum officinale*, Asteraceae), nettles (*Urtica dioica*, Urticaceae), and burdock (*Arctium minus* and *A. lappa*, Asteraceae). Sweating through exercise, saunas, and baths is also helpful in removing toxins via perspiration. Hydration is imperative, as well as daily bowel movements. If a person feels very nauseous, achy, shaky, or experiences headaches, that is a sign to slow down or stop the cleanse. The body cannot always easily metabolize fat-soluble chemicals, which enter the bloodstream when fat cells are broken down (through reduced caloric intake). One should never attempt a fast or cleanse when pregnant or nursing. Fasting is not appropriate for all people, and for many it can seriously worsen a pre-existing condition. On a final note, the support of long-term dietary and lifestyle goals should be one of the primary points of attention. After healthy patterns have been established, one may embark on fasting and cleansing.

25

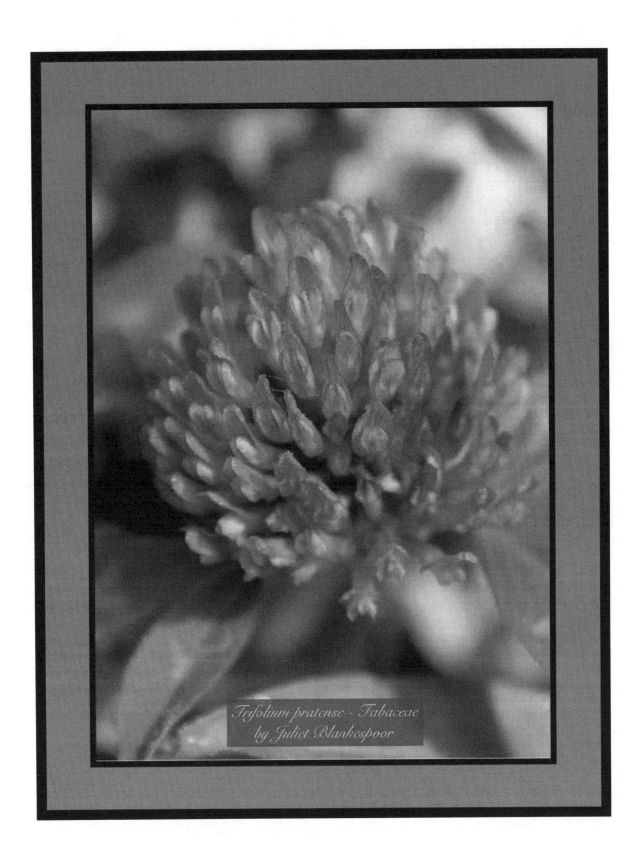

Trifolium pratense - Fabaceae
by Juliet Blankespoor

Most Americans have some control over reducing exposure to environmental toxins, but there are people throughout the world who do not have this privilege. Socioeconomic factors contribute greatly to accessing fresh food, and clean water and air. Pollution is typically higher in poorer areas. Endocrine disruptors do not observe political boundaries; air and water currents carry these chemicals far and wide. The decisions we make about how we live and consume have the power to affect the hormonal systems of all people and animals globally for generations to come.

The Liver breaks down circulating estrogen and progesterone and excretes the inactive metabolites from the body via the bile. If a woman's liver is impaired, hormonal metabolism and excretion can be slow. Her ovaries may be producing a healthy balance of estrogen and progesterone, but the liver is allowing the hormones to circulate longer in the bloodstream, resulting in increased estrogen levels. The relationship between the liver and female reproductive health has long been recognized by most, if not all, traditional systems of medicine.

Clinical Significance: With any female reproductive disorder, it is important to examine the health of the liver. Look for symptoms of liver and gall bladder disharmony, such as frequent headaches, pale stools, excessive anger, irritability, digestive sluggishness, constipation, and an inability to tolerate alcohol or digest fats. Often the person will describe feeling stuck or held back. Yellow eyes and skin is another indicator of possible liver distress. Is there a history of alcoholism, hepatitis, excessive NSAID use, exposure to solvents and environmental toxins, or intake of pharmaceuticals or recreational drugs known to be especially hepatotoxic? If possible, help to reduce any ongoing harmful inputs, such as the intake of excessive alcohol and fried foods, and habitual NSAID use.

Consider supporting the liver with traditional liver and blood tonics, such as dandelion root (*Taraxacum officinale*, Asteraceae), burdock root (*Arctium lappa* and *A. minus*, Asteraceae), red clover (*Trifolium pratense*, Fabaceae), reishi (*Ganoderma lucidum*, *G. applanatum*, and *G. tsugae*, Ganodermataceae),

Vervain (*Verbena officinalis*, *V. hastata*, and other species, Verbenaceae) and nettles (*Urtica dioica*, Urticaceae). If you suspect or know of liver damage, consider hepatoregeneratives, such as milk thistle (*Silybum marianum*, Asteraceae) and artichoke leaf (*Cynara scolymus*, Asteraceae). Bitters can also help to stimulate the flow of bile with the attendant excretion of estrogen. Many of the aforementioned hepatics have a bitter taste and can be taken 20 minutes before meals to optimize the bitter action. Note that most bitters are cooling and drying; you may need to add warming and or demulcent herbs to soften the energetic effects in people who run cool and dry.

Intestinal Flora imbalance is almost an epidemic in western industrialized nations. One in three babies in our country comes into this world through cesarean birth, and many are not breastfed; both factors contribute to the imbalance of intestinal flora. In addition, antibiotics are frequently administered to children, which also diminishes healthy populations of intestinal flora.

Our bacterial beasties help in the assimilation of phytoestrogens; intestinal flora convert lignans into their bioactive form and aid in the absorption of isoflavones. The repeated use of antibiotics and subsequent damage to intestinal bacteria has been linked to an increased risk of breast cancer, perhaps in part due to the lowered production of active phytoestrogen metabolites.[4] Intestinal bacteria also play a role in estrogen metabolism; certain bacteria produce an enzyme capable of converting the inactive estrogen metabolites in the gut back into a viable estrogen, which is then reabsorbed further down the digestive tract. It appears that supporting healthy populations of intestinal flora helps to reduce this "reinstatement" of estrogen, thus allowing estrogen to leave the body via the feces.

Clinical Significance: Support healthy populations of intestinal flora by introducing the use of bitters, prebiotics, and fermented foods. Prebiotic foods are not digested by intestinal enzymes, and instead are broken down and absorbed by intestinal flora. The best way to absorb prebiotics is in food, but tea is another delivery system.

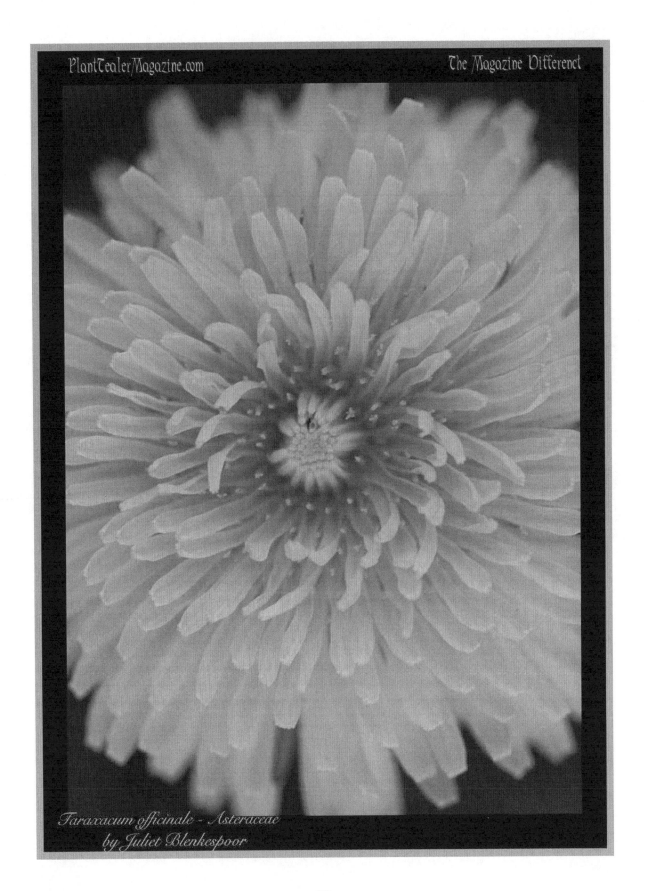

Taraxacum officinale - Asteraceae
by Juliet Blenkespoor

Herbal/Dietary prebiotic sources are: leeks, asparagus, and the roots of dandelion, chicory, burdock and Jerusalem artichoke. Roasting roots converts inulin (type of prebiotic) into sugars, and thus roasted root teas are less effective for supporting healthy intestinal flora. The ingestion of fermented foods is associated with a lower risk of breast cancer. Examples of fermented foods and beverages are: miso, live kimchi and sauerkraut, kefir (water and dairy), yogurt (dairy, soy or coconut), dosas, kombucha, and many others. Many of these items can easily be found in the aisles of health food stores, but it is much more economical to learn how to ferment at home. Probiotic supplementation may be indicated, but fermented foods should also be incorporated into the diet.

Dietary fiber intake reduces estrogen levels in the body, and is associated with a lower risk of breast cancer. [5] In addition, soluble fiber nourishes healthy populations of intestinal flora and reduces cholesterol levels in the body. A good way to remember soluble fiber is that both slimy and soluble begin with an S; soluble fiber binds with water to form a mucilaginous texture. Barley, oats, split peas, bananas, okra, and most beans are high in soluble fiber.

Clinical Significance: Incorporate ample sources of whole plant foods in the diet: fruits, beans, whole grains and vegetables. When a person is used to eating processed grains and little fruits and vegetables, the increased fiber intake can result in painful gas. Introduce these foods slowly while taking digestive bitters before meals. Carminatives can also help. Over time, the intestinal flora will adapt to the higher fiber intake.

Adipose tissue (Fat)

Pre-menopausally, the ovaries (specifically, the follicles and corpus luteum) are the primary producers of estrogens. In addition, some of the body's supply is derived from the conversion of androgens (male reproductive hormones) by the aromatase enzyme. This conversion (aromatization) takes place primarily in adipose tissue (fat) but also occurs in the brain, skin, muscle, and bones. After menopause, this secondary source of estrogen is particularly important as it provides for most of the body's estrogen. During the reproductive years, aromatization can account for a significant contribution to circulating estrogen levels; the powerful effect of aromatization is demonstrated in women who have undergone surgical removal of their ovaries without experiencing the symptoms of premature menopause. Excess aromatization has been linked to breast, adrenal, endometrial and prostate cancers.

High caloric intake has been linked to earlier menarche (onset of menstruation) and later menopause; this leads to a longer exposure to estrogen, and increases the risk of breast cancer.[6] Postmenopausal obesity has shown to be a strong risk factor for breast cancer, increasing the risk by as much as 50%. [7] Excess body fat has also been linked to uterine fibroids and endometriosis. [8]

Clinical Significance: Maintaining a healthy body weight can help keep the peripheral conversion of reproductive hormones in balance. If a woman has little body fat, she may experience amenorrhea (absence of menstruation), infertility, anovulation, or difficulty with menopause. It is important to rule out eating disorders, food allergies, digestive issues, depression, hyperthyroidism, body image issues, and over exercising as possible causes of low body weight. Often women are simply thin, due to genetics or constitution, without any underlying pathology. Inquire about the diet, and help to optimize the ingestion of whole foods, including high quality fats and proteins. Often, increasing wild or organic animal foods in the diet will help to build the body's reserve and build connective tissue (including adipose tissue) and blood.

If a woman is clinically overweight or obese, excess aromatization can take place, leading to higher levels of circulating estrogen. Look for any possible underlying causes of obesity, such as hypothyroidism, depression, and stress. Socioeconomic factors must also be explored: does the woman have access to fresh fruits and vegetables? Does she know how to eat and prepare whole foods? Help to strategize a plan for weight loss including exercise coupled with reduced caloric intake, focusing on fresh fruits and vegetables. Find out what exercises she enjoys, and help her to create an exercise plan that feels realistic to her. Social support is extremely effective in helping to change ingrained dietary and lifestyle habits. Who does the cooking in the household? The person who prepares meals needs to be on board with any dietary changes. Remember, for most people it is psychologically easier to add healthier foods, rather than subtract unhealthy items. A reasonable goal would be to add a fresh salad or cooked greens to lunch and dinner and to add fresh fruit to breakfast and/or snacks.

In conclusion, there are many factors contributing to each woman's personal estrogen ecology; these need to be explored in any female reproductive disorder. Often, herbal hormone balancers are indicated along with appropriate dietary and lifestyle changes. It is my hope that this information is part of a foundation for sustaining healthy reproductive systems!

Resources/ Suggested Reading:

Trickey, Ruth. *Women, Hormones and the Menstrual Cycle—Herbal and Medical Solutions from Adolescence to Menopause.* Fully revised and updated edition.
Romm, Aviva. *Botanical Medicine for Women's Health.*
Blankespoor, Juliet. *Phytoestrogens Demystified.*
http://blog.chestnutherbs.com/phytoestrogens
Steingraber, Sandra. Having Faith—*An Ecologist's Journey to Motherhood.*
Colborn, Theo and others. *Our Stolen Future.*

References:

[i] Julia R. Barrett, "The Science of Soy: What Do We Really Know?," *Environmental Health Perspectives* 114, no. 6 (June 2006): A352–A358.
[ii] Jillian Stansbury, "Gene Expression and Reproductive Health. Medicines from the Earth. Official Proceedings. June 4-7, 2010. P138-142.,".
[iii] "Linus Pauling Institute at Oregon State University," accessed April 26, 2013, http://lpi.oregonstate.edu/infocenter/phytochemicals/lignans/.
[iv] "Risk of Breast Cancer in Relation... [Pharmacoepidemiol Drug Saf. 2008] - PubMed - NCBI," accessed April 26, 2013, http://www.ncbi.nlm.nih.gov/pubmed/17943999.
[v] D. Aune et al., "Dietary Fiber and Breast Cancer Risk: a Systematic Review and Meta-analysis of Prospective Studies," *Annals of Oncology* (January 10, 2012), doi:10.1093/annonc/mdr589.
[vi] "Breast Cancer Research | Full Text | Does Diet Affect Breast Cancer Risk?," accessed April 26, 2013, http://breast-cancer-research.com/content/6/4/170.
[vii] Sandhya Pruthi et al., "A Multidisciplinary Approach to the Management of Breast Cancer, Part 2: Therapeutic Considerations," *Mayo Clinic Proceedings. Mayo Clinic* 82, no. 9 (September 2007): 1131–1140, doi:10.4065/82.9.1131.
[viii] Ruth Trickey, *Women, Hormones and the Menstrual Cycle,* n.d.

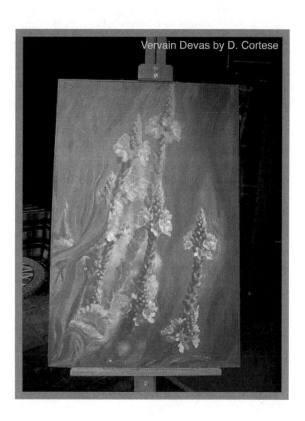
Vervain Devas by D. Cortese

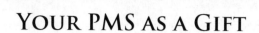

YOUR PMS AS A GIFT

Herbal Treatments For The Dosha Types

by Adrie Lester

PMS. The definition in Urban Dictionary says, "A powerful spell that women are put under about once every month, which gives them the strength of an ox, the stability of a Window's OS, and the scream of a banshee. Basically, man's worst nightmare." Other synonynms in popular culture include "about to ride the bull". "prehistoric monster syndrome". "bitch kitty", "tampire", "psycho maniac syndrome", "insta-bitch", "werebitch", "bitchuation", and "storm-a-brewin." Collectively, we fear PMS. Women fear it, feeling that it takes over their minds, their words, their emotions, and their cravings. Those who live with them fear it as well. Weeping, raging, outbursts, sensitivity, chocolate cravings - are the visible markers of PMS.

As a woman in my teens and early twenties, I didn't have PMS. Looking around at the cultural portrayals, I thought that women were using their "time of the month" as an excuse to complain and be mean. When I was 28, my second child was born. And when I weaned him at 29 and my menstrual cycle returned, I suddenly learned a lot about PMS. For the second half of my cycle, post-ovulation, I was filled with rage. Not anger, not bitchiness, but rage. My own PMS led me on a journey towards wellness that changed almost every aspect of my life. It forced me to examine how I was living, what I was avoiding, and in particular, the anger I had been stuffing for many, many years that was now uncontrollably spilling out.

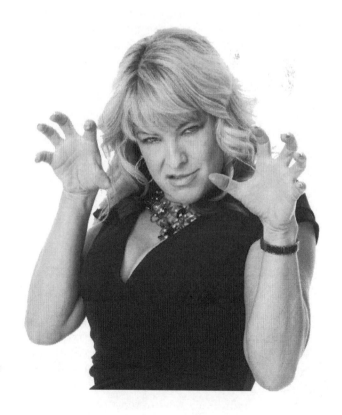

I once lived with a housemate who referred to preparing for PMS as "taking out the compost". In our kitchen, we had a large bucket we filled with food scraps, that we regularly emptied out into the compost pile in the back yard. If we didn't empty the bucket regularly, it festered and rotted. The food scraps began to break down and smell gross, and in theory, if we didn't empty it but just kept adding scraps in, it would have overflowed onto the floor and eventually filled the kitchen and house. I love her metaphor. When PMS time comes, if we haven't spent our month taking out the compost, our PMS will make that abundantly clear. All the tension we ignored, the rest we didn't take, the emotions we didn't take time to feel, now come up full force and all at once, so they feel incredibly

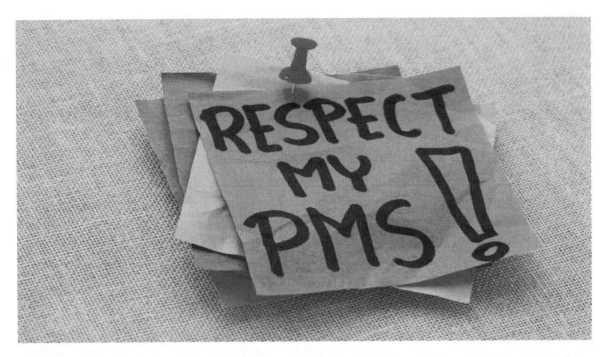

I view PMS now as a gift, as the body's incredible, beautiful intelligence. As we pass from accumulation and growth of blood and tissue (maiden phase), to the abundance of fertility (mother phase), we move towards release and barrenness - crone time.

Who is the crone? Culturally, she is feared, just as PMS is. She is the elder who has the wisdom of accumulated years. She is past her years of attracting mates - she has passed into the land of giving no fucks. She wants what she wants, dresses how she wants to dress, says what she wants to say, asks for what she wants to ask for. Already scorned by the culture and viewed as useless, she has nothing to lose. All too often, when these same impulses come up during PMS, we fight them. We are afraid to harness her power, to accept her gift. We fear the consequences of saying what we want to say, of not being nice, of telling everyone to go away so we can take a long hot bath. We are afraid that we are not allowed to take good care of ourselves, that there is not enough time, that we have not earned it.

The way I experience PMS now is not as anger but as a sense of heightened clarity. What I don't want to do and what I do want to do, feel clear in this time. What I want to say, and what I refuse to have others say to me is clear. The next few steps on the path illuminated. My refusal to do what isn't on my path strengthened. The strength of the willpower, the energy given by anger, burns within me. Not as not as a fire that burns those around me, but as a light.

Care of PMS, or PMS protocols almost always focus on herbs, diet, and exercise: *stop consuming caffeine and dairy and alcohol, move your body, use these herbs.* These are all completely valid recommendations, and they do help. With severe or long-standing PMS, it has been my experience with myself and with clients that while they help some of the symptoms get better, they will not budge the root of PMS. In the wise woman tradition, our dis-ease comes to us with a lesson to be learned. Until we have fully absorbed that lesson, the dis-ease will stay with us. PMS is a profound example of this. The most powerful shift we can make is to stop treating PMS as a set of issues that need to be resolved, and start seeing it as a profound offering that is getting our attention using these very unpleasant symptoms.

Early on in my own PMS healing journey, an acupuncturist asked me, "Do you take time to do things that you enjoy?" I thought this was a ridiculous and infuriating question. I was the mother of two young children and a small business owner - as far as I could see, there was no time and no one gave a hoot about what I enjoyed. As profoundly irritating as the question was at the time, it stayed with me and worked on me. *What do I enjoy*, I asked myself. *Why isn't there time for that? When do I think my to-do list will be complete enough that I will be "allowed" to do something I like? Who is doing the allowing?* Sometimes the questions we begin to ask our clients and ourselves are biggest gifts, more productive than telling someone what to do.

As I address the different types of PMS and specific indications for them, I urge you to not focus on those particulars and forget where we have begun. Lean in to PMS and listen closely. Why is PMS here? How does it change or move if you begin to speak up, speak out, pursue what gives you joy, say no to the things you don't want but think you're "supposed " to do? These changes are the biggest lever we have for PMS. And if we forget, she will return to remind us, never fear.

In Ayurveda, the tradition I'm trained in, PMS is not treated as a single issue, it's addressed according to the constitutions (doshas). Pitta, Kapha, and Vata all have their own types of PMS, and the treatments are different for each. It's important to note that while a person may have one dosha, their dis-ease (in this case, PMS) can be arising from an imbalance of another dosha. So a Vata person, for instance, can have Pitta PMS, and we would treat the Pitta, while always keeping in mind that their base constitution is Vata. (This is particularly worth noting because of the "Vata pushing Pitta" phenomenon, which I have seen present in many PMS cases.) Let's take a moment to review the different "flavors" of PMS, and the constitutions they align with.

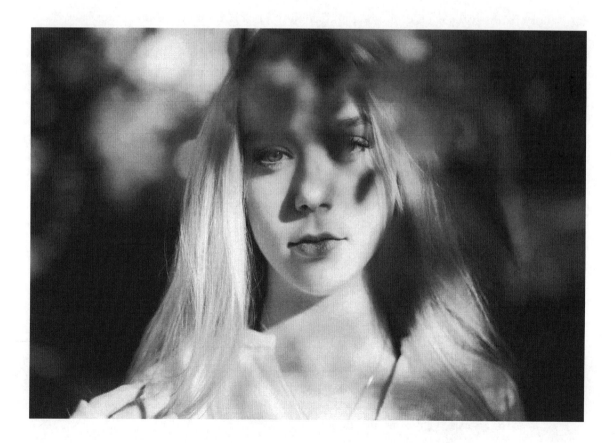

Since Vata rules the nervous system, Vata PMS is distinguished by anxiety, fear, depression, weepiness, and insomnia. Nerves include pain, so Vata PMS often has cramping pain, and since Vata rules the colon and is dry in nature, Vata PMS often includes constipation. Vata is changeable in nature (its elements are air and ether)- moods may shift rapidly and unpredictably. The emotions of Vata PMS can be extreme - the person may feel despair to the point of being suicidal, but will begin to feel better almost immediately when the blood begins to flow. The menstrual flow itself, when Vata is high, will be scanty, possibly brown, and lasts only a few days. Symptoms are aggravated at 2-6 am and 2-6 pm, sunrise/sunset (Vata times of day).

Pitta rules the blood, and its elements are water and fire. Pitta PMS is notable for fiery anger and temper, irritability, temper, argumentativeness. Sweating and feeling of heat in the body are often present. The person may have diarrhea, thirst, rashes, and acne is common. Menstruation may begin early. When menstruation begins, the blood is red, abundant (even excessive), and there may be clots. Symptoms are worse at 10-2 am and 10-2 pm (Pitta times of day).

The elements of Kapha are water and earth. Kapha rules the stomach, lungs, and chest. In Kapha PMS, we see bloating, lethargy, stagnancy, heavy feelings, crying, clinginess. The emotional changes are not likely to be as extreme, though, as with Pitta or Vata. There is increased likelihood of colds and more mucus is produced. Appetite may be lacking, there may even be nausea. Kapha also rules the lymph, and in Kapha PMS there is often swelling of the breasts or edema. Menstruation may be late, and the flow will be pale, thick, with large clots or mucus. Symptoms are worst in the 6-10 am and 6-10 pm (Kapha times of day). Treatments for the different types of PMS are similar in many ways to general treatments for balancing those doshas, with an emphasis on nervines, antispasmodics, and reproductive system tonics. I'll overview recommendations for each dosha, and then highlight some of my favorite herbs, including their effect on the doshas.

For Vata PMS, the focus is on grounding and calming - bringing the wind and ether back down to the earth. Foods that reduce Vata are recommended, especially cooked onions and garlic, and absolutely focusing on warm cooked foods with a generous amount of fat or oil, and avoiding raw or cold foods. As usual for Vata, it is recommended to avoid stimulants, including caffeine (coffee, tea, chocolate), alcohol, and drugs - these will greatly aggravate the mental anxiety of Vata. Self-massage is recommended, especially the lower abdomen and the feet (massaging the feet draws energy down from the head). For Vata, sesame oil is indicated since it is the heaviest, warmest oil, but over long periods it is drying, so I recommend a mixture of sesame-olive oil, or sesame-sunflower oil. (Vata is already dry by nature, we don't need to exacerbate that!). Oil can also be applied to the vagina. Yoga postures that are restorative, especially poses supported by bolsters, and forward bends, to support the nervous system and reduce the hyper-activity in the mind. Hot baths are recommended, as long as the body is oiled before or after, so the skin doesn't become dried out. Warm compresses on the lower abdomen and low back are also very supportive - either just a hot water bottle or a ginger compress.

For Pitta PMS, the focus is on cooling the aggravated fire, criticism (of self and others), and inflammation. Foods that reduce Pitta are indicated. Avoid hot spices (Cayenne, Ginger, Black Pepper, Cinnamon, Garlic), even though Pitta types may crave these. They have the strongest natural digestion of all the doshas, and can eat raw foods and cold foods. They should avoid fried or overly greasy food. Pitta types want to exercise a *lot*. Exercise is beneficial, but especially when working with PMS or high Pitta, it is very helpful to encourage Pittas to only exercise at 80-90% of their capacity. They are used to being competitive and love to push themselves - this is the time to hold back a little. In yoga, forward bends, to soothe the hyper-critical mind, are recommended. Also any poses that open up the side body (such as triangle pose and extended side angle) are beneficial, as they release heat from the body.

For Kapha PMS, the focus is on moving stagnancy and heaviness. Foods that reduce Kapha are best, so avoid heavy and oily foods, eat small and light meals with lots of vegetables and culinary spices. Kapha types need to *move* - go outside, breathe deeply, take a vigorous yoga or other exercise class daily. Heat therapy such as saunas or steams are recommended (especially dry saunas since Kapha tends to be damp). A hot Ginger compress on the womb area before and during bleeding is beneficial to warm the cold nature of Kapha, move stagnancy, and keep things flowing.

The following are specific herbs that I have used with benefit for treating PMS. All of these herbs have many beautiful potential uses that are not fully covered here - I'm specifically talking about their uses with PMS and how they affect the doshas.

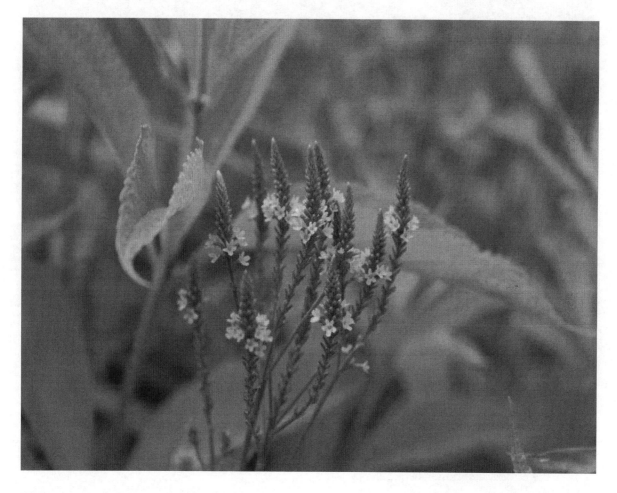

Blue Vervain (*Verbana hastata*) - this is not on the most common list of PMS herbs, but I love using it with Vata and Pitta type PMS. Blue vervain is an intense bitter, cooling and drying, a relaxant nervine, digestive stimulant, and endocrine/thyroid tonic. It is particularly suited for type A personalities (high Pitta) who can't slow down even when they know they're overwhelmed. It has an affinity for both the reproductive/hormonal system and the nervous system. Reduces Pitta. It is suited for Vata also, as it has a history of being used for nervous exhaustion and depletion. Since it is dry and cool, for Vata you need to be conscious of combining it with herbs that are warming and moistening. It is a very strong, powerful herb and I use it in small parts in formulas (usually ⅛ or 1/16 pt).

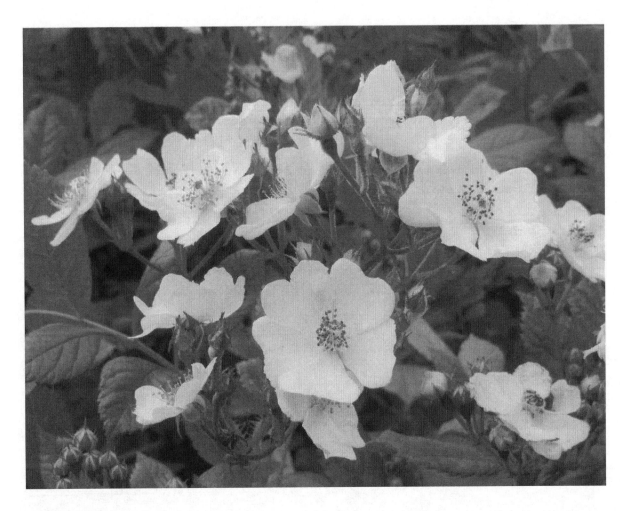

Wild Rose *(Rosa multiflora)* - I love using rose with PMS, and I usually use wild rose since I can wildcraft it freely, as an invasive species that grows profusely where I live. Cultivated (organic) rose could be used similarly here. Rose, with its open beautiful petals, luscious smell, and protective thorns, has good medicine for us in PMS time - reminders to communicate openly, receive love, and having solid boundaries and protections. (Yes, I include the thorns in my preparations.) Wild rose is cooling and drying. She has an affinity for the reproductive system, nervous system, heart system, immune and digestive system. In terms of PMS, the support is mainly targeted at the heart, repro, and nervous system. I usually use wild rose flower essence, rose petals in tea blends, and wild rose elixer. Reduces pitta. I also use wild rose for Vata type PMS, but since it is cooling and drying, make sure to balance your blend with warming, moistening herbs. (This is partly why I like wild rose elixer, the brandy and honey help balance.)

Licorice *(Glycyrrhiza glabra)* - Licorice is a classic PMS herb. Supportive to the nervous system and reproductive system, it is sweet and mildly bitter, its energy is cooling. Licorice reduces Pitta and Vata and increases Kapha with long-term use. As a muscle relaxant it helps with cramping, its moistening helps counter drying herbs in formulas, and it has a stabilizing effect on out of balance hormones. It is considered *sattvic* in Ayurveda, meaning it is calming and nourishing to the mind and the spirit. Often used as a harmonizer in formulas. I use licorice root in root chai blends for PMS, to balance taste when strong liver herbs like burdock and dandelion root are indicated. Also combines well with ginger.

Ginger (*Zingiber officinale*) - The energetics of ginger are pungent and sweet - hot if dried, warming if fresh. It reduces Kapha and Vata, and increases Pitta. Ginger supports the sluggish digestion of Vata and Kapha that is often exacerbated by PMS and menstruation, and also acts as an emmenagogue. Taken as tea, tincture, or made into a ginger compress (be sure not to apply directly to the skin, use a cloth). Ginger is also considered *sattvic* - calming and nourishing to both mind and spirit. It also relieves gas and cramping in the abdomen, including menstrual cramps (often caused by cold in the uterus area). A prime, wonderful PMS ally, and so accessible, since it's available in pretty much every grocery store, isn't expensive, and can be easily prepared by anyone with hot water and a grater. Can be used as a simple infusion, honey should be added to smooth the harshness and also mitigate the dryness (especially for Vata). Should be avoided during menstruation if there is prolonged or excessive or bright red bleeding. Excellent for spotty bleeding, brownish blood, clots, or delayed menses.

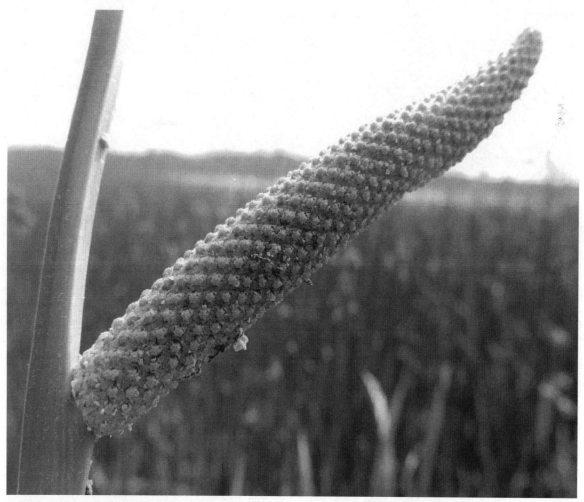

Calamus Root (*Acorus calamus*, also called Sweet Flag) - Calamus is pungent, bitter, and astringent. (Note: calamus was banned from use in food or as a food additive in 1968 by the FDA as a liver carcinogen.) Used for thousands of years in Ayurveda as one of the most renowned herbs. A rejuvenative for the brain and nervous system, calamus is primarily indicated for high Vata, and also for Kapha. Calamus also supports, warms, and strengthens the digestive system, is antispasmodic, and is also *sattvic*. Increases Pitta. Emetic in high doses.

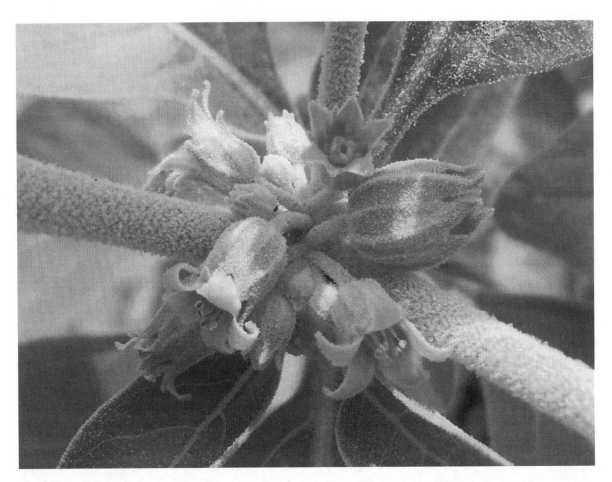

Ashwagandha (*Withania somnifera*, also known as Winter Cherry or Indian Ginseng) - the name in Sanskrit means "that which has the smell of a horse, gives the vitality and sexual energy of a horse". Ashwagandha is warming, bitter, and astringent, Vata and Kapha reducing. Ashwagandha holds a similar spot in Ayurveda that ginseng does in TCM, but luckily is not expensive (due to ease of growing). Prized as a rejuvenative herb, especially for Vata people or high Vata conditions that include depletion, exhaustion, tissue weakness, lack of sleep, and general burnout. When used as a regenerative tonic, the powdered herb (from the root) is added to warm milk with honey (for sleep disturbances, this is taken before bed). Supports and rebuilds the nervous system, reproductive system (also used with pregnant women), hormonal system, and promotes healing of tissues. Also taken in ghee, or as a tincture. I've started using ashwagandha in a sleep tincture blend for Vatas.

Burdock root (*Arctium lappa*) - Burdock root is primarily bitter and cooling, and also moistening/ oily. As a powerful liver supporter and blood cleanser, burdock is an important PMS ally for Pitta types. Pitta rules the blood, and if the liver is slow or cannot process all that it needs to, when the extra hormones leading up to menstruation come in, it overflows and can usually be seen as breakouts (acne) on the skin, particularly the chin. Since burdock is nutritive and moist, even though it is cool, it doesn't aggravate Vata as much. Can be used regularly for Pitta people, it is also a support for clearing out hot Pitta emotions such as anger and aggression. I use burdock in an herbal root chai (decoction) with dandelion, licorice, fresh ginger, and black pepper. The ingredients can be shifted and balanced to match the dosha. If there are a lot of skin eruptions, I find adding echinacea root to the blend is very effective. A favorite of mine, since it grows across the US abundantly and is potentially a free medicine anyone can find and harvest for themselves.

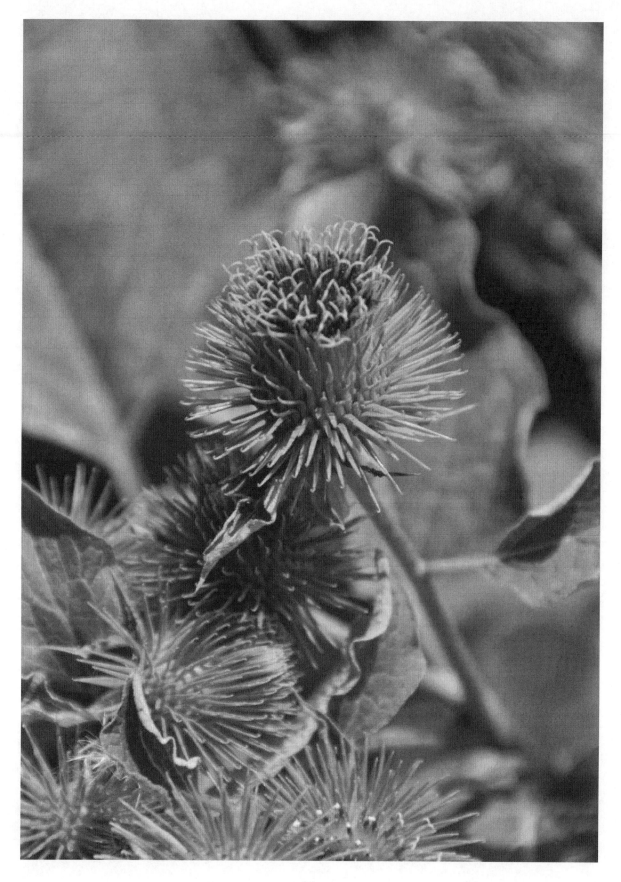

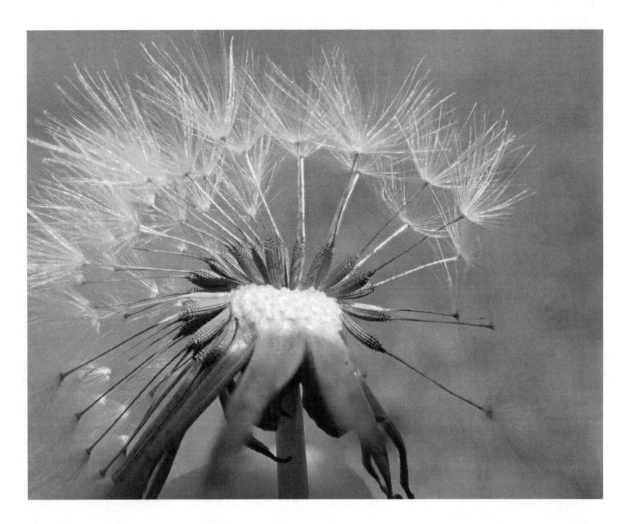

Dandelion root (*Taraxacum officinale*) - Dandelion root is cool, bitter, and dry. Pitta and Kapha reducing. Similarly to burdock, dandelion is a PMS ally for its detoxification of the blood, liver, and lymph. It clears and dispels stagnancy, supporting the elimination channels of the body. I used dandelion in an herbal root chai (see Burdock). Helpful for buildup from eating greasy or fried foods.

There are so many beautiful herbs that are allies to PMS, and not enough space or time to list them all here. The categories which are particularly beneficial are antispasmodics, hepatics, alteratives, emmenagogues, nervines, and tonics. Notable herbs that I have not covered in depth here are Skullcap, Shatavari, Rosemary, Chrysanthemum, Red Clover, Violet, White Pond Lily, St. John's Wort, Red Raspberry leaf, Motherwort, Mugwort, Myrrh, Nutmeg, Oatstraw, Passionflower, Lavender, Hibiscus, and Calendula.

I will say in closing that I find a combination of having herbal preparations for PMS be very simple and easy, and also having some participation from the person in their own care, is a beautiful part of the healing. For instance, I might make a supportive tincture blend and also give an herbal chai recipe - there is something that can be taken easily right away, and there is a part of their wellness plan that requires them to actively engage in taking good care of themselves in a new way. May these words reach you in peace and with blessings. May we all learn the profound lessons our bodies are bringing to us.

RIVER OF LIFE:

A Holistic View of Lymphatic Breast Health

By Anja Robinson

"To love life as much as you love water"
– The meaning of Lympha in Latin

The Lymphatic System: An Overview

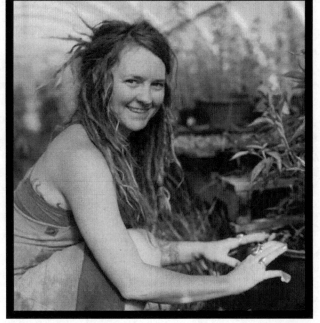

The lymphatic system is a beautifully complex and intricate circulatory system flowing throughout the body, intimately connected to our immunity and health, and yet it seems to be one of the least understood body systems. Why is that? What is the function of the lymphatic system, how can we recognize the quality of our lymph, and how does it interface with the immune system to create balance and homeostasis in the body? Often when speaking on this subject I open my talks with such questions, and even amongst herbalists and healers alike the answers are not always so clear unless one has gone deep into studying anatomy and physiology. Why are we not taught about such an important element of our bodies: the river of life and vitality that flows through us?

In Eastern medicine traditions, such as Ayurveda, the term for the Lymphatic system is *"Rasa"* meaning river of life. They consider this *Rasa* our life essence, our liquid vitality. This precious lymph, or life force energy also known as *Ojas* in Ayurveda, flows through our system and defends our bodies from invading pathogens, unfriendly bacteria and viruses. It is both a nutrient delivery system and a detox system without which life would not be possible.

How then, is it possible for us to be so disconnected from this aspect of ourselves and our immunity? If we think of our lymph as a river, we can begin to ask what is the quality of my river? Is it dry, or rocky? It is stagnant and pooling? Is it cold, or trapped? As we explore the terrain of our own bodies through the elements we will gain insight into the flow or lack thereof in our lives as well as our immunity and health.

41

The lymphatic system is the largest circulatory system in the body, and is an integral part of our body's immune system and defense against disease. It is a one-way river that runs from our feet to heart, hands to heart and head to heart. The lymph system is made up of an elaborate arrangement of drainage ducts, vessels and nodes that collect excess interstitial fluid and metabolic byproducts throughout the body, along with plasma—known as *lymphatic fluid*. The lymph system itself is made up of two distinct parts; the vessels, which branch like rivers throughout the body in a similar fashion to the cardiovascular system, yet hold a very different function, and the nodes, tissues and organs which are scattered in various places around the body. The lymphatic system is virtually everywhere in the body and serves as the primary vehicle for our immune function. It clears waste and accumulated toxins, known as *Ama* in Ayurveda, and is a key component in the development of healthy cells.

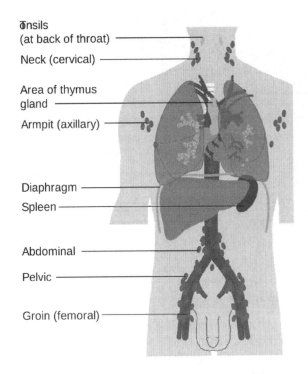

Tonsils
(at back of throat)

Neck (cervical)

Area of thymus
gland

Armpit (axillary)

Diaphragm

Spleen

Abdominal

Pelvic

Groin (femoral)

The Lymphatic - Immunity Connection:

"Human immunity is a vital component of the interface between the individual and the world. The role of the human immune system is not simply to resist the dangers present in the environment. Rather,

it is part of the complex and beautiful dance of elements flowing back and forth between the human body and the rest of the world. Seen within the context of ecology, both human and environmental, immunity is about harmony."
-David Hoffman

The immune and lymphatic system are intricately connected and designed to protect and cleanse the body from foreign invasion and the metabolic byproducts of infection. If you want to support your immunity you need to strengthen your lymphatic system. Our immunity is in essence our security system. It guards us from viral and bacterial antigens, or invaders in the body, and uses the lymphatic system as a means to seek out these antigens and cleanse the cells of the body. If we think of it terms of a battle, the warriors fighting the battle could be seen as our actual immune system, where the lymphatic system would be in charge of the cleaning up the aftermath.

Our immune system is comprised of two primary components, our *innate defenses* and our *adaptive defenses*. The innate defenses of the body primarily include our skin, or outer layer as well as all of the mucus membranes that coat our organs that come in contact with the outside world, such as the lungs, GI tract and urinary tract. Here we also see our immune cells which actually "kill" all the invading pathogens in the body such as our natural killer cells, phagocytes and anti-microbial proteins as well as our inflammatory & fever response. These are what is known as our *non-specific immunity*. The adaptive defenses, or our *specific immunity*, includes various specialized cells in the body which attack specific pathogens. These are known as our B and T cells and they are responsible for responding to invasions and building a memory of them, so we can be more prepared to mobilize and fight them in the future. B cells are the "defense" and produce proteins called antibodies that circulate throughout the blood and fight these foreign invaders, and the T cells are our "warrior" cells that attack the invaders directly and communicate to the B cells to begin producing more antibodies when needed.

When the immune system comes across an invader, it creates an immune response (also known as the *inflammatory response)*. Our bodies speak to us though symptoms of pain, swelling, fever and mucus production to buffer the inflammation that is occurring. These symptoms are our bodies way of communicating to us that it is working hard to solve the issue at hand.

As our blood is squeezed out of our capillary beds it enters the interstitial fluid, or the fluid surrounding our cells. The majority of this blood is picked back up by the venous system and returned to the heart. The fluid that is left behind along with all of our cellular waste and debris is picked up by the lymphatic vessels, cleansed, filtered and dumped back into the blood stream. As the lymphatic fluid moves through this elaborate system, the vessels gradually get larger in size, from capillaries to collecting vessels and eventually to lymph ducts. This is a one-way river that flows to the heart, and unites back into the blood stream via thoracic duct and the subclavian veins, which are located under our clavicles. The lymph drains waste from every cell and organ in the body, including the heart and the digestive system. Once reunited with the bloodstream, it travels to the liver where it can be sorted and recycled. The liver will reuse what it can to make more red blood cells (B & T cells) and delivers these to the *spleen*, which is our primary immune organ, the "headquarters" of the immune system if you will.

constantly mobile, moving between the blood stream & the lymph tissue so that they are ready to respond when needed. From the spleen, the lymph then reenters the lymphatic system once again searching out and scanning for any foreign invaders and providing an immune defense for toxins passing through the organs. Whatever does not get utilized and repackaged by the liver will leave the excretory stem as waste; through feces, urine or sweat.

The lymph nodes are the primary organs of the lymphatic system, and act as filters for the bloodstream via macrophages and immune components cleaning the lymph that will reenter the bloodstream. Foreign invaders are met by antibodies in the lymph. These antibodies surround the attacking antigen and move it into the lymph nodes where it can be digested, detoxified and then excreted out of the body. These lymph nodes assist the body in keeping the immune system active by constant screening for these invaders. One familiar way our bodies communicate illness to us is though the swelling of these lymph nodes. This happens in an acute infection due to congestion in the lymph node of newly produced lymphocytes as well as pathogenic material. A few other important lymphatic tissues in the body include the tonsils, Peyer's Patches, which are located in the wall of small intestine, and the appendix. All of these tissues are a part of our immune system as well as the lymphatic system.

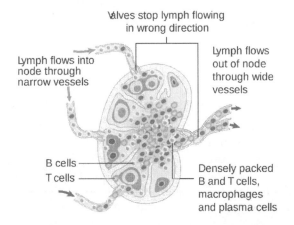

The spleen is also where lymphocytes are produced, one of the main cellular component of our immune system. These lymphocytes are

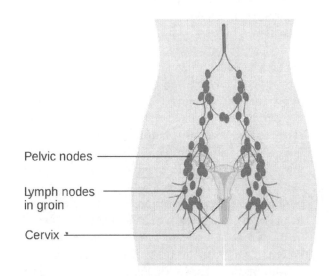

One important difference between the circulation of lymph and blood is that unlike the cardiovascular system, the lymphatic system does not have a pumping mechanism; it moves passively. This means its movement is based on the movement of the diaphragm via breathing and the movement of the physical body through exercise. Lack of exercise can congest the brain and the CNS (central nervous system) lymphatic channels. When the channels' drains become congested, a traffic jam of sorts occurs in your body, and it takes a toll on all of the organ systems.

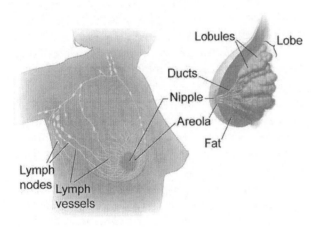

The Role of the Lymphatic System in Women's Health

As far as woman's health is concerned, at the beginning of a menstrual cycle, lymph drainage increases. In very simple terms, according to Ayurveda, when women menstruate, not only is the endometrial lining shed, but also much of the reproductive waste and hormonal metabolic byproducts are removed through the lymphatic system. If the lymph is congested, the menstrual cycle may become painful, irregular, overly heavy or missing completely. Congested lymph may bring with it typical PMS-associated symptoms such as breast swelling or tenderness, bloating, water retention, and breakouts (especially around the mouth and chin). Dis-ease in the lymphatic system can show up as edema, weight gain or weight loss, auto-immune conditions, increased viral load or infections, and inflammatory immune response. Other symptoms include but are not limited to: ovarian cysts, uterine fibroids, polycystic ovarian syndrome, fibromyalgia, fibrocystic breasts, cellulite, rashes or acne, edema, joint pain, weight gain & extra belly fat, swollen glands, frequent colds, fatigue, headaches, allergies constipation, diarrhea and/or mucus in the stool. This is quite a list of symptoms, and if you are a woman, I would wager that you (at some point in your life) have experienced one if not multiple of these symptoms. Again, I raise the question, why is this not something we are taught? How did such a crucial aspect of our health and immunity, as well as something so intricately tied into our menstrual cycles and reproductive health not get more spotlight or explanation?

Now that we have become more informed and aware of the function of our lymphatic system, let's take a deep dive into breast health. To start, I would like to shed some light and clarify some of the terms you may have heard from your doctor, mainly fibrocystic breast disease, benign cysts and tumors. Most knowledgeable heath care providers agree that the term "fibrocystic breast disease" should be abandoned in favor of a more accurate, physically based description. This term is often misinterpreted and causes a great deal of fear. This condition is rather common and is found in 60-90% of all women. Many women notice painful, sensitive and swollen breasts prior to menses. Women with this condition often describe their breasts as ropy, lumpy and tender. This is often attributed to more predominant estrogen than progesterone, produced late in the cycle, or irregular ovulation also known as an inadequate luteal phase. Essentially, women who have fibrocystic breasts have more fibrous breast tissue, and in that are more susceptible to cysts, which can occur within this fibrous tissue. There are some dietary and lifestyle factors that can be helpful in relieving symptoms of this "condition".

Painful swellings that flux with the cycle and do not change over time are not worrisome as cancer signals. As mentioned before, the lymphatic system speaks in pain as an inflammatory immune response. When there is inflammation in the body it is like leaving a fire unattended, as it can spread quickly. Thus, it's important that we listen to our bodies and the signals they are giving us. A good thing to remember is that if you feel painful lumps in your breasts, that is ultimately a good sign: it means there is work to do but your body and immune system are hard at work. What we need to really pay attention to is irregular shaped lumps, that have no feeling. A benign cyst will be painful, and will change with time by working the lymph and surrounding tissues. Cysts are formed by yeast that has been trapped and encapsulated in the lymphatic system. We can gently pump these cysts as they need to drain in order to leave our bodily systems through our lymph. This pain, and tenderness of breast tissue often occurs cyclically with menses, and is often referred to as cyclic mastalgia. There are however two types of worrisome lumps to be aware of. The first are small, hard irregular nuggets not connected to anything. They feel a bit like a piece of broken down pumice, and will not change over time, nor feel painful. The second are tight, rubbery water balloon feeling lumps that have "tentacles" attaching to the breast bone: these are often breast tumors. If you find one of these worrisome lumps, the best thing to do is contact your primary care provider immediately and look into further testing options such as mammograms and thermography graphs to gain further insight and information.

Ama & Stagnation: An Ayurvedic Perspective

In Ayurvedic medicine, both Ama and stagnation are contributing factors to poor breast health. *Ama* can be thought of as a sticky, toxic sludge that is formed from poorly digested matter and is a byproduct of a variety of pollutants. Ama can arise from toxic chemicals in our bodies and environments that have an affinity for breast tissue, or adipose tissue in general; this can be ingested chemicals, poor quality food or poorly digested food. In either case, Ama circulates the bloodstream and gets lodged in the breast tissue if there is stagnation present. As we will soon see, diet and digestion

are very closely intertwined from the perspective of Ayurveda. Healthy digestion and elimination can reduce the amount of Ama circulating in the bloodstream and reduce the chances of these toxins getting stuck in the breast tissue. Both Ayurveda and Western Medicine agree that diet plays a major role in breast health. A high fiber diet, one that contains a variety of fresh and organic fruits and vegetables, whole grains and very little processed foods, white flour and white sugar is recommended for women to care for their breast health. Tras-fats can also act as Ama in the body and should be completely avoided.

According to Ayurveda & TCM, there can be a stagnation of Qi, or nourishing fluids (think lymphatic fluid) in the breast tissue, and in the body as a whole. We can encourage this stagnation though holding our breath, breathing shallowly, and not having physical movement of our breast tissue. This lack of breath can occur for many reasons, but often happens because of stress. Lack of breath, according to Eastern Medicine, results in stagnant Qi, or Prana in the chest, heart, lungs and breasts. Stagnation of energy in the breast tissue fosters an environment where Ama can more easily lodge and fester, resulting in dis-ease. Our breasts are composed of mostly passive, adipose tissue (fat), therefor do not receive as much blood flow to bring nutrition and remove waste and debris as other muscles in the body do. Throughout our lives, our breast tissue remains mostly stagnant compared to our muscles, which experience pretty consistent stimuli. Not to mention the use of tight, possibly ill-fitting bras and bras with under-wires, which cut off the flow of prana and lymph in our breasts. We wear deodorant with antiperspirant; hindering our sweat as well as when we finally get massages, this area is wholly ignored. Aside from our own monthly breast checks, if we do them at all, foreplay and breastfeeding are the most action our breast tissues get. Sad, I know.

Contributing Factors

There are a variety of contributing dietary and lifestyle factors that influence our breast health, and becoming aware of how our daily choices affect our health is the first step to positive

45

change and personal empowerment. The *liver* is the primary site for estrogen clearance and metabolism in the body. Once estrogens makes it to the liver they are conjugated and sent over to the intestines for elimination. If our livers are comprised it can lead to a state of estrogen dominance, and this can cause texture and density changes in the breasts, or fibrocystic breasts. Supporting a healthy liver though nutritional and herbal support is the primary way we can make sure we are achieving proper estrogen metabolism. Our digestion and elimination are also fundamental factors involved in hormone-related health issues. The longer it takes food to move through the colon, the more waste products can pass into the bloodstream to be reabsorbed, causing a potentially toxic environment in the body. When intestinal reabsorption of these estrogens occurs, the estrogens become *de-conjugated*, which is essentially a toxic form, and they return to enterohepatic circulation. Enterohepatic circulation recycles metabolized and unmetabolized compounds which are absorbed in the gastrointestinal tract, then enter the portal circulation, then go to the liver to be returned to the gastrointestinal tract via bile excretion. When this intestinal reabsorption of estrogen into the liver occurs, we become predisposed to inflammation as well as estrogen-related cancer risks. The more we focus on a healthy, whole foods diet high in fiber, the more we can support healthy elimination and transit time in the body, which will have a positive, healthful effect on our hormonal system as a whole.

Caffeine from coffee, black tea, chocolate and medications contain a substance called *methlxanthines*, which studies have shown to be a factor in increasing a woman's risk of fibrocystic breasts and symptoms, as well as smoking cigarettes. Another factor in limiting lymphatic flow in the breast tissue is underwire bras. Although these have become a staple undergarment for most women, they are actually causing lymphatic stagnation as well as the matting of the lymph tissue to the breast bone. This cuts off the proper flow of lymphatic fluid in the breasts, which contain dozens of lymph nodes, acting as a natural process of detoxification for the body. The use of anti-presperant deodorant causes stagnation of prana, or life force energy in the body as well as discoursing sweat, another essential process of detoxification.

Lack of movement and exercise is one of the biggest contributing factors to breast dis-ease in women today. We need movement in our lives to keep our rivers juicy and flowing, reduce lymphatic stagnation and support our livers ability to detoxify hormones. The lack of touch and massage that we experience in our breasts directly affects our immune system and our body's ability to fight infection and detoxify properly. The more we can incorporate exercise and movement as well as manual manipulation of our breast tissue the healthier we will become. Taking charge of our health and touching our breasts regularly is a form of self-love and empowerment that can bring about radicle change for our bodies, minds and spirits.

Holistic Solutions for Lymphatic Health

So how can we care for our lymphatic systems to optimize our immunity and keep our lymph juicy and flowing? One of the simplest ways in which we can support healthy flow is through hydration. *Electrolytes.* In Ayurveda, electrolytes mean salt; I am talking about real, mineral rich, unrefined salt. Natural, unrefined salt contains trace minerals & electrolytes such as sodium, calcium, magnesium potassium, iron and zinc. Adding ½ tsp of electrolyte rich salt such as Atlantic grey salt, or Celtic sea salt can help you to restore your electrolyte balance which directly effects the flow of your lymphatic system.

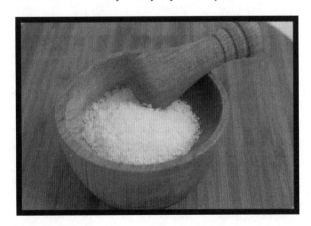

As far as nutritional considerations go, eating a diet rich in a rainbow of whole fruits and vegetables is one of the best ways we can naturally support our flow. Conversely, processed foods, food additives, excess sugar, refined grains and trans fats can have a negative effect on our gut microbiome and hormonal system. Eating hydrating and mineralizing vegetables, as well as leafy greens full of vitamins and minerals help to nourish the blood and build our immune system. Increasing dietary fiber with whole grains (unrefined of course!), legumes, and fresh fruits and vegetables is key. Adequate intake of dietary fibers aids in healthy transit time and elimination supporting our overall hormonal balance. Soaking and sprouting nuts, seeds and legumes helps to remove phytic acid (an anti-nutrient that binds to and blocks absorption of fat soluble vitamins and zinc) and makes them more easily digestible overall. Essential Fatty Acids found in raw, healthy fats help maintain the lymph, bones, nerves and skin tissues. It has been scientifically studied that EFA's, particularly *Evening Primrose Oil*, can alleviate pain and tenderness of benign breast disease such as cyclic mastalgia. Other EFA's are helpful as well, such as raw seeds, raw olive oil, flax oil, pumpkin seed oil, borage oil, black current oil and raw milk. Enzymatic rich spices help to motivate change as well as fuel many of the biological processes in the body, supporting our lymph such as rosemary, ginger, coriander, cilantro, basil, cumin and celery seed. Supplementation of essential vitamins such as Vitamin E and Vitamin B6 can also help us to support our overall immunity.

As far as botanical treatment is concerned, one of the primary classes of herbs we look to here are the *bitters* which help enhance liver detoxification as well as aid in digestion and assimilation. Dandelion root (*Taraxacum officinalis*), Burdock root (*Arctium lappa*), Licorice root (*Glycyrrhiza glabra*), Oregon grape root (*Mahonia aquifolium*), Motherwort (*Leonurus cardiaca*) and Blue Vervain (*Verbena hastata*) are just a few examples of herbs with bitter actions. Vitex, or Chaste Berry (*Vitex agnus-castus*) can be used to enhance hormonal regulation and hormone metabolism for cyclic breast pain as well as fibrocystic breasts and is often paired with bitters to support liver clearance. Dong Quai (*Angelica sinensis*) and Blue Cohosh (*Caulophyllum thalictroides*) are used to modulate hormone levels in the body. According to TCM Dong quai dissolves blockages and relieves blood stagnation. Lymphatic and diuretic herbs are a great choice here as well; to help stimulate detoxification though the lymphatic system and encourage the flow of the waters of the body. A few of my favorites are Cleavers (*Galium aparine*), Dandelion root (*Taraxacum officinalis*), Red Clover (*Trifolium pretense*), Calendula (*Calendula officinalis*), Yarrow (*Achillea millefolium*) and Poke root (*Phytolacca americana*).

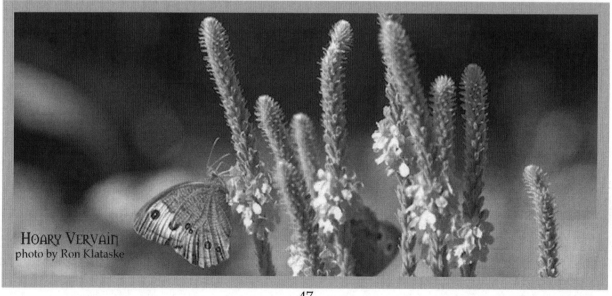

HOARY VERVAIN
photo by Ron Klataske

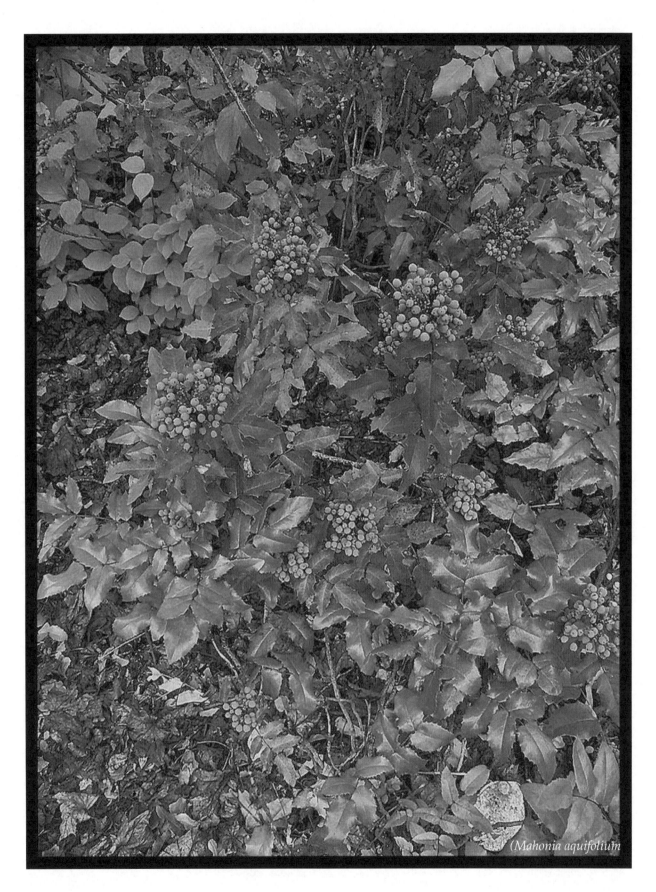

(Mahonia aquifolium

Of course, whenever using botanicals it is important to realize that every lymphatic herb will not work for every person, nor should it. Herbal actions, energetics and constituents are as unique and individual as the people themselves. In this regard, it is of utmost importance when working with our botanical allies, that we take into consideration their specific elemental correspondences and energetics, as well as the patient or client we are working with. In this way, we can honor the specific gifts of our herbal allies and really get to know the plants on a deeper level, not just what they are good for. An understanding of bio-individuality and constitutional theory are essential when working with botanical medicines so that we may find the remedies that will resonate and be the most effective for our clients.

Ayurvedic Self-Care

Within the Ayurvedic tradition there are many daily self-care practices, known as *dinacharya*

that help to support health and vitality on all levels, and are especially nourishing to the *ojas* and supportive of lymphatic flow. When performing these various acts of self-love and self- care it is important to remember to always move from feet to heart, hands to heart and head to hart, following the innate flow of the lymph itself. Dry brushing and salt scrubs are a wonderful and invigorating way for getting the lymph flowing.

Abhyanga is a daily body oiling practice for nourishing and grounding the body. It strengthens the tone and vigor of the tissues while simultaneously stimulating blood and lymph flow and brining about a deep connection to self. This is a beautiful practice on its own or can be done after dry brushing or a salt scrub.

In Ayurveda and TCM they use a tool for stimulating the lymph called a gua sha. The gua sha is a flat piece of wood or jade, used to "spoon or scrape" the lymph in the body. This

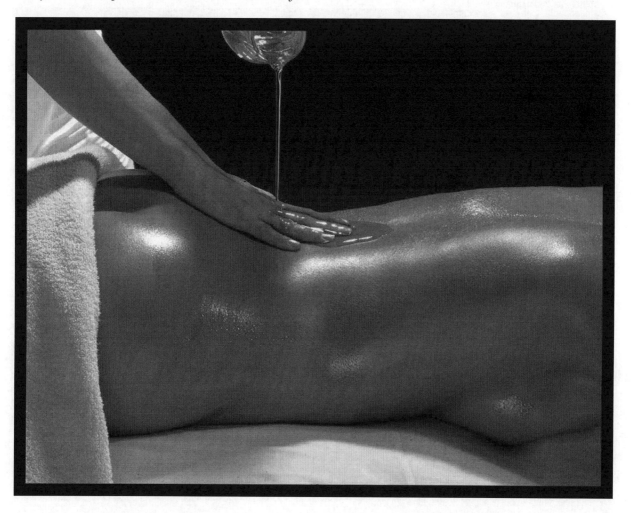

practice stimulates both blood and lymphatic flow as well as breaking down scar tissue and tenderizing muscles. Studies show it has an anti-inflammatory and immune protective effect. The edge of the gua sha is vigorously rubbed along the skin, as always, moving from feet to heart, hands to heart and head to heat. There is more emphasis on the stoke towards the heart, moving the lymph towards the main drains underneath the subclavian vein. The gua sha can be seen as an investigational tool used to map the terrain of our lymphatic health. It can be used with water in the shower, steam room, bath tub or used after Abhyanga, driving nutrients from the oil deep into the tissues. Using the gua sha dry on the skin can cause too much friction and be a bit painful so the use of oil or water are preferred. Creating self-care rituals and caring for your lymph through touch is an invaluable aspect of health, wellness and immunity.

Immunity, woman's health and the lymphatic system are intricately woven together in our bodies and it is imperative that we continue to bring awareness to the important role they play in our health. Exploring the symbiotic relationship of these systems is fascinating and brings so much of our current health experience into context. I believe that as a society we can begin to take back our bodies through body literacy and feel empowered in our decisions around health and wellness. Connecting with our innate flow, and tuning into our inner rivers we can become

so much more aware of the subtleties of our own immunity. There are so many facets to caring for the lymphatic system, and this article barely scratches the surface. In all matters of health, we must consider not just the physical but also the mental and the spiritual aspects of our selves so that we may truly heal on all levels. Movement of all kinds, a varied whole foods diet, botanical medicines and deep breathing are all important ways in which we can support our immunity, vitality and, ultimately, our rivers of life.

Parker, S. (2007). The human body book. New York, NY. Dorling Kindersley Limited

Romm, A. (2009). Botanical medicine for woman's health. St. Louis, MO. Elsevier.

Welch, C. (2011). Balance your hormones, balance your life. Cambridge, MA: Da Capo Press.

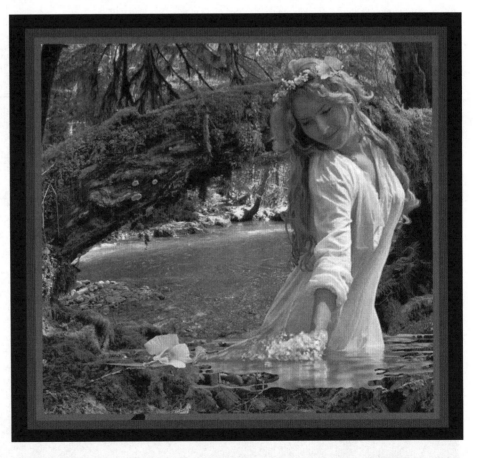

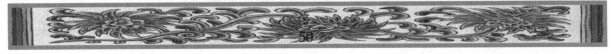

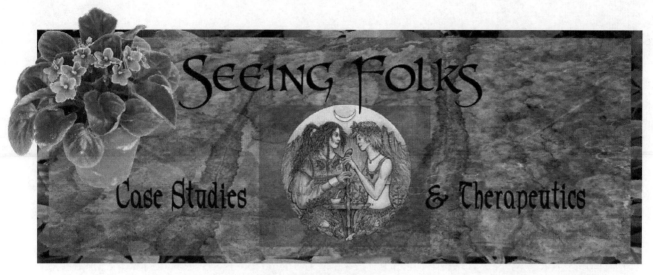

ADDRESSING SEXUALLY TRANSMITTED INFECTIONS
FROM THE HERBALISTS PERSPECTIVE

by Juanita Nelson

As herbalists, getting to know our client is an essential component in providing the best possible care. That means we've taken the time to gather the medical, familial, social, emotional, reproductive and sexual history of our client. We might be their primary provider or we might work in collaboration with other practitioners. We might order our own labs or depend on the results the client brings us. One thing we cannot ignore or overlook is the impact of both our client's overall health on the potential risk of STIs and the impact of STIs on their overall health.

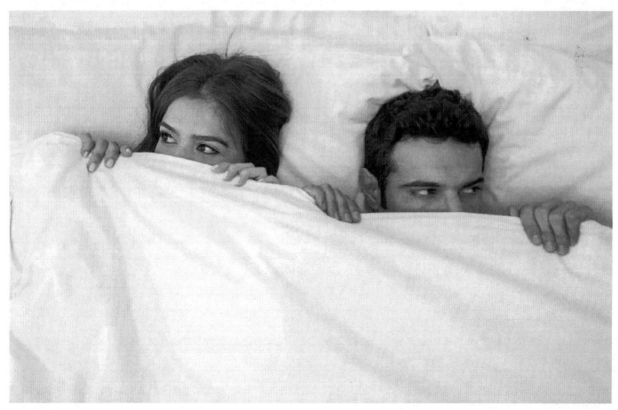

There is still a ton of stigma around STIs that can affect both the client's willingness to seek treatment and the way the practitioner approaches the client. While there my be certain populations that are at higher risk for STIs it is also true that they are equal opportunity infections affecting people across the spectrums of age, race, gender or sexual orientation. If you are a sexually active human then you are at risk of contracting a sexually transmitted infection. If we as the practitioner find we have prejudices or negative thoughts about an individual client or a certain population or group then I encourage all of us to acknowledge limitations and either refer that person to someone better suited or figure out how to work through our stuff. The history of patient blaming in the medical community is both inappropriate and unprofessional in this day and age.

If someone walks into your clinic and says, " I have been diagnosed with chlamydia," that's pretty clear. But if someone walks in and says, "I'm not sure what is going on and am in need of some help. I have this weird discharge." It's a different situation. As an herbalist you have to decide if you are going to do clinical diagnostics as part of your practice. Leaving the legal perspective aside for the time being, knowing how to examine someone's genitals is a valuable tool. Using a speculum is a skill-set that is not difficult to learn. Creating a relationship with a lab is important because you can send cultures to them or have them do blood draws and gain essential, invaluable information. Learning the difference between discharges, rashes, and lesions in conjunction with lab studies only gets you closer to accurate diagnoses and ultimately appropriate treatment.

Dealing with people's sexual habits and examining genitalia is fraught with issues that can be everything from awkward to abusive, so deciding ahead of time how you are going to deal with these issues is important. While many people feel more comfortable going to a provider who is the same gender identity as they are it is not always the case. Neutralizing any hint of sexual attraction is essential while verbalizing the exact sequence of your actions and getting permission to touch your client are not just good practice they are un-negotiable requirements.

This article is not going to teach you the skills of doing a genital exam. I am not going to discuss the viral infections that effect folks. I am going to talk about some of the most common STIs and the ones that are becoming epidemic level infections.

Organisms that cause sexually transmitted infections can be classified into four different groups.

1.Fungal
•Primarily yeast infections.
•Candida albacans (May be present without sexual contact)

2. Bacterial
•Bacterial vaginosis aka`non-specific vaginitis, gardnerella, (May be present without sexual contact)
•Chlamydia-parasitic bacterium`
•Gonorrhea
•Syphilis

3. Parasitic
•Trichomonas

4. Viral
•Herpes simplex type 2
•Human Papilloma virus•
•Hepatitis B
•Hepatitis C
•HIV

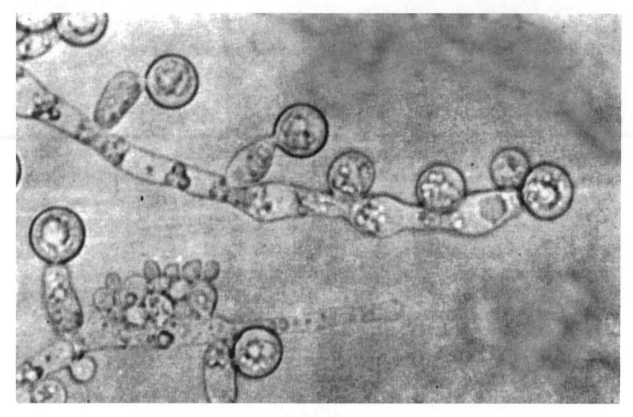

Yeast

Let's start with Vulvo-vaginal Candidiasis or Yeast. While not strictly a sexually transmitted infection it is one of the most common "infections." The reason it is not considered an STI is that it is caused by a fungus that can be present without engaging in sexual contact.

Yeast is essentially an imbalance within the body caused by an overgrowth of the genus Candida. Most common is Candida albacans but there are 20 different strains that can cause inflammation. It is usually found in the vagina but different strains can be found on the head and foreskin of the penis, in the mouth and throat, on the skin, and on the diaper area. Different candida species live in the gut and skin and due to an overgrowth can either migrate to the genitals. Changes in pH, hormonal changes like those during pregnancy, antibiotics which can kill off all the bacteria in your gut eliminating the "good" bacteria that keeps other bacteria and fungus in check, diabetes which can cause an imbalance in how sugar is regulated in the body, and immune deficiency are often instigators of the imbalance causing yeast infections.

Symptoms are fairly universal-in the vagina a yeast infection is characterized by a thick, clumpy, whitish discharge. It can irritate the vaginal wall as well as the labia, perineum and rectum. On the penis it can be identified by inflamed, red skin. Other infections can look similar so visual identification should not be the only diagnostic tool used here.

Medical treatment is most often with Monostat. Anti-fungals like Monistat will work for some strains of candida but not all of them. A person who has reoccurring bouts of yeast that are chronic or keep returning especially after using otc drugs probably has other strains that are not albicans and not being addressed. Treating yeast from an herbalist's perspective means treating the underlying imbalance. I have a standard three-fold approach.:

1. Put good bacteria back into both the gut and the vagina. A broad-spectrum oral probiotic can do that or a commitment to food-sourced lactobacillus. (Although there would need to be a BIG commitment to get enough into the system if it's already out of balance from say antibiotic use.) I recommend the probiotics Lactobacillus reuteri and Lactobacillus rhamnosis both orally and as a vaginal suppository. I have had folks use plain yogurt but the delivery system can get iffy and while yogurt can be soothing it is not often enough by itself to rebalance the system.

2. Eliminating what the yeast is thriving on, i.e. sugar. This includes all sugars in any form. Fruit, honey, refined sugars, overly refined carbs, alcohol.

3. Change the ph. The vagina needs to be more acidic which can reduce the growth of both bacteria and fungus. I like using boric acid suppositories. I recommend inserting a gel-cap of boric acid into the vagina for three nights, take a night off, and insert a cap for three more nights. It often makes the discharge runnier and profuse so make sure they are aware of that. If there is a break down of tissue as a result of irritation or scratching then the boric acid may be too burning for some. For those folks I recommend coating the outer labia with plantain salve before inserting the capsules for the first few nights and then trying it without for the next three.

You can use herbs orally and as an external wash especially if the yeast is on the penis or around the rectum. Penis soaks are highly effective in preventing passing excess yeast right back to your partner. Barberry, Oregon Grape Rt, and garlic are all good to reduce the fungus but I have found if you don't correct the underlying imbalance with reducing sugars, and increasing good bacteria it will come right back. Thinking imbalance as compared to infection often gets people moving in the right direction.

Bacterial Vaginosis

Bacterial vaginosis is another "infection" that is fairly straightforward to treat and like yeast is more of an overgrowth of bacteria rather than a true infection. BV will often present with a vaginal discharge that is often profuse, greyish, and has a very strong, "fishy" odor. Itchiness when present can be extreme. BV is often the culprit when I see erosion of the cervix. If I am also doing a PAP smear I will often treat the infection and then re-do the PAP or re-culture for HPV once it has been cleared up. Any erosion of cervical tissue increases the risk of both viral and bacterial infections. If left untreated it can ascend into the uterus, tubes, and ovaries causing PID. Pregnant folks with active BV can go into labor prematurely.

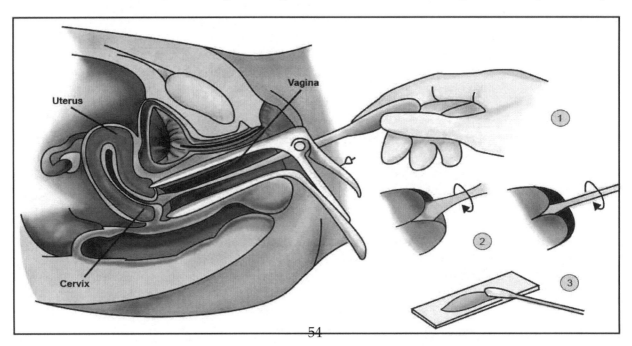

It is often tx with antibiotics taken orally. Get a sense from the client what they want to do. For some folks they want to get treatment over with and just want to do antibiotics and are asking for help in countering the side effects. For others, the idea of taking antibiotics is not acceptable and they are asking for help in treating the infection. Medical treatment is usually with oral or topical Metronidazole or clindamycin. My experience has shown that taking the antibiotics can create a vicious cycle of BV-yeast-BV-yeast and does nothing to treat the underlying imbalance. In general, if someone has recurring BV despite treatment it is often because their partner is not being treated and is giving it right back to them.

The same protocol that works for yeast works here. Three-fold approach:

1. Eliminate all dietary sugars including fruits and alcohol
2. Increase good vaginal and intestinal bacteria using probiotics, especially L. rhamnosis and L. Reuteri both vaginally and orally.
3. Acidify the vagina with boric acid suppositories.

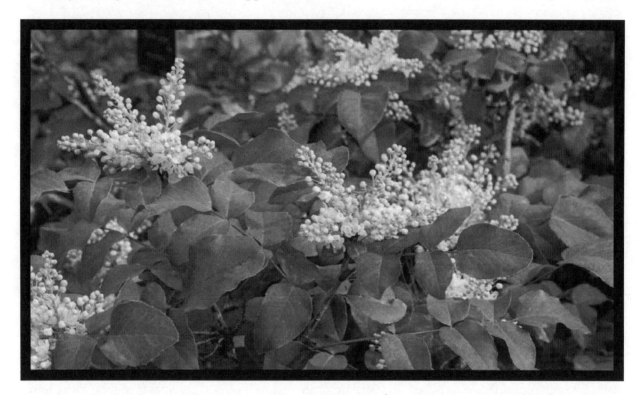

Partners really do need to be treated as well and following the same treatment to clear the vagina or penis soaks with antimicrobial herbs like Oregon Grape rt, garlic. I have used both tea tree oil and oil of oregano to clear these imbalances but the application can be a little tricky. Remember that both mouths and penises can carry different bacteria than the vagina and the body's response to these "different" bacteria is to create an increased response leading to more inflammation. Using a suppository to actually eliminate the excess bacteria is important. I have used the following formula many times with success.

Suppository for rebalancing vaginas:
½ cup cocoa butter,
½ cup coconut oil
1/8-cup calendula oil
8 drops of tea tree oil
8 drops of oregano essential oil

Suppository for rebalancing vaginas:

½ cup cocoa butter,
½ cup coconut oil
1/8-cup calendula oil
8 drops of tea tree oil
8 drops of oregano essential oil

You can definitely add powdered Oregon grape root or other berberine rich herb but be aware it will stain everything (underwear, bedding) it comes in contact with. You can use garlic but chopping it and putting it into these suppositories means you end up with small pieces of garlic in the vagina. Not pleasant. You can make garlic oil by chopping up several cloves and infusing them in olive or coconut oil. Add several drops to the above recipe.

Obviously don't use it if you have an allergy to garlic. You will smell like garlic for as long as you are using it. Gently warm until all ingredients are thoroughly mixed and liquid. Pour into pre-made molds and refrigerate until solid. Cut into 1inch sections. Insert one section into the vagina at night and let it dissolve. Treat for at least 7 days and repeat if necessary.

Penis soaks with yarrow, chaparral, barberry or Oregon grape root will stain the skin yellow but will also get rid of the bacteria. Try it both ways-with or without the berberine-rich herbs and see how it feels. This usually requires soaking every day for a minimal of 7 days.

Any time you use strong antimicrobial herbs to treat an infection you run the risk of decreasing or eliminating the good bacteria along with the bad. Replacing the good bacteria actively will help in avoiding the rebound of increased fungus or bacteria that you don't want. This means lots of plain yogurt, lactobacillus-rich fermented foods, or a multi-strain probiotic should also be added to your regimen.

Trichomoniasis

Trichomoniasis vaginalis is a flagellate protozoa that is typically caused by sexual contact with someone who is infected however, it can be harbored in any moist, warm place and actually transmitted via contact with toilet seats, towels, bathing suits etc. Multiple sex partners, smoking, and IUD's increase the risk of becoming infected. Untreated, the infection can lead to PID in the uterus, pre-term birth, and a potential for increased risk of acquiring HIV.

Those with vaginas often present with a thin, watery, green to grey discharge, inflammation around the vulva and vagina, a strawberry-like rash on the cervix, and a rash on the upper thighs. Those with penises may be asymptomatic but may have a thin whitish or yellow purulent discharge and urethritis.

Most often the infection is diagnosed by a quick wet-slide preparation and microscopic visualization but cultures and molecular-identification may be more reliable and available as home tests.

Medical treatment is effective 90-95 % of the time but only if both partners are treated. The most common pharmaceutical used in treatment is metronidazole either as a one time dose of 2 grams or a 500 my dose daily over 7 days. The drug has a long history of side effects and even though it is considered safe it has a KNOWN risk for both miscarriage and teratogenicity.

Herbal treatments can be somewhat frustrating but if both partners are treated the success rate goes up significantly. Anti-microbial herbs like Oregon grape Root, yarrow, chaparral, tea-tree oil, and oregano oil can be made into penis soaks and done every day for 10 days. Vaginas need to be acidified to decrease an optimal environment for thriving protozoa and/or bacteria.. I have found alternating boric acid suppositories with suppositories using the following formula is most helpful. The recipe can be made up and put into gel caps and inserted into the vagina:

¼ cup Slippery Elm powder
¼ cup Oregon Grape root powder
10 drops tea tree oil
10 drops of oregano oil
10 drops of Usnea tincture
Mix all together. You want the mixture to be more like a powder than a soft, oil-based suppository. Fill 00 gel caps. Alternate insertion with boric acid suppositories for 10 days.

The next couple of infections are becoming rampant in folks 18-25 but everyone who is sexually active is at risk.

Chlamydia

The number one STI that is being defined as epidemic is Chlamydia. There were 1.7 million cases reported in 2017. Chlamydia is a parasitic bacterium that enters through a cell wall and thereby 'hiding' within the cell making both it's recognition and treatment difficult. Most folks are symptom free but some will express symptoms like an abnormal, whitish vaginal discharge . Urethral discharge is whitish and irritating. Rectal discharge can be more yellowish and pus-like. When there are symptoms it is because the immune system has been able to detect it and the resulting inflammation is acute. But again most Do Not Have Symptoms, which is why it can cause so much damage.

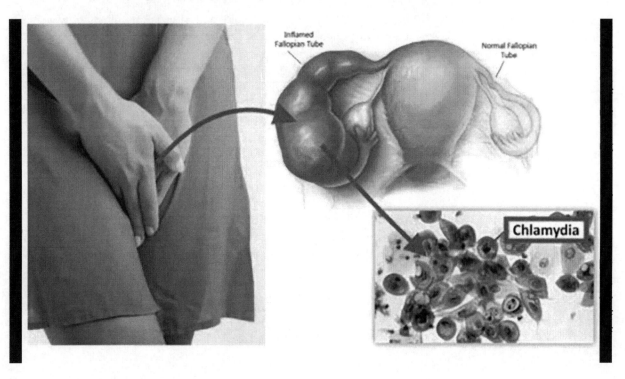

It can cause direct damage to the cervix, uterus and endometrium, fallopian tubes and ovaries and epididymis. It is the leading cause of both Pelvic Inflammatory Disease (PID) and infertility. It can damage both the fallopian tubes and the epididymis inhibiting the flow of egg or sperm. It can cause scarring in the fallopian tube increasing the risk of ectopic pregnancy. It can alter the cervical cell structure making that person more susceptible to HIV and HPV. Untreated in a specific population of white males (most common) chlamydia can lead to Reiter's disease or Reiter's Syndrome. It is a disease caused by an infection that leads to a triad of issues: arthritis in the large joints of the body, urethritis, and conjunctivitis. It is a leading cause of blindness and can be passed to baby in utero and during delivery causing both eye infections and chlamydial pneumonia that can occur 1-3 months after birth.

The standard way of diagnosing Chlamydia is through culture swabs of the cervix, urethra, rectum, or throat. This can be done routinely during a PAP exam, yearly, or during routine testing in pregnancy. Urine cultures are also used but are slightly less accurate.

Medical treatment for Chlamydia is with antibiotics. The standard is to give Azithromycin 1 gram orally in a single dose or Doxycycline`100 mg twice a day orally for 7 days. Because doxycycline is contraindicated in pregnancy the drug of choice is either Azithromycine or Erythromycin. However Erythromycin does not cross the placenta so the fetus is not effectively treated. The whole goal of aggressive treatment is to reduce the damage that is caused by long-term infection especially in light of the lack of symptoms.

As herbalists, it is important provide our clients with as much information as possible so that they can make decisions that work for them. How many times has someone said to you that they feel ok but were given this random diagnosis and don't want to do antibiotics based on how they feel? That to me is where it gets sticky. I have my own opinions about what I think is a good route of treatment but it's the client who needs to be onboard with their treatment first. Obviously not contracting the disease in the first place is the ideal but if you are already there then how to do counsel your client to proceed? I personally think you have to have a clear discussion about the "risks vs. benefits."

You need to have some basic information in order to help them make decisions. First, how was the infection diagnosed initially? Was it a routine check-up or were there changes in lifestyle that made your client want to get tested (new partner, partner with known infection, symptoms, geographical or cultural location that has been identified as higher risk?) If the infection has been present for some time has damage to organs already occurred? Are there concurrent infections for example gonorrhea or HIV? What is their medical history? What would the impacts of treating or not treating be on their health both to specific systems or issues and overall. Do they have the means to buy, prepare, and take the treatment? There are STI clinics all over the country and they often have ways of offsetting the cost of drugs but nobody is doing that with herbs. Because herbal treatment may take longer and requires a high degree of compliance does the client feel like they can be committed to that treatment? It's worth it to both you as the provider and your client to take the time and explore the answers to these questions.

The obvious benefit of treating with an antibiotic is that the infection can be treated and basically be done. (All partners must also be treated.) Follow-up testing needs to happen in a couple of months to be sure there is no ongoing infection or re-infection but you go on with your life. The risk of treating with an antibiotic is:

1. The potential for side effects,
2. The alteration of individual microbiome and
3. Potential future problems such as resistant bacteria both in this specific situation and in the overall response.

The risks of not treating because someone is asymptomatic are:

1.the infection could be severe even without symptoms
2. Damage can occur to your fallopian tubes and ovaries or your epididymis which may alter the ability to conceive.
3. The infection could be passed to a partner

Treating with herbs has the benefit of not using pharmaceutical antibiotics, which potentially allow you to avoid side effects, but runs the risk of:

1. Allowing damage to occur which is non-reversible
2. Herbs being ineffective prolonging the potential and/or real damage as a result.
3. The infection could be passed to a partner.

Counseling folks that it doesn't have to be either or is another approach. They can take the antibiotics *and* take herbs to enhance both the efficacy of the antibiotic and reduce the side effects. Being non-judgmental towards both our clients and their treatment choices is important. Treating with herbs either alone or in conjunction with antibiotics involves a multi-faceted approach.

Systemic anti-bacterial:
Equal parts Usnea, Oregon Grape Root, and Yarrow tincture 1 dropper full 3x/day
        d. Chaparral tincture 3-4 drops/day

Immune Boosting

Long Term:
- Reishi, shiitake, turkey tail mushrooms powdered extracts 2x/day
- Astragalus, eleutherococcus, tincture 2x/day
- Vit d 2000/mg/day, sunlight on exposed skin

Short Term:
- Vit c 1000 mg of Sodium ascorbate q 3-4 hrs
- Vaginal suppositories
- Calendula oil, garlic, oil of oregano suppositories1x/day
- Penis washes-3x/day
- antibacterial herbs like yarrow, barberry, Oregon grape root,
- Lifestyle changes
- Stress reduction
- Eliminate alcohol, excessive sugar intake, reduce red meat
- Increase sleep, water consumption,
- Lactobacillus-rich foods like plain yogurt, kim-chi, sauerkraut, kombucha

Things to watch out for are:
- Any allergic like responses, rashes, SOB, swelling
- Pain-either initial occurring or increased.
- Bloating or pressure in the abdomen.
- Fever
- Irritation or increase in quantity of discharge
- Diarrhea

Life-style changes
- Celibacy until verified free of the disease
- Condom use
- Identification of all partners so that they can be treated

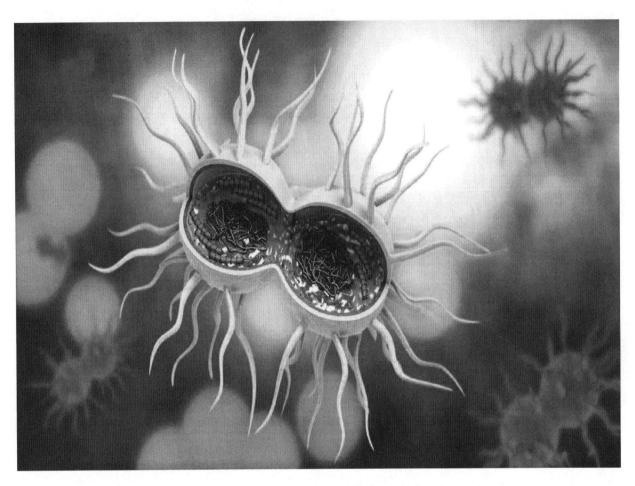

Gonorrhea

Gonorrhea is caused by a gram negative bacterium Neisseria gonorrhea. As an infection, gonorrhea has been acknowledged and identified since ancient times. Also known as the clap. Like Chlamydia, gonorrhea is dramatically on the rise. Cases are up 67% in the last five years. It is often times concurrent with a Chlamydia infection. Symptoms can range from none to urethral swelling and/or milky, yellowish, or greenish discharge from the penis or cervix. Typically symptoms show up 10-14 days after exposure. People with penises are much more likely to have symptoms-about 90%. While only 20% of people with vaginas have symptoms. If left untreated, gonorrhea can cause PID, tubal and epididymis scarring and infertility, mouth and throat infections, fever, bleeding during intercourse, heart, brain, and skin problems. Causes blindness in neonates born to mothers with active infection.

Diagnosing Gonorrhea is most accurately done with a swab of the urethra, the cervix, the rectum, or the mouth/throat and then cultured. Testing is also done on urine samples although slightly less accurate.

The standard medical treatment for Gonorrhea was initially with penicillin or tetracycline antibiotics but completely resistant strains are now prevalent. The next wave used ciprofloxacin or fluoroquinolones but those too have created resistant strains. The drugs of choice now are 250 mg of Ceftrioxone in a single injected dose in combination with 1 g orally of Azithromycin in a single dose. Because gonorrhea is a bacterium that has been able to adapt quickly the concern of course is that there will soon not be a viable pharmaceutical treatment option. The CDC's current recommendation is that if symptoms have not cleared up 3-5 days after treatment that they be re-evaluated.

This is a situation that can prove challenging to both client and practitioner. As more and more antibiotics are deemed ineffective and the bacteria continues to change and prove resistant the potential for treatment with herbs begins to look promising. The challenge of course is that nobody is studying how alternative methods can be effective so it is left to the folks using herbs to both figure out good treatment protocols and make sure folks are not put at undue risk if treatment fails. Of course one way to look at it is that if all the pharmaceuticals are failing why not go full force in using alternative treatment modalities. In the case I think there is good rational behind using herbs as compared to antibiotics. The only thing that must be considered is that the provider must provide full informed consent with the client so that they understand the pros and cons.

So, as an herbalist how can you approach treatment? Once again, knowing your client's history, and where they are in the process is essential. Included in that is the discussion about risks vs. benefits for all options. Knowing the status of any concurrent infections is very important-many people who have gonorrhea also have chlamydia increasing the risk of damage if left untreated or partly treated. If you have ruled out other organisms either through their testing or doing the tests on your own it will help you make some decisions about treatment.

Gonorrhea is a nasty infection. If the choice is to treat with herbs or to treat with antibiotics AND herbs then the same approach to chlamydia is used here. In this case, along with the antibacterial tinctures already recommended I would add Echinacea tincture given in large doses 90 gtts every 3 hours for 7 days. Garlic is really quite effective. Caution of course is appropriate because eating raw garlic several times a day if you are allergic is a bad idea. The suppositories with calendula and garlic can do wonders and doing penis soaks with garlic "soup" is helpful. It must be done several times a day to be effective. There is good research into using Mangosteen fruit and/or juice or powders. Xanthones can be quite effective as an antibacterial and anti-inflammatory agent. Mangosteen is sprayed heavily with pesticides so being aware of your source is important. There are some herbalists using small doses of Poke Root tincture but I would want to be very clear with my client about the potential for toxicity vs. benefits.

Anytime you're dealing with an infection with the potential for serious consequences, the herbalist must communicate that your clients' commitment to treatment, awareness of whether symptoms (if present) are improving or worsening, and retesting has to be a priority. It is unacceptable to give them recommendations for treatment and then say, "I'll see you in a month. The client needs to be seen frequently and the efficacy of treatment evaluated.

Syphilis (Trepenoma pallidum)

Syphilis is a systemic sexual infection that has been identified for thousands of years. It is transmitted from person to person through direct contact with the lesions or chancres of primary syphilis, through contact with the condylomata or mucosal lesions in secondary syphilis, or through a direct transmission from an infected mother to her unborn child.

The awareness of the disease seems to have been around for centuries if not millennium. The debate over the origin of syphilis and whether is was present in Europe prior to exploration of the Americas or was brought to Europe with the return of Columbus has been going on for centuries. It appears that after Columbus's return the virulence of the disease was much more intense than in later years. Based on reports it appears the disease moved through the different stages much quicker and the latent stages moved into the Tertiary stage within months to years as compared to decades. It was often confused with and perhaps misidentified as leprosy. Physicians in the 18th and 19th century went to school with a primary intent of determining which symptoms were a result of syphilis and which ones weren't. There are still researchers today who believe that Syphilis is at epidemic proportions and that most cases are underreported and undiagnosed. Historical treatments have been varied and intense.

The CDC keeps records of cases and in 2013 there were 16.929 cases of primary syphilis in the US. Of those cases the vast majority but not all where identified in 19-24 year olds. There were 15,861 cases identified in men and 1,500 cases identified in women. Four years later in 2017 there were 26,885 cases identified in men and 3,722 cases identified in women. Again, these were primary stage infections. In 2017 there were another 36,992 cases identified as secondary or latent syphilis. Remember, these are the cases of identified infection. The nature of the infection is that MANY cases go unnoticed or unidentified while transmission is still active.

Syphilis is categorized based on the presenting symptoms and the time since initial infection. Primary syphilis is identified by the presence of chancres-firm, round, small, and painless lesions. Lesions can appear on the penis, rectum, mouth, and vagina or cervix. Typically they appear around 3 weeks from the time of initial exposure (can range anywhere from 10-90 days.) Lesions typically heal on their own in a few days. The patient is highly infectious most likely to pass on the infection at this stage. Women who are pregnant are most likely to pass on the infection to their fetuses at this stage.

Secondary Syphilis symptoms occur averaging 6 weeks (3 wks. -6 months) after initial exposure and most often present as a rash on the torso, but rashes can be present on the hands and feet or anywhere on the body. About 25% of the time there are condylomata-rough, wart-like patches on the genitals or mucosal patches on the tongue. Rarely, folks present with patchy alopecia or neurological symptoms. Typically, symptoms disappear in 2-6 wks. but can take up to 3 months. During this time the patient is still highly infectious, especially if there is direct contact with a moist lesion. Transmission to the fetus is still high.

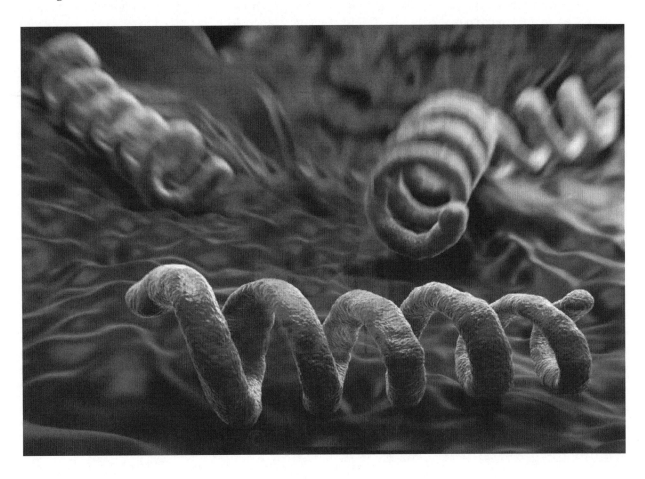

The infection then goes into a latent period that is identified in two stages. Early latent can present with no symptoms but positive blood tests within a year of that initial exposure or can present with reoccurring symptoms (chancres or rash) and the person is still able to infect others. Often the symptoms go unnoticed and the infection is then passed on to others. Late latent is identified by positive blood tests typically 1 year after the initial infection or if the initial timing of the infection is unknown but there are usually no symptoms. The patient is not infectious however in utero transmission can occur in the latent phase usually in the early latent phase.

Tertiary syphilis occurs in 30% of people who were untreated during the earlier stage and can occur anywhere from 10-30 years after initial exposure. This stage is classified into three key types identified by the location although it may present in all locations simultaneously. The first is cardiovascular syphilis. This is identified with inflammation of the arteries causing restriction and valve injuries resulting in aneurysm, heart attack, or death. The damage is permanent and debilitating. Symptoms are the same as any cardiovascular disease including angina, weak aortic valves causing heart failure and/or aortic regurgitation, blood clots, dry cough, back pain, hoarseness, trouble swallowing.

Neurosyphilis is the next form of tertiary syphilis. It can occur in two stages. Early neurosyphilis can present anywhere from a few weeks to a few years after the initial infection. It typically manifests as meningitis affecting the cranial nerves and meningovascular syphilis, which may present with stroke-like symptoms. Late nerosyphilis can present 10-30 years after the initial infection can present as chronic meningoenchephalitis leading to dementia, muscle weakness and paralysis and myelin sheath degeneration leading to general numbness and loss of motor function.

Gummatous syphilis is the third type identified and can occur 45 years after initial infections. It is classified based on the presence of soft, rubbery tumors of varying sizes that can occur on any of the vital organs including the liver, kidneys, eyes, brain, spinal cord heart and blood vessels, intestines, skin, and long bones. Often the "gummas" rupture and ulcerate leading to scars and permanent damage including arthritis, muscle pain, inflammation of connective tissue, breathing difficulties, liver cirrhosis, abdominal pain, sever cardiovascular and central nervous system problems.

Essentially, tertiary syphilis looks like many of the degenerative diseases that are so prevalent in our current society. If someone is actually tested and identified with syphilis the treatment at this point is to do IV penicillin every four hours for 14 days. It is rare for anyone who presents with, for example, a heart attack or dementia to be tested for syphilis antibodies partly because usually the infection has progressed to the point that damage is irreversible and also because it is not widely recognized as the underlying culprit.

Ocular syphilis is a specific manifestation of the infection and can occur at any of the stages of syphilis. It can present with vision loss, blurred vision, pain, or redness. Anyone at high risk of STIs with ocular symptoms should be tested for both Syphilis and HIV. Careful neurological and ophthalmological assessment should be made ASAP including lumbar puncture and MRI. It is recommended that treatment be initiated immediately even before test results are returned as permanent blindness can occur quickly.

Diagnosing syphilis has changed over the past decades but currently the most accurate determination comes from a combination of treponemal and non-treponemal tests. Essentially these blood tests are testing for the presence of syphilis antibodies (trepenomal) and the quantity of specifically IgM and IgG antibodies (non-treponemal.) Because the treponemal test cannot tell you the stage of the infection or whether or not it's been treated it is followed up with the non-trepenomal test to gauge where the patient is in the spectrum of disease. Because of the relatedly high false positive or negative results it is important to also have both a clear history of actual or potential exposure as well as a physical exam for determining the presence of symptoms.

Treating this infection has been the focus of innumerable experiments with often times tragic results. Historically, many of the herbs and substances used were designed to purge the body by inducing sweating, salivation, increasing urine output, and laxatives thinking that if the body were detoxed enough the infection would be cured. Mercury as both an elixir and an ointment for the skin was know and used at least as far back as Paracelsus in the 1500's.

It's interesting that even though the toxic side effects of mercury were well known it was considered the lesser of two evils and routinely administered. The side effects of mercury included mood changes and irritability, depression, numbness, tremors, muscle weakness, nausea and vomiting, kidney failure, severe ulcers of the mouth and skin, and loss of teeth, loss of language capacity. It was later altered so that it could be administered as a pill or injected. Many, many people died from mercury poisoning. As folks looked for alternatives they would create combinations that might include salicylates, ammonia, and arsenic.

In 1910, Paul Ehrlich, while doing research on creating anti-microbial drugs using organic compounds created a drug using arsenic that was heralded as a "magic bullet" and garnered him a Nobel prize. It was only 5 years earlier that spirochete Treponema was seen using dark field microscopy. Once visualized, the ability to create compounds to target specific organisms was possible. The drug was designed to kill Treponema pallidum and while unstable, difficult to use, and fraught with side-effects-it worked. It was 37 more years before the use of penicillin to target Treponema became available and marked the end of any other treatment.

Today the use of penicillin is still the treatment of choice for both primary and secondary syphilis: 2.4 million units of Benzathine Penicillin G given IM in a single dose. It is affective 98% of the time. If the infection has gone beyond those stages and is the patient is in the early or late latent stage the treatment changes to be 3 doses of 24,000 units Penicillin G IM one week apart.

The idea of treatment here is to prevent transmission from mother to child or to halt the damage caused by Tertiary Syphilis. Penicillin can eliminate the bacteria but if allowed to go on too long it cannot repair the damage caused by the way Treponema works on the body. Even folks who are actually diagnosed with a penicillin allergy are recommended to desensitize to the drug and use it anyway. Folks who live in a high-risk area or population for HIV, or who currently have HIV infection are recommended to treat both prophylactically and aggressively.

So, knowing some of the background of this infection and its impact on the body if untreated or under-treated it's challenging to recommend trying to treat this without using penicillin. This one disease has been plaguing humanity for thousands of years and the success rate for treating it without antibiotics has not been very good. At the very least, our record of successful treatment has not been overwhelming. In the event that penicillin stops being effective, stops being made, a major shake-up of standard care, or the patient is unable or unwilling to use penicillin then we have to work towards finding viable alternatives.

Because of Trepenoma's ability to change and become less visible to antibodies in it's latent and tertiary phases it becomes more essential to treat during the initial stages of the infection when 1. Spirochete reproduction is at its highest and 2. The inflammatory reaction allows the body's antibodies to recognize the invader and mount a response. Timing is everything! Overwhelming the infection in its early stages means that folks need to be willing to treat aggressively. This means large doses frequently for a minimum of 10-14 days. What antimicrobials to use is the hard part.

The following is a list of antibacterial herbs that may be helpful (Please be aware of potential side-effects, toxicity, and contra-indications especially if there are co-infections of HIV):

1. Poke Root: 1-4 drops fresh root tincture daily
2. Echinacea Root: infusion 2-4 cups/day, or tincture 1-2 droppersful every 4 hours
3. Chaparral leaves: fresh or dried leaf tincture 1 droppersful every four hours
4. Yarrow: infusion 2 cups /day or tincture 2 droppersful 3x/day
5. Geranium Root: Strong decoction 2-4 cups/day
6. Cryptolepsis sanguinolenta: Rt. Tincture, 20-40 drops 3-4x/day

Immune boosting herbs and mushrooms to keep the immune system functioning optimally is important here. Astragalus, Eleuthero, Turkey Tail, Maitake, and Shitaki mushroom extracts. Vitamin A as beta-carotene, 5,000-10,000 iu/day; Vit c. 1-2 grams/day, Vit E 400-800 iu/day, and zinc 15-25 iu/day helps.

The work that Stephen Buhner is doing with using companion herbs to enhance the actions of antibacterial herbs is promising in this case. Ginger and black pepper are two of the plants he is recommending to both increase the recognition of the invading organism by antibodies in the body boosting the body's natural immune response as well as enhancing the antibiotics to break through the cell membranes of the invader and destroy it.

If you are treating someone with Syphilis please be sure to gauge how well the treatment is doing and do frequent blood tests to see if the antibody titer is decreasing. Having the conversation about protecting themselves so they do not get re-infected is important.Treating folks with sexually transmitted infections is challenging as an herbalist. Much more challenging is to be the person fighting the infection. We have to remember how much the lives of our clients are being impacted and strive to support them with compassion, empathy, and facts. We have to search for viable treatments and be non-judgmental both in our approach to the client themselves and their choice of treatment.

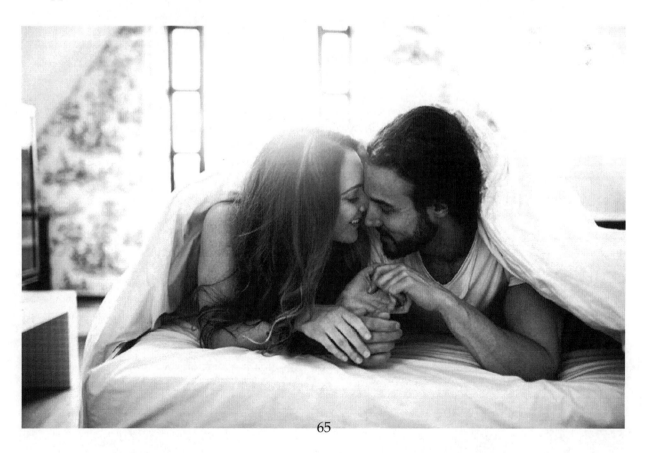

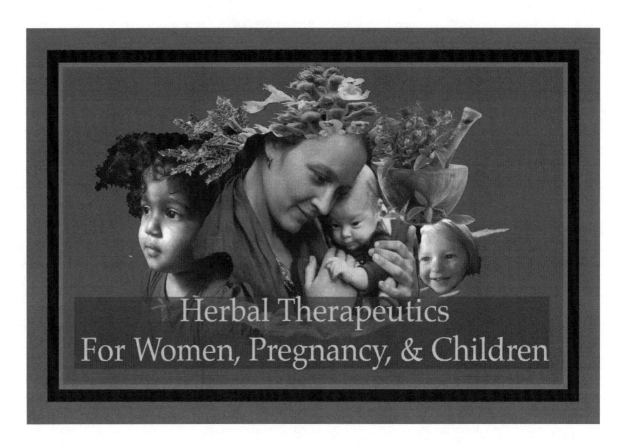

Herbal Therapeutics
For Women, Pregnancy, & Children

CANDIDA & YEAST INFECTIONS

by Phyllis D. Light

Candida and other fungal infections can be irritating, debilitating and take a long time to adequately treat. Under normal conditions, the yeast known as Candida albicans as well as other fungi live at a low level inside our digestive tract, mouth, bladder and genital regions. Under circumstances of stress, digestive difficulties, treatment with antibiotics and other conditions that limit the growth of probiotics, candida and other undesirable fungi can rapidly reproduce, causing discomfort and health problems. Fortunately, beneficial bacteria (probiotics) also live there and help keep a balance of microorganisms that promote good health.

In addition to the use of antibiotics, constipation and lack of stomach acid can also lead to candidiasis. Also, food which remains too long in the digestive tract can ferment which leads to nutritive substances that promote yeast growth. Under normal circumstances, levels of Candida are controlled by beneficial bacteria. However, antibiotics are not discriminate, killing off all bacteria while making the intestinal lining more susceptible to bacterial invasion, impacting the health of colon cells and disarming the immune system. With the good bacteria out of the way, parasites and fungi have the opportunity to flourish. This can lead to an overgrowth or superinfection of yeast which can lead to another course of anti-infective drugs creating a vicious cycle.

Location, Location, Location

For women, changes in the body prior to and after menstruation, during perimenopause, or while taking oral contraceptives, affect pH levels making conditions right for fungal infections. A diet high in processed foods and sugars and normal changes associated with aging also creates a higher risk for yeast infection both vaginally and in the intestines. Main symptoms of vaginal yeast infection are an itchy vaginal discharge, painful intercourse or urination and redness of the vulva and inner thighs.

Other symptoms of candida infection include swollen lymph nodes, depression, insomnia, carbohydrate cravings, abnormal fatigue, mood swings, mucosal deposits in the nose, throat and lungs, skin infections, oral and vaginal thrush, problems thinking, intestinal gas and strange feelings after eating.

Yeast colonies can also be found on the skin between the fingers, toes, and around the anus. An abrasion can also become the site of a skin fungal infection. Moisture can` contribute to infections and workers who have constantly wet hands or feet often develop infections around their nails. Skin folds can create moist environments encouraging the growth of yeast or fungus.

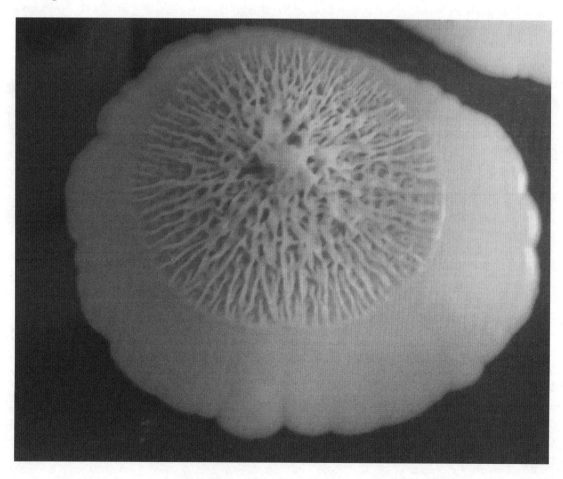

Back to Balance

From my experience, the best way to recover from chronic candida is not by killing off the yeast with strong anti-infective herbs or drugs, but rather by creating and building a healthy digestive system and bringing the flora and fauna back into balance. This can be accomplished through a combination of diet, supplements, and herbal remedies.

Diet is the essential tool I use for returning the digestive system back to a balanced state and fermented foods play a primary role in this process. Removing wheat and other grains helps reduce inflammation in the digestive track, helps heal leaky gut syndrome and improves gut motility. In addition to avoiding grains, avoid pinto beans, black-eyed peas, dairy, processed sugars, alcohol and caffeine, and corn, soybean and cottonseed oils. Eat clean by avoiding most processed foods, by eating fresh vegetables, locally grown when possible, and pastured or wild caught meat.

Good bacteria requires the same type of food for nourishment that yeast requires, sugar. For this reason, natural sugars can't be eliminated from the diet. However, the type of sugar or carbohydrate does make a difference. Using honey and eating fresh fruits, and starchy vegetables such as winter squashes, will provide adequate carbohydrate intake to build good, healthy bacteria.

Probiotic supplements should be taken on an empty stomach first thing in the morning. Pick a product that contains several different strains of bacteria for most beneficial effect. However, fermented foods such as yogurt, kefir, unpasteurized sauerkraut, tempeh, miso, some cultured cheeses, pickles, buttermilk, chutney, sour cream, and cultured butter are all excellent sources of food-providing probiotics.

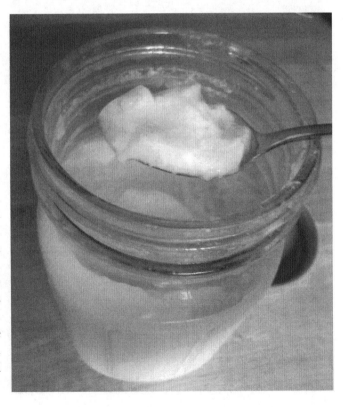

A caution here: don't overeat the fermented foods. It's best to begin with very small amounts and work your way up to larger ones. I generally recommend only about ½ teaspoon of fermented foods to begin, then after a week or so, try a whole teaspoon, and so on. The body seems bacteria as bacteria, not good or bad. So, any bacteria entering the digestive tract will initiate an immune response. Replenish slowly and surely to avoid feeling worse.

Supplement Support

Support the liver, when dealing with yeast, because it may be overstressed as it tries to filter out toxins. Herbs for liver support include Milk Thistle, Blessed Thistle, Dandelion, and Bayberry. Drinking plenty of water, getting exercise in the fresh air, and deep breathing also helps the liver function properly.

The amino acid glutamine helps rebuild the intestinal walls and helps eliminate leaky gut syndrome. And excellent, excellent supplement for this purpose. I've seen some amazing progress after adding glutamine to the regimen. Leaky gut, which can allow allergens and infectious agents to enter the blood stream through the walls of the intestines, occurs when the intestines become overly permeable. This condition is amenable to allowing candida and other fungi to spread from the intestines to other parts of the body such as the vagina. Glutamine may also be employed by the body to reconstruct sections of the intestinal villi and keep out microorganisms and toxins.

The complete set of B vitamins and the antioxidant nutrients vitamin A, C and E and selenium are important in supporting the immune system and reducing outbreaks of yeast. Healthy fats, such as the omega-3 fats found in fish oil, limits inflammation and reduces irritating symptoms of yeast infection. In addition gamma-linoleic acid (GLA), from evening primrose helps keep yeast from latching onto the walls of the intestines. Short chain fatty acids, which feed the cells of the intestines, are also important for improving the growth of healthy microorganisms in the digestive tract.

Herbal Aids

My herbal approaches for yeast fall into these categories: soothing herbs, building herbs, and anti-infective herbs.

My favorite herb for reducing yeast is Black Walnut, a traditional anti-parasite herb, that kills candida and other types of fungus. I generally recommend this herb be taken in capsule because its bitter taste is hard for some people to bear. I like Black Walnut because it will reduce yeast load without irritating the intestinal tract. As a matter of fact, Black walnut will help tone the intestines. If taking capsules, I recommend 2 capsules 2 times a day for about 7 days. I think it also helps reduces other opportunistic infections that can occur because the immune system is occupied trying to control the yeast overgrowth.

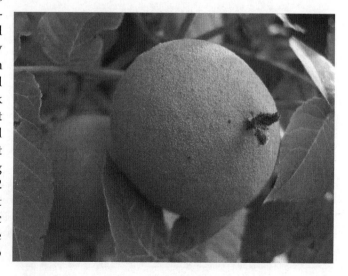

Herbs containing berberine such as Oregon Grape Root, Yellow Root, Goldenseal and Barberry are antifungal and can kill yeast but may be harsh on the tender, inflamed walls of the digestive tract. Cayenne helps stimulate peristalsis , relieve intestinal gas and reduce inflammation in the gut. I also can't say enough about Garlic for intestinal healing. Garlic kills parasites, boosts the immune system, and helps heal erosions and abrasions that can house colonies of yeast.

For topical yeast colonies, I've used both Tea Tree essential oil and Lavender essential oil with equal success. But I've found that a good quality yogurt or buttermilk applied topically is both soothing to itching, irritated skin and kills yeast.

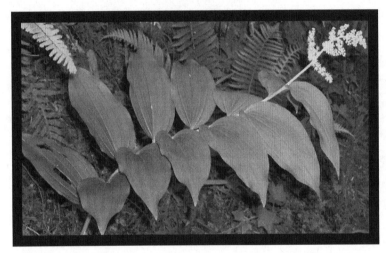

Solomon's Seal tea is my absolute favorite herb for soothing inflammation and helping maintain healthy mucosal layers in the intestinal tract. This herb is truly amazing for rebuilding the intestinal walls from any type of damage whether from yeast, leaky gut, or ulcers.

Marshmallow root and Slippery Elm bark tea also soothes inflammation and helps maintain healthy mucosal layers in the intestinal tract. They are demulcent, nutritive, slightly astringent and tonic. Slippery Elm tea also helps draw out impurities, promotes healing of intestinal walls and reduces effects of acidity.

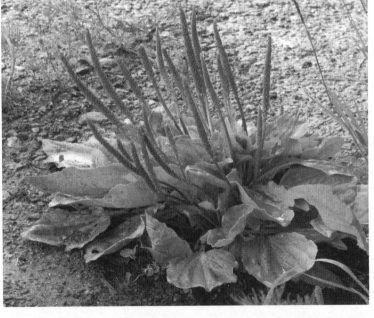

I would be remiss if I didn't mention the healing power of Plantain tea for the intestinal tract. It helps lift the yeast off the intestinal walls, soothes irritated tissue, reduces inflammation, and helps eliminate toxins from the digestive tract. One of my favorite herbal combinations is Solomon's Seal and Plantain tea.

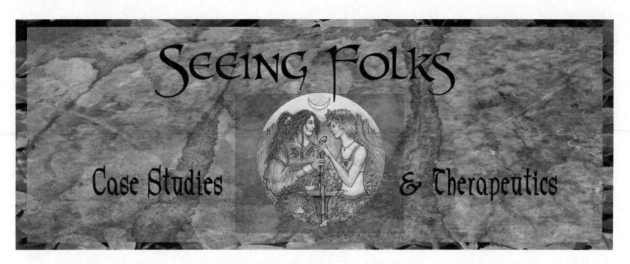

CERVICAL DYSPLASIA & ABNORMAL PAP TESTS

Treating Them Naturally

by Wendy Hounsel

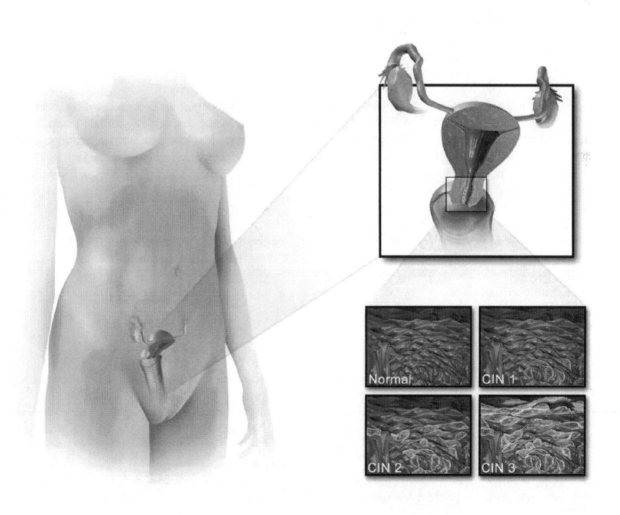

I was diagnosed with cervical dysplasia in 2009 and successfully healed myself with herbs and nutrition. Since then I have worked with and advised many women in healing themselves. All have had successful results. This is revolutionary work. Women have historically had little power in the medical system. I have never felt so powerless as when I was told blithely that I would have to have a chunk of my cervix cut out – and I have never felt as empowered as I did when, after months of herbal treatment, the doctor said, with some surprise, "Huh! It seems to have spontaneously resolved!" I went to multiple providers, searching for one who would listen to my ideas and goals non-judgmentally and support them. I was unsuccessful. They simply had no knowledge or context for women taking care of this themselves. There are no double blind or clinical studies for what we're going to learn today.

What is Cervical Dysplasia?

Definition

According to the Johns Hopkins University Kimmel Cancer Center, Cervical dysplasia is the term for abnormal cells on the cervix. If untreated, it's possible for the cells to develop into cancer. Cervical dysplasia affects between 250,000 and 1 million women in the US each year. It is most often seen in women between the ages of 25 and 35. According to the National Cervical Cancer Coalition, around 12,000 women are diagnosed with cervical cancer each year in the US – and 3,000 die -- but it's one of the most preventable forms of cancer due to our ability to screen for abnormal cells way before cancer has a chance to develop, through Pap tests. In developing countries, death from cervical cancer is much higher due to the lack of screening. Most cases of cervical dysplasia are caused by an HPV virus. There are scores of different strains. The HPV viruses that cause genital warts are NOT the types that cause cervical dysplasia and cancer. The strains of HPV that cause genital warts are termed "low risk," while the strains that cause cervical dysplasia and cervical cancer are termed "high risk." There are over 40 different HPV viruses. High risk strains include

16 and 18, which the cervical cancer vaccine protects against, as well as 31, 35, 39, 45, 51, 52, 58, and others.

These abnormal cells are very slow-growing. If the changes are mild, an allopathic clinician may simply monitor the situation by repeating the test in six months to a year. Many cases of cervical dysplasia resolve without intervention as the body clears the virus and returns to homeostasis. During this time, there are many ways to support our body's efforts with nutrition and herbs. The clinician may also recommend removing the abnormal cells with electro-cautery or surgery. Certainly, there are times in which this may be appropriate. However, because the cells are so slow-growing, it is most often very safe to try an herbal and nutritional approach first, considering a more invasive technique only if no progress is seen.

Causes

HPV is a sexually transmitted infection. Taking safer sex measures during and after treatment is advisable, as is testing and/or treatment of one's sexual partners. Other contributing factors to cervical dysplasia include nutrient deficiencies, early sexual activity, multiple sexual partners, smoking cigarettes, oral contraceptive use longer than 10 years, low socioeconomic status, and poor diet (Marshall, 2003), and never having had a Pap test. There's a lot to be extrapolated from this list, but it's clear that our economic system engenders widespread poverty and that the burdens of poverty, including lack of screening, nutrient deficiencies and poor diet, make avoiding cervical dysplasia harder for poor women.

Cervical A & P

The cervix is the lower part of the uterus, and is shaped like a doughnut. It's about an inch long, is mostly made of connective tissue and muscle and is made up of two parts: the endocervix is the inner part of the canal leading to the uterus; the exocervix is the outer part that protrudes into the vagina and that is visible with the use of a speculum.

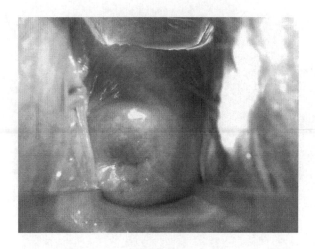

The canal itself is called the endocervical canal, or os. The exocervix and vagina are covered with a thin layer of flat epithelial cells called squamous cells. The endocervical canal is covered with column-shaped, mucus-producing cells called columnar cells. The area where the columnar and squamous cells meet is called the squamo-columnar junction, or the "transformation zone." It's a highly active area where the columnar cells are constantly moving down and turning into squamous cells. This is the area where precancerous changes are most likely to occur, because the increased activity in this area increases the likelihood of misshapen or mutated cells.

What is a Pap Test?

Definition

The Pap test is the screening test for cervical dysplasia and is the single most important tool for preventing cervical cancer. In a Pap test, cervical cells are gently scraped or brushed from the endocervix and the exocervix using a specialized brush or swab. They are then examined under a microscope for abnormalities.

Testing Guidelines

Guidelines for the frequency of Pap testing have recently changed. Older guidelines stated that a Pap test was necessary every year for all women but the newest guidelines released in 2012 by the US Preventive Services Task Force and the American Cancer Society recommend that Pap testing for women with cervixes begin having Paps at age 21 and no earlier. The reason behind these recent changes is that cervical cancer is very rare in young women and Pap testing has not been shown to be of any benefit – young women's immune systems are very effective in clearing the HPV virus that causes dysplasia and Pap testing leads to unnecessary treatment – the harms outweigh the benefit. After age 21, testing with cytology - the examination of cells under a microscope - should occur every three years. Women younger than 30 should be screened with cytology only, not HPV testing. After age 30, testing can be reduced to every 5 years if combined with high-risk HPV testing. After age 65, if there is no high risk for cervical cancer and if adequate prior testing has occurred, testing is no longer necessary. All of these recommendations differ for women who have a history of high grade precancerous lesions, and those who are immunocompromised, such as folks with HIV. In these cases, frequency is determined on a case by case basis. In the cases that I have worked on with women doing herbal treatment, Paps have been repeated every three to six months depending on the severity of the dysplasia at any given time, until the dysplasia has cleared and the person is HPV negative. After that, Paps are done every 1-3 years. Different practitioners have different ideas about how often Paps should be done in these cases.

Further Research

There is some evidence that the physical act of scraping the cervix when performing a Pap test stimulates an immune response that decreases the risk of developing cervical cancer. According to authors of a 2007 study documenting significant immune responses (specifically, markers of cell mediated immunity and T-cell regulation), having even a single Pap test reduces a person's risk of cervical cancer and high risk HPV infection. According to the National Cervical Cancer Coalition, 50% of women diagnosed with cervical cancer have never had a Pap test, and 10% of women diagnosed with cervical cancer have not had a Pap test in 5 years.

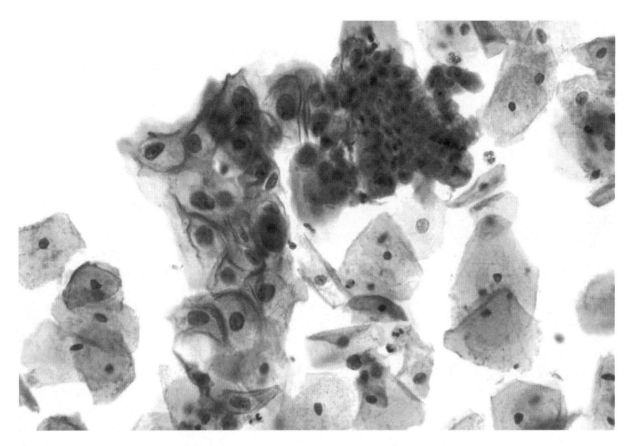

The Abnormal Pap Test: Medical Terminology for Abnormal Cervical Cells

A Pap test will detect patches of abnormal cell growth, called intraepithelial squamous lesions, or ISL. ISLs can be further designated as either low grade (LSIL) or high grade (HSIL). Many cases of ISL heal spontaneously, and all are slow growing. In cases of LSIL, treatment consists of observation by means of a repeat Pap test every three to six months. It may very well go away on its own, and it can be helped to do so with herbs.

Pap Test Categories

Pap test results are divided into the following categories:
- Normal

ASC-US: Atypical Squamous Cells of Undetermined Significance.

These cells may be normal, but they need to be monitored with repeat Pap tests, as it's possible for them to progress to more advanced abnormality.

- ASC-H: Atypical Squamous Cells, cannot exclude High-grade.

A step up from ASCUS. Still mild.

- LSIL: Low Grade Intraepithelial Squamous Lesion.

A bit more concerning but still often resolves spontaneously. Monitoring needed; colposcopy not needed.

- HSIL High Grade Intraepithelial Squamous Lesion.

You definitely want to keep a close eye on this. Still grows slowly and can be healed, but more concerning than the others. HSIL should be followed up with a colposcopy to discern the severity of the lesions.

Further Diagnosis

If the Pap test shows HSIL, the provider may suggest a colposcopy. A colposcopy is a visual examination of the cervix itself, done with a special magnifier called a colposcope. If the provider sees lesions with the colposcope, they will biopsy the lesion to determine the level of abnormality. A biopsy is a very small piece of tissue that is removed and examined microscopically. When done, the biopsy feels like a pinch. You may bleed a bit after the procedure. Biopsy results are categorized into CIN I, CIN II, CIN III, and carcinoma in situ. Carcinoma in situ is not yet cancer, but it is the last stage before the dysplasia is considered cancer. The difference between dysplasia and cancer: cancer cells penetrate into the deeper tissue layers instead of living only in the epithelial layer, and can spread throughout the organ and to other organs.

What are the medical solutions for abnormal Pap tests and cervical dysplasia?

LEEP:
Loop Electrosurgical Excision Procedure. This procedure uses a wire loop heated by an electrical current to remove abnormal tissue. Local anesthetic is used. The edges of the tissue are examined to ensure that all the abnormal cells were removed. Healthy tissue can then regrow and replace what was removed. The LEEP is the gold standard of care today.

Laser:
Abnormal cells can also be removed with a laser. Usually only for very small lesions.

Conization or cone biopsy:
The most invasive procedure. Performed under general anesthesia. A cone-shaped piece of the cervix is cut out with a scalpel or laser. More tissue is removed than with the other procedures. This procedure is chosen when there are abnormal cells in the endocervix to ensure that all cells are removed – LEEP cannot reach into the os.

Cryotherapy
This involves freezing off abnormal tissue. A device called a cryoprobe is inserted into the vagina and the metal end held to the cervix. Compressed nitrogen flows through the device, causing the metal to become cold enough to freeze the tissue. Healthy tissue can then regrow and replace what was removed. Cryotherapy is not used as much anymore because after it heals it may be harder to identify new areas of dysplasia. It's also not very successful at treating large areas of dysplasia.

Side Effects From Conventional Procedures:

Many women have only minor discomfort after these procedures and no permanent sequelae. Other women experience extended periods of bleeding after the procedure and/or pain during sex, as well as cervical scarring that can impair the ability of the cervix to dilate during labor and delivery. LEEP procedures are associated with an increased risk of overall preterm delivery, preterm delivery, and low birth weight. Women who are considering future pregnancies should be counseled about these risks during informed consent for LEEP. Regardless of these risks, LEEP or conization are sometimes necessary – cervical cancer is very serious in comparison to these risks. However, since the cells are very slow growing, there is little risk in trying an herbal approach first. The exception would be if carcinoma in situ or invasive cancer were present. Then, a conventional procedure would be the best idea, followed by herbal treatments and support.

Cervical Scarring:

Although many times, medical treatments do not leave cervical scarring, it can occur. Although the impact of cervical scarring on childbirth is not explored much in the scientific medical literature (that I have been able to find), there is a lot of knowledge about this among the midwifery community. Cervical scarring sometimes prevents the cervix from dilating during labor. In conventional medicine this is considered "failure to progress." Unfortunately sometimes it results in C-sections, but knowledgeable providers can often massage the scar tissue, allowing it to soften and release. A midwife I know suggests that pregnant women with a history of LEEP or conization request an initial cervical exam from the person who will be delivering the baby in order to establish a baseline for how the cervix feels, so they have more information if the cervix isn't dilating properly during labor. Midwives often use evening primrose oil to help the scarring soften and labor to progress naturally.

What are the naturopathic solutions for cervical dysplasia?

Naturopaths may use a variety of escharotic solutions to slough off abnormal cervical cells. This can include a bloodroot preparation and another using magnesium sulfate (Crawford, 1997) painted directly on the cervix. It is possible to use the magnesium sulfate solution oneself (see Crawford's book, Herbal Remedies for Women) – but as I have had success with less intense methods I can't really give advice on it. Do not ever use bloodroot for any DIY cervical treatment, or for any topical treatment of growths, for that matter. It can cause serious injury.

Male & Female Partners of Those Affected: Risks & Roles

Penis-having folks can incubate and transmit high-risk HPV, and they often show no symptoms. There is no screening test for males. This is partly because penile cancer is very rare, and also because it's hard to get samples of abnormal cells from penile skin because it is relatively thick. Vagina-having folks can transmit the infection to one another via hands and sex toys. So if one partner in a two-vagina relationship tests positive, the other should definitely get tested. There is no role for male partners in conventional treatment, but male partners can definitely participate in holistic treatment. HPV can also be transmitted through anal sex, and it can cause anal dysplasia. There is an anal Pap test that you should request if you have receptive anal sex.

Holistic Support for Healing the Cervix & Clearing HPV:

Holistic treatment of cervical dysplasia includes:
1) correcting nutrient deficiencies
2) applying herbal preparations topically to the cervix
3) building and supporting the immune system as it works to clear the virus.

4) An optional avenue you may want to consider is addressing any pelvic congestion that may be present.

Addressing Nutrient Deficiencies:

• **Folate Deficiency** (Butterworth, et. al, 1992)
Folate is a B vitamin, aka B9. Many people with cervical dysplasia are also folate deficient, and folate deficiency is believed to contribute to the development of CD. This is especially true for folks with cervical dysplasia who also take oral contraceptives, which have been shown to decrease folate levels. Oral contraceptives themselves are also a risk factor for cervical dysplasia regardless of folate levels. Some researchers think that many cases of cervical dysplasia in oral contraceptive users is actually due to contraception-induced folate deficiency rather than HPV infection.

Unfortunately, most studies show that folic acid supplementation does not help improve cervical dysplasia. This could be because folic acid and folate are not the same, the body doesn't react to them in the same way - although they are generally thought of as the same in the medical community. Another theory is that maybe folks who end up developing cervical dysplasia have a problem converting synthetic folic acid to a usable form. Folic acid supplementation can actually be harmful if taken long term, increasing risk of developing cancer. The mass enrichment of foods with folic acid was done due to overwhelming evidence that it reduced neural tube defects. However, its effects on the general population are untested and there is evidence that it increases rates of cancer.

What we can do instead is really concentrate on getting our folate through diet. Unlike synthetic folic acid, you can't overdo dietary folate, and it is really important. Excellent sources of dietary folate include vegetables such as romaine lettuce, spinach, asparagus, turnip greens, mustard greens, parsley, collard greens, broccoli, cauliflower, beets, and lentils. Some of the best food sources of folate are calf's liver and chicken liver.

You can supplement with folate if your dietary intake is inadequate. Chris Kresser, a functional nutritionist, recommends products that contain the Metfolin brand, or list "5-methyltetrahydrofolate" or "5-MTHF" on the label. Avoid products that say "folic acid" on the label. Make sure to check your multivitamin, because most contain folic acid and not folate.

Women planning on becoming pregnant should consume between 800 and 1200 mcg of folate per day for several months before the start of pregnancy. Unless you're consuming chicken or calf's liver and substantial amounts of leafy greens on a regular basis, it's difficult to obtain this amount from diet alone. If you're pregnant or trying to get pregnant, I recommend supplementing with 600-800 mcg of folate per day, depending on your dietary intake.

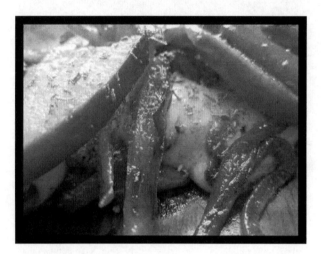

•**Vitamin A & Carotinoids** (beta-carotene):

Deficiencies of both of these nutrients have been associated with increased incidence of cervical dysplasia – but supplementation has not only been shown not to help, but to contribute to an increased risk of cancer. Do not supplement these nutrients. Instead, make very sure you are getting enough through food.

Foods high in Vitamin A: sweet potatoes, carrots, dark leafy greens, winter squashes, lettuce, dried apricots, cantaloupe, bell peppers, fish, liver, and tropical fruits.

Foods high in carotinoids: sweet potato, dark leafy greens, carrots, romaine lettuce, squashes, sweet red peppers, dried apricots, cooked peas, and broccoli

Foods high in vitamin C: bell peppers, dark leafy greens, kiwis, broccoli, berries, citrus fruits, tomatoes, peas, and papayas

•**Anti-inflammatory Diet:**

I suggest following anti-inflammatory diet guidelines: vegetables should make up 2/3 of every plate, protein and carbs should make up the remaining 1/3. Never eat carbs alone – always combine with a veggie or protein.

Topical Applications to The Cervix:

Suppositories:

Michael Moore's Recipe (with additions by Caty Crabb, and taken from the HPV zine by Down There Collective)

Ingredients:

1 oz (by vol) Echinacea fluid extract* (or 5 oz Echinacea tincture)
5 ml Yerba Mansa tincture** (Anemopsis)
5 ml Calendula officinalis tincture
6 oz (by wt) Glycerin
1 oz (by wt) Gelatin (pharmaceutical grade – cheap and easily purchased online)
5 ml Thuja occidentalis essential oil

*If you cannot find the fluid extract, you can make an equivalent by slowly evaporating 5 ounces of Echinacea tincture down to 1 oz of milk-grey liquid in a double boiler. Re-measure the evaporating tincture frequently as it reduces quickly at the end.

**If you cannot find Yerba Mansa, double the amount of Calendula tincture used to 10ml.

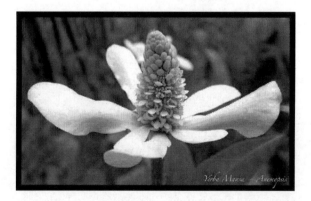

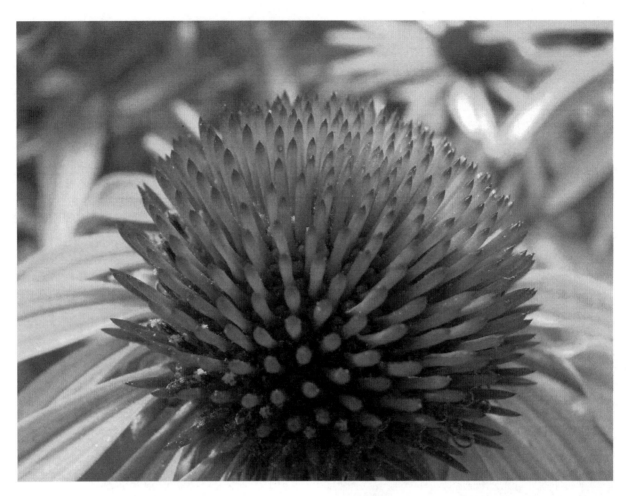

Preparation:

Heat the glycerin on a double boiler, add the Echinacea, Calendula and Yerba Mansa and maintain at a low temperature for at least 30 minutes to evaporate off some of the alcohol. Add the gelatin (preferably finely powdered) and whisk (or egg-beat) until the gelatin is thoroughly dissolved in the liquids. Don't leave any little gelatinous solids. Continue stirring until the liquid is a clear grey-brown syrup. Add the highly evaporative Thuja oil to the dissolved syrup just before you begin to pour into the molds. Stir right before pouring and even give an extra stir once or twice while pouring to keep the consistency even.

The original recipe calls for suppository molds, but I had a really hard time finding them and have made these numerous times by placing sheets of aluminum foil over empty ice cube trays, and making shallow, ¼ inch indentations over each hole. I pour the syrup into these and

allow them to set. I then take a long knife and split the suppositories down the middle to make them the right size, keeping them on the foil. To store, I roll up the foil with the suppositories inside and store them in the freezer. This makes them easier to insert, but I have kept them in my backpack for weeks while traveling, and I haven't had them go bad.

•Insert one suppository nightly into vagina, as close to the cervix as possible. The suppository will leak, so wear a pad. Do this for three months and re-test. Additional treatment time may be necessary.

•Echinacea: alterative, "blood cleanser", vulnerary, topical anti-infective, brings the immune system to the area and stimulates phagocytosis

•Thuja: anti-viral, anti-fungal, antibacterial. I pretty much use this in external applications only. Essential oil is very useful. May irritate very sensitive skin.

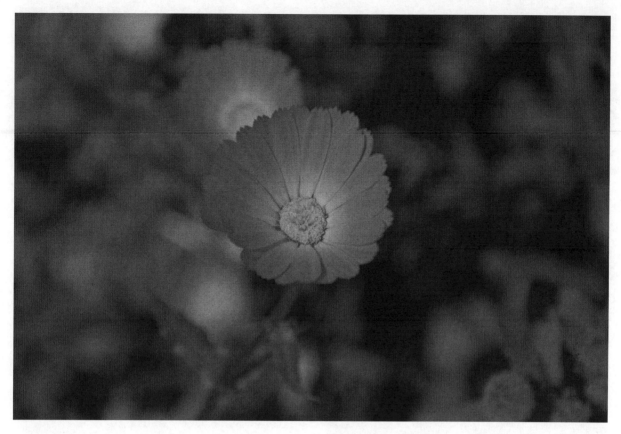

•Calendula, anti-inflammatory, anti-viral, vulnerary

•Yerba Mansa (Anemopsis): astringent, stimulating to the healing process, anti-microbial and likely anti-viral, traditionally used on ulcerations of the skin, mucosa, and GI tract. Yerba mansa is on the United Plant Savers watch list.

•Ghee suppositories: Kate Hirst, an Ayurvedic practitioner in Eugene, OR, uses licorice, turmeric, and bitter herbs soaked in ghee, strained, cooled, and rolled into suppositories. Licorice is an anti-viral and anti-inflammatory, while bitter herbs are cooling and drying. Appropriate bitter herbs here include Yarrow or Oregon Grape.

Bastis:

Amanda McQuade Crawford's recipe:
    4 oz Periwinkle (Vinca)
    3 oz Marshmallow (Althaea)
    1 oz Goldenseal (Hydrastis)
    1 oz Gotu Kola (Centella)

My recipe:
    3 oz Yarrow (Achillea)
    2 oz Marshmallow (Althaea)
    1 oz Cedar Leaf (Thuja)
    1 oz Calendula (Calendula)
    1 oz Oregon Grape Root (Berberis)

Instructions: Prepare a strong infusion by just barely covering the herbs with boiling water and allowing to infuse for several hours, until it is completely cooled.

Douche (Basti):

You can lay in the bathtub, use a douche bag, and try to hold in the infusion for several minutes before it comes out. Crawford recommends doing this 2-5 times weekly. My opinion is that 5x/week is too frequent, as bastis can be highly disruptive to the vaginal flora. I recommend 2-3x/week at the most. If at any time the vagina starts feeling itchy, dry, swollen, etc., this treatment may be too disruptive. Try suppositories instead. Always follow a douche with a probiotic capsule or plain yogurt inserted into the vagina to help repopulate the flora.

79

Wheatgrass Basti: Amanda McQuade Crawford recommends this in her book, and one of my case studies did this and felt it was an important part of her healing process.

Other herbs that are great for topical treatment:

Chaparral (Larrea):

A versatile herb having antibacterial, antifungal, anti-inflammatory, and antioxidant properties. Used against infections of all types and against malignant growths. This herb is used both externally and internally, but it is very strong and I consider it a medium-dose botanical when used internally. It is often recommended as a basti ingredient. Beware allergic reactions.

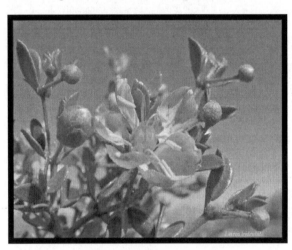

Turmeric (Curcuma):

Anti-inflammatory, antiviral, hepatoprotective, anti-oxidant; suppresses HPV in human cells and stimulates apoptosis in cervical cancer cells.

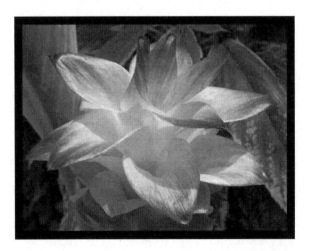

Immune Support

Deep Immune Tonic:

4 oz Reishi (Ganoderma)
4 oz Shitake (Lentinula)
4 oz Maitake (Grifola)

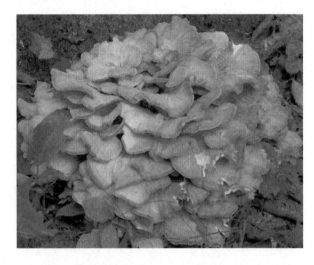

4 oz Chaga (Inonotus)
4 oz Astragalus (Astragalus)
6 oz Burdock (Arctium)
2 oz Licorice (Glycyrrhiza)

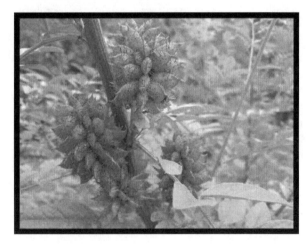

Preparation:

Combine the herbs in a crock pot or large pot on a hot plate. Bring to a boil, then reduce heat and simmer for three days. Because of the time needed, and the fact that your housemates or family may complain about the strong, mushroomy smell, you might want to cook this

80

outside. After three days, cool, strain, and freeze in ice cube trays. Store the cubes in a Ziploc in the freezer and take 1-2 cubes a day for 2-3 months.

Alterative Tea:

2 oz Astragalus (Astragalus)
2 oz Dandelion Root (Taraxacum)
1 oz Calendula (Calendula)
¼ oz Licorice (Glycyrrhiza)
2 oz Burdock (Arctium)

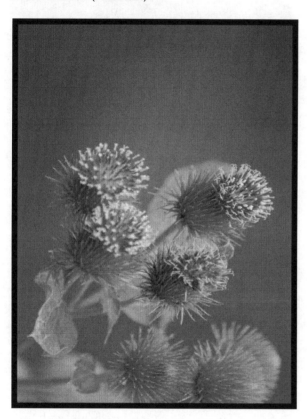

Preparation: Combine herbs with 2 ½ quarts of water. Bring to a boil, then reduce heat and simmer 20-30 minutes. Strain and store in refrigerator. Drink 1-3 cups daily.

• Burdock (Arctium): alterative, promotes detoxification, strengthens liver function

• Reishi (Ganoderma): adaptogen, enhances immune response to viral infection and has anti-tumor activity, and also down-regulates immune overactivity as related to autoimmune conditions. Other benefits include improved stress response, anti-inflammatory activity, strengthens the cardiovascular system and improves cognitive function.

• Chaga (Inonotus): traditional Russian and Eastern European medicinal mushroom; has been shown to increase apoptosis (programmed cell death) in cancer cells

• Maitake (Grifola): enhances both acute response to infection and long-term immune response; decreases inflammation and may inhibit the growth and spread of cancer cells.

• Shitake: immune-modulating, tumor-preventative

• Astragalus: immune-modulating, anti-inflammatory, anti-viral, hepatoprotective, promotes tissue regeneration

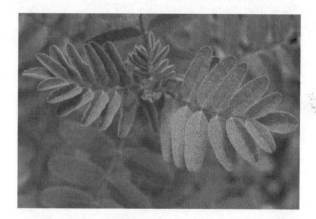

Other herbs of note:

• Olive Leaf (Olea): has shown antiviral activity in the lab, including against HIV. I can't find any evidence of traditonal use for viruses. Matthew Wood says it's active against over 100 viruses. Studies indicate it is safe.

• Lemon Balm (Melissa): anti-viral activity, both topically and internally

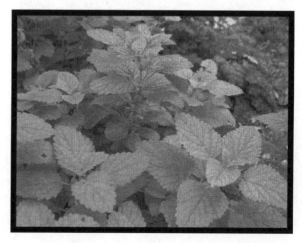

81

•Other medicinal mushrooms: Lion's Mane, Cordyceps

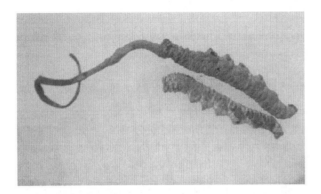

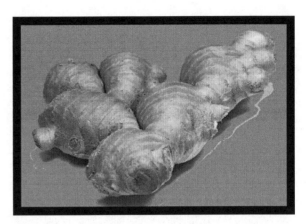

Pelvic Congestion

Address any pelvic congestion that may be present. Symptoms of pelvic congestion may include: a history of slow-to-start periods, brown or dark blood, a dull, aching discomfort before/ during bleeding, hemorrhoids, varicose veins or spider veins, aching legs/butt.

The following tinctures can be combined and taken, 1 tsp, 2-3x daily, as a tonic:

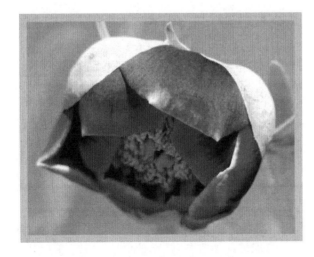

1 part Peony (Paeonia)
1 part Horse Chestnut (Aesculus)
1 part Ocotillo (Fouquieria)
½ part Ginger (Zingiber)

Case Study 1:

Pt A
March 2010: abnormal Pap. Last previous Pap 2006.
Colposcopy: CIN 2. Was advised to get a conization. Refused.
April 2010: Began herbal treatment
- Michael Moore suppositories every night except while menstruating
- Deep Immune tonic daily
- "clean" diet
- low to no alcohol
- folic acid supplements
- mushroom extracts
- alterative teas
- copious amounts of nervines
Repeat colposcopy in June: ASCUS.
Continued above treatment for another few months.
Pap: ASCUS. MD advised a "wait and see" approach.
Herbal treatment continued but with a lighter hand.
Spring 2012: normal Pap result

Case Study 2:

Pt B
2007: Colposcopy: CIN I cervical dysplasia.
History of multiple abnormal HPV+ Pap tests beginning in 2007 that varied between ASCUS and LSIL.
Patient preferred monitoring over an excisional procedure. The cells kept changing back and

forth, but not getting better. Her practitioner advised repeat Pap tests every 6 months.

Before she came to see me, she was taking:

- Natures Plus arra-larix (500mg) (aribinogalactan, a polysaccharide – immune stimulating – food for good bacteria)
- Olive leaf (Olea) extract 750 mg complex
- Anti-oxidant vitamins from Country Life: grapeseed extract, vit a,c e – I don't recommend

2011: She came to see me and began herbal treatment:

- Michael Moore suppositories x 3 months
- After 3 months: switched to using a douche 1x/week or 1x/2weeks and at minimum 1x/mo. We started with a formula from Amanda McQuade Crawford's book Herbal Remedies for Women: Gotu Kola, Periwinkle, Marshmallow and Oregon Grape. After about a month or so I changed the formula, mostly due to herb availability. I substituted Yarrow for the Periwinkle, Calendula for the Gotu Kola, added Cedar Leaf, and used Oregon Grape instead of Goldenseal.

Next three Paps: negative for cervical dysplasia but positive for HPV.

Most recent Pap (March 2015): negative for both the virus and dysplasia. Practitioner now advises Pap monitoring every year.

This client stated that she really struggled with improving her diet but did succeed in incorporating more veggies and fruits. She lost around 20 lb in the process. She felt that this was one of them most important parts of her healing process.

Case Study 3:

Pt C

Diagnosed November 2013 with CIN II with small areas of CIN I and CIN III. MDs wanted a LEEP.

March 2014: started herbal treatment

- Alternated the following as bastis 2-3 times/week for 6 weeks (from Amanda

McQuade Crawford's book Herbal Remedies for Women):

   o Formula 1: OGR (Berberis), Sarsparilla (Smilax), Calendula, Blue Cohosh (Caulophyllum, and Blue Vervain
   o Formula 2: Gotu Kola, Periwinkle, Marshmallow and Oregon Grape

- After 6 weeks, decreased basti to 1x/week and combined Formulas 1 and 2. Added wheatgrass basti 1x/week.
- Stopped using herbs in beginning of August 2014.
- Acupuncture starting in May 2014 2x/week x 4 weeks
- Started exercising, lost 15 lb, changed diet. Was working in restaurant and had been mainly eating carbs, meat, creamy rich food to eating more veggies, whole grains, less pasta, leaner meats.
- Supplements: multi-vitamin starting in Feb 2014 x 6 weeks.
- June 2014: started drinking kombucha 2-3x/week and wheatgrass shots 2x/week.

Re-tested colposcopy in May: CIN I and II, no III detected.

August 2014: colposcopy showed CIN I only. MD suggested to monitoring, and decreasing colposcopy frequency to every 6 months.

January 2015: colposcopy showed no dysplasia.

Patient believed that attitude, optimism, empowerment was really important. She stated she was determined to keep her cervix whole, and to heal herself on her own. She described herself as proactive with a positive outlook.

References:

American Cancer Society

Butterworth, C., Hatch, K., Macaluso, M., Cole, P., Sauberlich, H., Soong, S., Borst, M. (1992). Folate Deficiency and Cervical Dysplasia. Journal of the American Medical Association, Jan 22-29;267(4)

Crawford, A.M. (1997). Herbal Remedies for Women. Prima Publishing: Roseville, CA

www.healthline.com

Marshall, K. (2003). Cervical dysplasia: early intervention. Alternative Medicine Review, May; 8(2)

Katja Swift:

To Baby or Not To Baby
When & How Herbs Can Help

Probably some of you have IUDs, or use the pill, or the ring, or . . . It's worth noting that we all do what we've gotta do, taking whatever best option we can at the time. No one can judge the choices a woman makes about her fertility – and the truth is, we aren't presented with much in the way of good options. But as it turns out, we have more options than we've been led to believe, and with a little care, we can continue to change the landscape for future generations.

The Fertility Cycle

In order to understand birth control, we have to understand conception.

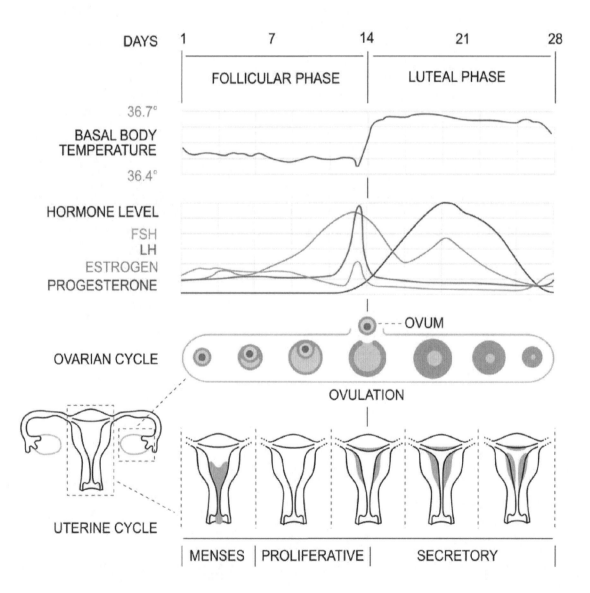

Follicular Phase

in the ovaries, the increase of FSH (follicle stimulating hormone) causes several follicles to develop; each contains an immature egg. typically, only one egg will become mature enough for ovulation, and will burst out of the follicle. in the uterus, first there is menses – the old lining is shed, and then the proliferative phase begins, which includes the build up of estrogen.

The Fertile "Moment"

a surge of luteinizing hormone, produced in the pituitary gland, triggers the actual ovulation, and subsequent development of the corpus luteum. the cervix produces fertile mucus, which reduces the acidity of the vaginal canal, providing a better living environment for sperm.

Luteal Phase

the corpus luteum produces progesterone until the placenta can take over the job at ~10 weeks. (women who repeatedly miscarry just before 10 weeks may have insufficient corpus luteum.) if the egg is not fertilized, the corpus luteum dies and progesterone production stops. a luteal phase of less than 12 days makes pregnancy difficult, because there is not enough buildup of progesterone, and the embryo is not able to implant.

And Along The Way, The Liver Clears The Hormones

If the liver is struggling, hormones don't get cleared out appropriately, instead building up and wreaking havoc – for example, unmanageable PMS symptoms. a healthy liver, and enough sleep during which the liver can do its job, are both critical to proper hormone levels!

*The key here is that the whole system depends on the *appropriate fluctuation of hormone levels*. this fluctuation causes the uterine lining to thicken in preparation for pregnancy, and to shed when one does not occur. if hormone levels do not fluctuate appropriately, the buildup and shed does not occur, or does not occur appropriately (abnormal menstrual cycles).

Conventional Birth Control Options: Unplanned Non-Parenthood

Non-Hormonal Options
These still contain toxic chemicals (except condoms without spermicide), but they do not contain hormones.
- •**Condoms** – widely available, fairly dependable, but in other countries they make better ones – thinner, stronger, more "feely". make sure to get spermicide-free condoms.
- •**Diaphragm** – hard to get in the States, and we only have a small number of options – so if one of those fits you, that's great. in Canada/Europe there are lots of size and style variations, and non-toxic spermicidal options too. new options are being invented and it is becoming possible to purchase European diaphragms in the US.
- •**Female condoms** – a lot of spermicide, expensive, not widely available. also, fiddly.
- •**Sponge** – not widely available, a very high dose of spermicide, unreliable.

In this country, the spermicide most frequently used is still nonoxynol-9, which is an irritant to cell membranes, causes sores and lesions that are often mistaken for latex allergy, and is banned in most other countries. Contragel, a very popular non-toxic brand of spermicide in use in Europe for decades, is now available in the US for purchase online. http://www.buycontragel.com

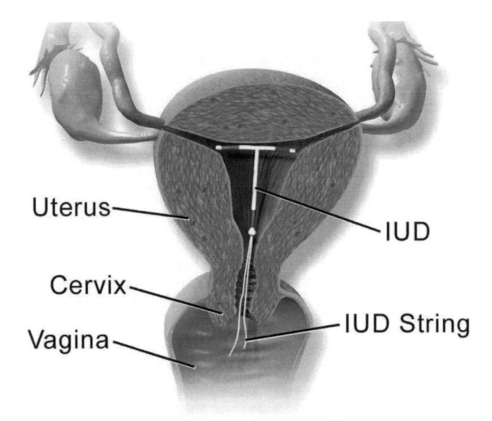

Intrauterine Device (IUD)

ParaGard, the copper IUD, fits into this category as well – no hormones. copper functions as a spermicide, though this is secondary to the actual purpose of an IUD, which is to cause irritation and inflammation so that the uterus is not capable of being implanted by a fertilized egg. however, prolonged localized inflammation leads to systemic inflammation. periods are typically heavier and more painful.

Hormonal Options

The Pill, NuvaRing, Mirena IUD, the patch, Depo-Provera and other injected birth controls, and implants. using hormones means you don't have a period, don't ovulate, etc - in other words, each of these options is intentionally disrupting your cycle, substituting cyclic fluctuation for a constant or near-constant unchanging high level of hormones in the body. there's no way to do that and not have negative endocrine effects, since our bodies expect a cyclic fluctuation. also please note, these are steroid hormones. (bleeding on the pill is not menstrual bleeding, it is withdrawal bleeding, as the body is exposed to the sudden drop in hormonal levels.)

Some common effects are B vitamin depletion, depression, brain fog, lowered libido, dryness, mood swings, hypothyroid symptoms, cholestasis (liver stagnation), fatigue, … but the biggest effect worth digging into is disruption of endocrine function (it's all connected!). you can't suppress the function of the reproductive endocrine organs without also affecting the thyroid, the adrenals, the pineal, the pituitary, the pancreas…

"But I do ok on the pill" – do you? or are there symptoms that are not being attributed to the pill? Or that are "less bad" than the horror stories? Will there be trouble in the future? What we do know is that it's an endocrine disruptor, and that's not without consequence. It might be the right option for right now, but it's important to know that there are effects so that they can be managed. even a right option isn't perfect, and knowledge is power.

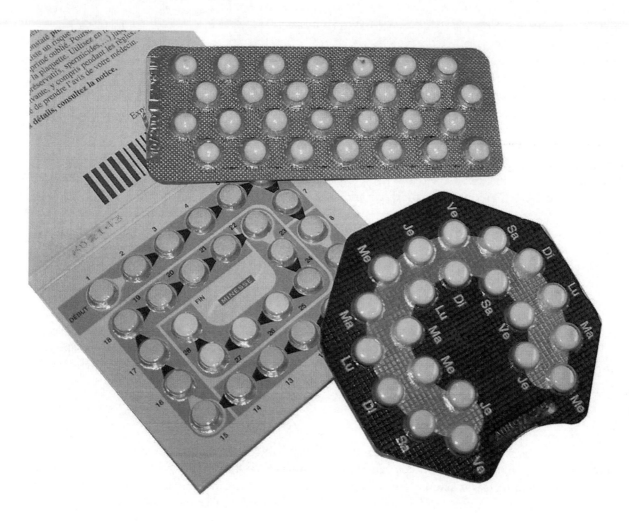

What About Taking The Pill To "Resolve" Problems In The Menstrual Cycle?

Hormones are all intricately intertwined: disruption in the menstrual cycle is an indication of systemic hormonal dysfunction. It's not appropriate to "smooth that over" by taking hormones that result in actually having no cycle at all – that's like saying "shut up kid, yer botherin' me". No problem has been fixed, you just stop complaining. This approach by the medical system is at once both using a sledgehammer approach to fix a fine-tuned problem, and more disparagingly, removing the power of women to understand their own bodies and take corrective action. most doctors don't educate women at all about menstrual problems – we are simply told "the pill will take care of that", without even understanding what "that" is! We could instead value menstrual disruptions as a kind of "early warning system" – a message that our bodies are not ok and need attention!

Natural Birth Control Options: Planned Non-Parenthood

The key word here is "planned" – for natural birth control options to work, there is some planning and thought involved. the process is simple: know when you're fertile, and if you are, use a barrier method. When you're not fertile, you're free! there's really nothing else to it.

First, we have to build a dependable menstrual/fertility cycle:

Eat Right

Foundational principles: eat whole foods. avoid processed, packaged food-products. avoid added sugars. eat meat from healthy animals, and vegetables from healthy soil. eat with the seasons. eat with intent, and gratitude, and enjoyment!

Eliminate – gluten, casein, sugars, soy, industrial seed oils (soy/corn/canola/"vegetable"), refined carbohydrates, caffeine, often corn, and sometimes legumes, nightshades, or other personal allergens. in other words, avoid modern food products and stick to ancestral foods.

Add/Increase – high quality fats (olive, avocado, coconut, and fat from healthy animals), high quality animal proteins, many vegetables in many colors, seaweeds, bone broth with roots and mushrooms, and some low-glycemic berries & fruits.

Sleep Right

Human adults require 9-12 hours sleep per night. Humans in puberty require 10-12+ hours sleep per night. Lack of sleep is an endocrine disruptor – increasing adrenaline and cortisol levels; melatonin & insulin levels are also affected. lack of sleep simultaneously decreases liver function – all of which leads to your whole cascade of hormones being quite a bit out of whack.

Lifestyle and Move Right

High stress levels increase adrenaline. being outside, spending time alone, allowing your head to get good and bored sometimes so that you have time to process the junk in the back corner is important. Lack of movement increases stagnation: walk more, play more, relax more. Natural movement is much preferable to time at the gym – go for a walk, climb a tree, hike up a mountain, play a game. Even if it's cold or rainy!

Charting: You Need Data!

It's not as hard as you think – you can download a chart with not only your just-woke-up morning temperature, but also other factors that can help you make sense of variations in your cycle – see example at http://commonwealthherbs.com/twhc - Every morning when you wake up, before you get out of the bed, take your temperature with a plain old digital thermometer, and mark it in your chart. on the day that your temperature shoots up, you are ovulating! (more on how to interpret the charts is at tcoyf.com.) you will be fertile five days before ovulation, and a few days afterward, so it's important to establish a regular cycle, and then to avoid unprotected sex for a window before and after your ovulation. ideally, your partner will take your temperature every morning and mark that part of your chart, so that you can share responsibility for the fertility of your partnership!

Knowledge Is Power!

Once you establish a regular cycle, then make sure it stays there for three months so that you know you can rely on it. when it is, hooray! you're ready to start. as long as you're in a time that is not fertile, you're good to go au naturel! When you are fertile (up to 10 days a month), use condoms or a diaphragm, and that's all there is to it. (order condoms from places like condomdepot.com – they don't sell any condoms that have spermicide.)

Understanding your fertility cycle is the first step, but to be really successful, also learn to understand your emotional cycles, and those of your partner. talk about them together. understand how you fit into the larger cycles around you. Use things that aren't sex to be intimate, so that you can expand your definition and practice of intimacy.

Cycles: Beyond the Fertility Cycle

We *all* need introversion time and extroversion time – it's ok and even good to have some nights where you just wanna crawl into your comfy baggy clothes and be alone! It's normal to sleep more in the winter and less in the summer. It's normal to be introspective (and not customer-friendly!) when you're bleeding. It's normal to howl at the moon when she's full. these things are natural and healthy. It's more convenient and fun when these times match up with your partner's cycle, but that's not always going to happen. Finding ways to communicate about these normal cycle fluctuations is key to a healthy sexual relationship.

Some History: The Real Red Tent

Historically, people had time every month to be away from each other during the dark of the moon while the women were bleeding – no manipulation, bribery, or big fight about "poker night" required! it's a cycle we evolved with – every month, the women went apart to bleed, the men went apart to be men apart, and the children stayed with the elders and the nursing mothers. a break from the daily work, from naggy irritations, and a nice bit of absence-makes-the-heart-grow-fonder.

It's not impossible to respect this cycle in our modern lives, it's just different. institute times each week/month to spend separately, and make sure that each partner gets time to be with the girls/guys. this time plays an important role in helping us understand who we are and process our experiences and emotions, so make sure to be conscious in making room for it in your relationships!

But Wait, There's More

This is all great, but it also isn't easy. how can a person decide? Is there a time when one answer is righter than another? everyone is in a different place on their journey with all this. It's a path, and there's no "good" vs. "wrong" place you can sit in – it's all a progression, with many factors involved. How can we see what factors were involved for us in our lives and pass to the next generation a scenario where the factors are different? Is there a way that we can create space for the next generation to grow in awareness of their own cycles, and to increase their mindfulness around sex? What roles do media, social structure, and culture play in our challenge to do this?

Political Influences

Saying no to hormonal birth control isn't simple – people have to have resources and education to eat well and understand fertility, and have a relationship committed to supporting the respect of cycle, as well as affordable access to safe and appropriate health care options. but what if those factors aren't present? What if a woman has an irregular cycle, or an irregular relationship pattern? What if the guy won't use a condom? And as a woman, would I rather have sole control over this in my own body? These are all really big issues, and they need to be discussed in order for change to happen. here are some thoughts to get you started:

Why don't men like condoms in America? in Japan and throughout Asia, condoms are preferred over the use of hormones. so how did other cultures fix the "condom problem"? They built a better condom! Why don't we do that here?

Why don't we have better diaphragms in America? in Europe they are preferred: they're not into hormonal options either, so instead they have a huge array of diaphragms available, AND they have non-toxic spermicide. Why don't we do that here?

In this country, hormonal options have eclipsed all other options. When women called for more options, we got more hormones, but non-hormonal methods continue to decline. (this is a good time to note that the same is true for abortion options: there is another option besides a surgical abortion and enormous doses of hormones: menstrual extraction in the first trimester is easy, quick, and can be performed in a regular doctor's office. Why isn't that more widely available? Find out more at www.earlyoptions.com!)

We, as a reasonably liberal chunk of society, tend to promote Planned Parenthood. In concept, this is good, but in action, Planned Parenthood often pushes hormonal birth control and harasses women who don't want hormones. They don't educate on non-hormonal contraception (though in some places they do have condoms). Planned Parenthood also is staunchly pro-vaccine. Limited accessible health care is better than no health care – or is it? Is there a way we can make this better? Planned Parenthood is a business, and they have business goals. Is there a way that we can promote access to full-spectrum reproductive health care that focuses on the goals of each individual client in a non-judgmental way? Groups like the Full-Spectrum Reproductive Support Network (reproductivesupport.org) are a start in this work.

How Does Our Culture Affect Our Sex Lives?

We teach our boys, in the locker room, in movies and media, and by example:
- That condoms suck and that they should abhor them
- That it's a woman's responsibility to suppress her fertility so that she can be available to him on his schedule (instead of him taking responsibility for his own fertility)
- To expect sex regularly, and that orgasm is what makes it sex
- That the only way to experience intimacy is through sex
- And we do NOT teach them to understand their fertility, or the fertility cycles of women.

We teach our girls, in the locker room, in movies and media, and by example:
- That if she doesn't put out, the boy she really likes won't like her
- That boys don't like condoms and therefore they can't be expected to use them

• That bleeding is bad, smelly, embarrassing, etc.
• That men's sexual needs come before women's, and that women's sexual needs are rarely acknowledged
• That it's not ok to talk about what we want or need
• And we do *not* teach them how to understand their own fertility!

A a society, much like everything else we do, we think more sex = good sex. As a society, we tend to believe that we're entitled to sex any time, whenever we can get it. We, as a reasonably liberal chunk of society, tend to think of sexual freedom as a good thing, and abstinence as a bad thing, because these things have become politicized (and because our culture is so sexualized). Separated from their politics, however, too much sex (or porn, or whatever) is like too much candy. Mindful awareness around sex – including choosing to have sex when you have time for it to be meaningful and with whom it is meaningful – yields "nutrient-dense" sex.

in order to have meaningful sex, we have to have meaningful things that form the foundation for sex: a safe relationship, where emotional needs are being met. Oh no! This is a point of disjunct – often emotional needs are met in two different ways in a relationship. It's not ok to hold sex hostage in order to get emotional nutrition. It's also not ok to withhold emotional nutrition and expect to get sex anyway!

Sex needs a "space", and I'll use the word sacred. You can't build that if one partner is feeling unheard by the other, if one partner is feeling unconsidered. You can't have it if one partner is stuck in some previous episode where those things were true, even if they aren't true now – and so in that case, building that space includes taking the time to bring that partner into the present. not to demand it of them, but to help them find their way here. This can be done by non-sexual touch, by story-sharing, or by something as completely un-erotic as doing dishes together.

What About Herbs?

You might have noticed, I didn't talk about any herbs for birth control. *That's because there aren't any.* Oh, you might have heard of Wild Carrot, and you've probably even heard some folks claim they're having success with it. There are a lot of factors to consider in these anecdotes, the first being: is the couple fertile to begin with? depending on the study you look at, between 2006 and 2012, 10-46% of all couples trying to have babies required fertility treatments to conceive – which means there's a pretty good chance a woman isn't pregnant because she (or her partner) isn't fertile, and wild carrot had nothing to do with it. in fact, in one poorly done but widely referenced study on Wild Carrot, women who did get pregnant were simply removed from the dataset and labeled "super-fertile". Were they, or were the unpregnant women simply infertile? The data on fertility in the general population suggests the latter, and a study that simply removes results that don't support the hypothesis is bad science.

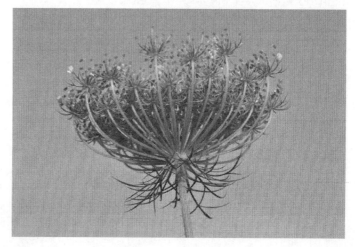

Regarding mechanism of action, one hypothesis is that wild carrot works like the "plan B" pill – a progesterone spike followed by a crash, which you can only do once a month, but your fertile window is about 10 days... That math probably isn't going to be very satisfying for most of you! Keep in mind, more frequent use of Wild Carrot has been used to *boost* fertility.

You might have heard of taking high doses of Tansy to dislodge a pregnancy; this does not work. If that would work, there would not be any children born to drug addicts, or children of alcoholics, or... a strong pregnancy is exceptionally difficult to dislodge. If a pregnancy is not strong, Tansy may seem to "dispel" it, but that pregnancy would have miscarried anyway. According to the march of dimes, 40% of all pregnancies miscarry, and of those, more than 80% occur in the first 12 weeks. 60% of those occur within a week of the normally expected date of menstruation. if you have a friend who tried Tansy and it "worked", is it possible that she was one of those 40% whose pregnancy wasn't strong enough to hold and miscarried, and the Tansy got the credit? seems likely! So, why not just try it? because it's teratogenic – it causes birth defects. Not to mention it'll make you *very* sick: you have to poison yourself profoundly to even attempt a Tansy abortion.

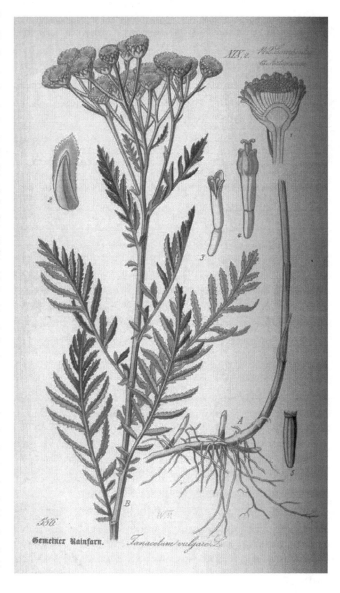

Other common herban legends for "natural abortions" include mugwort, pennyroyal, vitamin C, and even Ginger. Mugwort and Pennyroyal are great for a stagnant period, but they're not going to give you an abortion (and do not ingest the essential oils!). if you take enough vitamin C to get to the doses that are supposedly required to cause an abortion, your bones and teeth will ache and you'll end up with reverse scurvy. (and also, it doesn't work.)

Yes, there are many stories out there, and yes, lots of them are even being told by herbalists. remember: as many as 46% of couples are seeking fertility treatment and 40% of pregnancies end in miscarriage. yes, we want to believe that we can rely on plants for every thing, but you can't expect a cat to fetch; it's not in their nature. the nature of all beings is to reproduce: we can't expect plants to do something that is against nature just because we want it to be that way. so what to do, if you find yourself in that situation? Early Options in NYC, or some other clinic that performs menstrual extractions (MVA) – it's much much safer than a D&C, requires no anesthesia, it's fast and fairly painless.

92

But I'm An Herbalist!

Instead, use herbs to support cycle. Bleeding Tea, Nettle & friends. And what about Mugwort to support dreamwork with your partner – another kind of intimacy. Skullcap, Passionflower, and Damiana to come out of your work day and into your nice evening together. and also herbs and flower essences to support other parts of cycle...

Herbalism can be extremely useful in the quest to not baby! Look at the percentages of couples who are seeking fertility treatment, that reflects many women who actually need help in regulating their cycle, and bringing it back to a dependable place. herbs (and herbalists!) can also help women transitioning off hormonal birth control. In both cases, the real job is to get the cycle to a reliable place, so that a couple can know whether a barrier method is required or they're free to go *au naturel*.

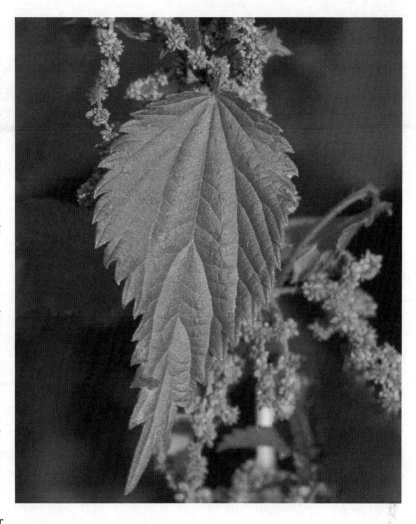

Some Herbs That Can Be Helpful Here, By Action:

Stimulate a stagnant and sluggish period: emmenagogues like Mugwort, Pennyroyal, or Ginger are useful. If a woman is typically stagnant, then consider Nettle, Raspberry leaf, and Red Clover (plus some Linden or Violet if the person is dry) to make sure the body is nourished, the uterus is toned, and the lymph is moving. Also, reducing sugar intake and making sure to walk: how does the pelvic area get stagnant? Sitting all day and having thick sticky sugar blood!

Amenorrhea: for women who don't cycle or who cycle rarely, causes could include lack of protein, extreme athleticism, PCOS, high stress levels, or other factors. Whether you know the reason or whether you don't, the first steps will be the same: a lack of cycle is the body saying "things are not right here". So make them right! Eat real foods, sleep real sleep, move more all day. Herbally, high-mineral nourishing herbs are a great support: Nettle, Dandelion, Red Clover, Violet, even Peppermint! if a person is dry, make sure to include plenty of Violet, Linden, Marshmallow, etc – not only do these prevent drying, but they are stress relievers, too!

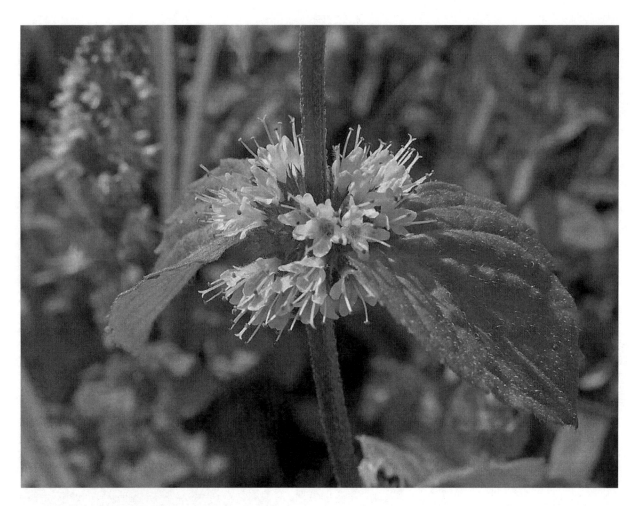

An over-heavy cycle is just as much an indication of imbalance as no cycle. Again, hormones are very touchy, and when the environment in the body is off, hormone levels will be off. There are various reasons for cycles that are too heavy or too long, and we will address it the same as no cycle: from the ground up. Eat real food, sleep real sleep, move more all day. consider herbs like Sage and Yarrow to help in the short term for heavy bleeding, as well as Raspberry leaf, Uva-ursi, and Mullein root to restore tone to the uterine walls.

Now What?

What Options Are There When Abortion is Necessary?

All politics aside, abortion is not an easy issue. Even when it's clearly the right answer, it is a very emotional experience, and depending on the methods available, it can be physically scary as well. in many places, abortion doulas are forming groups to make themselves available to women in need. abortion doulas can provide emotional and physical support during abortions, as well as assist in providing child care and abortion funding. Abortion doulas provide their services free of charge; you can find an abortion doula in your area at www.reproductivesupport.org, and for abortion funding in your state, check www.fundabortionnow.org.

When abortion is necessary, it's important to know you have options. Currently, there are several types of abortions available – a "traditional" sharp-curettage abortion, a medication abortion, electric vacuum aspiration, and a manual vacuum aspiration abortion. The MVA abortion is the least invasive, least likely to have side effects, least painful method, if it is available in your area. Early Options in NYC also provides national training for the MVA method, and may be able to help you find an MVA abortion in your area: www.earlyoptions.com.

As an alternative to abortion, in some states the "morning after pill" is legal over the counter, and can be taken up to five days after intercourse to prevent pregnancy. this is often also referred to as "emergency contraception". This pill is not without side effects, but is significantly less expensive than an abortion if you know at the time of intercourse that you might be pregnant.

Regardless Of The Type of Abortion That Is Performed, Herbs Can Help!

Abortions are stressful on the uterus, and on the whole reproductive system. After an abortion, make sure to give your reproductive system lots of love! Uterine tonifiers are important: Red Raspberry falls into this category, and Uva-ursi can be helpful as well. deeply nourishing plants such as nettle will also be handy – and Nettle's beneficial action for the kidneys is an extra bonus! Especially with medication abortions, the endocrine system will have a good deal of recovery, and working to the benefit of the kidneys is a foundational way to help the endocrine system rebalance itself. nourishing and support for the liver is also very important; consider Milk Thistle seed, and Burdock and Dandelion roots. Avoiding sugar and taking time to get plenty of sleep for a few months after an abortion are also important ways to help the body recover.

It's not just the body that needs nourishment and support post-abortion: nervines play a major role in helping women through a difficult time. some of my favorites are Wood Betony (*Stachys off.*), Linden, and Ghost Pipe (*Monotropa uniflora*). Hawthorn and Tulsi can be very good allies as well!

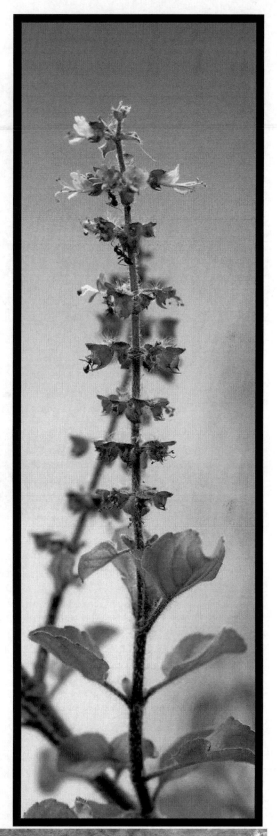

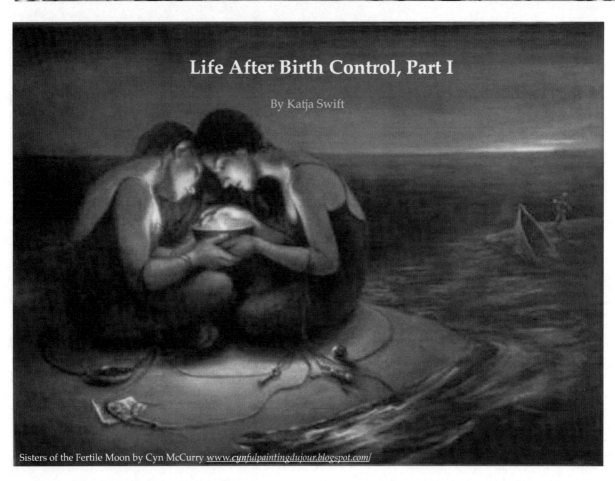

Life After Birth Control, Part I

By Katja Swift

Sisters of the Fertile Moon by Cyn McCurry www.cynfulpaintingdujour.blogspot.com/

One of the most powerful gifts we can give our clients is the gift of awareness. Helping a person to be conscious of their body, knowing how the pain Most likely some of you reading this have IUDs, or use the pill, or the ring, or . . . . I should note at this point that we all do what we've gotta do, taking whatever best option we can at the time. When I had Mirena IUD inserted, I knew there had to be a better way, I just hadn't found it yet. I left it in for years saying, yeah, I should probably take this out - but it's not an easy thing to do, and there are a zillion factors involved. No one can judge the choices a woman makes about her fertility - and the truth is, we aren't presented with much in the way of good options. But as it turns out, we have more than we've been led to believe.

The Project

It seems simple enough: remove hormonal birth control device, return to normal cycles, and employ natural or nearly-natural birth control methods successfully. It turns out, there's quite a lot to that!

First, there's the gauntlet of removing an IUD. The "return to normal cycles" part doesn't happen quickly, either. I had expected up to six months to become "normal", but it's hard to be patient. Then there's the daunting challenge of finding the bits and pieces of traditional knowledge about birth control, figuring out how to piece them together, and actually using them successfully. There's not *no* information out there, but there's not a lot, either, and there aren't many people who are willing to share the knowledge. Most herbalists I've met have been, outwardly at least, skeptical or even scornful

96

of natural birth control methods, and that was enough to discourage me for quite some time. But over time I came to believe that this outlook is rooted in our cultural disconnection from ourselves. For generations, women and men have been losing touch with the cycles of the earth, of the moon, of their place, of their bodies. Indeed, living as we do in a society that dumbs us down, mollifies us with sugar and boxfood and television - all we could ever want is available right down at our local Z-Mart! - we are also disconnected from Intent.

And so what started out as *I've had enough, I think I need to bleed again* (as I haven't done in 9 years) has become a 13-month project to reconnect to my body, my cycle, more deeply to Intent, and to learn new plants I haven't used before - or haven't used this way before. To delve deep into the sparse bits, a page here, a few sentences there, of information about a wisdom that was lost, or stolen, or forcibly removed - whatever your mythology calls it. (I don't know which it was, probably some of all of them, but the part that makes me sad is that I think a great deal of it over the generations was actually "given up" and "sold", for things of much lesser value made out to be grand, because "new" will always be made to look "better".) To gather up those bits, and carefully to weave them back into some whole something. To sit with these plants with whom women have had such deep relationships, but which have been forgotten, or marginalized, or repurposed, or stigmatized.

There are other women who are doing this work right now too, which is exciting. Together we might be able to revive what was lost, and learn a lot about ourselves in the trying.

Some Background

In January 2007, as my daughter was nursing less and my period was threatening to return, I had a Mirena IUD inserted. At the time, I had been in practice as an herbalist for several years, but had never really come across anything useful in terms of birth control, so I felt that an allopathic solution was my only option. Before getting pregnant with my daughter (June 2002, I was 28), I was taking the pill, in my case Ortho Tri-Cyclen, which I'd taken for at least three years, possibly four. I knew for sure that I

didn't want to go back on the pill, and that I wasn't interested in newer options like the NuvaRing, implants, or the shots, which also had relatively high hormone doses and about which I'd heard negative reports from friends. At that time, no one discussed diaphragms or sponges, and although I knew they had been previously available, I thought they weren't around anymore. (For some period of time, in fact, diaphragms weren't available, due to some changes in manufacturing.) I wouldn't have gone that route then anyway, because at that time, nonoxynol-9 was the only spermicide available in this country. Now there are natural spermicides based on lactic and ascorbic acid available from Canada and Europe.

At that time, it seemed to me that my least bad option was an IUD. There are two options for IUDs in this country, the "original" copper IUD (far from original, since IUDs have been in use for some considerable time - by which I mean, more than 100 years, and possibly much more - and in many different cultures; there's a whole museum about it in Toronto.) and the Mirena IUD, which is made of plastic and contains progestin. Progestin is a synthetic version of progestogen, which acts like progesterone in the body. It's a very low dose of progestin, described to me as approximately the amount in one birth control pill, but which is delivered locally and lasts for five years. The daily hormone dose is supposed to be approximately .02mg, which is significantly less than other options.

Beyond the progestin, it was less clear to me how IUDs worked. The copper IUD functions as a spermicide: copper in very high concentrations in the cervical mucus can impede the actual sperm migration, and sperm that do make it to the fallopian tubes are damaged and incapable of fertilization. At the time, I was told that the copper IUD is inert, but in fact, the copper leaches out. Elevated levels of copper can damage the liver and kidneys, among other things, and I wonder if that's one of the reasons that the copper IUD so frequently causes more intense cramping and pain in menstruation.

Besides the new hormone delivery aspect or the old copper spermicide, inserting a foreign object into the uterus causes an inflammatory response, which creates a hostile environment for sperm, and makes the uterine wall inhospitable to the implantation of an egg. In other words, an IUD causes an intentional chronic state of inflammation. An interesting note: often documentation fails to mention the inflammation, not because people are concerned about inflammation, but because people may consider it abortion.

The thing about inflammation is, it's not a local event. When there is inflammation in the body somewhere, there are stress hormones responding. When there is chronic inflammation, that's one long steady stream of stress hormones continually trying to respond. And while the body is in some ways amazingly fine-tuned, this isn't one of them: the inflammation and the stress responders cycle throughout the body. Chronic localized inflammation becomes chronic systemic inflammation.

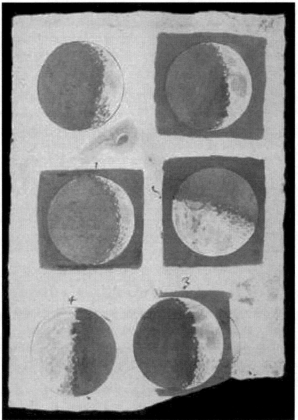
Art by Galileo Galilei

Regardless of the things I knew and didn't know, I went with it. Insertion was uncomfortable but manageable, the folks at Planned Parenthood in rural northern New England were very nice, and I had very few side effects that I noticed. Soon, as expected, I began to bleed a very small amount every day for several months, and eventually that dried up and I never bled again. At the time, I believed that that blood was somehow related to menstruation (why? I don't know. I think there was some selective lack of investigative thought going on!), but in fact I'm now quite certain that the bleeding was a result of the inflammation.

Many women have very serious side effects to Mirena IUDs, including nausea, headaches, vaginal infections, weight gain, acne, cysts, sudden lowered thyroid function, and emotional distress and depression, among other things. However, many women also have serious side effects to *removing* their Mirena IUD, which has been dubbed "Mirena Crash". In most cases, these effects seem to be emotional: mood swings (in some cases extreme), unexplained sadness, unexplained anger, brain fog, panic, etc.

So What Happened?

Once I got serious about taking it out, I planned to spend a month or two in research, and to have the IUD removed before my birthday in February. That seemed like a good deadline. But after about 10 days, in my typical fashion, I called Planned Parenthood and scheduled an appointment to have it removed (on December 17th). The decision was made, so why wait around? Also, I was very happy to have it out before the Solstice.

I was pretty nervous to have it removed; I was worried about Crash, I was worried it would hurt, and I was an emotional basket case: *Will I ever have sex again? Condoms are so evil! Oh no, this will ruin our relationship!* It went around and around.

I should make special note on the first and last concerns there that my partner is enthusiastically supportive of this work, and patient while I'm working through it. But I include the emotions because I think they're critical to the learning process: we're so backed into these hormonal options, they're so culturally ingrained in our emotions, even in an herbalist! I think that's actually the thing that should be at the top of the Practical Applications List: this work is emotionally challenging because we've been told for so long that The Pill (or other hormones) are our only choice, and in fact, we've enshrined them as Choice, that stepping away from them requires a great deal of support. Some women may make up their minds and never look back, and in fact, that's usually my style, but I completely fell apart here. I expect that actually, more women would share my experience, and probably be as surprised about it as I was.

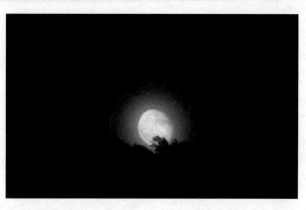

Preparation
So, the very first thing for a woman who is considering or who has made the decision to come off hormonal birth control is increased support systems, and nervines. If it's at all possible, make sure her partner is on board, and best if you can have a consultation with her partner or with them together.

At this point, there were already two things I had done to prepare my body to return to cycling, though I didn't plan it that way intentionally. In future protocols, I will absolutely include them. The first was that about 6 weeks before, we had transitioned from a gluten-free/casein-free/soy-free whole foods diet to a more specifically primal or paleo diet - adding grain-free, legume-free, and sugar-free to our list. This had the very fortunate impact of drastically increasing my consumption of

kale! We do eat farm-raised meats bought from the farm, and plenty of primal fats.

The second was that I had been working with David Dalton since May 2009 with flower essences. Like most people, I have some anger, fear, and hurt to put down, and that doesn't come easy. (I think it is particularly difficult to work on long-term emotional issues without a helper; it's hard to see yourself clearly.) I think that my work with the flower essences and David, though it was not in any intentional way targeted to help me get the courage to take out the IUD, absolutely yielded that additional effect. For women who are interested in doing that work, I would absolutely incorporate flower essences into their preparation protocol.

When I look back at how many times I thought about having it taken out and didn't, all of those times I said it was inconvenient, or some other excuse, I think actually I was just very afraid. If you can add flower essences to your protocol to work through the fear issues, it can be very helpful.

I would also have liked to have started drinking burdock and dandelion root about a month before having the IUD removed: the faster I cycle through whatever hormones are leftover in my system, the better, and that's all about the liver. I will definitely include that in my protocols for my practice, but in this case, there wasn't that much time. I might have drunk it anyway during the week between the making of the appointment and the appointment, but I was too busy being an emotional roller-coaster. Herbalists are not always the best in the compliance department!

Additionally, I would recommend what I call "Nettle & Friends": nettle, red clover, dandelion leaf, and a bit of licorice root, for kidney and adrenal support. I find this tremendously useful for preventing cramping and kidney pain in menstruation (both in my clients and from "way back then" when I used to bleed), especially when taken for the week or two before bleeding. I generally do have this a couple times a week anyway, but in terms of protocol, I'd make it a little more deliberate.

The Removal

The day came, and off I went. I asked additionally to be fitted for a diaphragm, now that there is a natural spermicide available. I'm not certain that I will use it ultimately, but for the short term while my body transitions, it seemed like a reasonable idea. (The spermicide is called ContraGel Green, and can be purchased online from Canada or Europe. Its ingredients are water, lactic acid, sodium lactate (a salt from fermentation), methylcellulose (a plant-fiber gel), and sorbic acid. There are also spermicide recipes, and I will probably fiddle with some of them, but not until I have a regular chartable cycle.)

First, they really questioned me about having it taken out. They could not fathom why on earth I would ever desire to do such a thing, and my explanations of "I'd like to use non-hormonal birth control instead" and "I'm uncomfortable not having a period" fell upon them as if I were trying to prove the earth was flat. They asserted strongly that there are no side effects to hormonal birth control, including emergency birth control (Plan B, as it's called in Massachusetts, which is available without a prescription in all pharmacies). It's not that they weren't nice, it's just that they were genuinely baffled by my decision.

This seems funny to me in retrospect, because when The Pill was first introduced, they included the placebo pills (or the week off, depending on the brand) not for medical reasons, but for social-acceptance reasons: women didn't feel comfortable not having a period. Times have changed, and to be honest, I had changed with them. For a long time I LOVED not having a period. But as I went through this process, I came to realize that never cycling meant that I was "always available". I was like the local 7-11. There was never any time to close, regroup, or be inside myself; I was always "open". Although this is convenient in our modern society, and certainly convenient in terms of sexual

relationships, I believe it has a very strong impact on us emotionally - where by "us" here I mean both women and men. It is one more thing that pulls us out of rhythm, that pulls us away from Cycle. It is one more thing that disconnects us from our bodies.

It was not their intent to harass me, but the ladies at Planned Parenthood, with best intentions in mind, strongly pressured me not to remove the IUD - another item for the Practical Application List: prepare your clients that they might need to stand up for what they want.

The actual removal process was much easier than I anticipated, and only painful in the moment that the IUD passed through the cervix. Then it was time to be fitted for a diaphragm, for which process the young practitioner seeing me had to go and get a 65-year-old nurse, because most practitioners are no longer taught how to fit a diaphragm. This was amusing to me, and the old nurse was earthy and gritty. I liked her. She did, however, really lecture about people who try to use Fertility Awareness Methods in combination with the diaphragm and how it never works out - I was very glad I had not offered any information about my own plans!

For the rest of the day I rested. I felt physically tired and a little wobbly, and emotionally tired and wobbly as well. I started a journal specifically for the purpose of documenting this information and sharing the long-term case study with some of my students, and the first many entries were deep emotional introspection. Although I had planned the journal for practical case-study purposes, it was tremendously helpful for me as I went through some pretty hefty emotions: add "keep a journal" to the protocol list.

The First Few Weeks

In the first couple weeks I was obsessed with bleeding. I bled tiny bits here and there, I had cramps sometimes, sometimes not, my kidneys were tender sometimes, I had headaches (quite unusual for me). But the one thing I thought about constantly was bleeding. I had originally planned to "do nothing" in the after-phase: I would leave my body to its own schedule, and only use herbs that were nourishing tonics - dandelion root, burdock root, nettle and friends, and whatever usually ends up in the soup (codonopsis, astragalus, seaweeds, maitake, calamus, among other things). For a while I had a strong desire to take higher doses of calamus, which I take a few drops of before most meals for the bitter aspect, but in talking with my friends and students in this learning circle, I finally agreed that even that was probably too much. I have a great desire to move very quickly, pretty much always, and to over-achieve: I'm about as type-A as it comes. It took some really perceptive students to point out that what I really needed was to get as far away from the driver's seat as possible.

But I was obsessed with wanting to bleed. Maybe because it was the pay-off to all the angst, maybe because I missed it, and in large part I think to get it over with: I wasn't even sure I remembered how! Whatever the reason, the new moon was coming and I'd decided this was the time to bleed. The new moon was exactly two weeks from having it removed, surely that was enough time to have waited for a good soaking bleed, right? I'd worked myself up to the idea of drinking tansy the night before the solstice, to induce bleeding, but fortunately, I didn't actually do it. Fortunately, not because I have any particular fear of tansy, but because I was letting my fear of my body run rampant. I was so afraid to trust my body, I was so afraid to trust my own healing process, I was so personally and culturally needful of control of this situation that I had given up my previous promises to give my body time to re-cycle on its own, with its own wisdom and its own timing. I think that another woman might be more patient with the process, but for all the type-As that want to go through this work, make a note: encourage patience!

I went through several rounds of the cycle of complete emotional basket case to feeling "much more" level-headed. I may still be going through those cycles, it's hard to tell. I have made many adjustments in my life since having it removed, and interestingly one of them is to speak up more, and to "be of service" less. I enjoy living my life in service, and I think it's a valid way to live. But there's appropriate service, and there's doormat, and sometimes that line is pretty blurry for me. I have been becoming much more aware of being *not* always available, in healthy ways. I've said "no" (in the healthy way) more often. It's not like someone

flipped a switch and I'm suddenly perfectly in balance, but I definitely can see that I'm doing things differently. My work with flower essences is tying into this, and in my last appointment with David, (which was the first since having it removed) we specifically worked it into our session.

I have noticed that I'm taking better care of my body now: there have been several things that I've been putting off working on that I have finally started, and not from any particular resolution or guilt-induced discipline, just finally easing into it naturally. To me this comes back again to the "always available" concept: when we are always open and available to others, when are we available to ourselves?

I also found in the first few weeks that I dreamt intensively, to the point of disruption. Any time I tried to sleep, even just for a nap, I was completely overcome by dreams, and very often they were intensely negative or unpleasant. Eventually this subsided, and I'm dreaming in a more normal way now, but it was very taxing while it lasted. I was not able to gather myself to resolve this issue in any way, because I was too tired, but I will watch for it in the future!

A lot of these things don't seem very big taken on their own. But I think it's worth making a point of them, for two reasons: the more practical, because if we as practitioners or we as women know what to expect, we can make the transition easier. But also because I would never have expected that I would have had dreams that interfered with my ability to sleep, and do so in a serious way. In this particular case, maybe it was years of dreams I hadn't had in all the inward cycles I had skipped. But each body will react in some strange ways, and if you know to watch for strange things, you may be able to provide comfort and relief where it's needed.

Intent
For me, reconnecting myself with Intent has become the core of this work, although I think that realization didn't come until I was into the process. I began working with Intent in direct relation to cycles. I began working my create-ive energy intentionally towards the things in the world I am trying to build. I began to look at my reproductive

cycles in a larger way, as create-ive cycles. This concept isn't necessarily new, but it's new work for me to put into practice, and a new way for me to think about Intent. I'm almost 37, I have a beautiful daughter, and my create-ability now can be channeled into the work I am doing in the world.

This is a very different way than our current societal norm of having intent around reproductive cycles: we see them as inconvenient, as interruptive. We have sex and in the back of the mind is the panic we learned from TV shows and movies and older siblings: *Oh no! Am I pregnant?* We dread the bother of bleeding, and we dread the consequences of not bleeding.

A central part of the work I am doing now is to move intentionally into these cycles, to see each part of the cycle as a necessary part of my own rhythm. I'm hoping to be able to translate that into a healthier, more relaxed lifestyle. I think it would be nice to allow my work to crescendo in my outward times, and to be comfortable with the turn inward that follows. I think that this type of Intent and awareness is probably a key in being successful with natural birth control methods, but more importantly, I think it is probably a key in settling more calmly into myself.

Practical Applications

Here is a condensed protocol for transitioning away from hormonal birth control. Each woman's experience will be unique, but these guidelines should help in all cases.

- *Be prepared to feel.* This work is emotionally challenging. Stepping away from hormonal birth control is counter to our culture's understanding of Choice. Be prepared for fears and anxieties to surface in spite of the conscious decision that this is the right choice for you.

- *Be prepared to fight.* You may need to stand up for what you want. Planned Parenthood and other organizations can not be expected to be supportive of women choosing to cease hormonal birth control (unless they are trying to get pregnant). Friends or partners

may question your decision. Be clear about your reasoning, your emotions, and your Intent, and you will be able to persist peacefully.

- *Be patient.* You are trying to come back into a natural cycle: try to let it happen naturally, without rushing or second-guessing. Try to observe, and even enjoy, the ride.

- *Emotional support.* Make sure any partners are informed and engaged. Consider flower essence therapy or other emotional work to formalize Intent.

- *Nutritional support.* Adopt a primal / paleo diet for as long a preparatory period as is possible. An exercise regimen is also a good idea. In essence, treat this period in much the same way as if preparing for a pregnancy.

- *Nervous support.* Use (and stock) appropriate nervines for your constitution and for symptoms of hormonal withdrawal ("Mirena Crash" and similar). This will vary from person to person, but some of my favorites are linden, chamomile, skullcap, lavender, and catnip.

- *Liver support.* Burdock and dandelion root, or other nourishing liver-supportive herbs to encourage the clearing of residual hormones.

- *Kidney and adrenal support.* Drink Nettle & Friends, or a similar blend. Sleep.

- *Keep a journal.* Having a record of your emotions and intentions is immensely helpful in trusting your decision, holding your Intent, and
- tracking your progress.

When last we met, I was feeling pretty Type-A about wanting to Just Bleed Already, but just before I took drastic emmenagogue action, I realized I was ovulating (so that wouldn't have worked anyway: emmenagogues won't make you bleed when you're ovulating!). And that was what I needed to feel like I had some kind of traction on what was going on inside my body. Fifteen days later, right on time, I bled. The bleeding itself was on the heavy side, and along with PMS I had a fever and was overwhelmingly tired, but all of those things can be reasonably expected, given I hadn't bled in nine years.

This was very exciting to me, in particular in its utter normality. But let's pause here for a moment to talk about what actually happens in a menstrual cycle: time after time, I sit with women who are having problems with PMS or other cycle issues, and they just don't have any idea how it's actually supposed to work.

The first thing I always teach them I learned from Brooke Medicine Eagle, and more than anything else, this teaching really changed my whole opinion about bleeding. Oh, I'd heard about the red tent – after all, I was schooled in Texas, and I knew all about the Indians. (You'll have to hear the sarcasm there for me.) Everyone knew that when an Indian (we didn't call them Native Americans yet, this was Texas in the early 80s) woman was bleeding, she was regarded as unclean and sent away from the rest of the tribe to sit alone in a red tent until she stopped bleeding and could rejoin her family.

But Brooke told me a different story. I learned that before electric lights, and when people still lived in

Life After Birth Control, Part 2

By Katja Swift

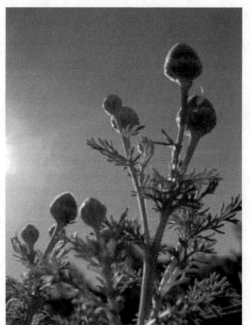

Matricaria discoidea © Rosalee de la Forêt

tribes and groups, all women bled at the same time. *Well, it happens in dormitories, so I suppose it makes sense*, I thought. That could mean that all the women in a tribe went to the red tent together, in community, not in penal isolation. She went on to explain that the time of all this togetherness was the New Moon. At the time I was learning this, I was under the belief that if you want to be *really natural*, you managed to bleed on the Full Moon, because of course, that's where the "power" is. But Full Moon power is about outward power. It's about howling-at-the-moon power, it's about ovulation and being fertile. Menstruation is about introspection, she taught, and the right time for that is the Dark of the Moon. At that time, I would not yet have recognized introspection as power.

The idea that menstruation was a time for introspection was fairly groundbreaking to me, and explained a great deal. Of course women get a little cranky when they're bleeding: there is a pull to be doing this quiet, deep, reflective work, and yet we are still required to live in our outward facing, ever producing society. We are a society of the Full Moon: of 24/7, of 365, of always available and always productive. I do believe that if we could find a way to do it, America would make the Moon be full all the time.

Brooke taught that the New Moon was a time when all the women of the tribes came together within their communities to do the emotional and spiritual work of their people. Guidance would be received in meditation or in dreams. The work of the women would be taken over for those days by the girls (with guidance, I suppose, from some crones), which would have provided the girls with wonderful training for the future. Food would have been simple, and the workload lighter, as this was not the time for starting projects. During this time, the men also had some form of retreat, though to be honest, I don't remember as much about what that was. Regardless, there is a beauty in this kind of cyclic separation, this monthly time apart to renew. Imagine if our society allowed, every month, three days for everyone to stop their daily lives and focus simply on meditation and spiritual work.

It was these teachings that finally helped me understand the concept of our cycle, what it really meant that bleeding was powerful.

Now with that in mind, let's talk about what's happening on a physical level during a woman's cycle. Moving forward, we can't make good decisions about birth control options unless we fully understand how fertility works.

A woman's cycle has two parts: the follicular phase, and the luteal phase. These phases are like inhalation and exhalation – in that moment in between there is a minute pause during which the body shifts from one action to the other. And yet, there's never really a moment that the cycle isn't in motion.

The very beginning of the follicular phase is menstruation, and we clear out the nutrients that had been prepared for a pregnancy, but which were not needed because no egg was fertilized. As we stop bleeding, estrogen levels begin to rise, slowly coming to a peak around day 14. A few little potential eggs, all of which we have been carrying around since our birth, begin during these first two weeks to mature into eggs ready to be fertilized. We develop a few, because the human body loves redundancy, but in the end, usually only one is released.

When the estrogen levels hit their peak, another hormone comes into play: luteinizing hormone. Luteinizing hormone does not build slowly like estrogen did, but instead is released in one quick burst. Its job is to cause the best of the candidates of maturing eggs to release, in hopes of fertilization. (Incidentally, men have luteinizing hormone as well, it is responsible for the production of testosterone.) Also at this moment, cervical fluid changes into a mucus that is more friendly to sperm, providing a

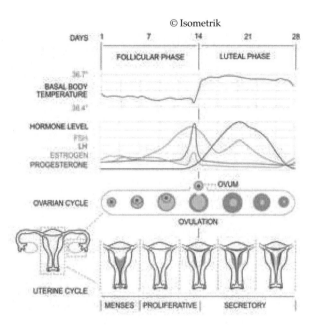

© Isometrik

less-acidic environment with a texture that is "good for swimming".

Once the egg is released, the corpus luteum, which is to the egg what the placenta is to the developing baby, begins to produce progesterone, and the luteal phase begins. The egg is only viable for fertilization for about 24 hours, although sperm can live within the woman for up to five days. This means that the window of fertility begins five days before ovulation, and may last for several days after, as it is possible for more than one egg to be released. (I have known some women to have extremely abnormal cycles in which they seemed to ovulate twice during each month, about a week apart, but this is not the norm.)

During the luteal phase, the body is preparing for implantation and the start of a pregnancy. There are some complications with the idea of pregnancy, which are what cause us to go through this monthly cycle to begin with. First, because a fertilized egg contains foreign DNA, the body wants to view it as an invader, and to fight it off. Second, a growing fetus very much resembles a tumor to the body, and the body would prefer to stop that growth if possible. How, then, can pregnancy occur? I envision the design process to have gone something like this:

> "Ok, and for pregnancy, we'll combine DNAs from the mother and the father, and implant in the uterus!"

104

"Wait – no, that won't work – foreign DNA gets rejected. Besides, the whole thing is going to look like a tumor…"

"Right. Ok, uh, no problem, we'll start to separate the uterine lining environment from the actual uterus, to buffer the rejection!"

"Yeah…that should work. Wait, no, what if the pregnancy doesn't take – the lining disintegrates…"

"Ok, no problem, we'll just make a new one, uh, every month! Sound good?"

"Great!"

(Obviously, this was a system designed by men!)

In order to allow the pregnancy to grow without being shut down as a pathogen or a tumor by the mother's body, the endometrial lining separates before the implantation occurs – but this means that if no implantation occurs, the lining just gets wasted, and has to be built up again next month. And so, we bleed.

Once the opportunity for fertilization has passed, but no fertilization has occurred, progesterone levels begin to drop, and the lining of the uterus prepares to shed. Follicle Stimulating Hormone increases and will stimulate the preparation of the immature eggs, and the whole cycle starts over again.

Remember, if a woman is on the pill, hormone levels remain constant, and these cyclic changes do not occur. Bleeding occurs only from the withdrawal of the constant hormones, and not because there is lining to shed.

When I decided to bleed again, I spent some time thinking about how to bleed naturally. I've worked with many women on this issue, but turning my advice around and thinking about it for myself was a new experience. Generally, I make the following recommendations to women about reclaiming their cycles:

Although it's hard in our modern society, try to give yourself time apart when you bleed. Don't book any social activities during this time. Take a break from your yoga class or your Tae Bo, at least for the heavy day of your bleeding. Do only what is absolutely needful in your schedule: go to work, and come home. If you can, prepare a large batch food ahead of time, so that you don't even have to cook for yourself. (Or perhaps your partner will cook during this time.) Use this time to be quiet at home, without television, and without computers if possible. Use the time to meditate or journal, or just to rest.

I found this advice to be the most challenging, as it's very difficult for me to give up what would otherwise be "productive time". Although I regularly give this advice, sincerely and convincingly, to other women, I am finding that making this shift in thinking about "productivity" is not entirely comfortable!

If it's possible, sleep alone, at least on the night of your heaviest day. A spouse or partner may want to take advantage of this time for himself: I encourage men to sleep outdoors on this night if it is possible. This allows both partners to re-ground themselves in what would have been a cycle that affected the whole community. Each may consider Mugwort, asking for guidance in dreams.

Whenever possible, use plain cloth for menstrual pads, instead of commercial pads or tampons. Even organic tampons cause irritation and can make cramping worse.

Many different cloth pads are available for purchase, but I have not found one that feels right for my body. Instead, I am using my daughter's old cloth prefold diapers on heavy days, folded the same way you would fold it for a baby and held in place with underwear – they don't tend to move around even if I'm walking all around town. With a little practice, they can be folded in such a way that they're really not noticeable under a skirt. On a light day, I use a folded washcloth, though this does need a safety pin to keep from slipping back if I'm walking any particular distance. (For those of you trying this at home, fold the washcloth on the diagonal – it's less bulky at the ends that way, so it won't show.)

One particular benefit of going without tampons is that you have to see and feel your blood. I absolutely am a recovering tampon addict. When I bled before my pregnancy, I even slept in tampons. I didn't realize it then, but a consequence of this behavior was that I really didn't know my blood. I never really saw it, I never felt it, it was as un-real as possible while still bleeding.

Now, when I bleed, I can feel the blood coming from me. I notice that I don't, actually, bleed all the time. I notice that there's a rhythm: I have a cramp, some blood comes out, then nothing happens for a while. Then I have a cramp again. I see the blood, and I can notice it: what color is it? What texture? How much is there, and when does it come? I've been very excited to see that my blood is not clotty, and has nice red color when it should – I wasn't certain that would be the case, after so long.

I've also noticed that although I was previously always afraid of "leaks", and paranoid I might have "something on my skirt", I am no longer afraid of my blood escaping. And surprisingly, it doesn't! I also used to be very afraid my period would start when I was unprepared. Now, I know I can just fold up any bit of cloth – a towel, a handkerchief, a sock – and I'll be fine. Familiarity, perhaps, breeds confidence.

Many people already have their favorite PMS and bloodtime allies. Next to my hot water bottle (a trusted friend!), here are mine:

Chamomile: Never confuse gentle with weak! A strong infusion of chamomile contains very powerful antispasmodic agents that relax aching, tense muscles and alleviate premenstrual pain. Better yet, anyone can get some. If you're using chamomile tea bags, I recommend brewing your tea with four bags, to make sure it's strong enough. Drinking strong chamomile tea regularly through the crampy time makes a huge, relaxing difference – not just on the body, but on the mind!

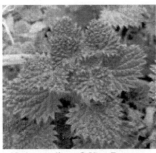

Nettle: I am particularly prone to the lower back/ kidney ache of PMS and bloodtime. I have found, however, that drinking strong infusions of nettle in the two weeks

Urtica gracilenta © Kiva Rose

before my period (or, during the luteal phase) makes a drastic improvement. I particularly like to blend nettle with some friends: dandelion leaf and red clover blossom (in roughly equal parts), and a bit of licorice root. I make it nightly – about an inch of herbs in the bottom of a French press or a mason jar, and filled to the top with boiling water. In the morning, it's ready to drink, as it is or reheated.

For someone who finds the flavor a bit on the "green" side, it can be cut – half hot water, half tea, which makes the strong flavor a bit more manageable.

Catnip: When you feel like your emotions are reeling out of control, catnip is a good friend. My favorite remedy for teething babies and cranky two year olds, catnip is great when PMS has us feeling like our own inner cranky two year old has taken control! Good on its own, or blended with nettle or with chamomile, as needed.

Ginger: I hate to be cold, anytime, but when I'm bleeding I seem to feel like I'll never get warm. (This might have more to do with living in New England than the actual bleeding!) Ginger tea is perfect for this! And ginger does it all: it gets your blood moving, whether it's your circulatory blood, or a sluggish period. It's pleasantly antispasmodic, and it tastes great (a key factor if you're feeling grumpy).

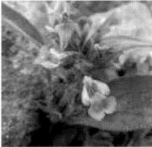

Salvia officinalis © Kiva Rose

Sage: In our house, sage is a special friend. Sage is wonderfully warming, and although I've never heard it used as a nervine, it certainly has that effect on me. Sage makes me feel like someone else is in control, like it's safe to rest. With specific regard to the blood, sage can help control heavy bleeding. It's great to blend with raspberry leaf to this end. For any woman who has experienced "lead uterus syndrome" – that feeling like your uterus suddenly weighs a ton and is trying to fall all the way out of your body – sage can pull you back together.

After my first bleed, I felt on top of the world. Look! Everything was going according to plan! I had expected months of irregularity and weirdness, but everything was instead progressing as if it were normal. I thought, this is great! (Uh oh, this can't be good…)

Life After Birth Control, Part 3
By Katja Swift

My cycle continued apace: that first blood stopping at an appropriate time, ovulation occurring right on time, and I was just amazed at how quickly my body was coming back into the swing of things. Given that it had taken me two years to get pregnant with my daughter, I didn't really believe that *everything* was back to proper functioning order, but I was thrilled that at any rate, I was lining up with the calendar right off the bat.

I waited a few days after ovulating (though not as many days as any of the Natural Fertility Awareness methods advise), and figured at that point everything was safe: eggs only live for 24-48 hours, and anyway, I had only just bled for the first time. The exercise of charting a cycle seemed more academic than real, given that it was so early in my process. What I was discounting was the drastic improvement in my health over the last eleven years: when I was trying to get pregnant with my daughter, I had not yet been diagnosed with Celiac (a diagnosis which Amber's father also received, after she was born, and which certainly played a large part in our fertility problems). At that time, I also still considered Cocoa Pebbles a viable food option. In the years since then, I have been very disciplined about maintaining a gluten and casein free whole foods diet, and for a couple months before having the Mirena removed, I'd given up grains and sugar entirely. So even though I didn't really think enough time had passed for me to be actually fertile, I had in fact given my body every opportunity to succeed – which is exactly what happened, though I didn't catch on until my cycle was late.

I always have been the kind of person, much to my own dismay, who has to feel the fire to know it's hot – the polite way to say that these days is "experiential learner". Even if I hadn't been, there was no one to teach me these things: I didn't have any generations of women before me to teach me how to understand my body or how to manage my cycles. So although this was definitely not how I'd planned things, I found gratitude for the experience. After all, you can't just wake up one morning and decide to drink quarts of Tansy just for the experience – it's just not the same.

By this time, I had done quite a bit of research on emmenagogues specific to this purpose, as well as other protocols. I was somewhat concerned for my own situation, because in my research I felt strongly that any of these options were best used *before* your period is late. I had missed that window of optimal opportunity, but I tried them anyway. Here is the research I did, followed by the protocols I used, and outcomes:

Wild Carrot, *Daucus carota*: There's quite a bit of information available on Wild Carrot (Queen Anne's Lace), and if you're interested in working with this plant, I would absolutely recommend you look up Robin Rose Bennet's work at her website, www.robinrosebennet.com

At this point in my experience, Wild Carrot is not a plant I considered working with. Given that Wild Carrot seems to work by temporarily increasing progesterone levels and is then withdrawn to cause an artificial progesterone crash, it's not the kind of thing you can use every day (in fact, every-day use of wild carrot may *promote* fertility!). Since I am specifically working to transition from my previous "always available" Mirena-controlled state to a time in which I can move appropriately through all parts of my cycle, and in particular since my cycle is brand new and may not yet be reliable, it doesn't seem like I'm in a place where Wild Carrot is the right choice. Also in this particular case, by the time that I realized the situation, it was too late for Wild Carrot. That said, Robin has done a great deal of work with this plant, and her work may be applicable to your situation, so do give it a read.

Pennyroyal (*Mentha pulegium*, European Tennyroyal and *Hedeoma pulegoides*, American Tennyroyal), Mugwort (*Artemisia vulgaris*), Sage (*Salvia off.*), and

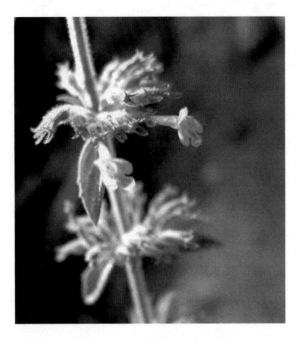

Ginger (*Zingiber off.*) are widely-known emmenagogues that I've had good success with for stalled menses, and they also have a history of use early in pregnancy. They went onto my list as worth trying.

Tansy (*Tanacetum vulgare*) is also an emmenagogue. Tansy is one strong plant, let me tell you. It is critical to note that if you want to attempt to prevent or dislodge a pregnancy with Tansy and you are not successful, keeping the pregnancy at that point is likely to result in birth defects, as Tansy is teratogenic. Ideally, as with all emmenagogues, you would want to drink Tansy tea or take the tincture in the time between ill-timed intercourse and when your period is due, but it does have a strong reputation for use in early pregnancy as well.

Tansy also has a history of being used to expel parasites, which I found to be darkly amusing, in this context.

Vitamin C (specifically *ascorbic acid*), while not an herb, does have some significant research around its use to stimulate menses in early pregnancy, specifically by interfering with progesterone levels. Doses need to be very high – between 6 and 12 grams per day, depending on the source reference. Also, it is important to use specifically ascorbic acid, and not the buffered vitamin C supplements with bioflavonoids added; the emmenagogue effect seems to be a "side effect" of using the isolated ascorbic acid.

Blue and Black Cohosh are often used as uterine contractors and often referenced in materials with information about terminating a pregnancy. Dosing information seems to vary widely. Dong Quai is also regularly referenced in this way.

The protocol I worked with shifted over the course of time. I did initially start to bleed, but it was scant and sluggish. The color was brown, but not as dark brown as one would expect in the range of the menstrual palette. I also felt breast tenderness, and although at first I thought I was imagining myself gaining weight and my breasts swelling, by this time, it was clearly not just an over-critical eye on my part.

After two days of the not-actually-bleeding, I started with European Pennyroyal tea, approximately 1 quart/day, taken hot. It tastes, by the way, delicious – I remember thinking, who wouldn't want to drink this tea every day!? Drinking this tea was enjoyable and uplifting, the sort of thing you do after a stressful day at work.

I have since used this herb in conjunction with Mugwort, Peppermint, Raspberry leaf, and Sage to stimulate sluggish-starting menses (in cases without any suspicion of pregnancy), with very good results. I feel that it is specifically suited to times when tension is involved in the stagnation of the menses, or when PMS is long and drawn-out, with (PMS-induced) depression.

But in this case, the Pennyroyal was not effective. Susun Weed recommends specifically the American Pennyroyal against the European Pennyroyal, although given my overall experience, I am not inclined to think that would make a significant difference.

I spent two days with Pennyroyal, after which, I began taking Tansy. I drank a very strong cup of tea (steeped for at least one to four hours, with oily resin visible), or three droppersfull of tincture, every two hours, continuing this dosing through the night. Tansy is a tremendously *strong* plant whose presence I felt quite immediately on starting with it. I felt cramping while I was still drinking the very first cup, and over the course of the first day, a strong "heaviness" in my uterus. In the beginning, I felt quite optimistic: I trusted that this plant would work. I felt fairly foolish for being caught unawares, but also very grateful for the experience: overall, I felt positive. I was meditating, and letting my body know that it was time to release. I dreamt a great deal during the night, and in my dreams, I was not able to relax my abdomen. By morning, my optimism was more like determination: this was work.

In the second day, I was feeling sicker. I felt heat in my middle, and cold everywhere else. I felt dizzy sometimes after drinking a cup of tea, which strangely was starting to taste rather appealing (and very much like drinking a meadow). From the start, although I wasn't exactly nauseous, I was absolutely not interested in eating: it seemed like the wrong direction. My body didn't want things in: I was very focused on the strange sensation of my outer reproductive parts looking expectantly at my inner reproductive parts as if they were waiting to catch whatever was coming. Every time I sipped the tea, I imagined (though not intentionally, more like "I could have sworn I heard") some kind of announcer in my innards yelling: "everybody out!" I felt very much like I was just about to bleed.

I was keeping a journal, and at some point I realized that I was writing in it every 15 minutes or so. Tansy was the only thing I could think about. I felt very aware that although no one was home to talk to, I very much wished someone had been. I noticed that when I was drinking the tea, I could feel my uterus moving, but when I stopped, it stopped. I was drinking tea (or taking tincture, or putting tincture into tea) every two hours consistently, and I wondered – is this too much? Is it too little? I started to realize that I was placing much more trust in this plant than I was able to trust my own body.

In the second night, Ryn started waking up for me every two hours, waking me only enough for me to take doses of tansy. This did help me sleep a little more, but it was still full of dreams.

In the third day, my body felt liquefied. I felt like I was drinking poison. I began to feel that nothing was real, and although I felt physically like I was going to start bleeding at any moment – crampy and heavy, and a very particular "raw" kind of feeling – I felt mentally discouraged. I was completely beset with self-criticism, not only for how I'd gotten into this situation, but for the actions I was currently taking. Why am I bothering, I kept thinking. Why am I doing this to myself? And with every sip, I was overcome with how very much *work* it was to just drink this tea. In fact, drinking tea and resting was about the only work I was accomplishing – otherwise, everything was mostly a haze.

By the end of the third day, I couldn't take any more, but I also couldn't take anymore because I ran out. I'm academically interested to know what might have happened if I'd taken the tansy for a third or more days, but I'm fairly certain that I could not have sustained it. Within four hours of the last cup of tea, although I felt as though I'd been wrung out, mentally and even physically I was feeling better.

I took one day off, to allow my body some recovery time. I promised myself that when everything was said and done, I'd drink burdock and dandelion and nettle till it seeped out my pores. That night I slept.

At this point, I really want to stress that I don't think it should be this way. I think that – or I want to think that – if you're going to successfully work with herbs to prevent a pregnancy, you and the plants should be working together. I think that taking plants until you're too sick to continue taking plants is NOT the right way to go about things: at that point, the plants just become a stand-in for RU486 (the "abortion pill"). There's the wise woman way, and the "heroic" way, and what I was doing was definitely the latter. I knew it, and I was going with it because I wanted experience with these plants, and I wanted to experience the protocols that I'd come up with in research. And in fact, a great deal of the research was saying specifically that you must make yourself very sick to achieve success. I don't feel like that can be right. We watch movies or read stories depicting women doing this and becoming sick, and we've heard all the modern cautionary tales. Were our original methods really so harshly purgative? I want to believe that they weren't, that there was more connection, more of the subtlety that can come from working in relationship, but there are plenty of examples of historical "brute force" methods, as well. Maybe I am romanticizing the issue – after all, people kept looking for better ways. Regardless, I do feel firmly that the ideal way to work with plants to this end is in awareness before your cycle is late.

When the Tansy didn't work, I was fairly certain that I was past the point of succeeding with natural options, and I would have to seek conventional methods to end the pregnancy. However, I was still interested to try the vitamin C protocol. I started this on "day 7" – my period was one week late at this point. I took 12-14 grams of ascorbic acid a day: doses I saw in research mostly gathered in the 10-12 gram range, but I weigh about 175 lbs, which I imagined to be more than most of the women we have data on (anecdotal and otherwise), so I dosed up somewhat.

I felt better with the vitamin C than I did on the Tansy, though the breast tenderness was becoming more and more aggravating. (It is possible that some of this was actually a lingering side effect of the Tansy, and not all just a result of the pregnancy.) I remember thinking how much easier it would be to just take the RU486 pill – it's just one pill, no lines, no waiting! Of course I was very aware how ridiculous that thought was: I have known women to take RU486, and their experiences were harrowing. As I watched my thoughts, I was surprised at how much society's "easy way" is simultaneously not at all easy, and yet completely manages to lull us into believing…

After 5 days at that dose (dosing every two hours and through the night to equal 12-14 grams daily), I did notice a significant reduction in breast swelling. The tenderness was nearly gone, and my breasts had reduced in size noticeably. I cramped regularly, but mildly. I was tired, and I was sad. I wondered whether the Tansy would have worked if I had been able to continue it; I wondered if I had given up too easily. I wanted to be able to say, "look! The plants work!", but I was certain I must have made some sort of mistake to cause them not to. I felt like I was letting them down.

Protocols for vitamin C generally call for a uterine contractor to be added into the mix around day 5. I added in various uterine contractors, starting with Dong Quai, by capsules. I was also drinking Ginger in warm water, more for the comfort than the contracting action. I considered adding in *Mitchella repens*, but I have conflicting data, and some of it noted that Mitchella can save a pregnancy from miscarriage. I decided better to not.

At the end of the first day with Dong Quai, I took Mugwort before bed and asked for guidance. I woke

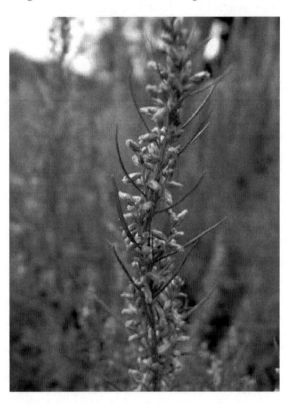

up with Black Cohosh, and going back to my research, I wondered why I hadn't gone with it before. I had plenty of cramping going on, and I felt like I was PMSing – what it seemed I needed was something to open the cervix. I started that by capsules, but I thought better of it and switched to tincture. After two more days, I added Blue Cohosh to the mix. The Blue Cohosh was quite intense. The particular preparation I had was made with grain alcohol. It was at this point that I started off on a tangent, questioning the use of not only grain alcohol, but distilled alcohol whatsoever in the making of medicinal preparations. I wondered, and am still exploring, whether wine and mead are not much more appropriate menstruums for alcohol preparations. In the case of Blue Cohosh, though, I'm not sure I can blame the alcohol for the vile flavor.

Once I started the Blue Cohosh, I was overcome with a very intense headache, and I was very nauseous. I had "period guts" – lower intestinal distress – and cramping.

After eight days with vitamin C (and the uterine contractor additions), I had very severe muscle cramping in my legs, and my bones hurt. I also began to have pain in all my teeth. This was upsetting! It was hard to find any information on these types of symptoms, and all I could think – as ridiculous as it seemed – was, well, gee, I wonder if *too MUCH* vitamin C would also result in scurvy? Although I never did find a good clear definition of what was going on (besides that I was wrecking my body), I did find some good information about "rebound scurvy", which is a condition where, after withdrawing from excessive levels of vitamin C, the body has scurvy symptoms until recalibrating to a normal level. None of the research that I found on using vitamin C as an emmenagogue mentioned titrating off the C, but at this point it was very clear that would be necessary, and probably sooner rather than later. It wasn't just the muscle cramping, though it was bad enough on its own, but I was also very nauseous. I continued to have menstrual-like cramps, and they felt so real that I believed that any moment I was going to bleed. I continued to have headaches.

On the ninth day, I was overwhelmed with "why am I not bleeding yet?". I have a fairly strong constitution, but still, I felt that I had done enough damage to my body, I couldn't imagine that there was any way anything could be left alive inside me. Maybe there wasn't, but if it wasn't alive, it also wasn't coming out.

That evening, I took Mugwort again before bed, and asked for guidance. Mugwort said "take less" (that was perhaps obvious advice!). I began to titrate off the vitamin C, and stopped taking the other herbs as well. I started drinking nettle, dandelion, and clover, and I baked a gluten-free cake. In retrospect, I might have been happy: it is not easy for me to dream for guidance, and here I'd done it twice in a short span of time. Instead, I was completely depressed. I was angry at my body, and I couldn't be "in" my body. I waffled for several days about whether or not I should have actually kept going – maybe I was *thisclose*, and if I'd just kept it up a little longer, it would have worked. I got a good raging head cold

and fever. I fumbled around for a couple more weeks, in which time I actually did some productive emotional work, but nothing particularly consistent or productive physically. It is interesting to me to note that the emotional work was all around release: there were some specific anger issues that I was able to put down, and that have stayed down.

I tried to make a deal with whatever may or may not have been alive inside me: "if you come out now, you can pick – you can go into my garden or I can release you in the ocean, wouldn't that be nice?"

I researched (again some more) the conventional methods of dealing with this. RU486 was pretty scary, but it seemed preferable to an abortion, especially given that I have a history of severe sensitivity to anesthesia.

Ultimately, I found a clinic that performs what is called Menstrual Extraction, which is not the same as a standard abortion, and does not require anesthesia, antibiotics, or any other drastic measures. The procedure is performed in a regular doctor's office, as opposed to a surgical clinic, and takes only about five minutes. The doctor uses an ultrasound to locate the implanted egg, and then inserts a very narrow flexible tube through the cervix into the uterus. There was local topical anesthetic used, and I didn't feel anything. The doctor then operates a small hand-operated vacuum pump, sucking endometrial lining and the egg through the tube. During this part, there was some very mild cramping, but it wasn't any worse than regular menstrual cramps. She let us see the pregnancy tissue, and then did a second ultrasound to make sure everything was removed. That was all – afterwards, we walked around the neighborhood and had a picnic along the water, where we could see the Statue of Liberty. I felt fine, and not at all fragile.

This procedure is not available in all areas, but there is a fabulous clinic in New York City that not only does the procedure, but also has started a non-profit to teach other doctors to do it. You can find them at www.earlyoptions.com. It is only available in the first 10 weeks of pregnancy.

Although the experiments with the plants were ultimately unsuccessful. I think there are several factors to consider, some of them are here below.

Related to the research and data that's available to us:

- First, fertility is in peril in this country. Statistics range from 25% to 60% of couples wanting to get pregnant are infertile (depending on how they break down ages, whether or not the couples ultimately sought fertility treatments, and the point at which infertility is diagnosed – sometimes as early as 6 months, in other cases one year). Any modern data about using herbs contraceptively needs to take into consideration that those women having success may not all actually be fertile, or may be only marginally fertile.
- In my experience (my personal experience and my collected experience), a fertile pregnancy is not easy to dislodge. Think of all the babies born to women who are actively using drugs, who are undernourished, who are in war-torn countries. If a pregnancy has taken hold, dislodging it is not easy. Any natural birth control must take this into consideration: it is far easier to prevent than to dislodge.
- Cycle is unfamiliar in our society. In order to have success with any natural methods of birth control, we need to be in relationship with our own bodies, and in connection with ourselves and the cycles in which we live. In my experience, and I am certain this will hold true for many other women, coming into a place of trust and relationship with my own body is very difficult. I don't think this work is likely to be successful for any woman until she is in that place.
-
- We only have parts of the story. This process, as it was practiced by women who were living in connection, who were healthy and fertile, and who were not subject to modern society's infringement on these things, is lost to us now. There may be some modern women who have been taught by their grandmothers, but on the whole, we have to understand that we are operating with only parts of the story. We need to be willing to recognize that it may take some generations of women sharing knowledge to build a complete picture again.

Related to the plants I worked with:

- My pregnancy with my daughter was difficult and tenuous: it was not an healthy pregnancy. I now have an entirely new appreciation for the tenacity of pregnancy, and in general I am now convinced that if a pregnancy is strong and healthy, I'm really not very worried about most herbs a woman might take.
- I definitely felt very strong effects from each of the herbs I worked with, even though ultimately none of them brought on bleeding. Although I'm not eager to reproduce the experiment, I feel that when used early in prevention, as opposed to after implantation, there's a reasonable chance of success with the options that I tried.

Related to my own journey:

- In this whole experience, the thing that I am having the most difficulty with is coming into trust and connection with my body. I know many women who say this comes naturally to them, but I am not one of them. I really do think that until I have resolved this part of the process, I am not a great candidate for relying solely on natural methods. That said, I can see that I've made significant progress in this area, for which I am grateful.
- As much as I hate to say it, it's probable that I needed to have this experience: my body forced me to slow down, which I was not doing very well on my own. I ended up dedicating the entire month of April to sleeping whenever possible, and I scaled back my schedule significantly to make it possible to sleep more often. Since then, I have been more and more successful in slowing down, and my cycle has come back in line again. I think that healing from an over-producing lifestyle is a fundamental part to finding and living in Cycle.

What does all this mean for our hopes for natural birth control? Stay tuned – that's coming next!

Life After Birth Control, Part IV

by Katja Swift

Through the last article, things were not looking so optimistic for proponents of natural birth control. Although I'm thrilled with how quickly my body recovered from hormonal birth control, the recovery was so speedy that unintended consequences were the outcome, and the herbs reported to be able to "fix" my problem weren't successful.

Not surprisingly (now that I know better what to expect), recovery from the menstrual extraction was also quick. In a month or two things were back to normal, and my cycle was back to 28 days. So what now?

Well, if at first you don't succeed, try again – just, a little more conservatively this time. I now have a model for natural birth control that relies a lot on knowing your body and where you are in your cycle, and very little on herbs. Why? Because, again, if a pregnancy is strong, even Tansy won't dislodge it. (If a pregnancy is tenacious, even alcoholism and crack doesn't dislodge it. Just for perspective.) So this protocol favors prevention heavily over "dislodging".

Before I jump in, I will say that there is a brief moment that hovers there, in between "prevent" and "dislodge" – it comes in that deciding point your body makes when deciding whether to implant a fertile egg or not. If you are a woman who wants to have a child (or another child) with your current sexual partner at some point, and "sooner" wouldn't be the end of the world, then you have more leeway to play with in between "prevent" and "dislodge". You have "don't-

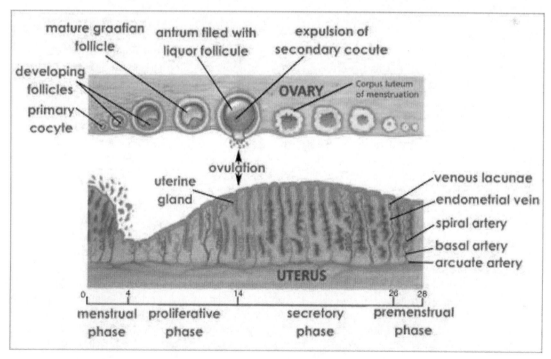

implant" as an option as well, because of course, if it does implant, it's not the end of your world. But if you're committed to having no (or no more) children, I recommend the stricter form of this protocol.

There are three parts to this protocol: charting your cycle, dealing with your fertile time, and bleeding on time. It helps tremendously to have a partner who is taking part in this work with you, and by taking part I mean, he is familiar enough with how your cycle works and where you are in it that you are not left alone to be responsible for whether or not you get pregnant. He needs to be able to know which days you are fertile and together you need to have agreed on a plan for dealing with those days.

First, charting your cycle. Many women mark on a calendar when their period starts, and many use that to loosely predict when their next period will begin. This is not enough for natural birth control – you will need to be a lot more detailed than that! There are two methods that I really like for this part of the protocol: Cycle Beads and the *Taking Charge of Your Fertility* (TCOYF) charting method. Both are methods of reliably keeping track of where you are in your cycle (for a concise explanation of what's happening during your cycle, see the second part of this series in Volume 1 Issue 3).

Cycle Beads are the simpler method, and as long as your cycle is reliably 26-32 days in length, you can use them. You can purchase them online from www.cyclebeads.com, and some people also make fancier versions – you can buy those on etsy, or make one yourself at your local bead shop. I recommend purchasing a bead set from Cycle Beads directly, though – even though they are not lovely, the proceeds go to support their work in the third world, providing a reliable method of birth control for women, especially in areas where contraceptives and abortion are either illegal or culturally unacceptable. Cycle Beads are based on the Standard Days Method, but provide you with a simple, tangible representation of where you are in your cycle. You move a small ring forward along your circle of beads each day, starting on the red bead on the first day of your period. There are ten white beads on the string: these represent days when you could be fertile. All the rest of the beads are brown (or another color – they have some different options now), and on those days you are not fertile, and don't have to use contraception, herbal or otherwise. Cycle Beads claim 99+% efficacy when used properly. If your cycle is NOT at least 26 days, or if it's longer than 32 days, or if it is irregular outside of the standard range, Cycle Beads will not work for you.

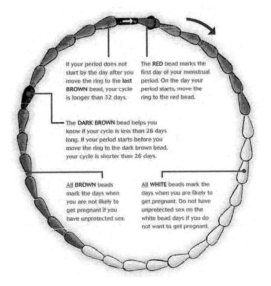

If your period does not start by the day after you move the ring to the last BROWN bead, your cycle is longer than 32 days.

The RED bead marks the first day of your menstrual period. On the day your period starts, move the ring to the red bead.

The DARK BROWN bead helps you know if your cycle is less than 26 days long. If your period starts before you move the ring to the dark brown bead, your cycle is shorter than 26 days.

All BROWN beads mark the days when you are not likely to get pregnant if you have unprotected sex.

All WHITE beads mark the days when you are likely to get pregnant. Do not have unprotected sex on the white bead days if you do not want to get pregnant.

Another method for knowing where you are in your cycle is to use a chart. I particularly like the charts provided with the book *Taking Charge of Your Fertility*, available free in PDF form at their website, www.tcoyf.com. I should note, both the book and the website are somewhat more geared towards getting pregnant than contraception, however, both issues are discussed, and regardless, both are simply two sides of the same coin: figuring out when you are fertile so that you can choose to have sex, or not to have sex without a contraceptive method. Charting is significantly more complicated than Cycle Beads, however, the data is more precise, which means that you can shave a day or two off your window of probable fertility. And although it's more complicated, it's certainly not difficult. Finally, this method can be used by anyone, regardless of how long the cycle is, or whether or not it's regular. If your cycle is regular, it can be a dependable guide for birth control, and if your cycle is not regular, it can give you valuable feedback as you work to resolve the irregularity.

The essential parts of charting are simple. Each morning before you rise from bed (even before you get up to pee), you take your temperature. This is best done if you have a reasonably consistent waking time (though there's no reason not to wake at your normal weekday time and take your temperature, then fall back asleep on Saturday morning!). The charts at tcoyf.com have a graph already set up so that you can easily chart your temperature graphically. This is particularly useful, because you're looking for the moment when your temperature suddenly jumps. This jump is small, maybe only a degree or a half a degree. That shift indicates that your luteal phase has begun, and at this point, your temperature will stay above that point until your next period begins. On the third evening after that shift, you are safely not-fertile.

You can also chart your cervical fluid, which has a great deal more variance than you might think! Cervical fluid charting by itself is not reliable as a guideline, but is great to validate your temperature data. Even better, it's just one more way of getting to know yourself, and I definitely encourage it. Every woman has vaginal discharge throughout the month, not just when bleeding – it's normal. As my roommate told me in college: "women leak". This discharge helps keep the vaginal canal clean, but can also serve other purposes at different times in your cycle. For example, when you are fertile, it becomes thick and slippery, very much like egg whites, to buffer the acidic environment of the vagina and to provide a better "swimming medium" for sperm. Charting your fluids can help you recognize the day or days that you actually ovulate.

Charting alone has one draw back, in that it's difficult to determine when you begin to be fertile. Since sperm can live in the body for up to 5 days, you need to have some kind of plan for dealing with that fertility for 5 days before you ovulate, the day or days that you do ovulate, and the three days after ovulation. When you're looking at only one month's chart, you can't see when the fertile period will start. However, by using your charts in the context of the previous months, you'll start to see a pattern; that you always ovulate at a particular time. With that information, you can work backward to find your window of fertility.

In the interest of knowing lots of stuff about your body, I advise using both methods simultaneously. Cycle Beads can give you at-a-glance confirmation about whether or not you are fertile, and charting can give you more detailed data. Someday, you may know your body well enough that you can just look inward to find this information, but for me, and I think many women who grew up in this culture, that "someday" is a very long way away.

So: now you have some information. What are you going to do with it? Well, on the days that you are not fertile, you've got it easy: no fuss, no muss, no worries. It's the fertile days you need to have a plan for. That plan can vary, based on your comfort zone. For me, right now, my comfort zone is pretty narrow: once is a learning experience, twice – not so much – and I am absolutely unwilling to bear any more children. For a client in my position, the only sure option that I see is abstinence or condoms during that fertile window. Abstinence isn't the end of the world, and this can be a time when couples can deepen their intimacy in ways other than actual intercourse (massage is a great option, though there are certainly many others!). As inconvenient as condoms can be, I do recommend having a supply on hand, because during your fertile time, your body really wants to have sex. His body does too, thanks to handy dandy pheremones you're giving off. Massage is great, but one thing can lead to another, and better safe than sorry.

For a client who knows they want to have a (or another) baby "someday" with this sexual partner, the issue is less critical. This client can try Robin Rose Bennet's research with Wild Carrot, or use a preventative cycle of emmenagogues, such as Mugwort or Pennyroyal tea taken a week before menstruation.

Again, regardless of which category you fall into, it is very important that you make your plan for dealing with your fertile days together with your partner. Ideally he is aware of your charting and/or your beads, so that he knows for himself whether you're fertile or not – that way, there's no last minute question, no after-the-fact "oh, I thought we were safe…". More importantly, you don't feel like you're carrying all the weight of the responsibility on your own.

Additionally, be clear with your body about what you want. This part may seem the hardest part – as I have already said, it is easier for me to trust the plants than to trust my body. You might be that kind of person as well. But tell your body anyway. Intent takes practice, and even if in the beginning it feels uncomfortable, every day that you communicate with your body, you are coming closer to working together in trust. And, Intent is cumulative: developing strength of Intent in one area will help you to define and develop your Intent in other areas of your life. Eventually, you will be a person who lives Intentionally, which is true Presence.

Finally, bleed on time. It seems that should come on its own, and most of the time it does. But I find that the act of participating in your on-time bleeding is a good way to build Intent. Two weeks before your period, start drinking Nettle tea. (I personally like a blend we call "Nettle and Friends" – 2Nettle, 1Dandelion Leaf, 1Red Clover Blossom, 1/4Licorice Root.)

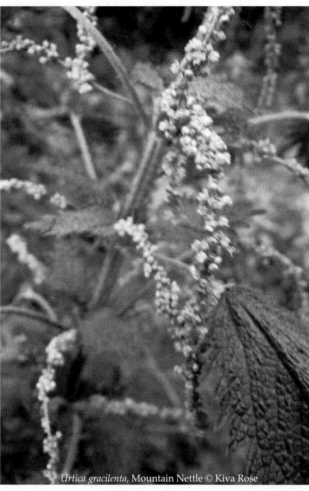

Urtica gracilenta, Mountain Nettle © Kiva Rose

Nettle is a great friend in PMS, and I have found in every single case that drinking Nettle tea throughout the luteal phase will ease cramping and kidney/lower back pain before and during menstruation. Several days before you should bleed, have a nice cup of emmenagogue tea before bed. I like a formula of equal parts Pennyroyal, Mugwort, Raspberry Leaf, Sage, and a bit of Mint. This tea is great for a period that is sluggish at the start (without any threat of pregnancy), and taken before bleeding starts, it's like bitters for your menstrual cycle: gets everything prepared and ready to go.

You might have other formulas that you like, but the key here is that you are telling your body what you expect. Of course, by this time,

116

you know you're not pregnant anyway, because you charted and you followed your plan for your fertile days, so all this is academic, right? Well, maybe it is and maybe it isn't. But the key here is that, especially for women who have difficulty communicating with their bodies, you now have a tangible way to let your body know exactly what you Intend. If you made some drastic mistake along the way and you are pregnant, this is probably not enough to dislodge it. But then again, you never know. Personally I wouldn't risk it on purpose, but maybe you slipped by one day – and so this last step is your safety net. That's well and good, but most importantly, it's communication of Intent.

Oh no, you think. This is not what you expected at all! You want to have sex any time, any day, without having to fumble with pesky condoms. You're not into "alternate" intimacy to accommodate your fertile days. I hear you; that's why I had a Mirena. But what I've come to realize is, that desire isn't Cycle. Nature comes in cycles, and cycles must be respected. If you want to be pregnant, you will respect this cycle in one particular way. If you don't want to be pregnant, you will respect it in another way. But the desire to be "always available" (or men, the desire for your partner to be always available to you) is just another in the homogenization of all cycles in our culture. We expect that workers will produce the same amount of the same type of work in July and in December. We expect that the things we want to eat or purchase will be available in all seasons. We expect that electric light will be available to carry our productivity late into the night (like when I'm writing this article!). But all these things have cycles, and coming back into observance of these cycles is what brings us back to our connection with Earth.

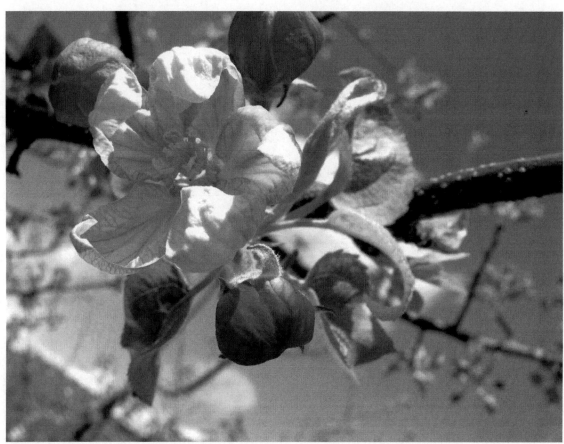

Malus spp., Apple Blossoms © Rosalee de la Forêt

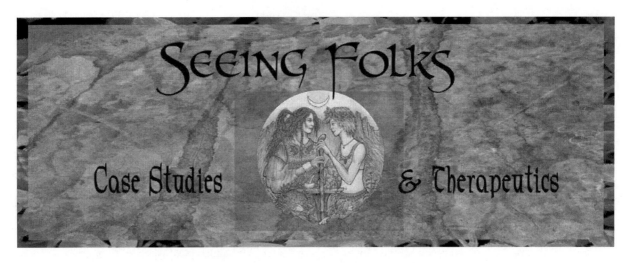

HERBS FOR ABORTION
& MISCARRIAGE CARE

by Julie James

Stories

Mine: I was 15 when I first got pregnant. My boyfriend and my mother were very supportive regarding my choice to have an abortion, and I still remember the discussion I had with my PE teacher whom I confided in: She told me that I didn't need to assign value to my choice as "good" or "bad", it was just the choice that I needed to make at that time. A simple lesson, and one I have remembered fondly for many decades afterward. We had a Planned Pregnancy clinic in our town that offered abortions. My boyfriend took me to the clinic, drove me home, cared for me (including an odd but well-meant gift of sexy lingerie post-abortion. I understood and was grateful for his intention, while shaking my head over the actual gift). It was as comfortable a process as I could have imagined, and though I experienced some grief and loss, the primary emotion was of relief. And for most of my life I felt that there were no repercussions. Until much later on, when I was actively seeking pregnancy and had numerous miscarriages, which were incredibly emotionally painful. At that time, guilt and recrimination became overwhelming, as I wondered if I had done myself damage with that abortion, if I was "paying" for having had that abortion.

Jo's: One of the most empowering moments in my life was in the back waiting room at Planned Parenthood--8 or so of us women, all different ages, different reasons

118

for choosing abortion, sharing our stories, what our families looked like. There was a teenage girl, too young to have kids; a mother with a young baby not ready for another; a mother with three older children who didn't want to start again; myself, easily the age I could have gone forward with motherhood, not choosing it. In the midst of a difficult day, a bunch of strangers, a bunch of women supporting one another. Plus a network of badass friends, who have all supported one another through the process.

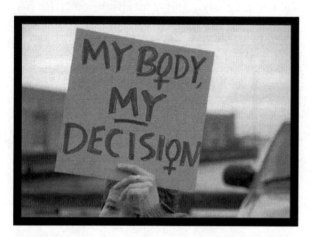

Chris's: I had an awesome abortion! And I'm so glad for the whole thing (yes, even the fact that I got pregnant in the first place). At the time, I qualified for free health care that covered the abortion fully. We had an excellent feminist abortion clinic right in the city where I live. (The feminist NP that I saw for the beginning of the visit didn't even blink when I asked for a photocopy of the ultrasound.) I had a fully supportive partner. My fantastic friend (a bit of a big sister figure for me) accompanied me to the appointment and emotionally cheered me on throughout. She was an important influence in my ability to be grateful to participate in something that so very many women go through.

The whole thing involved about five minutes of admittedly serious pain, but I was lucky to be pretty much pain-free for the healing period afterward. To celebrate, my partner and I threw an abortion party, with mimosas and a dyed-egg hunt (symbol of fertility and all that) and slightly bewildered but generally really supportive friends.

The only negative experience that I had around the abortion was not long afterward, when Operation Rescue came to the college

downtown. My partner and I made signs like "I heart emoticon my abortion" and "My abortion was awesome!" We arrived after the right-wingers had left and so we went to the feminist student union to ask if any other pro-choice stuff was planned. We were greeted by two condescending "feminist" women who were like "No, no, NO! Women don't feel that way about their abortions!" One went so far as to say that every woman feels sad about her abortion, and that some day I'd feel the remorse.

Seventeen years later, I'm so glad that I don't have a 16-year-old (or any kids, for that matter). And sadly that abortion clinic is long gone.

Pat's: I have had two abortions. One with protesters and one without. Having someone go with me was powerfully helpful. Also the second time I choose not to be put under and it was in many ways a better recovery but the doctor did not know how to deal with a 'live' patient that he could ask to scoot down the bed and in some ways it was more painful after. I would definitely choose to be present that way if I did it again though. It felt so much more complete and self affirming.

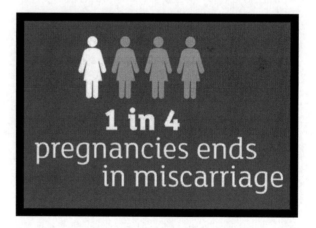

Nic's: Miscarriage is common enough in the medical world that it's basically routine. But when it happens in your personal world, it is anything but. We don't talk about it, so it's easy to feel isolated. Having so many people tell me that it had happened to them helped. Not having any guidance about physical or mental care afterwards (other than a routine check to make sure all was clear) did not. No one told me that postpartum depression is just as real with a miscarriage as a delivery, and without a child to focus on it can be worse. It was pretty much the

119

worst two months of my life. If it hadn't been for the healthy toddler I did have and a series of unrelated disasters that required my attention, it would have been much worse.

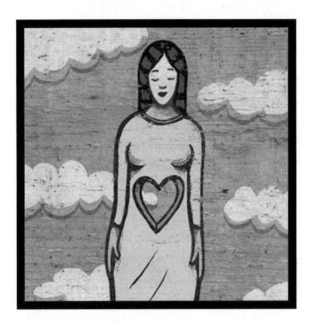

Dale's: I had a miscarriage just about 7.5 years ago. I recall feeling shame and embarrassment....like it was my fault, for being broken, or unworthy...

For the longest time it was so hard sharing my story and being open. It's just been in the last year or so that I've been open about sharing my experience. It's critical more women realize they are not alone.

Andi's: I've always been lucky enough to be surrounded by loving supportive people for all three of my miscarriages. It made all the difference. I was in pain, having mood swings and fits of tears. Since I was not prepared emotionally or financially to have children, it was good my body spared me the decision. In the first one my step-mom, an herbalist, made me "Strengthening Tea" --don't know what was in it, it was green and tasted awful, but I believe it was a blood replenisher. My dad and partner were also very supportive, making sure I got to medical appointments, etc. My second and third were with my current partner, and he took great care of me: medical appointments, feeding me iron rich food and painkillers, keeping me lying down, and doing what we later dubbed "riding the hormonal rollercoaster" (extreme mood swings). Emotionally it did help, the third time,

that we went to the Altar and made a small ceremony of telling the potential child that we were sorry but we could not be his/her parents in this life. I was depressed for several months afterward, and had dreams (good and bad) about my child's possible life.

Frances': On my 21st birthday, I was pregnant and scheduled for an abortion. I'm glad I could be honest with the people around me and I was never shamed. At first I thought I was going to see the pregnancy through, I went out with my boyfriend at the time to have a celebratory and legal beer for my 21st, and it was the worst tasting beer I had ever had in my life. Both coffee and beer taste horrible to me very quick when pregnant, which is what prompted me to go get a test because I knew something was way off. I read a story in "Hygieia, A Woman's Herbal" about going to a medicine woman (First Peoples if I remember correctly) where after the fetus was expelled (cannot recall if this was an induced abortion or a miscarriage), she would have the mother hold the fetus in her hands then say goodbye, and bury it. Not being a person that planned ahead, when I came to after the abortion, I asked the Dr. If I could hold the fetus and say goodbye...I think that was a bit awkward for him. I now know that there wasn't a way to tell my bits from anyone else's bits, even if he was amenable to my request.

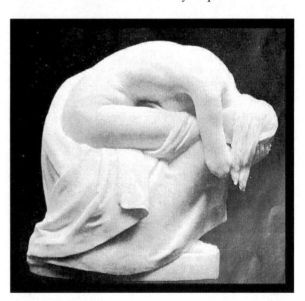

Jess': I grieve the loss of my unborn child pretty much daily. Occasionally do some basic math and realize where s/he would be in a life unimaginable and unrealized. I hope that when the scales are brought out, and my worth is measured, I will have done enough to strike some balance along the way. There has been absolute silence for decades; my family does not even know what happened to me, or why. Not likely much healing either, though I have learned to live with that particular type of scar. I'm guessing I'm not alone, though having company in this particular misery is no comfort. Someone once said the world was lucky that I didn't have children, because it left me free to love other other peoples' kids. Much as I wanted those words to sit in the loving way they were intended, the cut was deep, and I never truly understood before that day how much grief I carried for my childless status.

Gale's: We were all pretty "young" in experiences with magical energy. The day before my abortion my sister witches gathered to bless me and to say goodbye to the itty bit of new life growing inside me. I felt all of their loving care magnified by the healing energies of the Goddess. I was completely at peace. The procedure went well the next day. I did have lots of cramping and bleeding afterward, as is to be expected. But my poor sisters! They had been in pain all day! They hadn't thought to disconnect from me magically. Lesson learned.

If you cut off my reproductive choice, can I cut off yours?

I wanted to write about abortion for the same reason that I want to speak out about abortion: because it is a subject that people are silent about, and silence breeds shame and stigma. We must work to normalize abortion as part of reproductive health care. And while in this

article we will touch on other types of pregnancy loss such as miscarriage, the lack of information and the political climate around abortion require that we focus our attention there.

Gender Note: As we enter into this discussion, I am mindful of the beautiful complexity with which we humans can express our gender, and the limitations of our language in adequately identifying that complexity. The feminine pronoun will often be used in order to simplify a phrase, but I want to make it clear that there are other genders who experience pregnancy and pregnancy loss, and we understand and affirm this.

Abortion is an umbrella term for pregnancy termination. The word has many meanings, but for the purposes of this discussion, we use it to mean a deliberate medical intervention which stops a pregnancy from continuing. There are many forms it takes:

Medical abortion, an oral medication known as RU-486 or Mifepristone and Misoprostol. This is taken in-home, and is up to 95% effective when used during the first 50 days of a pregnancy. It block progesterone, stimulates contractions, and softens and dilates the cervix. Very effective, and quite safe, this medication is listed on the World Health Organization's model list of essential medications. It is legal and available in all 50 states, but distribution is restricted to specially licensed physicians.

Vacuum Aspiration and Dilation and Extraction are the two most common forms of abortion used in a clinic.

Menstrual extraction is a technique becoming more popular with more radical reproductive justice advocates in communities where access to abortion is limited. This is a DIY technique that, when done correctly, can be quite safe and effective.

Herbal abortions: Given that we have a class of herbs that are called abortifacients, there is considerable interest in the use of plant medicines for abortion. And while some people have had good experiences using herbs in this way, my experience has been quite different. I have counseled many people who wanted to follow this path, and I've not seen the effectiveness that many claim. And truthfully, there can be significantly more health problems associated with some of the herbal abortion protocols than with a safe medical or in-clinic abortion. I do not advocate herbal abortions.

Half of all pregnancies in the United States are unintended, with almost half of those ending in abortion. 43% of women in the United States have an abortion by the time they are 45 years old. Often the people experiencing abortion will not tell their partners, friends, or family if they are terminating their pregnancy. This points up the culture of shame and stigma that surrounds abortion.

Access to abortion is a primary aspect of reproductive justice: there are overwhelming systemic barriers to access for people with low income, as the out of pocket cost is very high with federal funding for abortion blocked, with limited exceptions. In addition, other barriers exist that restrict access. State laws banning abortion clinics (Most counties in the United States do not have clinics) can mean hundreds of miles travelled and many days of waiting in order to get care.

Abortions are expensive, too. The majority of abortions performed are paid for out of pocket, and vary tremendously in price as well as availability, from a few hundred dollars to several thousand, if they are available at all. For those with limited time, finances, or transportation, this systemic inequality creates socially unjust policy, a violation of human rights.

The story society and the media tell us is that poor, teenaged women of color are the majority of those who seek abortion. This is patently false, unsupported by readily available research. A 2008 study by the Guttmacher Institute shows that in the United States, of those who have had abortion, half are 25 or older, with only about 17% being teens. The majority of those over age 20 attended college. And while Black and Hispanic women are over-represented at 30% and 25% respectively, the majority of abortions, 35%, are experienced by white women .

So that we can see it is not only women of color, and it is not only the poor, and it is not only teens seeking abortion. The more typical picture of a person seeking an abortion, according to these figures, is an older, college-educated, middle class white woman.

At this time over 80% of counties in the United States have no abortion provider and 35% of all women in the United States live in those counties.   And the limited funding that is available for reproductive health care is often channeled from state budgets to "Crisis Pregnancy Centers". CPCs appear to meet the needs of women, but in truth fall far short. They provide limited information and much misinformation, and they have a history of manipulating women at a vulnerable time, encouraging them away from choosing an abortion and denying them adequate knowledge of options available. Where are there are abortion providers, the practitioners may perform as many as 25 to 30 abortions a day, averaging one every 20 minutes with little time to offer counseling and support to their patients.

In light of all of this it is heartening to see a new model of care provider emerging: The abortion doula. The idea of the abortion doula was realized in 2007 by 3 birth doulas and reproductive justice activists from New York City: Mary Mahoney, Lauren Mitchell, and Miriam Perez who created The Doula Project. Abortion doulas provide support to people choosing abortion, and those facing miscarriage, stillbirth, and fetal anomalies.

It is the job of a care provider, whether an abortion doula, herbalist, or other, to ensure that our clients feel supported and informed, to provide nourishment and healing in whatever way they need, and to realize that pregnancy termination is experienced by every individual differently.   Sometimes that experience is loss, sometimes a sacred ritual, and sometimes sheer relief. We want to avoid making assumptions as to how one will experience their pregnancy termination and to allow them to lead in placing this experience in their life in the way they need to. In addition the issues around choice are not easy, or clear, or even consistent--and they don't have to be. It is ok for both the client and the provider to have questions and to feel conflicted, and it is also ok to not feel conflicted. This last is an important issue. When we make assumptions that someone is grieving about their abortion, we are going to approach our work with them in a very different way. Our voice changes, our language changes, and the person in front of us, you can bet, will be acutely aware of those changes. If this person is relieved and happy about this abortion, then the sad look of concern in your eyes and the soft understanding voice may not be welcome, and may even be seen as an affront. Honor their journey and the way they need to experience it.

So what does it look like to offer care to those experiencing pregnancy termination?

Sometimes the most important job that we have is to support and affirm their choices, to hold their hands, to comfort and listen to them, and to bear witness to their journey. If that is all our client needs from us, then that is what we provide.

There are many other areas where we can offer support, however, and an experienced herbalist can be one of the best resources for a person in this situation.

The physical effects of pregnancy termination can be myriad, depending on the process and on the health of the client. Afterward, it is typical to see blood loss, which can be quite heavy at times. This is to be expected, and is, to a certain extent, desirable. There can be a tendency to reach for styptics (herbs that stop bleeding) right away, but as long as the client shows no signs of excessive blood loss (dizzy, pale, clammy, rapid

heartbeat, low blood pressure, confusion), such measures need not be implemented. Bleeding will slow and lighten over the course of a week or two, and cramping and pain will lessen even more quickly. A two-week follow up visit is recommended to verify that healing is progressing.

The herbs that will be of great benefit during this process are many. I will provide a few options here in each category, though you may have your own favorites or more commonly available alternatives. One of the many beauties of herbal healing is the abundance of choices in the plants we use.

Uterine Tonics strengthen the uterus and help to rapidly restore it to optimal health. My favorites are Partridge berry, Lady's mantle, and Raspberry leaf, and I find a combination of these three a very pleasing combination for a tea or tincture.

Blood Builders/Nutritives improve general health using deeply nourishing plants that provide a wide spectrum of readily absorbed nutrients. The usual suspects are still the best

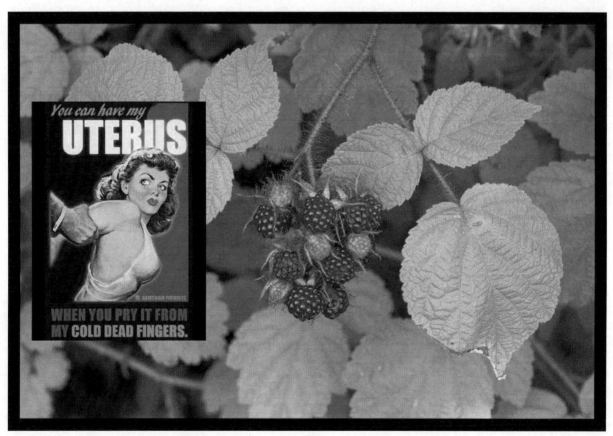

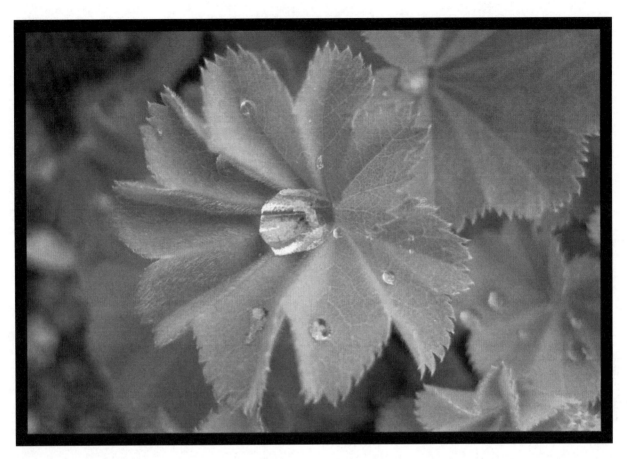

here: Nettle, Alfalfa, Horsetail, Red clover, Hawthorn, Rose hips, Yellowdock, Oatstraw-- whatever your favorites are, drink them abundantly, before and after, to restore lost nutrients and to improve tissue healing.

Styptics stop bleeding and while, again, we don't want to grab for them immediately, it's wise to have them on hand just in case of hemorrhage. My favorite is a blend of Shepherd's purse, Yarrow and Cinnamon, in

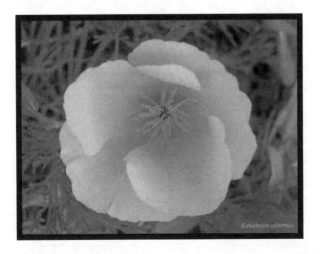

tincture form, administered in relatively large amounts relatively often on the way to the hospital.

Anodynes may be among the most gratefully received of the plant medicines here. Non-specific pain can be relieved significantly with the use of herbs such as California poppy, Corydalis, Jamaican dogwood, and Black cohosh.

Anti-spasmodics will relieve cramping, and many can be used both internally and externally. These include Black haw, Cramp bark, Wild yam, Kava, and Black cohosh. Kava and ginger hot compresses on an abdomen can be a little slice of heaven when dealing with a grumpy uterus.

Anti-galactagogues can be employed if the breasts begin to secrete milk. This is not often the case, however if the pregnancy termination is later, this can be very uncomfortable. Sage is my go-to herb to dry up breast milk production, used as tea or tincture, and applied externally, as well, as a cool compress.

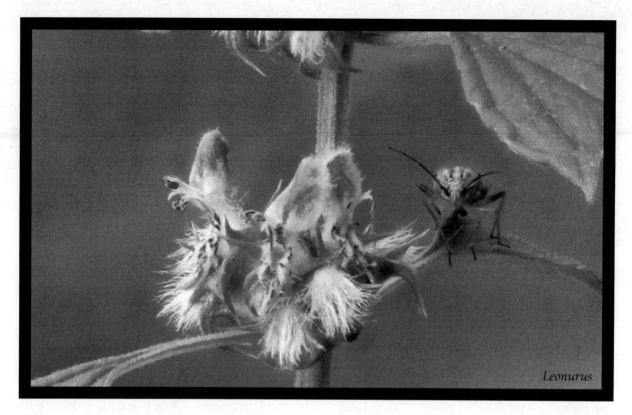

Leonurus

Nervines can be such a blessing here. Pulsatilla, for that heart-breakingly overwhelmed and fearful person, Motherwort (I wonder, depending on the individual we are working with, if it might be kinder to call her by her official name, *Leonurus*) for anxiety and depression (in small amounts, as she is a blood mover), as well as pain. Skullcap, Milky oats, Lemon balm, Vervain--we all have our favorites that we reach for time and again.

Hepatics are definitely indicated here, in order to assist in restoring hormonal balance. We can use one that offers other benefits discussed above, of course: Yarrow, Yellow dock, Dandelion, Motherwort.

Antimicrobials are another class of herbs to have on hand, which hopefully won't be used. Calendula, Echinacea, Yarrow (my how she pops up over and over again), Usnea. Again, to be used in generous amounts frequently on the way to the ER, in case of infection setting in.

Flower Essences may be profoundly helpful in this setting, however, I do not use them. If you do, I encourage you to use your knowledge, or seek out one of the amazing FE practitioners,

and look at how these energetic compounds can assist you.

Ritual can be another important aspect of healing. Assisting our clients in creating a ritual, creating one for them, or finding a resource for them if this is not something you offer or are comfortable with. And again, because I can't stress it enough, leave space for those who don't need ritual, who simply need their physical body to be cared for.

Providing care for all pregnancy termination situations, but especially for abortions, is critically necessary. The stories of the women at the beginning of this article--all true stories, modified only to the extent needed to provide anonymity--show that to be the case. They are crying to be seen and heard. We need voices raised. We need hands and hearts and minds opened wide. We need to stand up with our siblings who are even now walking into a clinic that they struggled to get to, where they are met with hate speech and violent images and trauma.

We need reproductive justice, and we need it now. And we can be an important, active and activist, part of that.

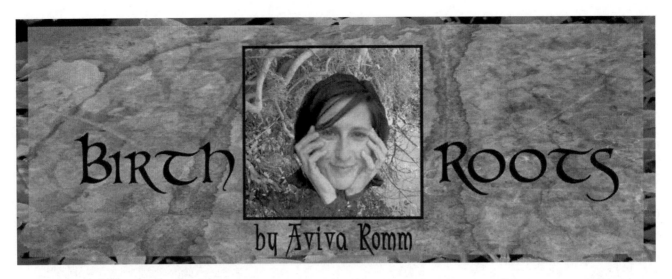

BIRTH ROOTS

by Aviva Romm

SaraLisa, 30 a year-old woman, is calling you on the phone. She is fourteen weeks pregnant and in emotional distress. Three weeks ago she had a few days of spotting so she went to her midwife's office for an evaluation. She had an ultrasound that showed that her baby had probably died at about 11 weeks of pregnancy. The midwife and back-up obstetrician told her she could wait a couple of weeks to see if the miscarriage happened naturally. Now they are recommended a dilatation and curettage (D&C), but Sara does not want to have this procedure performed. She would rather miscarry in the privacy of her own home instead of in a hospital operating room where the D&C would be done. The doctor told her that she is at risk of hemorrhage and infection. She has not had any further spotting and she is not having contractions. She is a friend of a friend and is requesting your assistance as an herbalist in completing the miscarriage. She has no major medical problems. What do you do?

Miscarriage is a life event that most of us will encounter amongst our women friends, relatives, and clients. In my practice, the above phone call is not uncommon. In fact, I receive more "thank you's" and miscarriage stories than any other type from folks who have read my books and attended my classes and have learned how to help themselves or someone else through a miscarriage naturally and herbally. A lot of what I offer is emotional support

Miscarriage:
Supporting Women Through Early Pregnancy Loss, Botanically

By Aviva Romm

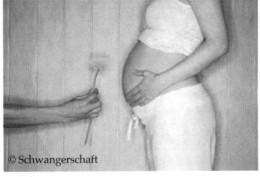

© Schwangerschaft

through my writing and words, but I also try to inspire body-confidence and intelligent, commonsense decision-making. I also provide information on the herbs that can help, and warning signs to look out for. Many women have written to me about feelings of abandonment by their midwife or doctor who was unable to recommend anything other than a D&C for treatment, and many herbalists and naturopaths have written, seeking my help in working with a client/ patient in the midst of a miscarriage or to thank me for protocols they've put together based on what they've learned using my books, to help someone miscarry without medical intervention. Women and practitioners have described natural miscarriage as a sacred process that allowed completion and resolution, rather than the trauma and grief so many find themselves with after a medically managed miscarriage.

Miscarriage can cause even seasoned midwives, herbalists, and naturopaths to feel uncertain about what to do and how to help –or even afraid of getting involved in miscarriage care at all. While miscarriage requires healthy respect, it is not something to be afraid of and it is an area where women greatly need help and guidance—and where botanicals can play a major role in facilitating the process. The medical model can be really useful for those times when a miscarriage just isn't completing itself effectively, when a woman feels like she just needs the process over and herbs aren't working quickly enough, or when natural approaches aren't adequate to control bleeding. Unfortunately, the medical model too often over treats women, while under acknowledging the psycho-emotional significance of a miscarriage in women's lives. The herbal-midwife model has healing to share on many levels—not only tending to the physical needs of the woman, but to the tender heart emotions that often accompany this experience of loss.

In this article I will share what I know from decades of experience and the countless women who have included me in the sacred passage of a miscarriage. My hope is to help you feel empowered to help women through miscarriage botanically, physically, emotionally, and spiritually, to change the culture of fear and shame for women and practitioners around miscarriage, and to know when medical management is needed.

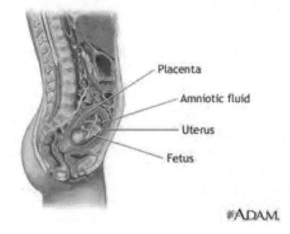

Placenta
Amniotic fluid
Uterus
Fetus

⬤ADAM.

What is a Miscarriage?
Miscarriage is pregnancy loss that occurs before the embryo (the baby before 8 weeks gestation) or fetus (the baby after 8 weeks gestation) has reached viability---which is when the baby is 500 g or less, which generally corresponds to a gestational age of 20 to 22 weeks or less. Most miscarriages occur by 13 weeks of pregnancy. Miscarriage is the most common pregnancy problem, with as many as 15% of all *known* pregnancies ending spontaneously before 20 weeks and many more ending before a woman even realizes she is pregnant. Chromosomal anomalies account for 50% of all miscarriages. Numerous other risk factors are associated with an increased risk of pregnancy loss including maternal age, previous spontaneous abortion, heavy smoking, moderate to high alcohol consumption, non-steroidal anti-inflammatory drugs, caffeine, fertility problems,

endocrinopathies, coagulation problems, autoimmune conditions, low folate levels, low or high BMI, infections, and untreated celiac disease.

This article will focus on strategies that can be applied to 3 major categories of miscarriage: *inevitable miscarriage, incomplete miscarriage, and missed abortion.* Unlike in threatened miscarriage, another major category, where the baby is alive and treating the causes may prevent miscarriage from happening in about 25% of cases, in these 3 categories*, the death of the embryo/fetus has occurred and the role of the herbalist is to help complete the process of emptying the uterus while addressing pain and bleeding. I present the 3 categories together because the process and protocols are essentially the same.

Definitions:

Inevitable miscarriage: this means that the miscarriage is not preventable—it's in process and about to happen; either the embryo/fetus has died, or there is an anembryonic pregnancy (no embryo formed after the pregnancy got established). There is vaginal bleeding of varying degrees and lower abdominal cramping or contractions of various magnitude. There is also cervical dilatation (a midwife or doc can provide this information). Bleeding is often heavy, though may start out with spotting. Miscarriage pain can be significant. Strategies to prevent miscarriage should not be used; rather confirmation that the baby is no longer alive should be obtained, for example, with ultrasound. Most women will miscarry spontaneously without complications or the need for any physical support, though emotional support may still be needed. Medically, a watch and wait attitude may be adopted, the woman may be offered medications to facilitate the miscarriage and ease pain, or she might be offered a D&C or suction abortion.

Incomplete Miscarriage: As with inevitable miscarriage, the baby has died or never developed, but part of the tissue is retained—in other words, the miscarriage has started but has not completed. It is accompanied by vaginal bleeding which can be quite heavy, cramping/contractions, cervical dilatation, and incomplete passage of the products of conception. A woman experiencing incomplete abortion will frequently describe passage of clots or pieces of tissue, and will typically report moderate to heavy vaginal bleeding, though there can be light to heavy bleeding that lasts on and off for even a couple of weeks. The products that remain in the uterus keep the uterus from clamping down effectively and thus the bleeding tends to be heavy. The cramping can be quite painful. Treatment focuses on helping the woman to complete the miscarriage process by expelling any retained tissue, controlling bleeding, treating pain, and providing emotional support. Medically, a watch and wait attitude is less likely to be adopted, though if the process of moving forward, this is reasonable, the woman may be offered medications to complete the miscarriage and ease pain, or she might be offered a D&C or suction abortion.

Missed abortion: the fetus that has died but is retained in the uterus, often with no signs of ensuing miscarriage. This condition may persist for several weeks before miscarriage spontaneously commences. In some cases, it will not commence without assistance, possibly persisting for weeks, in which case the role of the herbalist is to facilitate the miscarriage process. The medical options are similar to those above.

Miscarriage Symptoms

The most common symptoms of miscarriage include vaginal bleeding, low back ache, abdominal pain/uterine cramping or contractions, and many women report noticing a decrease in pregnancy symptoms (for example, they no longer feel nausea or breast tenderness goes away). Medical confirmation of whether fetal demise has occurred is recommended before starting a protocol to facilitate the miscarriage because any of the above symptoms can be present in a perfectly healthy pregnancy that does not result in miscarriage. Confirming miscarriage will prevent mistakenly using herbs that might be otherwise harmful to a healthy fetus or cause an herbal abortion in a healthy fetus. Miscarriage can be confirmed by cervical exam showing cervical dilatation, ultrasound demonstrating lack of a fetal heartbeat, lack of fetal growth, or even lack of presence of a fetus---all of which can be seen in miscarriage. Blood work can be done by a doc or midwife to check for hCG levels. Ultrasound and hCG levels can also help you to rule out an ectopic pregnancy. *Ectopic pregnancy is a life-threatening emergency and requires immediately medical attention! Signs include, but are not limited to, vaginal bleeding and abdominal pain.*

SIDEBAR: Miscarriage and Psyche

Feelings of loss, sadness, shame, grief, embarrassment, inadequacy, disappointment, and sometime even relief with or without accompanying guilt for feeling that way, are all in the range of what women experience during and after a miscarriage. Subsequent pregnancies where there has been previous pregnancy loss are usually accompanied by greater anxiety and stress than experienced by women who do not have a history of pregnancy loss, and repeated loss is especially emotionally charged for women (and their partners). A great deal of compassion and sensitivity is required when working with women in the vulnerable space of miscarriage, after miscarriage, and subsequent pregnancies after miscarriage, reassurance should be provided, and referral for ongoing emotional support given if needed. Ritual can help a woman heal emotionally and spiritually. I suggest creating a burial ceremony, writing a letter to the baby,

Botanical Treatment Strategies

Once you have established that the baby has, in fact died or that the pregnancy is otherwise not viable, and that you are not dealing with an ectopic pregnancy, you can put together a botanical protocol. Nature and women's bodies have nearly infinite wisdom. If the miscarriage is inevitable—cramping is becoming progressively more regular, bleeding is increasing, and the woman is passing embryonic or fetal tissue-- then simply letting nature take its course with cautious observation is completely appropriate—the woman's body will know exactly what to do, and generally, cramping, bleeding and emptying of the uterus will ensue, and the process will complete itself. In such cases, nothing needs to be done though botanicals such as cramp bark, black haw, motherwort, wild yam, Jamaican dogwood, and Corydalis can be used to ease pain. The first three of these are especially brilliant to use because their mechanisms of action include improving uterine tone while relaxing the uterus and easing pain---thus effective expulsion of the uterine contents is facilitated while painful cramping is minimized. Botanicals for pain control may be included at any time during the miscarriage.

If the miscarriage is incomplete or missed, herbs may be given to stimulate uterine contractions to encourage expulsion of the uterine contents.

Herbs to control bleeding may be part of a protocol, and after a miscarriage, herbs may be given to control bleeding and encourage uterine involution—it's return to the pre-pregnant state. Generally, these herbs are the same herbs that increase uterine contractility; for example, blue cohosh and cotton root bark tinctures. Raspberry leaf tea is a gentle uterine tonic and hemostatic that may be used, as an infusion for post-miscarriage support though is not generally strong enough to stimulate uterine contractions adequately to expel the uterine contents.

There is really no need to include herbs to prevent uterine infection---infection should not happen in a natural miscarriage. If a woman has fever, foul smelling vaginal discharge, or unrelenting abdominal pain at any time during or after a miscarriage, this can be indicative of endometritis or other infection. Uterine infections can be serious and life threatening and should not be treated at home; antibiotics are required.

Ideal botanical prescribing relies on the concept I call elegant formulating—this means using the fewest possible herbs with the most possible actions to create the most elegant, streamlined possible prescription. For example, motherwort is a uterine tonic, uterine antispasmodic, and mood-enhancing herb---you are feeding many birds from one feeder. The herbs in the table below are consistently reliable and allow you to select from a few possible choices to combine into an elegant formula.

Key Botanicals for Women with Inevitable or Incomplete Miscarriage, or Missed Abortion:

What to Expect When Facilitating a Miscarriage
Typically, once a miscarriage gets underway, it will start slowly and pick up in intensity over the course of several hours to a day. Initially, there is light to moderate bleeding and cramping, both of which become increasingly heavy and are eventually accompanied by the passage of some solid tissue through the vagina. The further along the pregnancy is, the heavier the bleeding and cramping will be. If the miscarriage is occurring very early in pregnancy, the tissue may simply look like clots; after about 8 weeks gestation, fetal tissue may be apparent in the form of a very small rudimentary placenta and a small sac that looks a bit like a thin grape skin. Sometimes you will see material that looks like wet toilet paper covered in more or less blood coming from the cervix if it is being examined, or the vagina —this is part of the membranes. Saving the tissue that comes out to show to a midwife or doc can be really helpful in determining if everything has cleared out of the uterus. After about 12 weeks of pregnancy, actual fetal parts may be discernable and the woman should be prepared for this. However, a good sign of this is that after the solid materials have passed, the bleeding and cramping begins to subside to more like a regular period, suggesting that the miscarriage is probably complete.

Sometimes a miscarriage will begin with a fury---heavy bleeding right from the start. In most cases, the bleeding will be accompanied by cramping and will also lead to passage of the products of conception and then will abate as described above. Anytime the bleeding is heavy enough to soak 2 large menstrual pads in 30 minutes, or 2 large pads an hour for 2 hours in a row, or if the woman feels weak or faint, medical care is necessary. It's important to have the woman wear some sort of pad that allows you to estimate blood loss---there can be a lot of blood and this can be scary and cause people to overreact. If the bleeding is within these guidelines and the woman is stable, then things are usually going just fine. the woman may Note that a woman may feel faint if she's been lying down for awhile and suddenly stands, or if she has lost a lot of blood suddenly as can happen at the peak of the miscarriage, so some amount of on-site judgment is necessary. See **Warning Signs!** (below).

Action	Goal	Botanical Name	Common Name
Uterine stimulant/ contractant	Stimulate uterine contractions; Expel uterine contents; Prevent excessive bleeding; Promote uterine involution	Gossypium Caulophyllum thalictroides	Cotton root Blue cohosh
	Uterine tonic and hemostatic for post-miscarriage support	Rubus idaeus Mitchella repens	Red raspberry leaf Partridge berry
Uterine spasmolytic	Promote coordinated uterine contractions to assist in effectively expelling uterine contents; relieve painful uterine cramping	Actaea racemosa Dioscorea villosa Viburnum opulus/ Viburnum prunifolium Leonorus cardiaca	Black cohosh Wild yam Cramp bark/ Black haw Motherwort
Analgesic	Relieve painful cramping	Leonorus cardiaca Actaea racemosa Viburnum opulus/ Viburnum prunifolium	Motherwort Black cohosh Cramp bark/black haw
Uterine hemostatic	Prevent excessive bleeding, slow heavy bleeding	Achillea millifolium Erigeron Cinnaomomum spp Myrica cerifera Capsella bursa pastoris	Yarrow Canada fleabane Cinnamon Bayberry bark Shepherd's purse
Nervine	Support emotional wellness and relieve anxiety	Leonorus cardiac Melissa officinalis Hypericum perforatum Passiflora incarnata Avena sativa	Motherwort Lemon balm St John's wort, Passion flower Milky oats

Sometimes a woman will just want to "get it over with"---herbs can be very effective but are not as strong as the medication misoprostel or as direct as surgical interventions for completing a miscarriage. Sometimes you try and try with herbs and no go; occasionally, the bleeding will be so heavy that medical intervention seems sensible. In all such cases it is important to give the woman "permission" to seek medical care---this is sometimes an emotional obstacle for folks who feel they have to do it only naturally. There is a time and place for everything and it is appropriate for the woman to do what she feels best doing, as long as she's making an informed choice.

Sample Botanical Protocol
Let's return to SaraLisa's case. SaraLisa has just shared her story and you would like to help her achieve her goal of completing her miscarriage at home if possible. What are some of the questions you will ask?

• How far along is your pregnancy?
• Have you had confirmation of pregnancy loss? If yes, how? (i.e., ultrasound?)
• If there is bleeding, exactly how much?
> Bleeding is normal and expected with a miscarriage—it is part of the process of the uterus emptying its contents of the products

of conception. Typically, there is initial spotting that picks up in intensity, and eventually there is bleeding on par with a heavy period with passage of clots and fetal tissue, which may or may not be recognizable as such. Soaking 2 large pads in 30 minutes is considered a hemorrhage and requires immediate medical evaluation. If a woman is bleeding continuously she should contact her medical care provider and in most cases she should go to the emergency room. If she is weak, faint, or losing consciousness, an ambulance should be called!

• Are you cramping or contracting?

    If yes, how often, how intensely, how long are the cramps/contractions lasting, are they regular or increasing in frequency? Increasing frequency and intensity, or regularity, *might* mean an inevitable miscarriage.

• Do you have any medical problems? Any bleeding problems?

• Is your midwife or doctor aware that you are going to complete this miscarriage at home (it's optimal for herbalists to have good relationships with other health professionals in the community)

• Do you have a support person who can be with you through the miscarriage? A working phone in case of emergency and for us to reach each other?

The initial goal is to stimulate uterine contractions and promote the actual expulsion of uterine contents. Your formula should contain primary uterine stimulant herbs; I recommend 60% of the formula with this action. Additionally, include herbs that will support the physiologic process uterine contraction and relaxation, and that will provide some pain relief, as miscarriage contractions can cause significant discomfort.

A sample tincture formula would be:

Gossypium herbaceum	40 ml (1:4)
Caulophyllum thalictroides	40 ml (1:4)
Actaea raccmosa 10 ml (1:4:)	
Viburnum prunifolium	10 ml (1:4)
Total	100 ml

An alternative formula might be:

Caulophyllum thalictroides	40 ml (1:4)
Gossypium herbaceum	30 ml (1:4)
Leonorus cardiac	20 ml (1:4)
Viburnum opulus	10 ml (1:4)
Total	100 ml

Instructions: Beginning in the morning take 3 mL of one of the above tinctures *every hour* for 4 hours to stimulate uterine contractions, then discontinue. If no contractions ensue, repeat the next day. Contractions usually begin after the first 24 hours, but it may take as long as 48 hours. The process can be repeated for a third day; if I ever have to do this I usually allow a one day break between the second and third days of using the protocol. There is no risk in waiting as long as the woman feels well and wants to wait. I have often done home care during a miscarriage, being at the woman's side while she was at the peak of the miscarriage through its completion. If I am not able to be there, I keep in close contact with the woman. One of my requirements for helping with a miscarriage is that the woman has a partner or close friend with her who can keep an eye out for her safety. Most of the time the process goes really smoothly; there can be a lot of bleeding. Strong yarrow infusion can be kept on hand and taken in cupful doses for 30 minutes as long as the woman is stable and blood loss is within the 2 pads/30 minute or 2 pads/hour for 2 consecutive hours rule. Tinctures of equal parts bayberry bark and shepherd's purse can be used for heavy bleeding; another reliable formula is Cinnamon and Erigeron tincture. This is an old Ellingwood formula produced by HerbPharm.

Warning Signs!

The following warning signs mean that medical care is needed:

During a miscarriage
    • Heavy vaginal bleeding/ hemorrhage (>/= 2 pads soaked in 30 minutes)
    • Sustained abdominal pain
    • Loss of consciousness
After a miscarriage
    • Elevated temperature (> 100.4 degrees F)
    • abdominal pain
    • Foul smelling vaginal discharge
    • Persistent vaginal bleeding greater than the amount and duration of a menstrual period

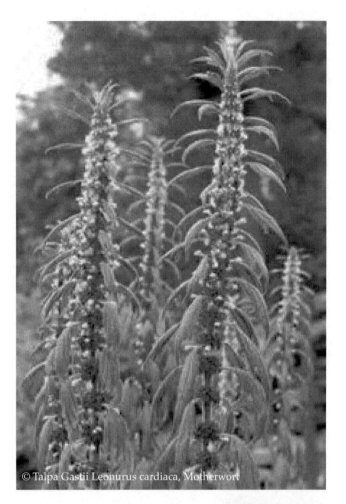

© Talpa Gastii Leonurus cardiaca, Motherwort

feelings and again, acknowledge the loss. Many women say that the hardest part of a miscarriage socially is that their partner, friends, or family don't know what to say so they say nothing. Acknowledging and honoring the loss can be the most important first step in healing. The herbs can be the common language you use to hold space with the woman. I love to give infused motherwort honey in chamomile tea for post-miscarriage women, motherwort tincture, lemon balm tea for gladdening the heart, St John's Wort, passion flower, milky oats---all of these nervine allies can be part of the support and healing.

After a miscarriage some amount of spotting or even moderate bleeding may persist or recur intermittently even for a few weeks or up to the next menses.

The next menses is also usually more heavy than usual. Most women will ask when they can try to become pregnant again---believe it or not, if they want to they can try as soon as they feel like it---and for unknown reasons, fertility is actually increased in the month after a miscarriage. Having a miscarriage does not affect future fertility so the woman can be reassured of this as well.

Emotional support is a big part of the miscarriage process. Supportive talk and listening are really important. Create time and hold space for the woman to share, grieve, and let go. Learn about supporting women through miscarriage and rituals that can help with the transition. Some women will move on without skipping much of a beat; more often a period of grief occurs. Acknowledge the loss for the woman---too often she is going through the process alone because she hasn't yet told people she was pregnant. Many women struggle with whether they are moms or not since they were pregnant. Explore their

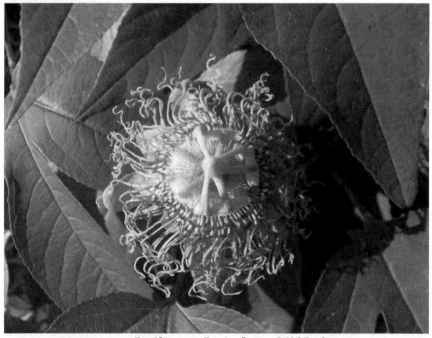

Passiflora spp., Passionflower, © Val Paul

Supporting women through the Change of Life

Between the ages of 40 and 60 women undergo a change of life as their fertility declines and their monthly cycles stop. This natural cycle of life manifests differently for all women. Besides the physical changes, women also may find themselves going through life changes. This may include new interests and a new direction or purpose in life. This time can be challenging yet positive and enlivening.

I want to give voice to the powerful and positive transition that can happen during this time. This article, however, is more focused on the physical changes that some women experience and how to assess these changes individually from a traditional herbal perspective. I'll be drawing mainly on a differential diagnosis from Traditional Chinese Medicine (TCM). However, my goal is that those with no understanding of TCM will walk away better understanding the nuances involved during this change of life. My overall goal is to help people move away from treating symptoms to addressing patterns and underlying imbalances.

Let's begin by defining a few terms. The term menopause is often used in common language to describe many years of this transformative experience. The term menopause literally means the stopping of the monthly cycles. Thus, menopause refers to a particular moment in time, the last menstrual cycle. Menopause is officially declared one year after the menstrual cycle has stopped.

Perimenopause refers to the years leading up to the last menstrual cycle. Some women experience more noticeable changes during this time, including erratic menstrual cycles, fatigue, hot flashes, etc.

Post menopause refers to the time after the last menstrual cycle and is declared a year after the last cycle.

The Change

by Rosalee de la Forêt

In Japan, these peri-menopausal years are referred to as konenki, translated as the "renewal years." I think the english language could certainly use some better terminology for this transition. For this article I'll use the term menopause as it is used colloquially.

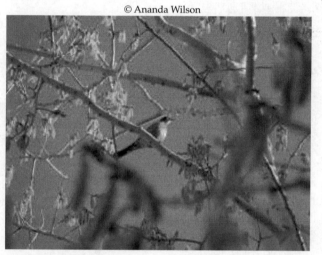
© Ananda Wilson

In recent years a lot of sensitivity has gone into reframing menopause, not as a disease, but as a natural process. "Hallelujah!" say many women as this is obviously important to recognize. However, it is just as important to recognize that the severe symptoms that some women experience during this time should not be ignored or dismissed because it's "natural".

We understand that menses is a normal cycle for most women. It's not a disease. However, heavy bleeding, severe pain from cramping, tender breasts and mood swings are not "natural". These are symptoms of dis-ease and should be addressed. The same is true for perimenopausal symptoms. The cessation of menses is normal. Excessive menstrual flow, hot flashes and night sweats, mood swings, hair loss, insomnia, fatigue and irritability are not "natural". Instead, they are symptoms of an underlying imbalance and should be addressed.

Common menopausal complaints

In the western world many women experience the following during this time of transition: hot flashes, erratic menstrual cycles (both in length of cycle and length and flow of bleeding), lowered libido, increased headaches, dryness (notably dry vaginal

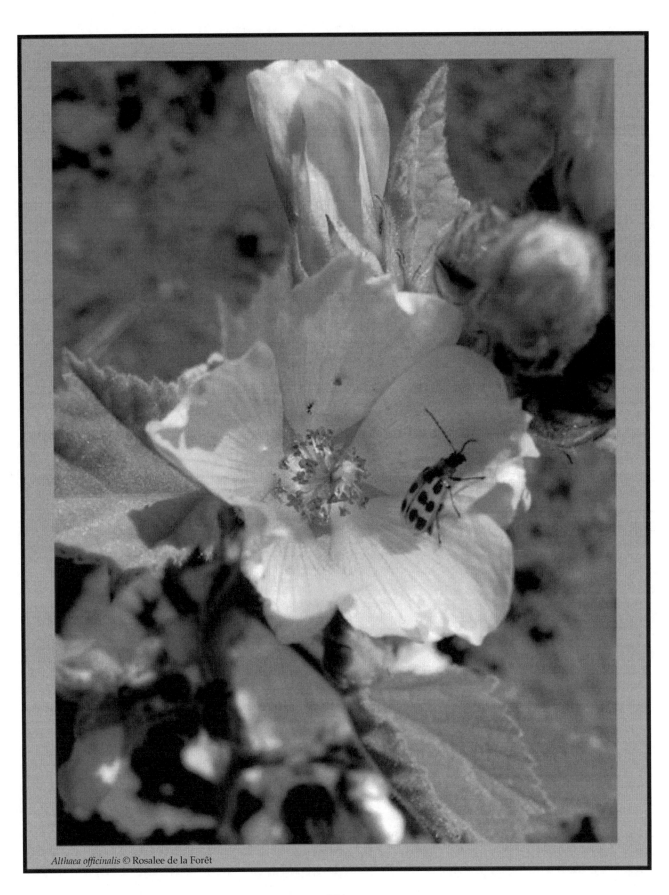

Althaea officinalis © Rosalee de la Forêt

tissues), insomnia, palpitations, irregular heart beat, fatigue, hair loss, bone loss, mood changes and changes in memory.

The most common treatment for these in western medicine is hormone replacement therapy, otherwise known as HRT. There is a lot of debate about HRT in the alternative health world, but this is beyond the scope of today's article.

Some practitioners of western herbalism approach these menopausal complaints with a western medicine mindset. They give herbs that contain phytohormones with the goal of balancing a woman's hormones. Black cohosh, wild yam, and vitex are mainstays of these types of protocols. There are many excellent resources for this type of approach. Amanda McQuade Crawford, Aviva Romm and Jillian Stansbury are herbalists who write and lecture about using herbs for their phyothormone content.

This article is going to focus on evaluating the individual and assessing common energetic patterns associated with menopausal complaints.

Proactive solutions

Of course, the best ways to ensuring a breezy time of transition is living a consciously healthy life well before the time of transition appears. Furthermore, actively consulting with someone trained in traditional herbal medicine can help correct imbalances *before* they are pathologies. Traditional herbal medicine excels at recognizing imbalances before they are entirely problematic. Prevention is key and women in their 20's and 30's who are actively engaged in creating vibrant health for themselves will benefit from this foundation for the rest of their lives.

It is often touted that other cultures have fewer menopausal complaints than the women in our western culture. Diet and lifestyle are frequently the reasons given for this difference and many reasons are given in a *soup du jour* attitude. One study claimed that increased amounts of soy in the diet was *the* reason that asian cultures have fewer menopausal complaints. Another study showed that dietary seaweed was *the* reason women in other cultures have an easier transition. Another study showed that cultural perceptions were *the* reason.

I think we will be hard pressed to find *the* reason. Furthermore, we hopefully realize by now that there is no *one* diet or lifestyle for the whole population. Approaching people individually and constitutionally from the beginning of life will help us recognize and correct imbalances easily to promote a lifetime of vibrant health.

Addressing menopausal complaints

Easily half of the people I see in my herbal practice come to see me because of menopausal complaints.

In this article I will cover the three most common patterns that I see. Please keep in mind that these patterns are portrayed in a very broad and general way. There are many distinctive patterns involved with this life process and much more specific ways of looking at it through particular organ meridians. A great resource for these are *Healing with the Herbs of Life* by Lesley Tierra.

Excess

Let's begin with a pattern that is more excessive in nature. This is by far the easiest pattern to address.

An excess pattern has many signs of true heat.
- Hot flashes. In particular these hot flashes are intense. Lots of heat and lots of sweating is involved. This is the person who has to change their clothes after a hot flash or change their sheets after having night sweats.
- Loud voice, red tongue and possibly a red face, not just red cheeks, but the whole face (important distinction).
- A lot of thirst.
- Fast pulse
- Possibly frequent headaches or headaches associated with menstruation.
- Excessive menstrual flow. They keep bleeding and bleeding, going through many pads and tampons in one day.
- This pattern often has heat in the digestive tract as well. This may manifest as cold sores, mouth ulcers, sensitivity to spicy foods, ulcers, irregular bowel movements.

To address an excess pattern

There are two main strategies with this type of pattern. First we want to use cooling therapies (herbs and lifestyle). Often referred to as eliminating and draining, this includes many of our bitter herbs.

Herbs I frequently recommend for this:

Fresh chickweed (*Stellaria media*)
Dandelion root (*Taraxacum officinale*)
Shepherd's purse (*Capsella bursa-pastoris*)
Rose (*Rosa spp.*)
Black cohosh (*Actaea -formerly Cimicifuga-racemosa*)
Motherwort (*Leonorus cardiaca*)
Wild Yam (*Dioscorea villosa*)
Licorice (*Glycyrrhiza glabra*)

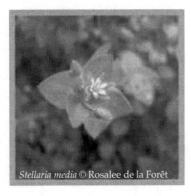
Stellaria media © Rosalee de la Forêt

Secondly, we want to support the adrenals using adaptogen herbs. We don't want these to be too heating in nature.

Herbs I frequently recommend for this include
Nettle leaf   (*Urtica dioica*)
Shatavari   (*Asparagus racemosus*)
Milky oats   (*Avena sativa*)

Astringent herbs can be applied for this pattern as well. Rose (*Rosa spp.*) and schisandra (*Schisandra chinensis*) are ones that I frequently use.

Deficiency

Deficient patterns are what I see more commonly in people I work with. This pattern is much harder to correct. In general it is always easier (in terms of duration and type of treatment) to eliminate and drain than it is to nourish and build.

Deficiency patterns usually arise after many years of draining the system through bad diet, excessive stress, improper movement, etc. If a menopausal woman is showing signs of deficiency after 48 years of not nourishing herself, it's going to take some time to correct this!

Deficiency patterns include:
• Hot flashes with little sweating
• Lethargy, fatigue, especially from 3 to 5 in the afternoon. This person may start off strong and then peter out quickly.
• Red cheeks and/or red nose (not a red face)
• Heat in the soles of feet, palms of hands or chest
• Tinnitus
• Cold hands and feet
• Pale tongue, slow or weak pulse
• Sore lower back, weak knees
• Copious and clear urination

To address a deficiency pattern

In this pattern we want to nourish and build and many times restore moisture as well. Here we are thinking about moisture building herbs (demulcents and blood builders) and adaptogen herbs.

My favorite herbs for this include
Shatavari   (*Asparagus racemosus*)
Ashwagandah   (*Withania somnifera*)
American ginseng   (*Panax quinquefolius*)
Dang gui   (*Angelica sinensis*)

As always, diet is important to address as well. Although we all have different needs, people with deficiency patterns benefit from focusing on cooked vegetables, grains (if tolerated), organic and pasture-raised meats, and warm foods. Raw fruits and vegetables, along with iced drinks and fruit juices, are usually contraindicated.

Liver Qi stagnation

Liver Qi stagnation is a Traditional Chinese Medicine pattern that is frequently seen in today's populace. This pattern can be in addition to either of the patterns above.

Symptoms include
• poor appetite
• mood swings
• quick to anger
• irregular menstrual cycle
• cysts that come and go, fibroids

- digestive complaints
- wiry pulse
- tongue may have curled edges or red edges
- alternating diarrhea and constipation
- fatigue and lethargy
- difficulty swallowing

The classic formula for this is a Chinese formula, Xiao yao san. It is made up of

Bupleurum	6-9 grams
Dang gui	6-9 grams
White peony	8-12 grams
Poria	9-15 grams
Dry-fried atractylodes	3 grams
Baked licorice	3-6 grams
Mentha	1-3 grams
Fresh ginger	1-3 grams

In western herbalism, liver-moving herbs would be indicated: dandelion (*Taraxacum officinale*), calendula (*Calendula officinalis*), St. John's Wort (*Hypericum perforatum*), etc. Lymphagogues and alteratives will also be important. I have the most experience with the above formula.

Dryness vs. Dampness

Most women I see during this transition have symptoms of dryness. Dry skin, dry mouth, dry hair, dry vaginal tissues (very common complaint). Dryness can manifest "false heat" symptoms. These include red cheeks or red nose, heat in the soles and palms and chest, night sweats, anxiety, dry stools, thirst, scanty and dark urine.

Using moisturizing and building herbs like shatavari (*Asparagus racemosus*), prepared rehmannia (*Rehmannia glutinosa*), marshmallow (*Althaea officinalis*), licorice (*Glycyrrhiza glabra*), etc, can help to balance the moisture in the body. Likewise, healthy fats and oils can be optimized in the diet. Lots of high quality olive oil and coconut oil can be added to the diet. Fish oil and evening primrose oil can be supplemented.

For administering these herbs I especially like using them as powders stirred into ghee and coconut oil and, if appropriate for the individual, a little honey. Decoctions also work well.

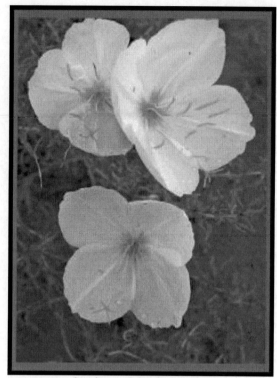

Oenothera sp. © Rosalee de la Forêt

For symptomatic treatment of dry vaginal tissues a vitamin E capsule can be pricked and then inserted vaginally at night, and as needed.

Signs of dampness may include edema, loose stools, thick coating on tongue, swollen tongue, heavy vaginal discharge and nausea. For these women we want to remove dampness using eliminating and draining herbs such as nettle or dandelion leaf. Warming the digestion is also a common solution and may include adding warming herbs and spices to cooked and warm foods.

Conclusion

My hope is that this article helps the reader to understand that there are no herbs for "menopause" and no herbs for "hot flashes". Instead, we want to evaluate the individual and then come up with a customized analysis (excess, deficient, stagnancy) and then a customized plan based on that analysis. Using this model we can move away from treating symptoms with herbs and move towards working with people to help to address underlying imbalances. The results can be radiant health for women preparing, entering and living through this powerful time of transition.

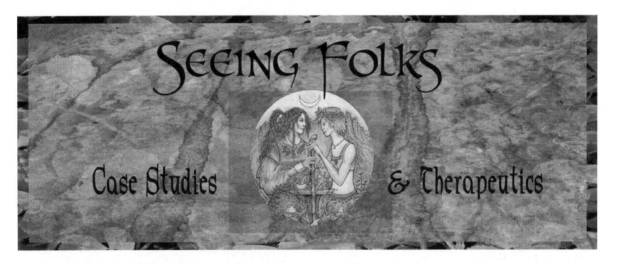

SERVING MENOPAUSAL/PARENTING WOMEN IN CONTEXT

Address the System & Assess

by Jennie Isbell Shinn

No matter if you know it from print, cartoons or the movies, if you are a fan of Spiderman, you know that the power of Peter Parker's transformation from nerdy high schooler to powerful superhero comes over him in an instant. He gets bitten. And then, wow. Webs shoot out of his wrists, his vision and other senses change. He's caught between wanting to literally swing from the rooftops and the urge to hide the fullness of his marvelous transformation from prying eyes.

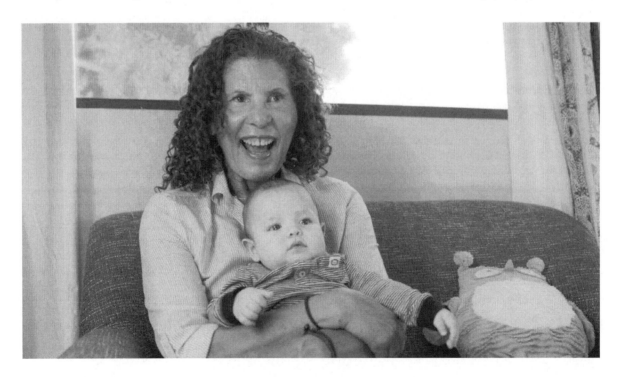

In spite of his identity crisis, Spiderman has a strong urge to use his post-transformation giftedness and newfound courage to help others. Me too. The truth is that I don't believe in the instant identity change of menopause, and I'm trying to engage my discomforts and my changes in a spirit of curiosity, and in the context of the bigger pictures I live in. I am trying to share from my transformation as it's underway, which means beginning in the middle, and in the past, with inherited misconceptions and fears.

I gave birth to my son the same year I turned 43. It was my second pregnancy, but my first full-term, live birth. Out beyond the indescribable joy of initiation into motherhood, the lack of sleep, and two years of postpartum reorientation*, I found myself sliding into another initiation— what conventional medicine calls peri-menopause. I love and hate that peri-menopause is defined as the time before menopause. It's literally true, but that's like saying to a married person that singlehood was the time before committing to a partner. Or that adulthood is the time that follows childhood. Um, yes. Once a woman has been 12 consecutive months without a moon cycle, she is considered to have reached menopause. Then poof. It's done. In common use, the term menopause is often used to refer to a stage spanning between six months and 10 years during which a variety of symptoms arise including mood swings, hot flashes, disturbed sleep, unstoppable weight gain, vaginal dryness and decreased libido.

As the change is coming my way in fits and starts, I find myself questioning the common wisdom, not just theoretically but personally and concretely. It's been an eye-opening five years for me, since five years ago I was eight-months pregnant with my child. I wondered then as I cataloged my own symptoms, which were related to peri-menopause (not helpfully defined as the time leading up to the cession of reproductive capacity), which were pregnancy related, and which were related to the general aging process, grief over my father's recent death and my own unrelated relocation. I think I knew it before, academically— that considering symptoms and complaints in context were merit-worthy things to do as I claimed to be a holistic practitioner, but living the confusion of overlapping causes helped me grok it. Context matters, a lot.

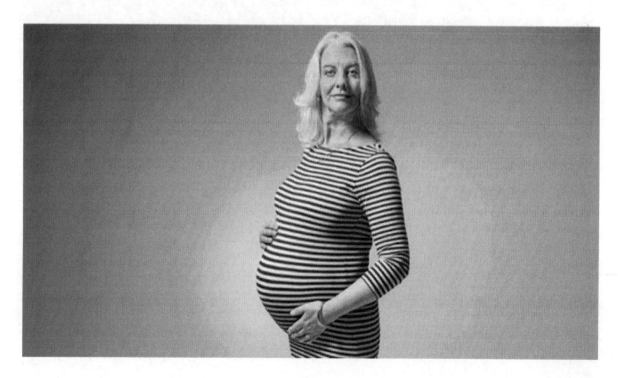

139

As an older first-time mom myself, it is no surprise to me that I have a lot of conversations with older women raising young children. As I consider herbal advice for the complaints these women bring, I listen deeper (than I used to) for each woman's attitude toward her symptoms. How much of the complaint relates to an internalized diminished self-regard based on the cultural norm of valuing women for reproductive capacity (i.e. women's use value as determined by patriarchy)? I listen for this and hear it more clearly as increasing numbers of women of the baby-boom are landing in post-menopause and are changing cultural values by their response. When it comes to older mothers, and grandmothers who are parenting, it seems as though the "bite" that has brought on their own Spiderman-like transformation to (s)hero-hood brings about initiation to power and re-framing ... sometimes reframing everything.

For example, vaginal dryness may seem to be derailing to a woman's sense of sexuality and perhaps even attractiveness, but what if dryness is a pause point, or an invitation to ask, "What really makes me juicy these days?" It could be an herbal moistening oil for lubrication, or it could be that one's sexual appetites are changing. Given the focus on defining women's life cycles by their reproductive cycles, finally the clitoris may have center stage. An organ whose primary purpose is the woman's pleasure is a source of moisture if it is pleased. And more than one woman I know has chosen a to leave heterosexual relationships behind in menopause.

My unfolding call to support women who are parenting while also navigating peri/menopause has firmed up and confirmed some "best practice" guidelines for viewing clients holistically, for looking (with clients) for invitations to initiations, and also for holding consideration of the broader context of modern life (and even politics, which I am not writing about here). I come from the perspective that whichever modalities I am working in from the several that might bring a client to my office, my persistent across them all is 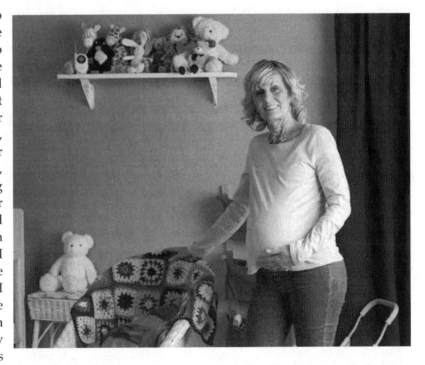 encouragement, lens shifting and practical care. Lens shifting has much to do with helping someone see possibilities for themselves or their circumstances. Sometimes all it requires is loosening one's grip on one thing, one diagnosis, one reality, to allow something else to enter one's field of view.

The work of all my modalities (bodywork, herbal support, and spiritual companionship) relies upon an open assessment process that reaches interim conclusions, but stays open to unfolding insights and change. Part of being in the business of encouragement is believing (and advocating) that change is possible. All the better if this is contagious to those whom I serve.

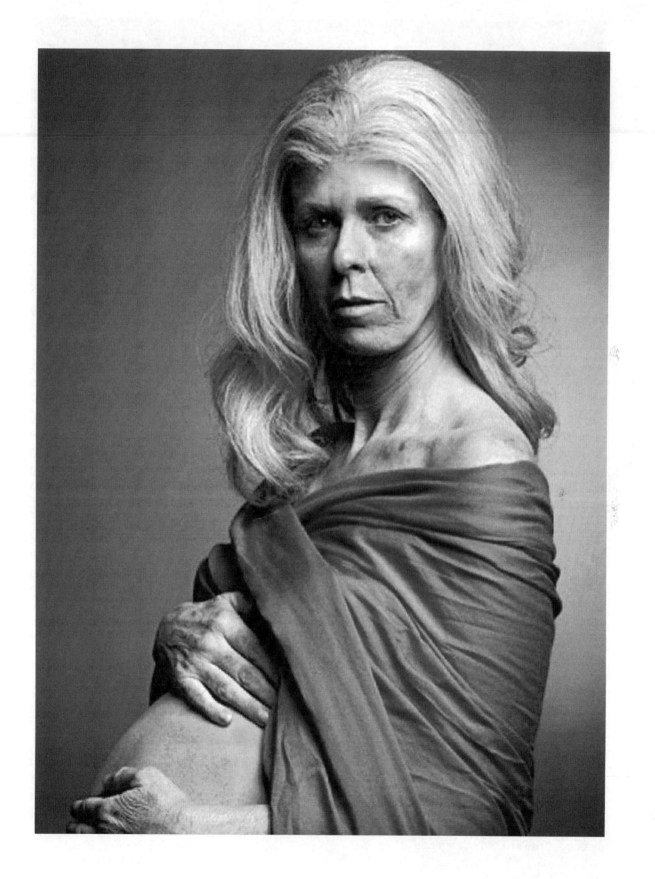

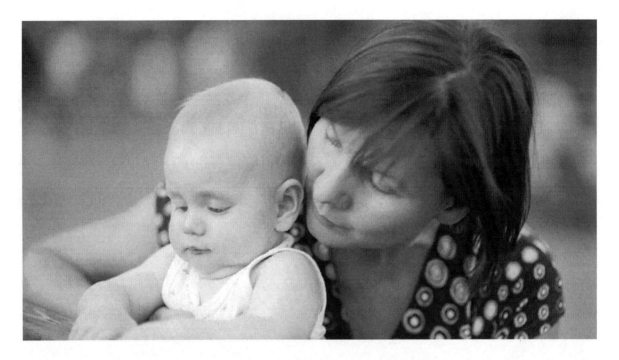

Living into the complexity of my own search for the cause of symptoms — was it grief, aging, pregnancy or peri-menopause that led to my complaints?— my mental spin was blessedly halted by the insight of the design/thinking methods of Permaculture (permanent agriculture or permanent culture, depending on whom you ask) which note the most fruitful places are where two zone or ecologies meet. The overlapping edge of forest and field can benefit from the two systems without being wholly like either of them. Very concretely, the edge of forest and field can sustain more diverse plant and animal life than the field or the forest. Traveling backwards through this metaphor, one might say that assessing the health of the places of overlap can get to the heart of healing what could be the most diverse and productive places. For menopausal parents, this means addressing the woman, the child and the system in which they co-exist (and everyone that is in the overlapping edge).

On a very practical level, "home" influences what resources are available for healing and sustenance. For example, multigenerational, co-housed family structures are not nearly as common as they once were. As the model of two adults with their off-spring = family has become the norm, the available supports for healing, and the problems family units face are also different. Addressing the system itself, in addition to the individuals who comprise it, can help.

Here is my list of five things that I now use to work with all clients. Whether I make notes according to this model or just hold it in my mind as I work the intake process, these are my primary areas of interest in addition to what has brought the client in for a consultation:

1. Name and address the System. When I am working with women— mothers and grandmothers raising children in particular, I try to include care of the whole home system, which may include blood relations as well as others. When the desired outcome can be achieved through multiple means, a nourishing infusion or tea that mother and child can share as an afternoon ritual is better for the system than an alcohol-based tincture for only the adult. If the home system includes multiple people, the ripple effect of the woman and child sharing plant medicine may extend even beyond those around the tea pot.

2. Nourishment includes food and other sources of vital in-flow. When making a wellness plan with a woman who is also parenting, conversations about meal planning often include the difficulty of planning and preparing two or more parallel meals because of food preferences and aversions. Finding a list of universally agreeable ingredients and recipes can be a huge boost to the wellness of the home system. Also in the frame of nourishment are non-food things like time, activities, rest, body care. I like to ask what would be nourishing to the woman (usually the client), what would be nourishing to the child, and what would be nourishing to the woman and the child, and to others in the home system. Mothers need alone time. Children need independence. Maybe what rises is a question for the client to carry— what would nourish her need for alone time and also the child's need for independence while keeping the child safe and the mother's vigilance in check? I find that women know the answers. They also know the difficulty with implementation and problem-solving, so this is where deep listening and holistic perspectives can bring healing to a system.

3. Body-dwelling. I use this term instead of movement or exercise because I find it casts a more inclusive net. Body-dwelling includes movement, but also body image, sensory awareness and pleasure, and body wisdom/instinct. Because my client base is largely female, I witness internalized misogyny and the fruits of patriarchal values on a daily basis. Personal dislike of one's body can range from vocally expressed hatred to subtle attempts to change for appearance' sake because of external feedback. (There is another desire to change one's body that I see that is not guided by an external mirror.) Many women I encounter who are in addictions recovery, or considering it, became distanced from physical pleasure and sexuality before the onset of their addiction. Sobriety brings a lot of fear and uncertainty to some women who have literally never engaged in sexual behavior while sober. And, another reason to consider body-dwelling is to tap into sub-rational resources, which I call body wisdom, that are somewhat protected from critics of the inner and outer nature. Helping people connect with their gut instinct can save, and certainly change lives as women reclaim their self determination and power.

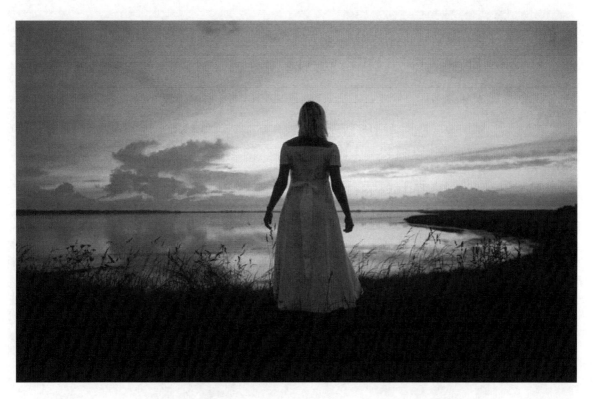

143

4. Herbs and nature as a category for me includes specific remedies and also encouragement of connection with nature. I do actually recommend herbs to clients! Why is it it number four on my list? Because numbers 1-3 help me connect with the client more deeply, so that the recommendations I offer are very particular to the person in front of me, in the system she lives in. My own walk with plant medicine convinces me of the multi-level effects of taking plants into my body and using them outside my body. Sometimes I don't know in advance what the whole body effects will be versus what I might calculate from an internal dose for a specific condition. How is a foot soak with Yarrow (*Achillea millefolium*) while drinking Yarrow tea effective in different ways that just tea or just tincture in hot water? Where two remedies might be good choices for their energetic effects constituent effects, I find that one is usually a stand out over the other based on something about the client's home system, the kind of nourishment the person needs or prefers, and her connection with body and pleasure. For example, a woman with addictive eating impulses who is in recovery with this addiction could use a an alcohol-based tincture of Tulsi (*Ocimum sanctum*) to curb sugar-craving impulses. She could also use a oxymel of the same herb.When possible it is good encourage and equip clients to make their own remedies, by providing recipes and sometimes herbs or seeds and plants for longer term use.

5. For my intake purposes, rest includes sleep, an honest self-assessment of one's sleep-hygiene, down time and also differently-paced time. This has been a significant area of expanded understanding in my practice, for me and for clients. When sleep is assessed only as night time sleep from feet-in-bed to feet-back-on-the-floor time, a woman with a child who wakes six times a night can believe that sleep is an illusive aspiration. Helping clients see the value of down time and differently-paced time as aspects of restoration and balance can give hope and encouragement with profound effects. Down time can be reading, resting, a quick meditation break or something of the like. Differently-paced time is a place where home system members can be engaged as well. For the work-at-home computer user, moving around, going outside, even folding laundry with others can be a support to the system.

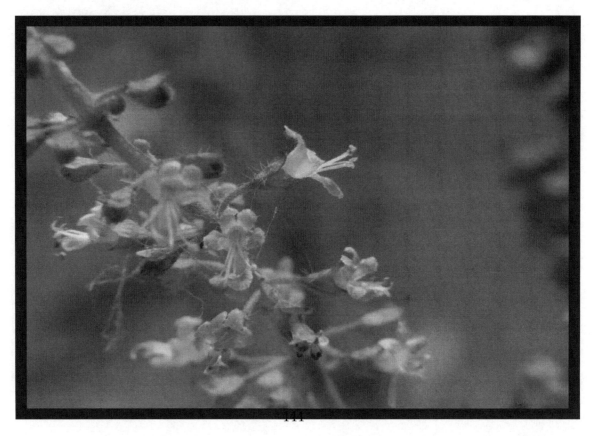

5. For my intake purposes, rest includes sleep, an honest self-assessment of one's sleep-hygiene, The care I offer begins the moment someone sets an appointment with me. I find that encouraging a durable commitment to self-care is better than any recommendation I offer, and the client's commitment to self care is in the gesture of setting an appointment. Simply, she said Yes to herself before she called me.

When developing the treatment plan, even in my mind as I am gathering information form the client, I prioritize by 1. greatest discomfort, 2. easiest fix and 3. best ripple effect. And don't forget the home system in which it's all happening. The intake process is really, really important. Assessment happens in it and healing also happens in it. The client has my undivided attention and can tell her story. Being heard is healing. Absence of judgment is healing. Ally-ship is healing.

Grief is common, and it is a process that includes finding a new normal after multiple attempts. Grieving sometimes takes on the shape of a spiral, in which one can visit the same territory over and over from a slightly different perspective, and feel like she is not making progress. Even talking to someone who is expecting a straight line of progress from themselves about seeing the spiral they are walking can be a relief.

Normalizing life stages and the accompanying life stage changes is key to normalizing human-being-ness. To accomplish this, I don't say "That's normal." I say, "That's common." Normal is too limiting and too-sought after. And besides, as the late baby-boomers and the rest of us crest the hill, and can see menopause for ourselves, even what's common is bound to change as more of us see the bite of initiation for what it is.

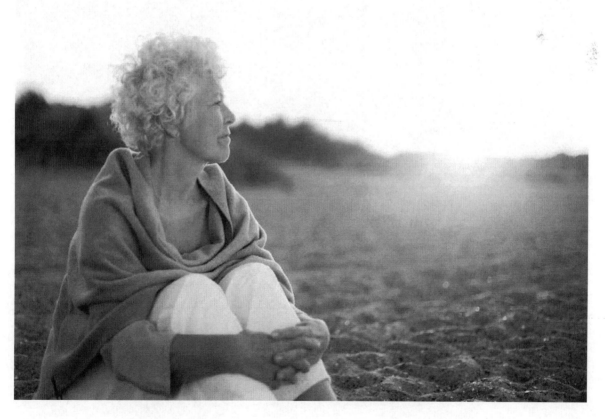

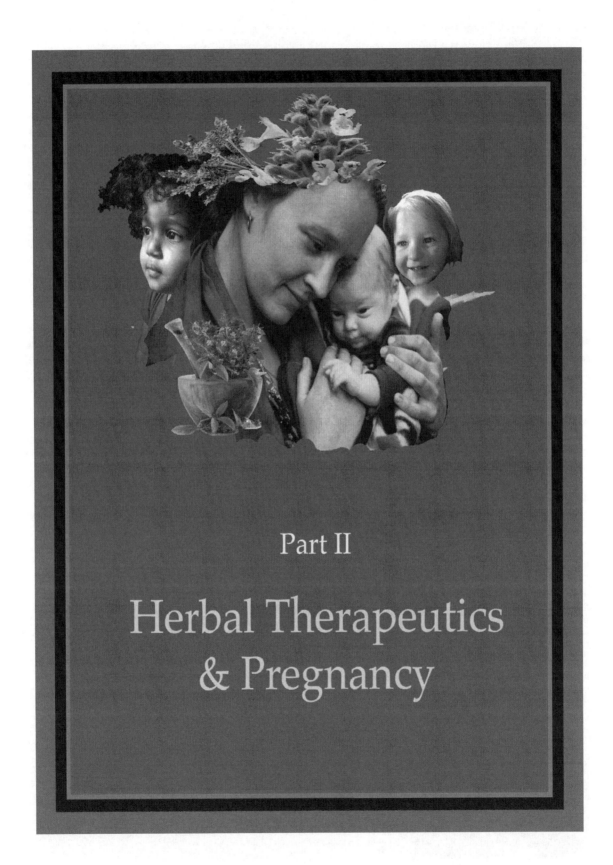

Part II

Herbal Therapeutics
& Pregnancy

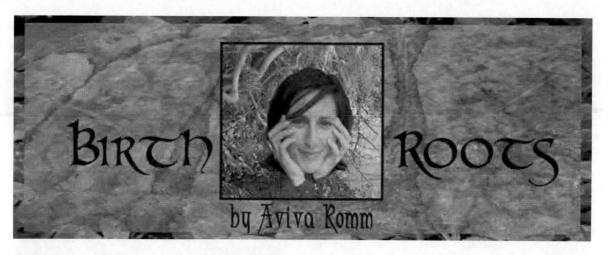

BIRTH ROOTS

by Aviva Romm

This column is dedicated to the memory of Jeannine Parvati Baker

Opening...

Welcome to *Birth Roots: Radical Herbalism in Women's Health and Childbearing*, a new column that Kiva and Jesse graciously invited me to create. The focus of this column will be empowering women to self-care and empowering herbalists to women's care through herbal medicine, women's healing knowledge, experience, and wisdom.

Whenever I pick up a new book sent to me for review or that catches my eye, when I see a documentary or hear a news story, the first thing I always seem to want to know is who it is that is sharing the information. Perhaps it's that I'm just very humanistic in my approach---a quintessential "people person"—and want to know the story behind the story. Or perhaps it is the part skeptic-part rebel in me that is asking, "why should I listen to you?" Really, it's all of the above. I do want to know if the person telling me something has walked that talk. So I thought the best way to start this column to is tell you who I am, where I come from, what my talk is and how I walk it, why you might listen to me (or not) and what I hope to share through this column. Most folks tell me what they love most about my books is that reading them is like hanging out with me and having a chat over a cup of tea. So I'll just work with that vibe right from

Radical Herbalism In Women's Health & Childrearing

by Aviva Romm

the start. Sit back and enjoy the hibiscus, raspberry, lavender and mint iced-tea I've just poured on this balmy July day.

My Roots...

My journey began in 1966 amidst the turbulence of the Vietnam War against the backdrop of the best rock and roll ever written. My parents were college-aged; my dad was able to avoid the draft because my mom was pregnant with me... and so my life began. My mother went into labor with me at my great-grandmother's funeral, several hours after playing in a neighborhood softball game—a start and story that taught me that birth is part of the natural flow of life, part of the cycle of life and death, and that a woman can play softball and then have a baby! I was born in Harlem, NY at a hospital called Flower and 5th, now long burned down (incidentally, herbalists Brigitte Mars and Janet Zand were also born in this hospital---must be something about the Flowers part of it...)and I was raised in a housing project in Queens, a borough of NYC (I'm a "home girl"). My mom was a single working mom at a time before divorce was acceptable and I learned a lot of mad survival skills from her. My deeper roots are Russian and Austro-Hungarian Jewish. My great grandparents left Eastern Europe to escape the pogroms. True to the classic immigrant experience, they arrived in NYC via Ellis Island and variously set up shop in the Lower-East side of New York City ("The

147

Village") and Brooklyn. They were tailors, pharmacists, vegetable cart peddlers, and machine shop owners. My Hungarian great-grandmother Bertha was an herbal healer, known in The Village for her topical burn creams, mustard plasters, and cupping skills. She made bathtub gin during the Great Depression to make ends meet. I knew her well when I was very young, and though I did not learn her herbal remedies I did pick up her imminently practical wisdom such as keep your head warm in the winter, use Epsom salts for sprains, boric acid for certain topical irritations, witch hazel for just about everything, and stay home from school to convalesce 1 day for every day one has a fever. Her chicken soup truly was medicine. She was also known in the family for being a psychic and I suspect my own deep intuitive knowing comes from her lineage. Sadly to me, the herbal remedies she knew had long been abandoned by her children in favor of modern medical practices by the time I was born. Once, when I was in my twenties, when my great-uncle, her son, learned that I practiced herbal medicine, he said, "Well at least you don't use those barbaric mustard plasters my mother used." I told him that, in fact, just a week before I had treated someone with bronchitis with a mustard plaster—and it worked! My great-grandmother herself avoided doctors whenever possible. She and her two sisters, my *tantes*, baked challah on Fridays and brought the old world into my early childhood which was otherwise something like that Tupac song Old School, filled with stoop games and all things urban.

My respites were summers at my grandparents' small home on Long Island where I spent my time reading and imagining under a giant willow that my mom and uncle had planted when they were small children, collecting rocks, and pressing flowers I "appropriated" from neighbors' gardens during the long bike rides I relished.

From the earliest age I can remember I was a science geek. I think being 2 years old and seeing the lunar landing (Apollo 11—one small step for man, one giant leap for mankind and all that...) left an indelible imprint. Those rocks I collected? I usually split them open looking for hidden treasures and then tried to classify them, emulating the rock collections at my favorite haunt—the Museum of

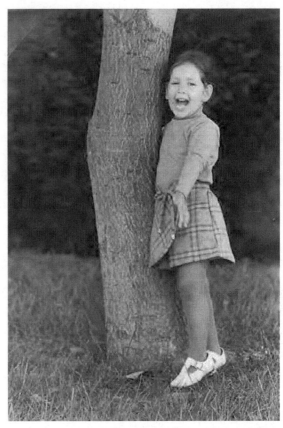

Little Aviva with a willing tree friend.

Natural History; I similarly organized my flower pressings. I won science fairs and planned to become a physician, the idea first geminating in me at age 9. I went to the famous NY public high school Bronx Science, riding the train under the watchful eye of the Guardian Angels, the self appointed youth group that patrolled the NY Subway system, on my daily bidirectional trek from Queens to the Bronx and back again. But I wanted something different than high school had to offer with its cliques and pressures, so I applied to a small liberal arts college for gifted and talented (or just plain rich) kids called Simon's Rock and at age 15 found myself with a scholarship starting college in the Berkshire Mountains of Western Massachusetts.

There I started my road less traveled. And so in 1981 part 2 of my journey began. I discovered midwifery, herbal medicine (all kinds of herbs including the psychedelic variety comprised those early explorations of plant medicine), and I discovered myself. I devoured *Spiritual Midwifery*, *The Autobiography of a Yogi*, macrobiotic, raw foods, and self-healing books, and the few herbs books that were published at that time (*The Way of Herbs* was just about the be published and the only major published books aside from the arcane and *The Web that Has No Weaver*, and *The Yellow Emperor's Inner Classic* were *The Herb Book*, *Swiss Nature Cure*, and *Jeanne Rose's Herbal Body Book*).

I left school at age 16, moved to a coop house in Cambridge, MA, and began studying with a midwife in Roxbury. Midwifery and herbal medicine became my life. My midwifery training came through apprenticeship; my herbal training through self-study and real life. I hiked, camped, swam naked in quarries and lakes, went organic, grew dreads, grew gardens, and eventually grew a family with the love of my life. Together we've had 4 born-at-home kids---three born with just the 2 of us and our kids present. I breastfed for something like 13 consecutive years. We homeschooled our kids –two up to college, two up to high school, and raised them in an earthy, socially conscious way, trusting in nature when healing was needed. During those years I midwifed a few hundred babies into the world, using herbal medicines throughout all phases of the childbearing cycle as needed, and found myself called upon to provide instruction, information, guidance, and healing for all manner of children's ailments from common colds and infections to dog bits and pertussis. I have stood side-by-side with women as they have gone through everything from normal, triumphant birth to pregnancy losses and serious illnesses during, before, and after the childbearing years. I wrote a half dozen or so of books to bring the principles and practices that were keeping my own family healthy and out of the doctor's office and hospital to others.

...and Branches

During all of those 20+ years, my midwifery practice was illegal. I watched as women, mothers,

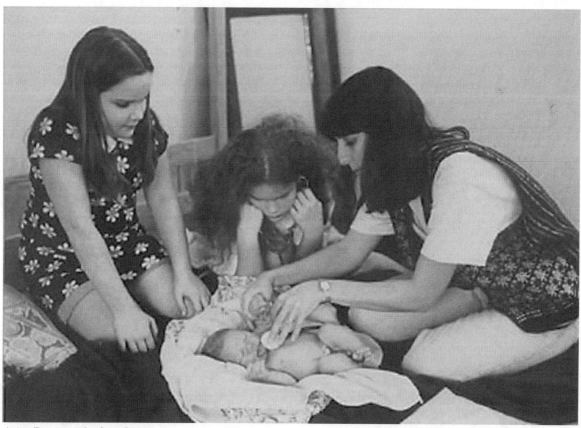

Aviva Romm midwifery, C.2004

and midwives struggled to find compassionate medical care when it was needed, and assisted in finding it when possible or providing an alternative when not. I watched midwives be abused by state laws and I watched birthing women be verbally accosted in the hospital for their homebirth choice if a hospital transport became necessary. I once told a doctor that if he was going to cut an episiotomy in my birthing client's perineum he was going to have to cut through my hand. He put the scissors down and looked at me with mouth agape. No episiotomy was cut. Those were some days. I knew of families that had been mistreated by the medical establishment over vaccination choices, co-sleeping, and homebirth; I saw antibiotics doled out like candy even when not medically indicated. I knew what it was like, from first-hand experience, to wonder whether the police were going to show up at my door, arrest me for practicing midwifery without a license, and detain my kids should my partner not be home when the axe fell. It was profound work. It was also tremendously stressful and I do not tend to remain silent in the face of injustices.

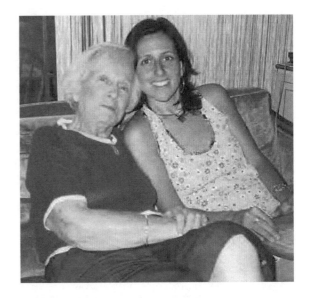

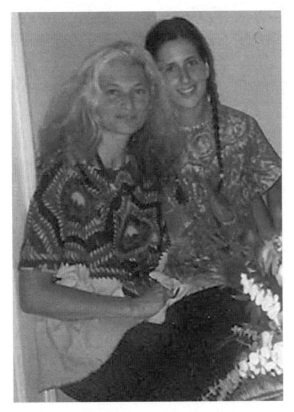

While the herbs and natural living and practices had never failed to serve, at some point I thought "enough is enough" about the medical abuses I was witnessing. I decided that I had to get to get inside the medical system and make some changes, that folks like us (all folks, really) need doctors they can turn to safely and comfortably when medical care is needed—and that medical care needed some major radicalization (radical=roots=back to basics and

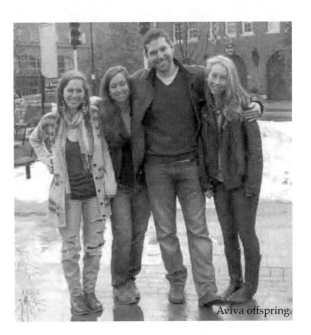

Aviva offspring.

herbs). I held my nose and jumped into the cold water of medical training.

The Dark Side and the Light at the End of the Tunnel

As you are reading this I am entering my final year of medical residency in family medicine—what I feel is the light at the end of a very long tunnel of medical training. It's not been an easy road as an herbalist---not so much from the medical side of things, but because a lot of folks in our own community haven't understood why an herbalist-midwife would, as some have said to me, "go over to the dark side" and become a doctor. But I've had my reasons and these have been about bringing more access to what herbalists and midwives do to more people, while expanding my own understanding, knowledge, skill set, and power to make a change. True to my life-education style of learning, I did my entire undergraduate degree via distance learning, creating and completing a major in Women's Health Studies. I completed my medical training at Yale and I got an amazing education in the process. The receptivity to what I had to bring was surprising and refreshing and I created what has become a required second year medical school course in integrative medicine. I learned that true scientists—whether herbalists, medical docs, or purely academic --are eternally curious and open-minded sorts and that the true healers from all traditional are eternally receptive to what might benefit their patients, suspending limited viewpoints. I've had an incredible depth and breadth of opportunity beyond what I'd previously experienced as an herbalist and midwife, diagnosing

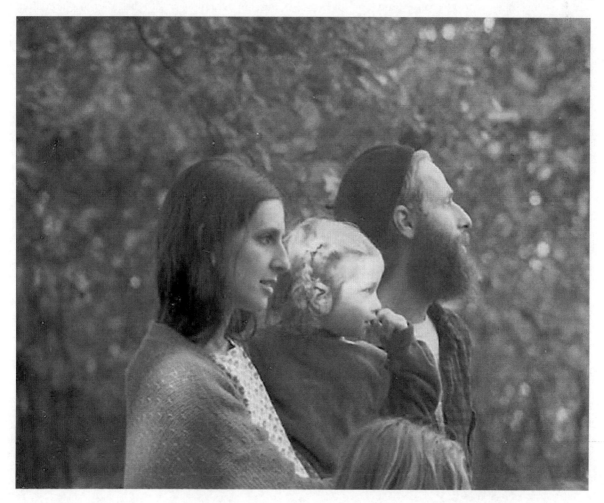

151

and treating everything from preeclampsia in pregnant women to tubercular meningitis in a Nepalese immigrant, and have gotten really comfortable with the day to day medical problems faced by so many Americans and the most serious illnesses that lead to hospitalizations. I am in the position to tell my patients that I understand their medical issues, and as often as not can say, "No, you do not need a medication (or surgery) for that." My training has deepened my already great respect and appreciation for natural healing approaches and herbal medicine, particularly when it comes to the prevention of chronic diseases such as cardiac disease and diabetes. Most profoundly I've realized that every culture has a story it tells about healing. The mainstream modern post-industrial story is about drugs, bugs, and surgery. It is about survival of the fittest. Conquest over nature. Over women. But it is just one story. Herbalists and midwives have another story to tell. It is about trusting and working with nature, symbiosis, nurturing.

I've Looked at Birth from Both Sides Now, or The Reasons We Need Radical Herbalism in Women's Health and Childbearing

While western medicine has started to adopt more integrative approaches such as mind-body medicine, use of some nutritional supplements, and even the inclusion of some botanicals, for example cranberry for preventing UTI in elderly nursing home patients, for the most part, the landscape of women's health has not improved much over the past couple of decades and the birthing situation in the US has become downright bleak, with an all time high rate of interventions. Amnesty International has declared birthing practices in the US to be a human rights issue---1 in 3 women will have their baby delivered by cesarean and most will experience a host of other interventions including labor inductions, antibiotics in labor, epidural or other anesthesia, continuous fetal monitoring, and some sort of assisted delivery (ie vacuum extraction). Hysterectomy remains one of the most frequent (and over-utilized) surgeries; its use is known to vary regionally and even from one hospital to the next, suggesting that the decision to do a hysterectomy is not based on firm medical evidence but on other considerations including profit driven motives. Young girls and grown

women are starving themselves to look like airbrushed women they see on magazine covers. Internationally, women still die literally every minute of septic abortions and lack of adequate care during birth and the postpartum.

Can herbalists and midwives prevent and solve all of these problems? No. Can we make a hearty contribution? Absolutely. Particularly if we embrace our healing work not just as a return to simpler times, but if we take it on as a political mission. Every woman has the right to safe health care options for all issues ranging from the prevention and treatment of acne to heart disease, from nausea in early pregnancy to postpartum depression. All women have the right to choice in health care including choosing natural approaches in conjunction with or as an alternative to conventional treatments without fear of reprisal or recrimination. It's going to take a posse of "barefoot" herbalists, midwives, and doctors to bring about these changes.

Looking Forward

I've learned a great deal in becoming a physician. But at heart I remain a midwife and herbalist. Midwifery and herbalism aren't just something one "does"-- they are what one "is." Conventional medicine has a role---it is sometimes a necessary response to modern medical problems that have arisen as a result of *life out of balance*. But for the most part in this case like does not cure like. Conventional medical tools offer patients very little in terms of true "health care" and disease prevention. Life has become terribly medicalized as a result of fear of nature, of life's cycles. To some extent this medicalization—or "sickifying" of life is the inevitable product of a model of western life that is separate from nature. But it is not inevitable that women continue to suffer as a result.

This column is about realigning women's health care with nature. It is about life in balance. It is about helping you, as herbalists, to embrace the confidence to educate women about their health care options—herbal and otherwise. Through this column I hope to share stories, clinical pearls, and practical wisdom gleaned from my now 30 years as an herbalist-midwife-mom-doc on how, when, and what can be done with botanicals to prevent and heal common—and even not so common—women's concerns throughout all of women's lifecycles. How to know boundaries. When medical care is needed. When it is not. And how to have to humility and respect for life to know the difference. In each column I will do two things: one will be to present a major article on a specific topic. In the next issue I will be discussing miscarriage. This is an oft overtreated and overmedicalized process leaving so many women feeling alone and confused rather than supported and cared for. The article will help you learn how to recognize different types of miscarriage, when medical care is needed, compassionate approaches to helping women with the psychoemotional aspects of this type of pregnancy loss, and of course, the wealth of botanicals we have for helping women on every level through miscarriage—prevention, treatment, completion, and healing—physical, mental, emotional, and spiritual. It is one of the topics I hear most about from readers of my book with thanks because they felt that it was a compassionate botanical approach that helped them get through what was otherwise a potentially lonely and under-recognized and medically mistreated process. I look forward to bringing you on that healing journey.

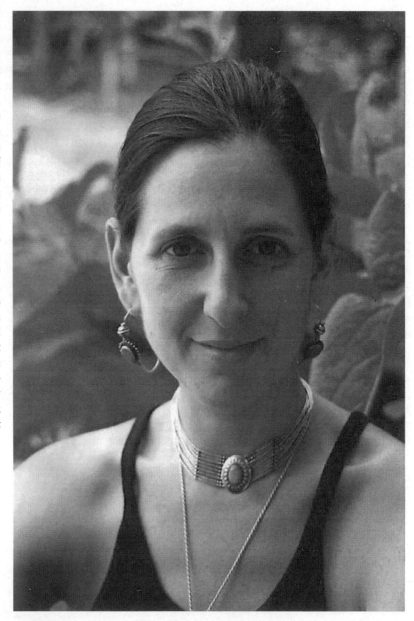

FERTILITY FOR EVERYONE ELSE

How To Get Pregnant Like a Lesbian

by Alanna Whitney

Fertility for everyone else. There's a lot that's often left out of "female repro" classes in herb school, in herbal texts, and therefore, in the way that we train herbalists to think about fertility. Instead of assuming that all baby.having people are straight cis.ladies partnered to straight, cis.men, this class will address the many multifaceted experiences of baby.having, cause queer folks, trans folks, and single parents also have babies! We will cover how to think about fertility and parentage in a more inclusive way that makes room for all kinds of folks to show up as their whole selves.

Thinking about fertility like a lesbian (homo, queerdo, uterus.having.person, etc.) often means treating sperm like a precious and limited resource, so we get really good at timing and at watching for the perfect crescendo of many different indications that the time is right. We will cover broadly

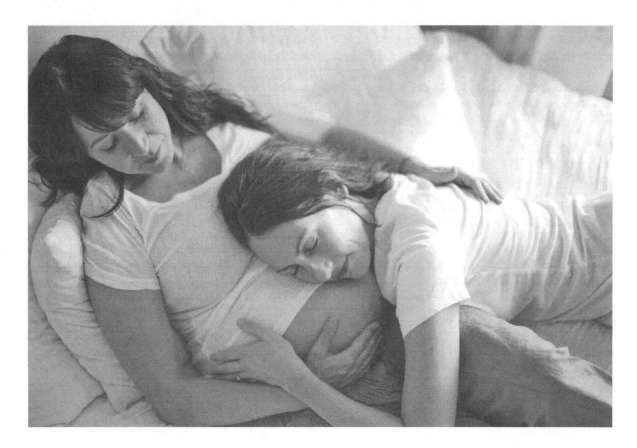

applicable methods for improving fertility and optimizing chances, including nutritional interventions, assessing for important nutrient deficiencies, Vitalist practices, and herbal therapeutics. We'll talk about the basics of charting alllll the different fertility signs (mucous, temp, sex drive, etc.) and the foibles of some of the tools of the trade (ovulation tests, drawbacks, how to not rely on them exclusively) as well as weighing some of the ways of accessing sperm (banking, known donors, friends, family, etc.). We will also touch briefly on pro.tips for navigating legalities of parentage.

Why?

My goals are twofold: first, how to get pregnant if you're having a hard time with that, but also I want to introduce new ways of learning, teaching, and speaking about fertility and pregnancy that make room for everyone. For most folks who want and have not yet been successful in having babies, the thing is fraught with frustration, fear, anxiety, and more, and what worse time is there to sit down to the onerous task of educating your care providers about your life ("no, I don't have a partner" / " no 'he' didn't leave me, I chose to do this on my own" / "no I'm not doing IVF" / "no I don't have a husband").

I am so grateful for all the ways in which the herbal world is changing, and most especially grateful to the work of Kiva & Wolf for making space for new, younger, and more diverse folks to come to the fore and share their wisdom and experience. Those efforts make it possible that herbal education can serve more folks, including people who are often left out of conversations about health and wellness – that is, people who aren't middle or upper middle class, white, partnered, cisgender, straight, citizens, and on and on.

Talking about queer fertility is important to me because I'm queer and I have rarely seen myself represented in herbal literature, books, and classes. I want to point out, too, that as a college educated, white, cis-femme lady, I am super used to seeing myself represented in the world 'cause I move with a lot of privilege. So the rare moments of invisibility I've felt suck, and are a reminder of how much representation I'm accustomed to having/ seeing. Anyway: in a world where discussions and education about fertility & baby.having have long been accompanied by requisite broomstick skirts, fertility goddesses, and visualization instructions to "get in touch with your wombspace", I want to offer something else.

Teaching Fertility & Generative Systems

Lots of people *other * than straight, cis-folks having penile-vaginal sex have babies. Queer folks have babies (that is, uterus.having queers and queers without uteruses, but for the sake of simplicity and time, we're sticking with uterus.having.folks today), single people have babies, and trans folks have babies. Teaching and writing about baby.having in a way that recognizes the existence and reality of more people makes our work accessible for those people! And this is a big shtick of mine, but I think that the radical, life.giving, connection.building, heart.felt work of herbalism should be accessible to as many people as possible, because connection to earth and knowledge of plants is birthright. Working to make our work and teachings representative of all people means that those folks who are most commonly left out, invisible, and ignored, don't have to do the arduous work of educating and advocating for themselves.

How to start:

•Use better language! It's weird to think about if you haven't had to before, but conception, birth, and parenting aren't inherently gendered experiences. A really easy fix for "pregnant mamma", which is super reflexive for a lot of people, is "pregnant person".
○Don't "mom" people! Don't "ladies" folks!
○Don't assume a dad, second parent, etc.
○Other options: parent, gestational parent, non-gestational parent, partner, birthing person, breast/chest feeding person, etc.
•Not all women have vaginas, not all men have penises, ad infinitum. Equating genitalia or generative organs is called gender essentialism and excludes folks whose assigned gender at birth doesn't coincide with their gender identity.
•I love Dave Meesters' recent suggestion that we shift our language from "reproductive system" to "generative system". Check out his blogpost here: http://www.medicinecountyherbs.com/blog/venerable-new-language-for-the-human-reproductive-system
•Talk about queer fertility! In discussions of pregnancy, sex, fertility, contraception, and sexually transmitted infections—how are those things different for queer folks? This could be as simple as not reflexively equating pregnancy as something that happens when you have sex (this is true even for straight, cisgender folks!)

Accessibility in Clinical Work

All the above suggestions for how to teach fertility & generative systems are also applicable to clinical work! There are other pitfalls common to clinicians, though. Curiosity is a big source of discomfort and presumption on the part of clinicians, especially those who haven't worked with trans folks/ queer folks/ single folks before. The clinician – client relationship creates an inherent power differential that we must actively work against. We sit in session with folks, expecting that they give us unfettered access to what are sometimes deeply personal histories, traumas, as well as other super personal information (like how they have sex, who they have sex with, what their poops look like, etc.).

In our defense, a lot of that information is helpful, even necessary to ensure that I'm going to make the most badass herbal formula & protocol recommendations. And yet, if we're working with folks whose lives and realities are new to us, it's easy to allow that position of power to get the better of us. We might ask the single-parent-to-be *why on earth* they would choose to have a child alone – won't it be expensive? Won't it be difficult? Certainly that information isn't critical to our clinical work, nor to our understanding of the case. Being curious about other people's lives isn't a problem, but it becomes one when we unwittingly or unknowingly use it in a position of power. We might wonder about the pregnant queer couple – where the sperm came from, what decisions they might have made about how to navigate complex relationships with donor, or how they plan to explain the process to an eager 3 year old. Again, this is legitimate curiosity that doesn't have any place in our clinical sessions (but thank goodness for Google!).

What else? Learn about queer fertility and teach it! At least touch on it, speak to the fact that there are different ways of making babies and different kinds of families.

How to Get Pregnant Like a Lesbian

The greatest advantage of trying to get knocked up as a uterus.having.homo is also the greatest inconvenience – when you don't have a steady supply of sperm, you get really meticulous about timing. Easy access to sperm is a great benefit and in many cases, major money saver! Most people are born from simple, time tested penile-vaginal sex! But because of the idea that having sex is *the* normal and natural way to get pregnant, it can create a feeling that having more sex can solve fertility issues. Of course, there are many issues that can be solved by having more sex, if you like that, but infertility isn't *necessarily* one of them. Folks who *don't* have ready access to sperm instead have to treat sperm like a precious resource and get really diligent about ensuring that the timing is just right. So if you *treat* sperm like it's a limited resource, you get more strategic about how to use it, which increases your chances.

Ways to Get Knocked Up When You Don't Have Easy Access to SPERM

Step 1: Procuring sperm
•**Fresh sperm from a known donor.** You basically get sperm in a container and then insert it into the vagina.
o**Advantages** of using fresh sperm include vastly improved success rates, ease of use (not having to time shipment of cryogenically frozen sperm to match up with unknown future ovulation date…), and cost. In most cases using a known donor is free. Many couples may incorporate their families – using a sibling or other relation of the nongestational parent as a donor so that they may maintain a genetic connection to the baby-to-be – or communities this way.
o**Disadvantages** include legal considerations – in many states, known donors could theoretically sue for parental/ custody rights. For this reason, it's advised to hire a lawyer and have the donor relinquish parental rights / legal parentage (this gets more complicated if the state you live in requires relinquishment to a person). If the known donor isn't local, the cost and timing of travel can be overwhelming and difficult to arrange. Navigating the complexity of existing and future relationships can also be a deciding factor for many people—if the known donor is a member of your community, how do relationships and expectations pan out for parent/s involved? The cost of things like genetic testing, sperm count testing, and sti testing, if the parent/s decide to pursue it, is an additional cost (whereas these costs are built into the fees one would pay for banked sperm). Fresh sperm can only be used for intra cervical insemination (ICI) and not IUI (intra uterine insemination), so if there were cervical factors preventing pregnancy, IUI would be the course of action.
•**Banked sperm:** banked sperm is cryogenically frozen for at least 180 days (quarantine) and can purchased either washed (for IUI) or unwashed (for ICI). Because it's frozen, banked sperm is shipped overnight in a huge canister that is generally good for 48 hours, so tracking and anticipating ovulation is even more crucial. Most banks have a variety of options around the identity of the donor, and include donors who will remain forever anonymous and donors who are "willing to be known" when the child has reached adulthood and wants to reach out.
o**Advantages** of banked sperm include the vast vetting process for all donors and a great deal of medical testing of the donor and samples. These almost always include genetic testing for common heritable diseases (cystic fibrosis, sickle cell anemia, and more, as well as other tests for donors of Jewish ancestry, including screening for carriers of Tay Sachs and other genetic risks). Cryo banks are licensed by the board of health, require a quarantine period on all sperm, and include a detailed medical history, STI scans and physical examinations for donors. Banks require donors to relinquish

parental rights, which eliminates the obstacle of having to hire legal counsel to sort out parentage. The simplicity of using someone's genetic material and *not* having to navigate personal relationships, roles, parenting or co-parenting decisions, can be really appealing, as well.

o**Disadvantages** include cost that can be prohibitive (often $500 to $700 per vial, which may or may not include overnight shipping). Because the sperm has been frozen, it is also less viable, so most fertility consultants recommend using 2 vials per ovulation cycle, making the cost of sperm astonishing. Depending on the regulations and practices of the individual sperm bank, there may be many, many other families who use the same sperm, meaning that there may be scores or hundreds of donor siblings out in the world. While ICI is easy to do at home, pursuing IUI may require the services of a doctor / midwife / nurse, depending on individual state regulations and personal preferences.

Getting Sperm Into Your Uterus

The time-tested method of "natural" insemination or vaginal-penile sex, sperm is inserted into the vagina in slurry of seminal fluid. Sperm swim out of the seminal fluid, and into the vaginal fluid (cervical mucous), following it up to its source, through the cervix, into the fallopian tubes, and finally into the uterus. There are a few different options for getting sperm up there, and some depend on the type of sperm you're using. Fertile cervical mucous can help to filter out poorly performing sperm, as well as protecting sperm from the acidic environment of the vagina. The cervix is a magical safe haven for sperm, and fresh sperm can stop there and release slowly for up to 3 days (for frozen sperm, that's about 24 hours).

•**Soft cups** are used to basically place sperm as close to the cervix as possible and to keep it from leaking out. The Instead cup (a disposable menstrual cup) is a better choice than something like a diva cup because it is shallower and more flexible, so it keeps the sperm closer to the cervix.

•**Intra Cervical Insemination (ICI)** uses a tomcat catheter (not a turkey baster!) to insert sperm directly into the cervix, which shortens their journey. Chances are around 25% with this method. Note that ICI often isn't the best choice for someone who has known fertility issues.

•**Intra Uterine Insemination (IUI)** uses the same catheter as in ICI, but instead of stopping in the cervix, it is actually threaded all the way up into the uterus. IUI bypasses all the cervical mucous and it's filtering capacity, so sperm used for IUI has to be "washed" – that is, you can't use fresh sperm for IUI. IUI sperm is also about $100 more expensive than ICI sperm. Plenty of folks do IUI at home, but depending on your level of comfort with a speculum and catheter, etc., it can be a little tricky. Many people choose to do IUI with a doctor or midwife.

•**In Vitro Fertilization (IVF)** is a method in which an egg and is placed in a lab dish with sperm to ensure fertilization. The embryo (with 1 or 2 fertilized eggs) is then placed in the uterus. Sperm for IVF is less expensive, but the total cost is astronomical (a single cycle can range between $8,000 and $20,000 and medications required for IVF are also wildly expensive.

Some A&P
•**Ovaries** produce sex cells, secrete hormones (estrogen and progesterone), and are home of the cycle of development and maturation of follicles ("eggs-in-waiting"[1]). Several-to-many follicles develop simultaneously, and between days 8 and 12 of the follicular cycle, one of them becomes primary. That follicle continues to develop and grows the ovum, which is released into the fallopian tubes and travels down to the pelvic cavity at ovulation.

•**Corpus luteum** means "yellow body" and is what remains after the ovum has been released. The corpus lutuem directs the second half of the cycle (the luteal phase) and is responsible for much of the hormonal production and orchestration, as well.

•**Endometrium** – 2 layers of tissues – basal layer lies underneath, is unchanging. Functional layer grows and is expelled in response to hormonal changes throughout the cycle.

○**Proliferative phase of the endometrium** happens alongside the **follicular phase of the ovarian cycle.** In response to high levels of estrogen, the endometrium proliferates. Under this influence, the endometrium thickens, develops glandular structure to conduct its own hormonal processes, and vasculature to deliver nutrients to developing tissues.

○**Secretory phase parallels the luteal phase of the ovary.** Once ovulation has occurred, the corpus luteum secretes large amounts of progesterone (this is why we talk about the second half of the cycle being progesterone dominant). There are still high amounts of estrogen alongside progesterone, and the dual effects of these hormones cause the endometrium to become *secretory tissue*. The glandular structure of the endometrium enlarges, arteries begin to develop, the endometrium thickens even more, and the endometrium itself begins to secrete glycogen to nourish a fertilized ovum. If no fertilization occurs, progesterone production drops off, and the endometrium degenerates, and menstruation begins.

○**Menstrual phase** happens approximately 14 days after ovulation (in the textbook 28-day cycle). The corpus luteum begins to break down if fertilization doesn't occur, and since the corpus luteum is the main source of hormone secretion at this point in the cycle, progesterone (and estrogen) also decline rapidly. Prostaglandins contribute to the breakdown of the endometrium's blood supply as well as triggering uterine contractions.

•The **Hypothalamus** secretes **GnRH** (gonadotropin releasing hormone, which signals to the pituitary to release **FSH** (follicle stimulating hormone), which is responsible for beginning the growth and maturation of the follicles in the ovary.

○As follicles develop in the ovary, they secrete more and more estrogen, which stimulates proliferation of the endometrium

○Eventually high estrogen triggers the hypothalamus to secrete more GnRH, which triggers simultaneous surges of **LH** (luteinizing hormone) and FSH in advance of ovulation.

▪This rise in LH is what's detected on ovulation predictor kits or OPKs. LH signals the final development of the egg, and finally signals the follicle to release the egg.

○**Ovulation** is the release of the egg from the corpus luteum

▪After ovulation, FSH levels drops fairly quickly and LH levels decline more slowly

•Estrogen is responsible for the development of secondary sex characteristics – growth of breast/ chest tissue, pubic hair, genitals, female pattern fat deposition (hips, chest, butt)

○Stimulates growth of endometrial lining

•**Luteal Phase**

○After follicle releases egg, what remains becomes corpus luteum – yellow body

○Corpus luteum produces progesterone, which helps to sustain pregnancy, and estrogen

○Right after egg is released, you see a rise in temperature – direct result of higher progesterone in luteal phase. Charting temperatures for a few cycles can really help to hone in on when ovulation is about to happen, as well as to get a look at progesterone activity.

○Progesterone stimulates proliferation of epithelial lining (proliferative phase)

Tracking/ Charting

•**Day 1** of your chart is the first day of menstruation (full flow). If you have spotting, that should be charted at the *end* of the previous cycle.

•**Temperature** – because basal body temperature rises in direct response to the spike in progesterone that happens right after ovulation, charting temperatures for a few months can give you a retrospective look at when the rise in progesterone happens in relationship to other fertile signs. Essentially the rise in temperature marks the end of the fertile window.

○Don't wake up just to take your temperature! This is one of the hugest sources of stress for folks trying to conceive and the world is stressful enough without having to get neurotic and hypervigilant about taking your temp at the right time everyday. Just make a note of when you take your temp.

○If you get up in the morning to go to the bathroom and head back to bed, take your temp when you get up and just make a note of the time.

○The number of days that temperature stays elevated also shows the length of the luteal phase and the relative strength of progesterone compared to estrogen. Short luteal phases can be indications of estrogen excess.

•**Cervical mucous** – check before you go to the bathroom. Clean hands – put a finger or two inside the vagina before you pee, feel the consistency of the mucous. It's important to check 1-2 times a day in the days leading up to ovulation.

○It isn't super important to check cervical mucous throughout the whole cycle, but it *is* important to check frequently around ovulation.

○Mucous progresses from dry to gummy / sticky to creamy / milky, then to egg white mucous

○The most fertile mucous is what's called egg white mucous – slippery, clear, stretchy, thin, gooey, and copious

○Egg white mucous can last for several days, so track *how* stretchy (e.g. 2 inches of stretch, 3 inches of stretch)

•**Cervical quality** - Standing with a leg up, use two fingers, reach into the vagina. The walls of the vagina are ridged tunnel of muscular tissue, and the cervix is the round, smooth thing you feel with the small dimple in the middle. The dimple in the middle is the os, the opening of the cervix.

○Sometimes there's a change in position in response to ovulation—often the cervix is lower, easier to reach, but the position of the cervix can vary from person to person.

○Low, firm, closed – nonfertile (before ovulation, and closes up again after ovulation)

○High, soft, open – the cervix opens to make it easier for the sperm to swim up! It's important to chart during the period of openness so you know the point at which the cervix is the softest and most open

○Can use a speculum to track changes to cervix, as well.

•**Other things**

○Ovulation sensation – chart any cramping, pain, sensation, fullness, twinges, with ovulation (and R or L side)

○Mood – people often feel a shift in perception with ovulation, either feeling more creative, more spiritually connected, inspired, elated, etc.

○Sex drive – often higher at ovulation

○Sleep

Other Tools

•Ovulation Predictor Kit (OPK) – The OPK measures LH. Recall that high levels of estrogen trigger release of LH, then the ovaries pick up the signal of the LH, which triggers the final development of the egg and, finally, the release of the egg from the follicle. By the point at which the OPK registers LH, ovulation is likely to occur in the next 12 to 48 hours, which is quite a large window, especially for anyone using sperm that they worked hard (traveled, paid of a lot of money for) to get. Because the predictive window for ovulation is so large, it's important to test at least twice a day. You want to be able to register the first point at which LH is high. That is, if you only test once a day at 8am, your LH could spike at 10am, and by the time you test the next morning, you're already 22 hours into your 12-48 hour window.
○Clear Blue Brand (classic, not the Digital Advanced) with the smiley faces is recommended. One fertility specialist I know turned me on to this pro tip: if you look at the test line (the one that turns blue so you know the test is working), there will often be a faint line before you get the smiley face. The test instructions say to not pay attention to this, but it's got valuable information! It shows when your LH levels are rising, even if they aren't yet high enough to trigger the smiley face. So pay attention to those early faint lines and chart them!
○Because of the changes that happen in LH production, OPK's aren't as reliable for folks over 40.

•Apps are not super useful. Ovulation predictor apps rely on algorithms, averages, and 'norms' of people who are not you. They also don't tell you anything about your other fertile signs, like how long *your* fertile window is, or which point in the fertile window is the *most* fertile, so they can really lead you astray.

Improving Fertility

It turns out that regardless of your sexual orientation and your access or lack of access to sperm, many therapeutics for enhancing fertility are the same for all uterus.having people (thank goodness). The foundation of fertility enhancement should be, naturally, optimizing diet. Throwing 'fertility herbs' at a protein or EFA deficiency doesn't work and can mask a serious issue that has downstream effects in every single body system. Dietary regimens should focus on improving nutrient density, assessing for and removing inflammatory foods and lifestyle factors, assessing and addressing digestive dysfunction, addressing nutrient deficiencies, and stabilizing blood sugar. Phew. It feels important to say, however, that removing food allergens can be a lynchpin in some fertility cases – if you think of it in terms of just immune system activation and subsequent inflammation – an unidentified food allergy is enough to keep the immune system on high alert and inflammation at a low boil, all of which has serious impact on reproductive function. Food allergies can cause chronic elevation of stress hormones, which wreaks havoc with hormonal communication feedback loops, as well as contributing to liver tension and stagnation, which in turn increases the circulation and reabsorption of hormones from the hepatic system, increasing hormone levels in the body.

While I'm not sure if there is in fact an increased incidence of estrogen excess (either frank or relative) these days, it often seems like estrogen dominant hormone imbalances are the norm rather than the exception. But again, the sample size of folks that I see isn't random (obviously, because most people are coming to see me for a specific reason or health challenge). In any case, some changes in the physiology of modern uterus.having people may contribute to higher incidence of hormonal imbalances. We see increasingly early menarche, people having fewer babies later on in their potential baby.having careers, and returning to work earlier than parents of the past might have needed to. Combine these factors with vast amounts of processed sugars and dietary carbohydrates, xenoestrogens in the food supply and everything.supply, greater chemical load, etc., and you can start to understand how these imbalances would be so common.

Considerations in Fertility Enhancement

Development of egg relies on healthy development of corpus luteum, which relies on healthy development of follicle, which relies on, among other things, appropriate hormonal firing and a nutrient rich diet.

Specific nutrient recommendations:

- Good quality multivitamin
- EFA supplementation (or eating a pound or more of good quality, deep sea, cold water fish per week – more if you have inflammation)
- Antioxidants – eat berries! Drink herbal tea!
  ○ CoQ10 – 100mg 3x day. CoQ10 is an important cofactor for mitochondrial health, and naturally the formation of human life is a very energy-demanding process.
  ○ Green tea, turmeric, rosemary, gingko, hawthorn berries and other brightly colored berries, purple foods (purple potatoes, eggplant, purple cabbage).
- B vitamin

Liver clearance – estrogen is cleared through the CYP450 system in the liver (this is the same system that clears many-to-most pharmaceutical drugs, exogenous hormones, and more). Enhancing liver clearance can go a long way toward shifting hormonal imbalances, but only in someone who is nutritionally replete. Enhancing liver clearance without first building the baseline of nutrition can make people feel awful, and also lose their trust in you. Liver function requires myriad nutrients, including a slew of amino acids (so assess for adequate protein and digestion of protein), essential fatty acids, B vitamins, and minerals (selenium, zinc, magnesium, molybdenum being the most important), so starting with nutritional assessment is important.

- Brassicaceae – the cabbage family contain a potent upregulator of CYP450, indole-3-carbinol (also available as an isolated supplement). Of course, green vegetables also contain so many other

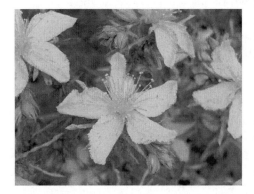

important nutrients and good fiber, so increasing these foods in the diet benefits baby.having people in myriad ways. Brassicas include cabbage, Brussels sprouts, arugala, kale, kohlrabi, mustard greens, collard greens, cauliflower, and on and on…

- **St. John's Wort. Hypericum** is a potent inducer of liver clearance (CYP450) and while contraindicated with many pharmaceuticals, can help tremendously in improving clearance of endogenous hormones through the liver. It is especially useful where there is a downcast, dark edge to cyclical mood changes before menstruation (often an effect of estrogen excess). It can also help to shift feelings of stuckness that can accompany hormone imbalances. Note that St. John's wort as tea or tincture is generally pretty gentle, but concentrated or standardized extracts can sometimes move things too quickly through the liver, and can have some side effects like skin eruptions.

•**Bitters** – most bitters enhance liver function (specifically phase 1)

•**Dandelion, Berberine containing plants, Milk thistle**

•**Liver tension:** liver tension is a common and subclinical presentation that is relatively common, especially accompanying sedentary lifestyle, pharmaceutical use, food allergies, etc.
oSymptoms include cold periphery (hands or feet) and heat signs in the middle (diarrhea, menstrual cramps or irregularities), often includes some psychosocial / spiritual symptoms (tension, irritability, frustration, anger, depression, loud voice). May develop into more overt symptoms, including red face, headache, or acne (again – look for heat symptoms in the middle), allergies, or high blood pressure.

o**Liver relaxants:** Mints, Citrus, Rosemary, Lavender, Peony, Fennel, and Rose. Note that many of these herbs have simultaneous actions on the digestive and nervous systems – many are relaxant nervines, relaxant to smooth muscle and/ or skeletal muscle, as well as aromatic and carminative. Many also have an affinity for the spiritual heart.

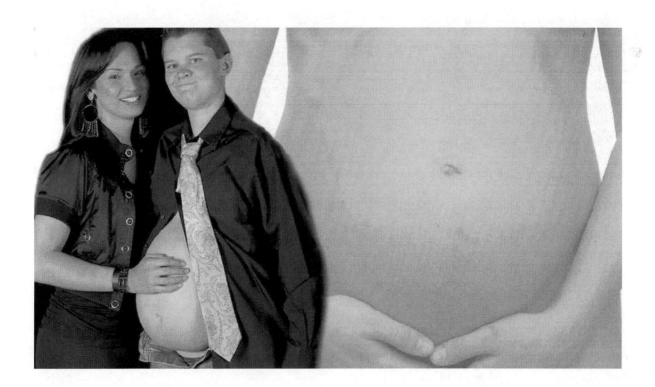

Herbs

•**Uterine tonics** – Raspberry leaf (*Rubus idaeus*) is the most well known, well tolerated, and safe uterine tonics available. I've seen astounding things happen with the addition of a raspberry leaf based fertility tea, including regulation of irregular cycles, elimination of menstrual cramping, relief of PMS, and more. When in doubt, using raspberry leaf is probably a good idea. Because of its tonic and astringent action, it can aggravate dryness in some climates and people. Combine with Shatavari (or Marshmallow if more demulcent action on the gut is required or linden if more emotional heart support is needed).

•We don't have time here to go into specific indications for these, but I almost always use specific indications for fertility differentials, if not in formulatory strategy for other systems.

•**More stimulant uterine tonics as necessary.**
•**Astringents**
•**Antispasmodics**
•**Emmenagogues**
•**Pelvic decongestants**
•**Nervines**
•**Circulatory stimulants**
•**White Peony** (*Paeonia lactiflora*) is among my most used herbs for progesterone deficiency or relative estrogen excess. Peony helps to relax liver tension while also enhancing progesterone production and helping to lengthen the luteal phase. Can help to reduce prolactin levels (often elevated in celiac disease, by the way). Peony also nourishes blood and acts as a smooth muscle relaxant, so can be helpful for menstrual cramps and blood deficiency.
•

•**Vitex** (*Agnus castus*) is quite reliable for correcting relative progesterone deficiency and estrogen excess. In my own practice, I have had varied results with tinctures, so it is one of the few botanicals of which I generally recommend a standardized concentrated extract. Standard Process MediHerb and Gaia both have excellent products with which I've had great success. It is also important to note that Vitex generally works as long as it's taken, and many people are disappointed to find that their previous hormonal milieus shift back to 'normal' once they cease using it. For this reason98 , it is always important to attend to underlying cause.

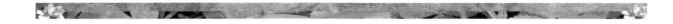

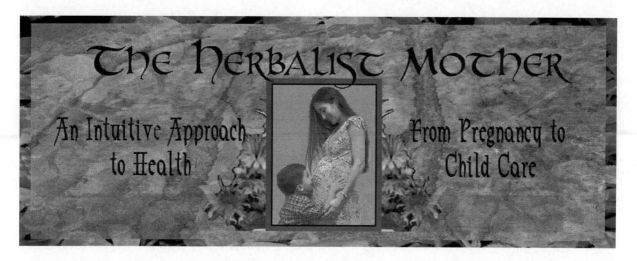

The Herbalist Mother

An Intuitive Approach to Health

From Pregnancy to Child Care

A woman's belly grows with child, expanding not just physical flesh but psyche and spirit as well. Her bones and joints may ache from the pressures and weight. She knows her body was built for this. Yet the seeming impossibility of it circles around her mind. Stories from the ancestors and from well-meaning family, friends, and caregivers fill her and drive her to think so many things. Some of them built on truth, many on legend. Strength, fear, holiness, these emotions fit congruently together in her brain, the very organ that is now shape shifting more than her body. Her mother mind is forming. Yet what it whispers to her may be confusing in the face of all the authority, well-wishers and storytellers out there. She needs a safe space to help her call forth her new self. The self yet to be completely born until her child is decades old. This support needn't come from educating or teaching. It can be in the form of trusting what this mother already knows. To celebrate and make holy a space for her to emerge, to be still and listen to her own story, an ongoing commitment to creating this space is really important and must not just be saved for a few hours at the end of pregnancy during a blessing way or baby shower.

Anointing & Adorning
The Awakening Mother

by Sabrina Lutes

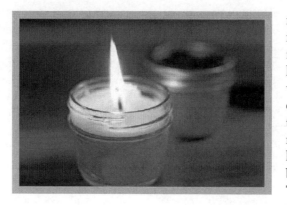

The plants lend themselves to this process so very seamlessly. The scent of flowers can calm and center. Growing a garden can strengthen and focus. Collecting wild plants hones our gratitude and willingness to trust. These are effective in tuning into our yet to be born babes and children.

As I carried my babe in my belly, I would take miles long walks in the forests surrounding my home. The Florida heat was buffered by the great oaks and pines. I used these hikes to strengthen my legs and pelvis and to help my child get into the best position for our birth. The soft, sandy earth cushioned my foot fall as my feet grew and widened as they so often do in pregnancy. These were the times I felt most strong in my mothering mind, times where the trees and the earth and my partner were all that surrounded me. My mind and body focused on the task at hand. Walking…breathing…vital processes. My belief now, after attending many, many women in their pregnancies and births, including my own, is that women tune into the nature of what's before them much more easily when they are not bombarded with information. When they have been nurtured with symbols,

165

hands on touch, art, and surrounded by the natural world, both by heading outside and by immersing adorning their bodies and home with earth, water, and the green beings.

How can we as healers and caregivers, lovers and friends help nourish that instinctual knowing in mothers? First we must trust birth. Trust that it is a very raw process. That women experience it in so many different ways and in so many different cultural constructs. Trust that while we may have an educated knowledge we cannot make a woman hear that information. She must feel into her innate knowing and only in her own time.

As I attended more births as a birth doula, the less I carried with me. My birth bag became lighter. The more I began listening and honoring the space the woman was creating in her birth. I became quiet and used the elemental tools when needed (water, candlelight, simple herbal infused oils, soft spoken word). The items I initially packed so carefully went unused or felt burdensome.

I love that the plants and elements can convey more than our words or even stories can. Words often become misinterpreted, muddled, or sink deeply into psyche and change thoughts and feelings within the listener. Often this is healing, but just as often it is not. Towards the end of my active practice as a doula and in the last few years opening and softening into my own mothering, and community building I have found that intentions conveyed through gentle actions reach much further into someone's heart. It bolsters them in ways wordy education or teachings cannot. So, to the caregivers, I feel that this way of working with woman, particularly women in their pregnancy and later parenting, is such an important ally in our healing modalities.

Some of the things that I began doing, felt so very, very simplistic. My ego would get in the way and question the very essence of what I was trying to convey. I felt childish. Yet, what slowly became apparent is that the child self was what was very necessary for me to do the work that needed to be done. I chose to approach my tasks

with as much innocence as I could muster. I needed to lay down the part myself that needed to be recognized as the expert, the one who was certified and educated. This brought humility to my soul and gave me the ability to speak from an authentic place. I began asking questions. Questions about what the woman felt soothed her, where she felt the best. What she could do to bring those things front and center into her pregnancy, her birth and later how those things could help her in mothering.

By asking these questions and simply allowing her a moment to recognize the small ways in her day she could give herself care and realizing that practicing these routinely can carry her in those tough moments during and after birth. I would also suggest we as caregivers, while engaging in these conversations, to actually show the woman how to integrate her knowing into a physical, anointing form. If you are visiting, go ahead and bring a small muslin bag of dried rose petals and draw a foot bath. Have a cup of tea with her and sew a rice sock filled with botanicals that are pleasant (while you're at it, make a plain one in case scents are too much in labor). This can be heated in a microwave (check for hot spots before placing on the mother) to soothe an aching back and straining muscles. Go for a walk together and gather flowers and botanicals to create labor and postpartum treatments. Sing together as you work. Listen to her as she shares her thoughts, fears, expectations and dreams. Listen deeply to her. Fill her mothering cup with a softened expression and open heart. A small blessing after each trimester would be a wonderful way to tune in to the awakened mother she is becoming. Allow her to grieve if she needs to, to weep, to shed tears of joy. Her body is changing and aching and growing. Give her permission to feel all that she is feeling. Brush her hair, rub her hands, scrub her feet with ground flower petals. Drape a rose bead necklace around her neck. Paint her belly with clay or henna. Create dried herb mandalas. Dig in the dirt, dance. When we celebrate as well as deeply listen we create those anchors for a woman in a time where she is both deeply in the physical world, but also absorbed in an otherworldly place.

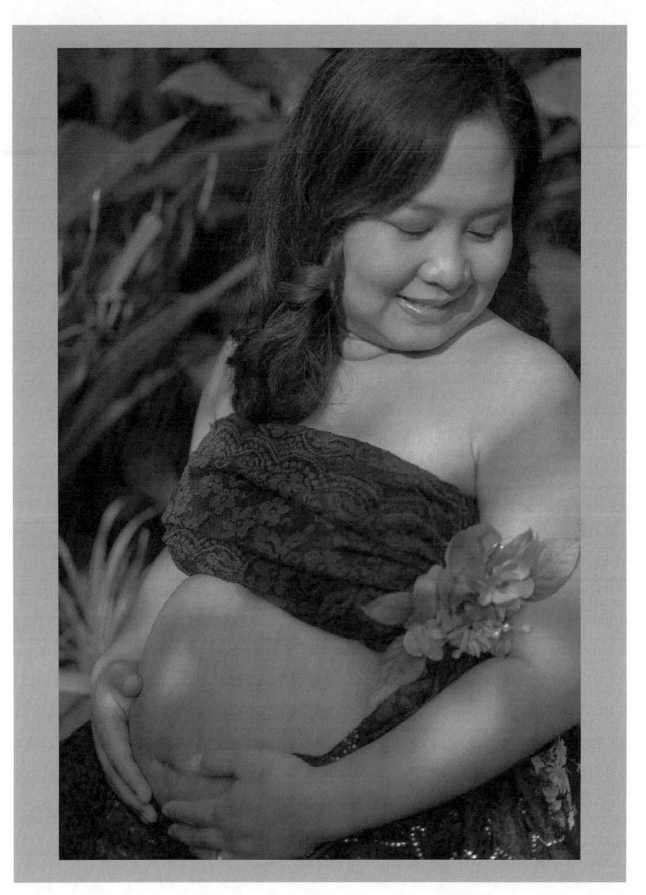

A List of Ideas

•Milk and honey-nourishment, tenderness-use in bath or foot bath

•Rose beads for a necklace

•Ground flower pedals for a scrub: A lovely recipe for this is ground and sifted rose or lavender petals that are mixed into a paste with honey.

•Float flowers in a bath

•Muslin bag of herbs for foot bath or bath- calendula, rose, chamomile, lavender, milky oat, sea salt

•Candlelight- beeswax is my preference, especially when working with mothers and babies

•Teas- nettle, red raspberry, oat straw, hibiscus, any that are not contraindicated in pregnancy

•Henna

•Clay body paint

•Infused oils, skin soothing herbs like calendula, aromatics like spearmint, lavender, amber, vanilla

•Mix an herbal tea formula for pregnancy, decorate the jar with a beautiful label, add a prayer or symbol that catches the mother's eye to remind her to slow down and think about her growing baby

•Begin formulating postpartum blends for her, with her.

•Pot up a few plants for her to tend during pregnancy, possibly one that she could plant along with her placenta if she chooses to do so.

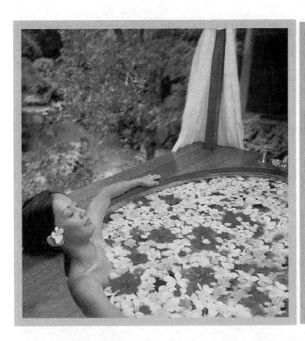 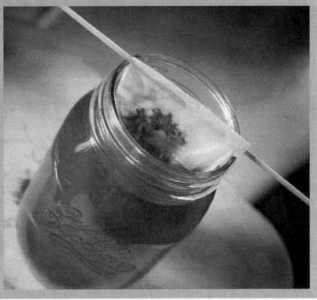

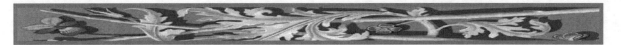

SO YOU'RE HAVING A FREEBIRTH
PART I:

Herbs to Have on Hand

by Astrid Grove

Some families are finding themselves disillusioned with the way in which modern obstetrics is medicalizing birth. Some women and birthing people are choosing to birth at home unattended. Some call this an "unassisted birth" or a "freebirth". This essentially means they will birth without a trained birth attendant- be it midwife or obstetrician. She is autonomous, birthing in her own way, with her own rhythms, unobstructed. This looks different for every woman. Some women want to be completely alone while others may hire a birth photographer, a doula, have all her other 5 kids there and her husband and her mother and her best friend! Some women will receive prenatal care, and birth unattended. Some women will do their own prenatal care without ever seeing an OB or midwife.

As I bare witness to what seems to be a fairly clear rise in unassisted births, it leaves me wondering why women are not able to find a midwife to support them to birth their way. I could launch into a long monologue about the history of obstetrics and the persecution of the wise woman that has been happening for thousands of years, but I will not do that...not in this article anyway. I see this rise in unassisted

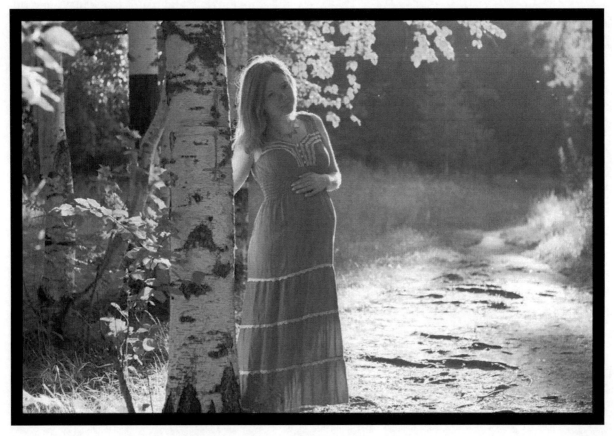

births as a reclaiming of the divine feminine. Women and families are starting to wake up and see that the "system" of birth, the "business" of birth does not have their best interests in mind. The system finds value in money, regulations, protocol. It is not based on evidence, it does not consider what may be best for the family, the birthing woman, or the baby- as individuals. It is based on fear, instead of trust. I say trust…I do not mean blind trust. I mean educated and evidence based trust. Trust grounded in her inner knowing which is supported by evidence.

The birthing woman finds value in being heard, being honored, being respected, and being held lovingly in what is certainly one of life's most powerful transformations. Not only that, motherhood at its finest is VITAL to a thriving human race. It is essentially one of the most important acts to support! A woman who is supported to become a mother through her own unique and divine way, has more potential to become a fierce mother, a bonded mother, a devoted mother.

This article is specifically addressing families who are choosing a planned unattended and out of hospital birth. It may also be helpful for herbalists that are working with families choosing this route. I hope that it can offer some herbal advice that may prevent harm or injury for the birthing person.

I am a part of several Facebook groups for freebirth and there is often discussion of what someone could have on hand in case they need a little more support in the birthing process. Of course, if one is experiencing an emergency it's best to call 911! Luckily, for the healthy woman childbirth risk is quite low if she is supported to listen to her body and her baby and surrender into her primal birthing rhythm. That being said it is my wish and prayer that we can have more midwives who are trained and called to support women to birth on their own terms. If this were the case I imagine some women who are choosing unassisted birth would instead choose a midwife who supports her autonomy.

I have decided to split this article into four parts. We will start with pregnancy, then birth, then postpartum and then a final article on preconception. Also, this topic is incredible rich and there is a lot I could share from many perspectives. I will be focusing this series of articles on herbal medicine specifically.

Let's start with prenatal care. First, I recommend daily nourishing herbal infusions. This brings a solid foundation of nutrition. Some people take prenatal vitamins, others do not. For the woman who has a whole foods diet rich in protein, fat, and vegetables along with nourishing herbal infusions, I would not necessarily recommend a supplement. Of course, it is every woman's personal choice.

Making an Infusion

You will need dried, cut and sifted herbs. (Mountain Rose is a wonderful company to purchase bulk herbs from). You will also need a quart jar with a lid, a chopstick or a similar object for stirring, and a quart of water. First put the kettle on the stove and boil the water. While the water is heating up, weigh one ounce of the dried herb and put it into the quart jar. Generally one ounce by weight of dried and sifted herb is equal to one cup by volume (this is not the case for red clover blossoms). Pour the boiling water over the herb filling the jar, and using your chopstick poke at the herb making sure it is all immersed in the water and add more boiling water if need be to fill the jar. Put the lid on and let sit for 4-8 hours.

I usually make the infusion at night before going to bed and then strain in the morning. To strain, I usually use a metal bowl and a mesh strainer. I pour the water and herbs into the mesh strainer with the metal bowl underneath. Be sure to vigorously squeeze all of the infusion from the herb. Compost the herb and drink the infusion. Be sure to refrigerate what you don't drink right away.

Here are the infusions I recommend:

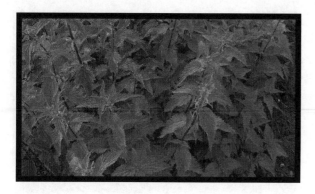

Nettle leaf and stem (*Urtica dioica*)

Nettle is my first choice of infusions to encourage a healthy pregnancy. Nettle contains every mineral needed by the human body including 1000 mg of calcium in each quart of infusion. Drink freely and enjoy this green drink rich in chlorophyll, protein, antioxidants, carotenes, linoleic/formic/linolenic acid, vitamin E, glucoquinones, and phytosterols.

Nettle leaf increases the iron carrying capacity of the blood (anti-anemic). Nettle leaf also helps the body stabilize blood sugar, regulate weight, reduce fatigue and improve stamina, increase vitamin K in the blood, improve thyroid function and restore adrenal functioning.

Comfrey leaf (*Symphytum uplandica*)

Comfrey leaf is rich in minerals, proteins, vitamins and alantoin. Alantoin helps to make tissues more elastic. Comfrey leaf helps to strengthen uterine muscles, perineal tissue, uterine ligaments, bladder, and yoni. Comfrey leaf also helps to prevent complications like pre-eclampsia, helps pelvic bones be more flexible, and increases the iron in blood.

Oatstraw (*Avina sativa*)

Oatstraw is rich in calcium and also the minerals and vitamins needed to help the body assimilate calcium. Oatstraw infusion stabilizes blood sugar, helps one to have a more restful sleep, and helps one to be more emotionally resilient. Oatstraw provides steroidal saponins which nourish the pancreas, liver and adrenals. This infusion also helps to make blood vessels more elastic thus reducing hemorrhoids and varicose veins. In addition, this herb strengthens the tissues of the bladder, urethra, and yoni.

Red Clover (*Trifolium pratense*)

Red Clover is rich in protein, iron, chromium, B vitamins, and phytoestrogens. Red clover increases energy, helps to normalize the thyroid gland, nourishes mucous membranes, relieves cystitis, calms the nerves, strengthens the immune system and prevents cancer.

Note: Red Clover contains coumarins, a blood thinner, and therefore can increase the risk of hemorrhage if overconsumed. I recommend drinking no more than a quart of infusion 1-2 times per week.

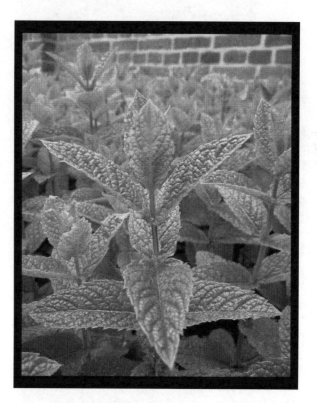

Peppermint (*Mentha piperita*)

Peppermint is a delightful herb, as most of us have experienced. It is soothing to the stomach and discourages flatulence, increases body temperature and therefore is healing when a cold is present. Peppermint contains B1 (Thiamine) which strengthens nerves and eases emotions; B2 (Riboflavin) which increases energy, decreases cancer, and lends to healthy skin; and B6 (pyridoxine) which improves immune functioning. Peppermint also contains folic acid, carotenes, calcium, iron, phosphorus for strong and flexible bones and more energy, and potassium.

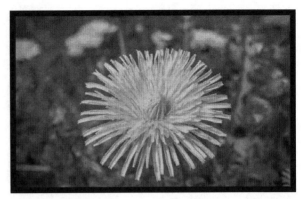

Liver Support

In addition to nourishing herbal infusions, it is important to take measures to support the pregnant woman's liver. I prefer Dandelion root over all other liver support herbs for its gentleness, it is easy to access, and cheap or free if you harvest this amazing weed yourself.

There are many ways you can consume Dandelion root. My personal favorite is the product Dandy Blend, available on Amazon. It is a coffee substitute drink like Cafix or Pero, though I don't use it to substitute coffee... because coffee is essential to life! I do enjoy some dandy blend in hot water, a teaspoon of raw and local honey, and a few tablespoons of raw and organic goat's milk. It is gluten free, but not grain free (it has barley and rye).

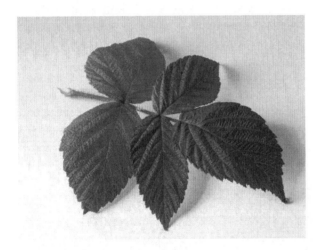

Raspberry leaf and stem (*Rubus species*)

Raspberry leaf is second to Nettle in beneficial aspects for the pregnant woman. The leaf can be brewed as a tea or an infusion. Because the tannins in the leaf are intense on the palate, I usually choose to brew nettle and raspberry leaf together.

Raspberry leaf is rich in minerals including phosphorus, potassium, calcium and iron and vitamins including vitamin A, B, C and E.

Raspberry leaf helps to tone the muscles of the uterus and thus reduces the intensity of the sensation during labor and after birth. The leaf also helps to facilitate the birth of the placenta and to prevent miscarriage and hemorrhage. Some herbalists do not recommend the use of raspberry before the end of the first trimester in order to prevent early miscarriage.

I also quite enjoy Dandelion vinegar. In the spring I harvest whole, tender Dandelion plants...roots, leaves, buds and flowers. I chop up the whole plant, put it into a jar, and cover with apple cider vinegar. I let this steep for at least 6 weeks. I use the vinegar for salad dressings and to put directly on cooked greens. I love the pickled Dandelion plant to eat with just about anything.

You can also just buy Dandelion root tea bags. I actually just did this for the first time recently and it's quite enjoyable. Sometimes a dropperful or two a day of the tincture can suffice as well. It's also very easy to make tincture, the same process as making vinegar, except instead of using apple cider vinegar, I use 100 proof vodka.

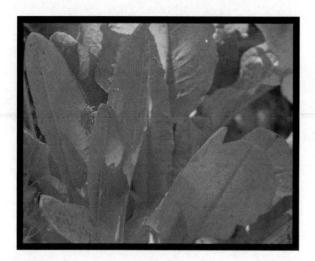

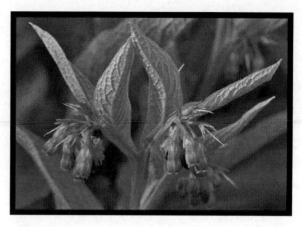

Anemia

A common complaint of pregnancy is anemia. The best way to treat anemia is to avoid it! Eat a diet that includes plenty of iron rich foods (including but not limited to egg yolk, liver, dried fruit, leafy greens), cook in cast iron, drink Nettles. For some women, extra measures must be taken. If you start to feel dizzy, faint, tired, under your bottom eyelid is pale…you are probably anemic. If this is the case, Yellowdock root tincture can be very helpful. If you take 2 droppersful up to two times per day about 15 minutes before you eat an iron rich meal it will help your body to absorb the iron. You can also make a syrup.

Iron Syrup

• Equal parts of Yellowdock root, Dandelion root, Nettle leaf (dried)
• 1 quart of water
• 1 cup of honey
• ½ cup of molasses

Put about 2 cups of herbs into pot with a quart of water. Bring the mixture to a boil, then turn to simmer. Simmer until the liquid is reduced by half (decoction). Strain and add a cup of honey and ½ cup of molasses (or to taste, this may be too sweet for some and not sweet enough for others). Keep in the refrigerator. Take 1-4tbl per day.

Yeast Infection

Another common complaint is yeast infection: Yeast (*Candida albicans*) is naturally present in 5-20% of healthy women's yoni's. Yeast flourishes in a warm, moist mucous surface in an acid environment. When the acidity of the yoni drops, the yeasts thrive. Lactobacilli are healthy bacteria that prevent yeast overgrowth and thrive in acidic vaginas. You will notice that you have yeast overgrowth by the sweet smelling cottage cheese like secretions. You may also notice itching and irritation.

If you are having the symptoms of a yeast infection, one simple and effective remedy to ease the discomfort is a nice herbal bath. There are several different herbal infusions I have found to be effective. Comfrey leaf infusion added to a bath is very soothing due to it's mucilaginous nature. Oatstraw infusion calms the tissues with it's soothing quality. You can either pour a quart of infusion of one or both of these into you bath and soak for 20 minutes.

Now that your tissues are soothed, let's address the overgrowth. I have found that taking an oral probiotic and using a probiotic suppository daily is most helpful. I like Femdoph brand. Insert two capsules into your yoni tucked up by your cervix every other day for 14 days. You may want to wear a panty liner as this can be leaky. You can also simply use yogurt that is free of sugars and any additives. A simple, organic yogurt like Stonyfield is best. You can scoop a tablespoon or so onto you fingers and gently swipe it up into your yoni, daily. This will help to re-establish healthy bacteria.

If after 14 days of this daily treatment you are still suffering, the yeast infection might be bacterial in nature. In this case I would insert an unknicked garlic clove at night, tucked up by your cervix, and remove it in the morning. Do this for 5 days at most. You can follow this up with another round of baths and probiotics.

Urinary Tract Infection (UTI)

If you feel you are brewing a UTI, don't hesitate to treat right away. Symptoms are commonly burning with urination and mild discomfort or even mild cramping in the bladder. Sometimes UTI's can be asymptomatic in pregnancy. First thing to do if you suspect a UTI is to stop eating all sugar and simple carbohydrates. Hydrate! Drink lots and lots of water and infusions! 100 oz. a day is not too much.

Remember that an untreated UTI can lead to contractions and preterm labor so it's good to be proactive. Avoiding antibiotics is possible if treated right away and with the following remedies. It is best to avoid antibiotics in pregnancy so as not to kill healthy bacteria or stress the kidneys, but if the herbal remedies don't work it may be necessary.

Unsweetened cranberry juice- Drink up to 8 oz every hour for the day that you first begin to feel the UTI. Cranberries create an inhospitable environment for the bacteria. You can also munch on cranberries and blueberries.

Tea of Uva Ursi (*Arctostaphylos uva-ursi*)- Uva ursi can kill the bacteria if used correctly. Make an infusion with the leaves. Drink one cup per day for 7-10 days, not to exceed 10 days. Be aware that because Uva ursi is diuretic we must be sure we are well hydrated so as not to become dehydrated. Also be sure to continue taking it even for several days after symptoms abate.

If the infection is still present after these remedies, I would move on to Echinacea root tincture (*Echinacea purpurea or Echinacea angustofolia*) taking 2 dropperfulls every 2 hours for 7-10 days and no longer.

Miscarriage Prevention

A possible miscarriage can be a frightening and intense experience for some in early pregnancy. I have found a simple remedy that will help keep a pregnancy that doesn't want to let go. Of course, some pregnancies are not meant to come to fruition.

If there is spotting in the first trimester, accompanied by some cramping this remedy can be very helpful. Of course, pelvic rest and rest and hydration in general is important.

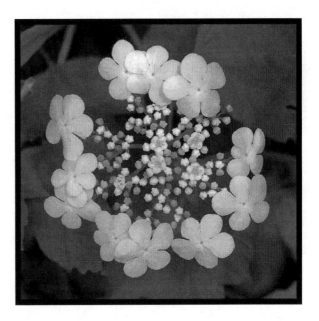

Early Miscarriage Brew

- Handful of Crampbark (*Viburnum opulus)* or
- Black Haw (*Viburnum prunifolium*)
- 2 Cinnamon sticks
- 2 tbsp Hibiscus flowers
- honey

Place the herbs into a pot of water (3 quarts of water). Bring to a boil and then cover and simmer for 20 or so minutes. Strain and sweeten with honey. Sip throughout the day. This is enough for a full day and night. Brew another batch the next day if the symptoms continue.

174

Postpartum Hemorrhage Prevention:

Postpartum hemorrhage is one of the main "concerns" in the freebirth community that I have seen...and for good reason! Postpartum hemorrhage is the number one way that women die in childbirth around the world. In the next article I will give some herbal remedies for stopping hemorrhage, let's focus here on prevention.

Diet! Eating a diet rich in nutrient dense foods is of utmost importance. Limit sugar and white flour. Eat bone broths (or veggie broths), eat 75-100 grams of protein per day, eat healthy fats, and lots of green leafy vegetables. Drink nourishing herbal infusions daily. Exercise gently every day. Relax, enjoy pregnancy as much as possible.

Be sure you are not anemic. If you don't know and are doing your own prenatal care and you are curious to know, you can buy a Tallquist and access your iron levels yourself. As a midwife I like to see my clients at 11.5 g/dl and above at birth. I have attended women with a hemoglobin as low as 9 g/dl.

Remember the lower the hemoglobin, the less blood you can safely lose at birth. If you have higher iron levels, you can lose more blood and still feel okay and heal well postpartum. Also every woman experiences blood loss differently. We will talk more about this in the next article.

Red Raspberry leaf infusion is especially recommended to tone the uterus. Strong uterine muscle will help your uterus to birth effectively, birth the placenta, and clamp down on the open blood vessels and prevent excess bleeding. If you have a history of miscarriage, I would avoid it in the first trimester. I personally find that my cravings for Red Raspberry leaf increase in my third trimester and especially the last 3-4 weeks of pregnancy. I sometimes drink a quart a day for days on end at that time.

Mood Stabilizing:

Pregnancy can certainly be a roller coaster ride of emotions! Hormones are surging, and this is another reason to support the liver (see above). By supporting the liver, we can help process the hormones and have less "stuck" energy and stuck emotions. Like I mentioned above, Dandelion root supports the liver. That being said, sometimes we just need to take the edge off. I have a few favorites that I recommend.

Motherwort tincture (*Leonorus cardiaca*)- The tincture is my go to for any stressful situation, or distress. I take 9 drops- 1 dropperful of motherwort tincture as needed. This plant works directly with our heart and our uterus (also a uterine tonic).

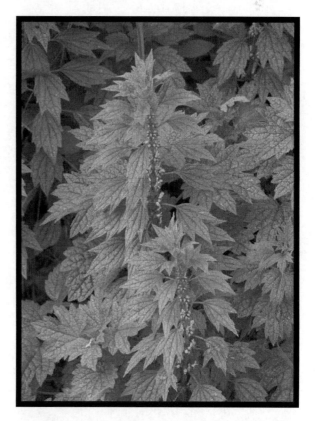

Add to your tea or water, and take a deep breath. Motherwort is here to soothe you. (Not recommended in first trimester or in general if there is a history of miscarriage).

175

Rose glycerite is a go to favorite calming remedy. Lemonbalm tea is the same. The glycerite is quite lovely as well.

Rescue Remedy- 5 flower essence. You can make this yourself or buy it.

Scullcap tincture- The dosage is 10-20 drops (not dropperfulls!) of fresh plant tincture. It can be very relaxing and even sleep inducing so best to take before bed or a nap.

Oatstraw infusion is also a nice calming herb to use in times of intense and fluctuating moods. Nettle infusion works with the adrenals and also can be helpful in this instance. If our adrenals are nourished, we will react less intensely to the mood swings. Another reason to drink your nourishing herbal infusions daily!

I hope this has been helpful! I have used every single one of the remedies mentioned above countless times when serving in my community as a midwife and in my own pregnancies. I will be offering virtual consultations soon via my website to women and families choosing an unassisted birth and wanting some support beforehand!

Blessed birthing!

Resources:

Healing Wise by Susun S. Weed
The New Menopausal Years by Susun S. Weed
Down There by Susun S. Weed

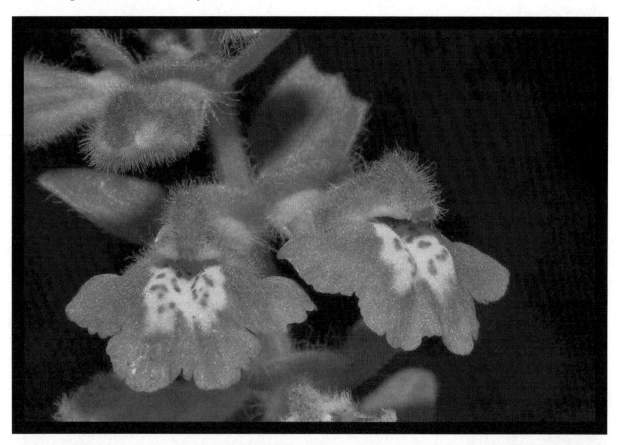

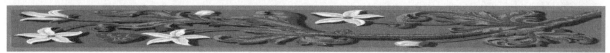

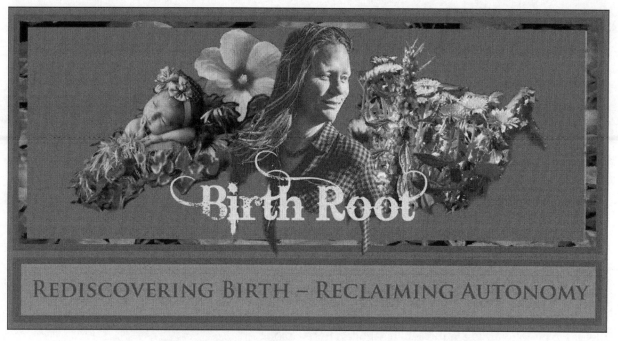

Birth Root

REDISCOVERING BIRTH – RECLAIMING AUTONOMY

SO YOU ARE HAVING A FREEBIRTH

Herbs to Have on Hand – Part II

by Astrid Grove

The Birthing Time

I am in strong support of autonomous birth. When listening to freebirth stories, I often see simple problems with simple solutions end up in an unnecessary transport to the hospital. With this segment of the series on freebirth, I strive to share with the birthing person and family simple tools to help support a healthy birth. In this way, I hope that more families can stay home and stay confident and healthy and enjoy the beauty that staying home can bring. I also honor that every birth unfolds in it's own special way and have no particular judgement about your birth story. Again, I stand in support.

I also want to mention that I am focusing on herbs in this series. This is a short article that will cover some true basics. Please don't take my authority, but instead do your own research and feel in your body what is true for you. In my experience, freebirthing people, birthing women, largely know their bodies and are in deep connection with their babies. There is an empowerment in this connection that triggers a deep sense of intuition and knowing. It is not a blind trust in birth, but instead an instinctual knowing that women have been birthing babies forever, and that both women and babies have the intrinsic knowing deep in their DNA...we know how to birth, we know how to be born. There are very few obstetric emergencies (namely cord prolapse, ruptured uterus, prolonged fetal distress, advanced infection). Most births are normal and uneventful, while simultaneously amazing and beautiful.

Many families are choosing freebirth so as to avoid an unnecessarily medically managed pregnancy and birth. Some families are choosing this way to birth because they feel comfortable and safe without outside support. Some families choose freebirth for religious reasons and others for financial reasons. I encourage all freebirthing families to really be clear about why they are choosing this route, so that they can have the best and most clear birth possible.

Below you will find some common complaints and some ways in which I have personally found helpful in moving through or alleviating the difficulty.

Preterm Labor

If you are having contractions before 36 weeks, there are a few methods you can use to support slowing everything down. First, drink a few glasses of water or nourishing herbal infusion to hydrate. Often dehydration causes contractions. Sit, put your feet up and rest for 30 minutes. If you are still feeling contractions coming and going, draw a bath with 2 cups of Epsom salts and soak for 20 minutes. The magnesium in Epsom salt is absorbed through your skin and then it binds with the serotonin in your brain, helping you to relax. Often this will be enough to slow everything down. If still things aren't slowing down, take 4 droppersful of either crampbark tincture (*Vibernum opulus*) or black haw tincture (*Viburnum prunifolium*). You can take up to 12 droppersfull per day of these tinctures to calm your uterus.

Sometimes a urinary tract infection can cause contractions. If all of the above remedies are not working, you may want to see if you have a UTI. If you have urine dip sticks then you can check for nitrites and leukocytes. They actually make a UTI dipstick now that you can just get at the drugstore. If they are high, then you may want to screen for an infection. You can order your own labs at HealthOneLabs at healthonelabs.com. You would want to order a urine culture.

(If you do in fact have a urinary tract infection, I wrote some simple cures in my last article in this column.)

If none of this is the case, and you are still experiencing preterm labor symptoms, you may want to rule out a vaginal infection (gonorrhea, Chlamydia, bacterial vaginosis, monilia, etc.). The lab has swabs to detect if there is an infection. I will not get into ways to treat vaginal infections here, that could be a whole article unto itself (and maybe it will be).

Prodromal Labor

Sometimes there are lots of contractions in those final weeks of pregnancy, especially if you have already had a baby. These contractions can be exhausting and can keep women up for days and sometimes weeks! Sometimes it's difficult to tell if it's the real thing. What makes this pre-labor/false labor/ or prodromal labor is that the contractions are not getting longer, stronger and closer together. These contractions are doing some work and helping with some cervical change. It's basically labor prep! The most important piece of advice I have is to rest as much as possible while also going on with life as normal as much as you can. There are four things you may want to do if you are experiencing disruptive and ongoing prodromal labor.

1. Relax the uterus- My favorite way to do this is with a relaxing bath. Make this your nightly ritual. You can add herbs to your bath that you find soothing. Some examples are lavender (*Lavendula species*), chamomile (*Chamomilla recutita* or *Chamaemelum nobile*)) and catnip (*Nepeta cataria*). I prefer to brew a strong tea and then add that to my bath as opposed to using essential oils. It's up to you!

2. Eat something high in tryptophan. You can google charts that show which foods are high in tryptophan, but dates are a good one as well as bananas, oats and milk. This is the wisdom of warm milk for kids before bed.

3. Drink a calming tea. I recommend chamomile and catnip (catnip is bitter and best mixed with chamomile with a spot of honey as well). I also really like rose (*Rosa sp.*) and Tulsi (*Ocimum tenuiflorum*) in this scenario, as a tea or as a tincture or glycerite.

4. Motherwort (*Leonorus cardiaca*) tincture and St. Johnswort (*Hypericum perforatum*) are both wonderful additions to your warm tea. I would put an entire dropperful of each into the cup of tea, and repeat as needed. Motherwort (*Leonorus cardiaca*), while toning the uterus, also calms the uterus and St. Johnswort (*Hypericum perforatum*) helps with pain relief.

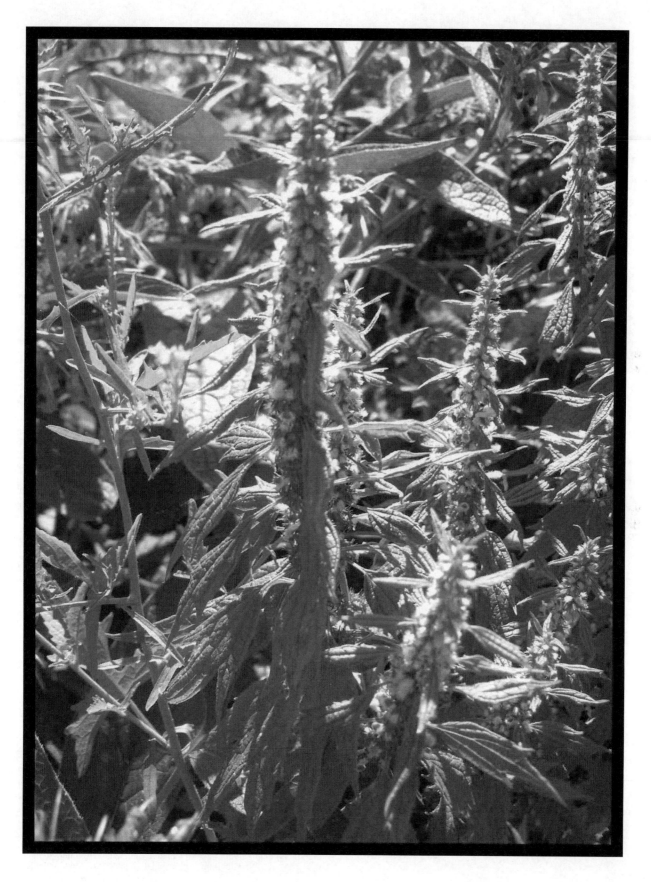

179

Also if you happen to be drinking a lot of red raspberry leaf (*Rubus species*) tea or infusion, you may want to stop and see if that helps. For some women the alkaloid fragrine found in red raspberry leaf tea can irritate the uterus.

Premature Rupture of the Membranes

Premature rupture of the membranes happens when the amniotic sac releases before the onset of regular contractions. With my first pregnancy my water broke 104 hours before my daughter was born, breech, at home. The main thing we focus on here is preventing infection. This is what I did and what I recommend to mamas:

1. Nothing in your vagina, no baths.

2. Stay home as much as possible (I only left the house to walk), to keep your uterus away from contaminating bacteria. The safe environment of your uterus is now opened up to the world with the release of the membranes.

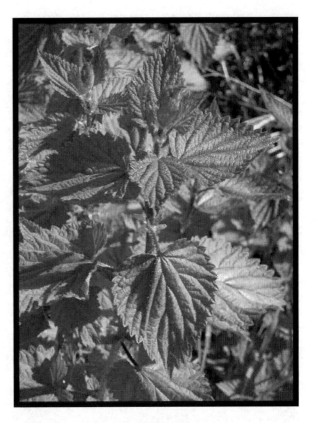

3. 250mg of vitamin C every 4 hours as an immune system enhancer.

4. 2 droppersful of Echinacea root (*Echinacea purpurea* or *Echinacea angustifolia*) tincture every 2 waking hours as an antibiotic and immune system enhancer

5. Increase fluid intake as your body is continuously making amniotic fluid as needed. Nettles (*Urtica dioica*) infusion is perfect!

6. Write birth affirmations, like: I trust my body and my baby to birth in perfect timing. My uterus is healthy and strong, and my baby will come when she is ready.

7. Also writing out exactly what you want can be helpful like: We will stay home and birth our baby healthily into our waiting arms. My body and my baby are healthy and well through the duration. We will stay home and rest and heal for 30 days after the birth with the support of our community and family. etc.

8. It is best to wear cotton undies and change your pad often, wipe front to back.

9. You may also opt to do some blood work at some point to be sure you are not brewing an infection. Again you can order your own bloodwork at the website above. Some labs and some hospitals also allow walk ins.

10. At some point you may decide you want to stimulate labor, which I will talk more about below.

11. I also kept a record of my temperature (every 4 hours or so), as a reassurance that I wasn't having a fever which might alert me to potential infection.

Also, sometimes the outer sac of the amniotic sac ruptures, but the inside stays intact. You can encourage the outer sac to heal by drinking Comfrey leaf (*Symphytum uplandica*) [Editors Note: please be sure to research liver toxic PAs in Comfrey before deciding to ingest intenrally) infusion. Positive affirmations are helpful here as well.

180

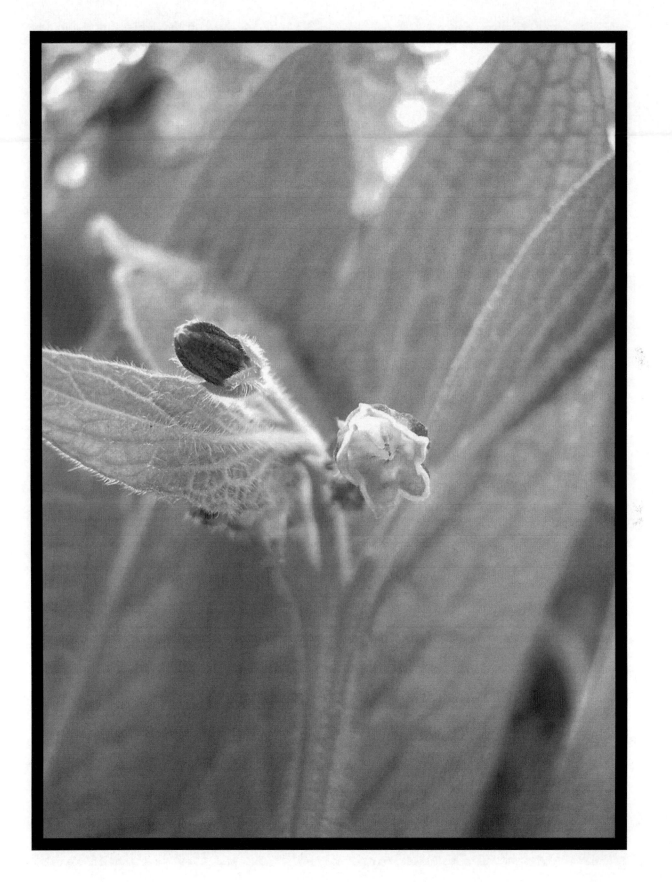

181

Stalled Labor

If you find that you have been in labor but you don't seem to be progressing or changing, it's time to take a step back. The best first step is to create an environment in which you can rest and reset. I have seen this support women in their birth process countless times. These are some techniques I have found helpful:

1. Take a nice, hot shower.

2. Tincture of California poppy (*Eschscholzia californica*)- 2 droppersful is likely sufficient to deeply relax you. Try 2, if you aren't feeling it in 15 minutes take 2 more droppersful. This may be all you need. If not you can keep dosing. Stop dosing at 10 droppersful.

3. Go to bed. Turn off the lights, shut the blinds, light some candles, play calming music.

4. Do the Texas Twist, alternating sides in case the baby is in a funky position:
   a. Lie on one side, with your bottom leg as straight as possible
   b. Bend your top leg, raising your knee as high as you can toward your chest.
   c. You can prop your leg up with pillows or a peanut ball if you have one.
   d. Roll over as far as you can, toward your bottom leg, and try to get as close as you can to a stomach lying position. Stay in this position as long as you can 10-20 minutes. This will help to open up your pelvis so baby can change position of she wants to.
   e. Alternate sides.

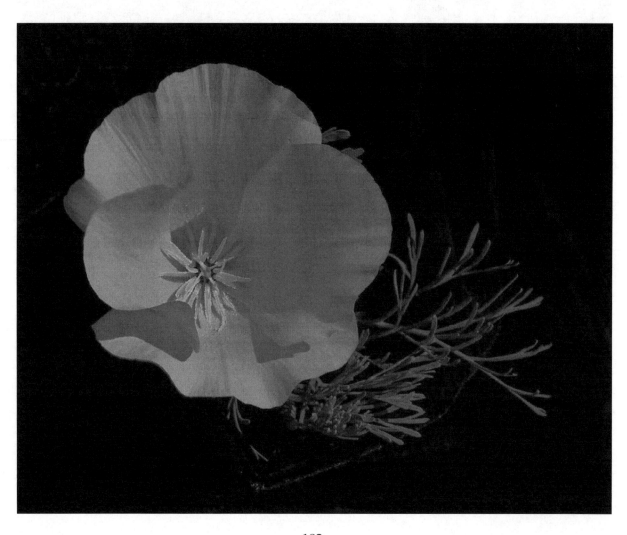

If you have a relationship with Marijuana, (*Cannabis sativa*) this would be a great time to enjoy some. I prefer tincture in labor, but it is important that you are familiar with how your body responds to this medicine and in which form. Cannabis has the amazing ability to start and strengthen uterine contractions while relaxing muscles and the mind. Truly a perfect labor herb, if used wisely and with great care.

Maternal Exhaustion

Some women have long labors. Even if we have implemented the techniques above for "stalled labor", she may still become exhausted. If you are experiencing a long labor, and you have already tried to relax and nourish and hydrate, etc. it may be time to stimulate. You can start with some Ginger (*Zingiber officinale*), which is warming and stimulating. A tea is great, with some honey for the sugar energy. Also Ginger candy is a good easy way to take in ginger in labor. I also have seen great success with Ginseng (*Panax quinquefolius* and *Panax schinseng*). You can by those little bottles in Asian markets or online.

Acupressure massage can also be helpful. Learn more at: https://acupuncture.rhizome.net.nz/. She has a great handbook with lots of great points.

Labor Induction

You may decide it is time to induce. Some reasons you may decide to induce are, If your membranes released many days ago, or if you are exhausted and you have tried resting and stimulating in other ways. If this is how you are feeling, it may be time to use some stronger herbs to get things going.

There are many herbal combinations to try when stimulating a labor. A nice and simple first herb to try is r=Red Raspberry leaf (*Rubus idaeus*) infusion, warm with honey. Drinking half a quart of infusion in half an hour may result in a stimulation of the uterus. I also quite like the flower essence of Birthroot (*Trillium sp.*). Since Birthroot is an "at risk "plant it is best not to harvest this plant's root to make medicine .The root is a very potent uterine stimulant. I find that the flower essence used with other labor stimulants can prove quite affective. To learn more about what plants are at risk , go to www.unitedplantsavers.org.

If you want to try something stronger, this is my preferred method, tried and true many times including my first birth.

Cottonroot bark (*Gossypium hirsutum*) and Black Cohosh (*Actaea racemosa*).

1. Take 10 drops of black cohosh tincture every 15 minutes.

2. Take 6 droppersful of cotton root bark every 30 minutes.

3. Do this for 6 hours.

4. Add in hot showers, nipple stimulation, and walks. Some women enjoy adding in sex and orgasms as well. So you could start the herbs and for the first hour, take a hot shower and then have some orgasms. Take a rest. Then for the next hour go for a nice walk. Take a rest. Then for the next hour do some nipple stimulation. Do what works for you.

> a.Some women prefer to use a breast pump for nipple stimulation. If you choose this route, here is my recommendation: Stimulate one breast with the pump for 15 minutes, and then switch to the other breast for 15 minutes. You can continue doing this for an hour. This technique encourages your body to release oxytocin which help contractions start.

I hope you have found this helpful for your freebirth or for someone you know who will be birthing unassisted. The next column will focus on the postpartum time, beginning with the immediate postpartum.

Until next time, blessed birthing!

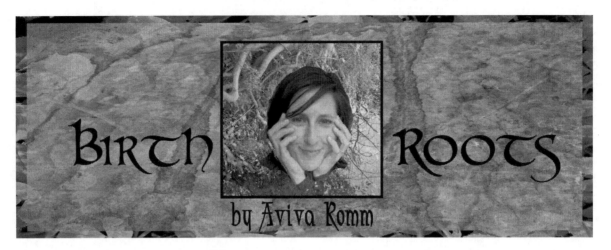

BIRTH ROOTS
by Aviva Romm

Leah is a 26 year old woman, 22 weeks pregnant with her second baby, and the mom of an active 4 year old son. She had her first outbreak of genital herpes two years ago. Her current partner, a different one than with her previous pregnancy, has genital herpes. She's pretty sure that's how she got it; she does not think she had it prior to their relationship.

Leah started receiving prenatal care about 4 weeks ago. Her midwife told her that if she has a herpes outbreak at the time of labor, she would not be able to have a home birth, which did previously, and that she would, in fact, have to have a cesarean section. Because she did not have herpes in her first pregnancy she did not know much about the risks. This news really terrified her, as she'd been having somewhat regular outbreaks every few months prior to becoming pregnant, and has already had on in this pregnancy.

Her midwife suggested she consider going on preventative antiviral medication to prevent further outbreaks during this pregnancy, or at least do this closer to when she is due, but Leah is really

Herpes:
Botanical & Nutritional Prevention, & Treatment During Pregnancy & Beyond

by Aviva Romm

uncomfortable with this approach. She lives a natural lifestyle and uses herbs as her primary medicine. Her midwife knows that you specialize in women's botanical medicine and refers Leah to you.

What is Herpes Simplex Virus (HSV)?

HSV is a recurrent viral infection that remains dormant in the nervous system, with periods of reactivation when it becomes symptomatic. It is characterized by single or multiple clusters of fluid-filled vesicles ("blisters") at affected sites. The vesicles rupture, leaving small, often painful, ulcers, which generally heal without scarring, though recurrent lesions at the same site may scar. It is highly contagious. Some individuals may rarely have a recurrence; others may have recurrences even several times each month. Recurrence rates are highly variable even in an individual.

Two members of the herpes simplex virus (HSV) family that commonly affect human health are HSV-1 and HSV-2. HSV-1 is referred to as *Herpes labialis* due to it primarily appearing on the lips (labia = lips in Latin) in the form of "cold sores." HSV-2, *Herpes genitalis*, typically appears on the genitals and less commonly, the skin. Oro-genital sex can lead to cross-contamination of these sites, with oral herpes more likely to be transmitted to the genitals than the other way around.

Who Gets It?

Herpes infection is *very* common, and I generally reassure patients of this and give them some statistics: 75% of folks in the U.S. are infected with HSV-1, and about 25% with HSV-2. That boils down to an estimated 500,000 to 1 million new cases annually. Consistent with this, 20-25% of pregnant women have genital herpes.

Factors that increase the likelihood of contracting HSV include:

- Sex -- women are more likely to become infected and have more frequent outbreaks; men are more likely to transmit infection
- Race -- rates are higher amongst African-Americans and Mexican-Americans
- Multiple sexual partners
- Cocaine use
- Co-infection with HSV-1 increases the frequency of HSV-2 outbreaks

How Does Someone Contract HSV?

HSV virus is spread through contact with the sores and through viral shedding. Sexual contact is the most common mode of transmission, however, kissing and even more casual contact, including sharing beverages or cigarettes, even with an asymptomatic person with herpes, can lead to infection.

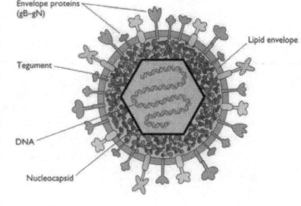

Asymptomatic viral "shedding" is common and occurs in cycles. Therefore, transmission of infection is possible at any time regardless of the presence of active lesions. The possibility of transmission between an infected and uninfected person in a monogamous relationship increases at a rate of about 10% each year.

What Happens in the Body?

Once contracted, HSV travels along the peripheral nerve axons to the nerve cell bodies in the dorsal root ganglia. It can exist in the paraspinous ganglia indefinitely, sometimes in a completely inactive state. The virus can be reactivated and begin replicating in response to such factors as stress, depression, and anxiety, trauma to mucosa, fever, sun exposure, menstruation, poor sleep, poor nutrition, spicy food, immunodeficiency, and other unknown factors.

When activated, the virus migrates to the mucosal surfaces back along the peripheral sensory nerves, leading to often pain superficial lesions.

Symptoms

Symptoms of initial HSV infection are typically much more dramatic than in recurrences. The first episode of herpes after initial infection is known as the *primary outbreak*. The incubation period -- that is, the time of exposure to the time of initial symptoms -- for HSV-1 is 3 to 7 days and 3 to 5 days for HSV-2. The primary outbreak is characterized by flu-like symptoms such as fever, headache, and swollen lymph glands in the groin. Primary outbreaks can last 2-3 weeks and can be severe enough, in rare cases, to require hospitalization, however, they are much more likely to be relatively mild and dismissed as "just a viral infection." Most infected people never realize that they are having a primary herpes outbreak, particularly if they did not realize they were exposed.

Recurrent herpes outbreaks are commonly heralded by a *prodromal stage* with tingling or itching sensations in the genital area, pain and tingling in the groin, and possibly in the buttocks and backs of the thighs, or around the mouth, depending on whether it's going to be an oral or genital outbreak. Virus is already present on the skin in the prodromal phase, so this is a contagious phase though blisters are not yet visible. The prodromal phase typically lasts 1-3 days and is followed by vesicles, lesions, and scabbing lasting for up to 10 days.

Recurrent outbreaks are often mild. Small sores or vesicles can occur anywhere on the skin or mucous membranes of the mouth or anogenital region, and are most common around the lips and genital area. The vesicles break open, become wet, and eventually crust over. Healing is complete when new skin is formed under the scab, which then falls off. It is rare for more serious local reactions to occur.

Ninety percent of people with herpes are unaware that they have it, with up to 60% to 75% having unrecognized signs and symptoms of genital herpes. Symptoms are falsely mistaken for other common urogenital conditions including irritation or discomfort from:

• Vaginitis
• Contact dermatitis from toilet paper, sanitary pads or other menstrual products, soaps, condoms, shaving or feminine hygiene products
• Vaginal dryness
• Frequent sexual intercourse
• Tight jeans, thongs, bicycle seats
• Urinary tract infections
• Shaving burns or reactions to hair removal
• Hemorrhoids or anal fissures

Antibodies to HSV-2 have been detected in about 20% of pregnant women, with only about 5% aware they have herpes.

Herpes in Pregnancy

Immunologic changes of pregnancy appear to make pregnant women more susceptible to a number of viral infections, including HSV. The stresses of pregnancy may increase the rate of outbreaks in some women.

Primary herpes infection during pregnancy is associated with miscarriage, premature labor, intrauterine growth restriction, and neonatal infection. Any woman with a primary infection during pregnancy should be referred to an obstetrician specializing in Maternal Fetal Medicine (care of women with high-risk pregnancies) for evaluation, treatment, and follow-up.

Infection in the newborn is most likely to occur via transmission during labor if the mother gives birth vaginally when there are genital herpes lesions. It is associated with increased neonatal death, brain damage, seizures, cerebral palsy, blindness, and deafness. Because 90% of cases of neonatal herpes are a result of direct contact with lesions in the birth canal, cesarean section is the recommended mode of delivery in active herpes outbreaks at the time of labor.

Keep in mind that herpes sores may occur on the vulva where they may cause pain and be visible, but they can also be present on the vaginal walls or cervix, where they might not be obvious. Therefore, women with a history of herpes, and particularly if they have had outbreaks during pregnancy, should have a thorough vaginal exam about a week before the anticipated time of birth to make sure no lesions are present.

Also note that either parent with cold sores or active genital herpes lesions can pass the virus onto the newborn through hand contact if they have touched an area with active virus or kissed the baby on the mouth or eyes; therefore, hand and general hygiene is important for prevention of neonatal herpes infection.

What's the Big Deal about Herpes if a Woman *Isn't* Pregnant?

Herpes infection may predispose women to cervical cancer. Recent research suggests possible long-term consequences of harboring chronic HSV infection, for example, development of rheumatoid arthritis. HSV-2 infection significantly increases susceptibility to HIV infection.

Conventional Medical Treatment

Antiviral therapy is used for both the treatment of active herpes outbreaks, and prevention/suppression of recurrences in folks with frequent outbreaks or prior to birth in late pregnancy. Acyclovir, famciclovir (Famvir), and valacyclovir (Valtrex) are the commonly used drugs. Treatment has been shown to reduce recurrences after a primary infection and reduce asymptomatic viral shedding.

Studies suggest that prophylactic administration of acyclovir during pregnancy can reduce the cesarean rate, though studies have been small and inconclusive. Teratogenicity has not been demonstrated, even with first trimester use. They are generally well-tolerated medications.

Side-effects of HSV antivirals are generally mild but may include nausea and vomiting, diarrhea, headache, dizziness, fatigue, skin rash, edema, inguinal lymphadenopathy, anorexia, leg pain, medication taste, and sore throat from short term oral administration, and nausea and vomiting, diarrhea, headache, dizziness, insomnia, irritability, depression, rash, acne, hair loss, arthralgia, fever, palpitations, sore throat, muscle cramps, menstrual abnormalities, lymphadenopathy for long term use.

The Green Approach

Like Leah, many folks are looking for safe and effective non-pharmaceutical methods for preventing and treating HSV infection. Pregnant women are especially likely to seek alternative therapies to pharmaceuticals due to concerns about exposure of the baby to medications in utero.

Prevention is always the best treatment. Practicing safe sex on all occasions regardless of whether lesions are visible, and avoiding direct and indirect contact with active lesions (i.e. don't share towels, drinks, etc., with folks with active lesions) is key. Condoms do not guarantee protection from transmission, but do significantly reduce HSV-2 transmission, especially to women. The virus is commonly passed by folks who do not know they have it because they may never have had symptoms. Women with vulvovaginitis, for example, from *Candida* (yeast) infection, who have HSV exposure are more susceptible to contracting the infection via fissures in the vaginal tissue, so keeping the vaginal tissue healthy is important in prevention.

Unfortunately, though a number of botanicals have demonstrated anti-herpetic activity *in vitro,* there are few well-designed human clinical trials looking at the effects of herbs in HSV infection. Substantial clinical experience has shown me that outbreaks can be reduced in frequency, severity, and length with a combination of interventions including stress reduction, nutritional approaches, immune support, and symptomatic therapy. Botanicals play a role in all of these. The information below is applicable to anyone with herpes, however, given that this is a pregnancy-related column, I have limited the recommendations to those herbs that are generally safe in pregnancy. For a more comprehensive review of botanicals for HSV prevention and treatment, including a review of the evidence, please see my book *Botanical Medicine for Women's Health.*

Nutritional Support
Nutrition plays the central role in the body's ability to resist and fight infection and is the cornerstone of an effective botanical plan. Review of dietary habits is particularly relevant for those patients with frequent illnesses and HSV recurrences. Phytonutrients are evolutionarily designed to provide us with key nutrients, thus botanicals – in the form of our plants foods – are important at this most foundational level of health. While foods are the optimal sources of nutrients, it can be difficult to get therapeutic levels of nutrients from foods alone, therefore supplementation is also recommended.

Zinc
Supplementation with 25 mg of zinc daily has been shown to inhibit HSV replication *in vitro* and clinically has led to complete suppression of an outbreak or resolution within 24 hours. Zinc stimulates cell-mediated immunity, decreases frequency, and reduces severity of outbreaks. Supplementation is suggested for 6 weeks with 250 mg Vitamin C. Topical use of zinc sulfate solution (0.01% to 0.025%) improves healing of HSV-1 blisters and prevents recurrence.

Examples of foods rich in zinc: oysters, beef shanks, crab, pork shoulder, lobster, chicken, yogurt, chickpeas, and kidney beans

Vitamin C

Adequate daily intake of vitamin C and bioflavonoid-rich foods is necessary for optimal immunity, prevention/reduction of chronic inflammation, and for wound healing. Vitamin C supplementation of 4000- 5000 mg/day during active outbreaks has been shown to speed healing time of lesions. The maximum recommended daily dose for supplementation during pregnancy is 4000 mg/day, beyond which rebound scurvy can be seen in the infant.

Examples of foods rich in Vitamin C: (this assumes uncooked foods): guava, red sweet pepper; kiwi fruit,
oranges, green pepper, grapefruit juice; fresh vegetable juice cocktail, strawberries, Brussels sprouts,
cantaloupe, papaya, broccoli, raw, tomato juice, pineapple, raw, kale, mango

Reduce Arginine and Increase L-lysine

Lysine and arginine are amino acids. Arginine is involved in replication of HSV; it may actually stimulate cell replication whereas L-lysine blocks arginine activity. L-lysine is shown in studies to decrease the severity of outbreaks and reduce recurrence, though it does not necessarily have an impact on healing time. *In vitro* evidence supports increasing dietary lysine and decreasing dietary arginine to prevent recurrent herpes outbreaks. Supplementation of 1 gm daily is recommended preventatively or 1 gm three times daily during an outbreak in additional to dietary modification. Due to concerns over prolonged lysine supplementation and the risk of developing atherosclerosis, dietary adjustments may be preferable to regular lysine supplementation, which can be reserved for acute need. However, nuts provide important and healthy fats to the diet, therefore it is not desirable to eliminate them entirely, especially during pregnancy. Therefore, moderation is advisable. Lysine supplementation is not contraindicated during pregnancy.

Food Sources of Lysine and Arginine
Lysine-rich Foods (Emphasize)
Fresh fish •
Canned fish •
Turkey
Milk
Beef
Cooked
beans
Eggs
Cheese
Soybeans

Arginine-rich Food (Minimize)
Chocolate
Nuts and nut products, for example:
    Brazil Nuts
    Hazel Nuts
    Peanuts
    Walnuts
    Almonds
    Cashews
    Sunflower seeds
    Peanut butter
    Gelatin
    Brown rice
    Wheat
    Oatmeal
    Raisins
    Coconut

Vitamin E

Topical use of vitamin E oil shortens healing time and significantly reduces pain associated with HSV-1 lesions. Apply 2-4 times daily with a cotton swab.

Stress reduction

HSV episodes are known to be precipitated by stress. Chronic stress has the most significant impact on recurrent HSV, even more so than acute stress. Nervines, particularly trophorestoratives (nervines), are an important part of the treatment protocol in patients in whom stress is a chronic underlying factor which is the case for many individuals. A combination of adaptogens and nervines is excellent for both short-term and long-term tonification of the nervous system.

Regular practice of mind-body therapies that help to relieve stress are important in the prevention of recurrent HSV for many patients. Examples include meditation, yoga, biofeedback, and massage.

Herbal Adaptogens to Improve Stress Response

Eleuthero, *Eleutherococcus senticosus*
Ginseng, *Panax ginseng*
American Ginseng, *Panax quinquefolium*
Rhaponticum, *Rhaponticum carthimoides*
Rhodiola, *Rhodiola rosea*
Schizandra, *Schizandra chinensis*
Ashwagandha, *Withania somnifera*

Herbal Nervines to Relieve Stress

Milky Oats, Avena sativa
California Poppy, Eschscholtzia californica
Lavender, Lavendula officinalis
Motherwort, Leonorus cardiaca
Lemon Balm, Melissa officinalis
Passionflower, Passiflora incarnata
Skullcap, Scutellaria lateriflora
Damiana, Turnera diffusa

Immune Support
When I think of immune support for individuals with HSV, I consider both their host status – that is, what is their fundamental immune substrate, and I consider the organism itself. Is this someone who has overall robust health and has an outbreak perhaps once or twice a year or less, and only during stressful times or under specific circumstances (i.e., travel, illness, preparing for a major event such as a wedding), or is this someone who is sort of chronically inflamed or sick frequently with colds, allergies, urinary infections, vaginal infections, or recurrent herpes outbreaks, for example, several times a year or more. (Individuals with frequent HSV recurrences should have an HIV test to make sure this is not a reason for frequent recurrence).

For the heartier host, I may recommend simply pre-treating with immune boosting and stress reducing herbs prior to and through an anticipated stressful time, and ensuring optimal nutrition and rest during those times, with no need for chronic ongoing therapy. For those with less optimal health, I emphasize ongoing use of anti-inflammatory and immunomodulating herbs to quiet immune reactivity while emphasizing a nutritional approach, plus adaptogenic herbs to boost immune health.

Pregnancy can be considered a time of ongoing stress, and thus some form of chronic treatment is needed for those women who tend to have frequent or even semi-frequent recurrences. If one is choosing to use botanicals for prophylaxis it is recommended to take them daily during the last half of the third trimester to prevent outbreaks at the time of labor. The efficacy of this approach has not been measured, and therefore cannot be compared to the relatively known efficacy of anti-viral drugs for prevention -- in other words, there is less certainty that the herbs will prevent a late pregnancy outbreak.

While herb safety in pregnancy has largely remained unstudied, many herbs have a long history of safe use, and have safety and constituent profiles that strongly suggest that they can be used with reasonable safety during pregnancy. Their efficacy for suppression and prophylaxis has not been compared to antivirals and cannot be guaranteed. If a pregnant woman continues to have outbreaks while using the herbs, this would be a time to consider switching to pharmaceutical agents.

Herbal Adaptogens to Improve Stress Response & Increase General Resistance

Eleuthero, *Eleutherococcus senticosus*
Ginseng, *Panax ginseng*
American Ginseng, *Panax quinquefolium*
Rhaponticum, *Rhaponticum carthimoides*
Rhodiola, *Rhodiola rosea*
Schizandra, *Schizandra chinensis*
Ashwagandha, *Withania somnifera*

Antivirals

The following herbs represent a selection of botanicals commonly used by herbalists for internal and/or topical antiviral therapy. Antivirals are used to control the degree of infection. All have shown some measure of antimicrobial activity in various studies and are a promising area of research for herpes treatment. Specific studies of the effects of herbs on HSV are presented below. These herbs may be used singly, but more commonly are used by herbal practitioners in combination with other antivirals, or in comprehensive, multi-herb, multi-effect formulae.

Antivirals to Reduce Systemic Viral Replication & Inhibit Viral Attachment to Cells

Aloe, *Aloe vera* (topical use only in pregnancy)
Calendula, *Calendula officinalis*
Echinacea, Echinacea spp.
Reishi, *Ganoderma lucidum*
Licorice, *Glycyrrhiza glabra* (topical use only during pregnancy)
St. John's Wort, *Hypericum perforatum*
Lemon Balm, *Melissa officinalis*
Sage, *Salvia officinalis* (topical use only during pregnancy)

Symptomatic Therapy

A number of herbs have shown analgesic effects with topical application, as well as ability to speed the healing of lesions and relieve discomfort associated with recurrent episodes.. Two studies specifically looked at topical pain management with herpes zoster, a relative of HSV that causes painful outbreaks along nerve dermatomes and often leads to significant postherpetic neuralgia. Both 100% geranium oil, applied directly to the affected area, and peppermint oil have demonstrated analgesic effects in a clinical trial and a case report, respectively. Geranium oil relieved pain dramatically in 25% of patients whose pain following shingles had lasted for three months or more and was not relieved by standard pain medications such as acetaminophen (Tylenol) or meperidine (Demerol). Fifty percent of patients showed some relief, and 25% did not benefit. Most herbs are safe for localized topical use in pregnancy

(thuja is an exception and should never be used, even topically, during pregnancy!). Essential oil (EO) rich herbs, for example, thyme (*Thymus vulgaris*), tea tree, and lemon balm, and anthraquinone rich herbs such as aloe and St. John's wort all contain antimicrobial activity, some specifically against HSV.

Wound-Healing Agents to Promote Granulation of New, Healthy Tissue

Aloe, *Alove vera*
Calendula, *Calendula officinale*
Comfrey, *Symphtyum officinale*

To Relieve Local Pain

Topical Analgesics:
St. John's Wort, *Hypericum perforatum*
Peppermint, *Mentha piperita*
Kava Kava, *Piper methysticum*

Anti-Inflammatories:
Licorice, *Glycyrrhiza glabra*
St. John's Wort, *Hypericum perforatum*
Lavender, *Lavendula officinalis*
Chinese Skullcap, *Scutellaria baicalensis*
Comfrey, *Symphytum officinalis*

For Weeping Lesions

Astringents:
Witch Hazel, *Hamamelis virginiana*
Plantain, *Plantago spp.*
White Oak Bark, *Quercus alba*

Antimicrobial Powder:
Myrrh, *Commiphora myrrha*

Discussion of Several Specific Botanicals with Known Effects on HSV
(and safe for use in pregnancy)

Aloe (topical)
Two studies were conducted examining the efficacy of topical aloe vera treatments on men experiencing primary outbreaks of genital herpes. In the first study 120 men were randomized into 3 parallel groups receiving either 0.5% in hydrophilic cream, aloe vera gel, or placebo three times daily for two weeks. The shortest mean duration of healing

occurred with aloe vera cream, followed by gel and then placebo, with healing times of 4.8 days, 7.0 days, and 14.0 days respectively. Percentages of cured patients were 70%, 45%, and 7.5% respectively. In the second study 60 men were randomized into 2 groups receiving 0.5% aloe vera extract in a hydrophilic cream base or placebo. The trial had comparable favorable results to the previously discussed trial. Additionally, in vitro testing has demonstrated virucidal effects of anthraquinones and anthraquinone derivatives such as emodin, a component of aloe.

Echinacea (internal and topical)
In a five-month uncontrolled clinical study of 4,598 patients, a salve prepared from the juice of the aerial portion of *Echinacea purpurea* was reported to have an 85% success rate in the treatment of a number of inflammatory skin conditions, among them Herpes simplex eruptions. Echinacea is used by herbalists during pregnancy for the prevention of herpes outbreaks. Longitudinal use of echinacea in pregnancy was evaluated for safety and outcomes by Gallo et al. In prospective study, 206 Canadian women, already taking echinacea-containing products, were compared to a matched cohort not taking echinacea. Products mostly contained *E. angustifolia* and *E. purpurea*, though one respondent took *E. pallida*. Thirty-eight percent took tincture (38%) at a dose of up to 30 drops daily and 58% took tablets or capsules at a dose of 250-1000 mg/day. Echinacea use was primarily in the first trimester (54%); 8% used echinacea during all three trimesters. There were no statistical differences between pregnancy outcomes in the two groups nor were there statistically significant differences in the neonates.

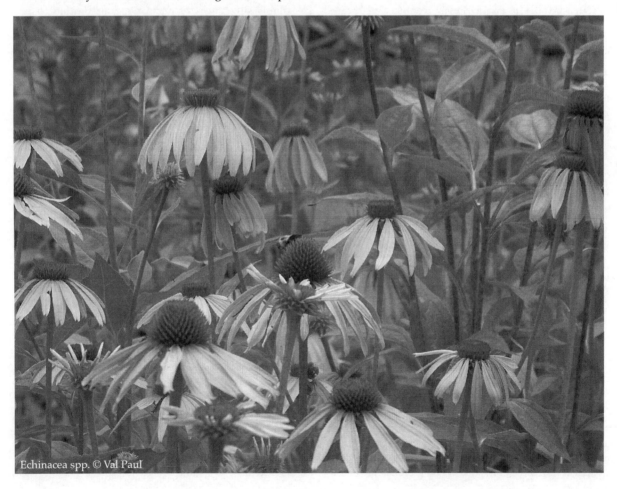

Echinacea spp. © Val Paul

Lemon Balm (internal and topical)

Lemon balm has classically been used as an uplifting herb for the treatment of stress and anxiety. Rich in volatile oils, *in vitro* and clinical research conducted for a little over the past decade has demonstrated impressive results using lemon balm ointment as a local therapy in the treatment and prevention of herpes outbreaks. In one study, four different concentrations of volatile oils extracted from lemon balm were examined for the effects against HSV-2. At concentrations of 200 µg/mL replication of HSV-2 was inhibited, indicating that the M. officinalis L. extract contains an anti-HSV-2 substance. Another study, a double-blind, placebo-controlled, randomized trial, was carried out with the aim of proving efficacy of standardized and highly concentrated lemon balm cream for the therapy of herpes simplex labialis. Sixty-six patients with a history of recurrent herpes labialis (at least four episodes per year) in one center were treated topically; 34 of them with lemon balm cream and 32 with placebo. The cream had to be smeared on the affected area four times daily over five days. A combined symptom score of the values for complaints, size of affected area and blisters at day 2 of therapy was formed as the primary target parameter. A significant difference seen in the combined symptom score on the second day of treatment is of particular importance because symptoms are usually worst at that time. In addition to reducing the duration of the healing period, the treatment led to prevention of spreading of the infection and had a rapid effect on common herpes symptoms including itching, tingling, burning, stabbing, swelling, tautness and erythema,. Some indication exists that the intervals between the periods with herpes might be prolonged with balm mint cream treatment. There is little reason to expect the development of resistance to treatment. Commercial lemon balm extract concentrated creams for topical use are available over the counter and in herbal pharmacies.

Licorice (short term internal; topical use)

Numerous *in vitro* and *in vivo* studies have shown licorice preparations to have antiviral, antiherpetic, anti-inflammatory, antiulcer, and a wide variety of immunomodulating effects. The herb is known for its inhibitory effects on HSV, its anti-inflammatory effects to reduce pain and swelling of lesions, and its immunomodulatory effects to enhance host resistance and reduce episodes of active lesions. Glycyrrhizic acid inhibits the growth of several DNA and RNA viruses in cell cultures and inactivates Herpes simplex 1 virus irreversibly.

Reishi

Considered an adaptogenic and immunomodulating herb, a number of studies have demonstrated activity of reishi against HSV. One study, looking at the mechanisms of action of reishi against HSV-1 and HSV-2 found that the *Ganoderma lucidum* proteoglycan (GLPG), obtained by liquid fermentation of the mycelia, works by inhibiting viral replication by interfering with the early events of viral adsorption and entry into target cells. Two protein-bound polysaccharides, a neutral protein-bound polysaccharide (NPBP) and an acidic protein-bound polysaccharide (APBP), isolated from water soluble substances of reishi were also found to be effective against HSV-1 and HSV-2. APBP was found to have a direct virucidal effect on HSV-1 and HSV-2. APBP did not induce interferon (IFN) or IFN-like materials in vitro and is not expected to induce a change from a normal state to an antiviral state. APBP in concentrations of 100 and 90 microg/ml inhibited up to 50% of the attachment of HSV-1 and HSV-2 to cells and was also found to prevent penetration of both types of HSV into cells. These results show that the antiherpetic activity of APBP seems to be related to its binding with HSV-specific glycoproteins responsible for the attachment and penetration, and APBP impedes the complex interactions of viruses with cell plasma membranes. Virucidal effects of reishi extracts have also been identified by other researchers. Reishi has also demonstrated beneficial effects in the treatment of herpes zoster, reducing post-herpetic neuralgia. Reishi is usually taken as a decoction or in tablet form. Though tinctures are also available, the polysaccharides are likely more bioavailable in whole or water-extracted forms.

Sage and Rhubarb Combination

A combination ointment containing sage and rhubarb extracts, the former EO rich and the latter anthraquinone-rich, and a product containing sage alone, were evaluated for their efficacy against HSV. A total of 149 patients participated, and 145 patients (111 female, 34 male) of whom 64 received the rhubarb-sage cream, 40 the sage cream and 41 Zovirax cream could be evaluated by intention-to-treat analysis. The dried rhubarb extract used was a standardized aqueous-ethanolic extract according to the German Pharmacopoeia and the dried sage extract an aqueous extract. The reference product was Zovirax cream with the active ingredient acyclovir. The mean time to healing in all cured patients was 7.6 days with the sage cream, 6.7 days with the rhubarb-sage cream and 6.5 days with Zovirax cream. There were statistically significant differences in the course of the symptoms. For the parameter 'swelling', at the 1st follow-up visit there was a significant advantage for Zovirax cream compared to sage cream, and for the parameter 'pain', at the 2nd follow-up visit there was a significant difference in favor of the rhubarb-sage cream compared to the sage cream. The combined topical sage-rhubarb preparation proved to be as effective as topical acyclovir cream and tended to be more active than the sage cream.

St. John's Wort

Hypericin and related compounds have been shown to have selective activity against viruses, both *in vitro* and *in vivo*, including HSV-1 and HSV-2 in a number of studies. A prospective double-blind placebo controlled study of St. John's wort extract compared to placebo was conducted on 110 patients with herpes genitalis. Patients were given a 90-day treatment protocol of 300 mg t.i.d., and 600 mg t.i.d. on the days of herpes outbreaks. Symptoms were significantly and equally reduced compared to placebo, including severity of episodes, size of affected area, and numbers of vesicles. Herbalists include St. John's wort in protocol for both internal and topical use for its positive effects on the nervous system, antiviral activity, and topically in tincture or salve, for its mild vulnerary and anti-inflammatory actions.

Tea Tree

Tea tree oil (TTO) has broad spectrum antimicrobial effects *in vitro*, and is specifically active against HSV. One *in vitro* study looked at the effects of both tea tree oil and eucalyptus oil (EUO) against HSV-1 and HSV-2. At non-cytotoxic concentrations of TTO plaque formation was reduced by 98.2% and 93.0% for HSV-1 and HSV-2, respectively. Non-cytotoxic concentrations of EUO reduced virus titers by 57.9% for HSV-1 and 75.4% for HSV-2. Virus titers were reduced significantly with TTO, whereas EUO exhibited distinct but less antiviral activity. In order to determine the mode of antiviral action of both essential oils, either cells were pretreated before viral infection or viruses were incubated with TTO or EUO before infection, during adsorption or after penetration into the host cells. Plaque formation was clearly reduced, when herpes simplex virus was pretreated with the essential oils prior to adsorption. These results indicate that TTO and EUO affect the virus before or during adsorption, but not after penetration into the host cell. Thus TTO and EUO are capable to exert a direct antiviral effect on HSV. Although the active antiherpes components of Australian tea tree and eucalyptus oil are not yet known, their possible application as antiviral agents in recurrent herpes infection is promising. A clinical trial by Carson et al. focused on the effects of topical application of tea tree oil on recurrent herpes labialis (RHL). Patients aged 18-70 years (n=18) with a self-reported history of RHL completed the study. Patients who had antiviral therapy in the previous month, long-term steroid therapy, immunocompromised status, pregnancy, lactation, or known TTO allergy were excluded. Participants presented as soon as possible after onset of a herpes outbreak and randomly received and applied either 6% TTO in an aqueous gel base or placebo gel 5 times daily and recorded treatments and any adverse effects in a diary. Subjects were assessed in the clinical daily except Sundays, with swabs collected for culture and PCR evaluation for HSV. Visits continued until vesicles were completely healed (re-epithelialized) and PCR was negative for HSV DNA on two consecutive days. Investigators were blinded to which patients were using which gel. Parameters measured included re-epithelilzation time, time to crust formation, duration of detectable virus by lab methods, and virus titer. While most of the parameters did not reach statistical significance, re-epithelialization time was reduced comparable to other common topical treatments. The authors state that the study size may have been too small to draw complete conclusions, and that the study may have been confounded by the fact that eight of the nine patients in the TTO group began the study in the vesicular stage compared to only six in the placebo group. Nonetheless, they concluded that TTO may be a useful and more affordable acceptable alternative to patients and poses little risk of causing resistance.

Eleuthero

Eleuthero is an important traditional medicine in China and Russia, used to stimulate the immune system, for prophylaxis of infectious diseases, and to enhance stamina and performance. It is mentioned repeatedly in the literature for its antiviral effects. An *in vitro* study by Glatthaar-Saalmuller et al. demonstrated specific activity against HSV virus. Given the ability of this herb to support general immunity, it is recommended in the prevention of recurrent herpes outbreaks, particular for patients exhibiting general susceptibility to infection, and when fatigue or stress precipitate episodes. It is regularly given in tincture or encapsulated forms, most often combined with other adaptogens, antivirals, and nervines.

Reishi

Reishi is an important adaptogen and immunomodulating herb. It was discussed extensively above for its specific activities against HSV. The combination of immune supportive and anti-HSV activity makes this herb especially important to consider for patients who have recurrent herpes infection in the context of overall susceptibility to infection, fatigue, and general depletion.

Sample Botanical Treatment Protocol for Recurrent Herpes Simplex Virus

Combine the following botanical therapies both for internal and topical treatment, as appropriate for specific patients' needs.

Immune Supporting/Anti-viral Tincture

For patients prone to regular recurrent outbreaks, give the following formula as a prophylactic agent to boost the immune system and for its antiviral effects, for use daily. For patients with only periodic and predictable outbreaks, for example, during periods of stress such as after the holidays or during exams or deadlines, give the following formula for 6 weeks prior to the time of anticipated stress and continue for 2 weeks after the stressful event or period. For women susceptible to herpes outbreaks at the time of menstruation, give daily until recurrent outbreaks become infrequent, and then take 2-3 times weekly.

Echinacea	25 mL
St. John's Wort	25 mL
Lemon balm	20 mL
Reishi	15 ml
Ashwagandha	15 mL

Total: 100 mL
Dose: 5 mL twice daily

Antiviral Formula for Use During Pregnancy

Prepare the following herbs as an infusion:

Echinacea root	3 parts
Lemon balm	2 parts

Steep 28 g (1 oz)/liter of boiling water for 1 hour. Strain and drink 2 cups daily during the second and third trimesters.

Nervine formula

For patients with stress induced HSV outbreaks also give the following formula either daily on an on-going basis, or for several weeks prior to and during times of anticipated stress.

Milky oats	30 mL
Passion flower	30 mL
Lemon balm	20 mL
Lavender	20 mL
	Total: 100 mL

Dose: 3-5 mL 2-3 times daily, based on severity of stress.

Topical Treatment

Herbs from the following topical formulae can be combined or treatments can be alternated for various effects, for example, using tincture to heal lesions twice daily alternated with topical application of herbs to dry lesions.

For Painful Lesions:

Mix the following combination in a 1 oz. amber or cobalt glass bottle. Shake hard before each use to mix the tinctures and oil. Apply using a cotton swab, 2-4 times daily:

Kava kava tincture	10 mL
Licorice tincture	10 mL
Peppermint or geranium oil	20 drops

To speed healing and as a topical antiviral:

Mix a combination of equal parts of the following tinctures in a 1 oz. amber or cobalt glass bottle. Apply using a cotton swab, 2-4 times daily:

St. John's Wort (Hypericum perforatum)
Licorice (Glycyrrhiza glabra)
Lemon balm (Melissa officinalis)
Calendula (Calendula officinalis)

Alternatively use lemon balm or St John's wort ointments, available over the counter in shops that retail herbal products, or simply use witch hazel extract available at regular pharmacies.

For weeping lesions:

Option 1: Mix equal parts of powders of myrrh and goldenseal and apply several times daily by packing the powder onto weeping ulcers. Note that goldenseal powder may will stain clothing so caution should be taken to avoid contact with garments, i.e., by using a panty liner in the underwear.

Option 2: Apply witch hazel extract onto weeping ulcers using a cotton swab, repeating 2-4 times daily.

To heal tissue once sores have begun to crust over:
Use a vulnerary containing comfrey, lemon balm extract, calendula, and an essential oil such as geranium or peppermint salve to quickly heal tissue.

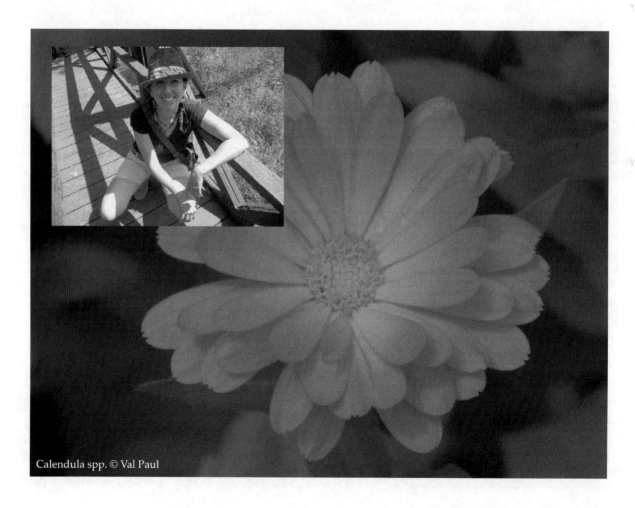

Calendula spp. © Val Paul

195

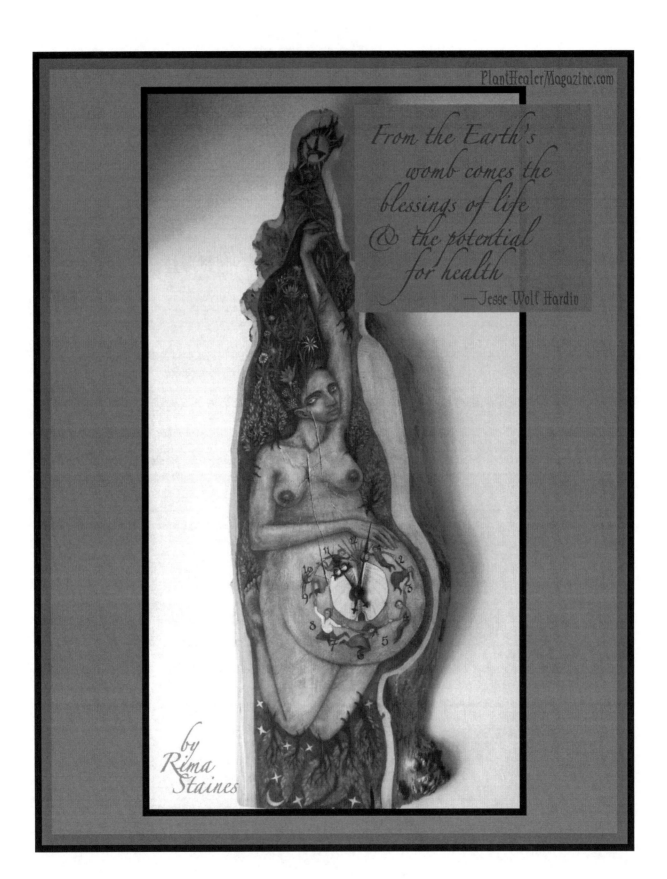

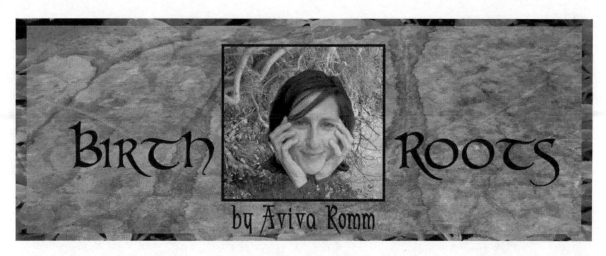

BIRTH ROOTS
by Aviva Romm

The Cannabis worked so miraculously that at first I thought my mind was playing tricks on me, as if I was being deceived by some placebo effect. In order to test, I stopped taking the Cannabis three times, and each time the uncontrollable and violent retching returned. Finally, my son, who was three years old at the time, begged me: "Mommy, please go take your medicine!" That was when I knew that Cannabis is truly an efficacious medicine, and that yes, I could look forward to enjoying a well-nourished and dignified pregnancy.
-Lin Curry, <u>Women & Cannabis</u>

Retro Intro

Cannabis Use
In Pregnancy & Birth

Why you let yourself suffer so?

By Aviva Romm

"Eh sista, why you let yourself suffa so?" were the words my old Rasta friend and reggae musician from Jamaica, Horace, said to me one languid August morning in 2003. I slid my nauseated, 9-week pregnant self deeper into the cool brushed cotton fabric of the futon sofa in the living room of his house on a quiet street in Cambridge, MA. The temperature at 10 am was already well into the 90s and the air was sticky-humid. My stomach was doing flips and I was about 30 minutes from embarking on a 20-hour car ride to the Deep South (read: hot and humid) in a tiny Honda, pregnant with my 4th

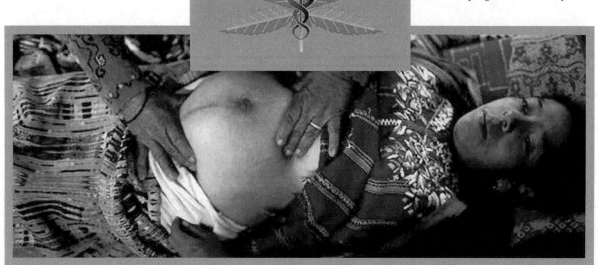

child, my 3 other kids in tow. Even not pregnant, I was someone who suffered from mild carsickness and I was uneasily anticipating the journey.

Horace (or Irace, as we called him, in true Rasta style), not missing the green around my gills, suggested I smoke some "kali weed" before the car journey: "*Women in Jamaica do it all the time for stomach problems when they are with child.*" I was well aware of the literature on *Cannabis* use in pregnancy and knew that limited use posed no hazard to the tiny fetus growing in me. Another good friend, a Harvard grad and pioneering homebirth mom, had just written a paper on the topic. I was several years into my herbal studies and well versed on many herbs, among them, marijuana. The article, rejected by parenting magazines at the time as too controversial, was a brilliant, well-researched piece peppered with anecdotes from well-educated women we knew who had used Cannabis to relieve pain in childbirth.

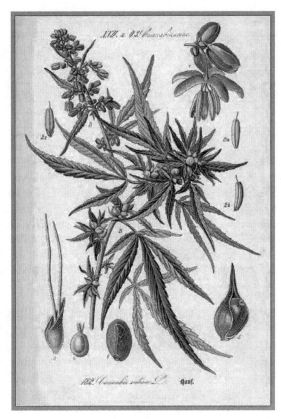

In spite of being someone who really dislikes the "high" from marijuana, I was less comfortable with the idea of taking a pharmaceutical for nausea while pregnant than with the safety profile of Cannabis, so I took a few small puffs off of a "pin joint" (a very thinly rolled marijuana cigarette) and shortly after got into the car (passenger seat, of course!). The small amount I'd smoked was just enough to ease my nausea and allow me to get several hours of sleep without making me "high." Some people, like me, actually do not enjoy the high from using marijuana, but appreciate the medicinal benefits, of which there are many.

"Jamaican women knew…that smoking…ganja [Cannabis] was good for the mother and the baby because it relieved the nausea of pregnancy, increased appetite, gave them strength to work, helped them relax and sleep at night, and in general, relieved the 'bad feeling' associated with pregnancy."

(Dreher, Nugent, Hudgins, 1994)

Cannabis Medicine: Credibility and Practicing Good Medicine

I've been a proponent of *Cannabis* medicine for decades, first as an herbalist, now also as a physician. I am less enthusiastic about the recreational use of *Cannabis*, especially by adolescents, though recognize that there is a fine line between recreation and self-medication for stress and anxiety, both of which are rampant in society, as evidenced by the large number of people in the United States using antidepressant and antianxiety meds. As with anything, moderation and appropriate use are key with *Cannabis*. In this article I focus strictly on acute medicinal use.

Cannabis is one of the oldest, most widely used, safest, and broadly applicable medicines. For pain no other herbs come close in efficacy, and it rivals many pharmaceuticals. It is similarly effective for appetite loss and cachexia of cancer and AIDS, and in pregnancy it is very effective in nausea and vomiting, including the more serious condition *Hyperemesis gravidarum*. During my intern year in internal medicine at Yale many of my patients confided in me that they smoked pot for pain relief, often using it instead of or as an adjunct to pharmaceutical pain relief, particularly opiates. They commonly reported that its use in conjunction with prescription narcotics allowed them to titrate down the amount of narcotics they needed to achieve pain relief. This phenomenon has been well-documented in Canadian research on *Cannabis*; patients who are opiate dependent for pain relief report using significantly lower doses of narcotics when they combine narcotic therapy with *Cannabis*. The safety profile of *Cannabis* is far better than that of opiates, and combined use with opiates allows patients to decrease the need for escalating doses of opiates that occurs as a result of the drug tolerance that naturally occurs over time.

Unfortunately, many medical clinics have a "zero tolerance" policy regarding the use of marijuana (as well as other illegal drugs and also inappropriately used pharmaceutical drugs) along with prescription pain meds; patients are "kicked off" of pain contracts, that is, they will no longer be prescribed narcotic pain meds if found to have marijuana-positive urine on routine drug screening. I often had to take a 'don't ask/don't tell' policy with my patients to protect their interests. I consider this practicing good medicine.

Cannabis and Gynecology

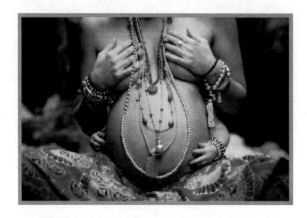

Cannabis is a powerful medicine with an enormous range of applications in women's health from dysmenorrhea (painful menses) and the pain of both acute and interstitial cystitis, to fertility and childbirth problems, to pelvic pain and other discomforts in menopause, to the treatment of pain in gynecologic cancers. It has an extensive written history to attest to its use in duration and scope. References in the written literature date back to ancient Mesopotamia and it was discussed in the *Ebers Papyrus*, the oldest known complete medical text. It has remained in the Egyptian pharmacopoeia since the time of the Pharaonic Dynasties, and its range of ancient use extends from the Africa and the Middle East to Asia and India. It was employed by the famous 13th century Persian physician Avicenna. Its uses are described in Arabic and Ayurvedic medicine traditions. The Kama Sutra extolls its virtues as an aphrodisiac, as well as an aid to sexual enlightenment. The flowers were used in ancient Chinese medicine for the treatment of menstrual problems (Russo, 2002).

Its earliest mention in European medicine is found in the *Old English Herbarium* where its use is recommended for sore breasts in the form of a poultice. Inhalation of the smoke of burning *Cannabis* was said, in a German text dating from 1564, to help women stooped over with uterine disease (presumably from pain) to "stand up straight again." By 1839 it was available in the form of solid extracts and tinctures and in 1849 it was first mentioned in Western medical literature in Dublin, Ireland for the treatment of uterine hemorrhage.

By the late 1800s its gynecologic and obstetric uses were quite widespread in then conventional European medicine. It was well regarded for its ability to check menorrhagia and uterine hemorrhages, control pain in dysmenorrhea, and to regulate menstrual function. In 1883 the *British Medical Journal* published two letters attesting to its efficacy in treating pain and bleeding associated with menorrhagia, one letter stating that there was no comparably effective medicine. Both ovarian pain and endometritis were also believed to be effectively relieved with *Cannabis*. The tincture was most commonly used.

Unsurprisingly, its used extended into medical practice in the United States as well. An Eclectic medical preparation taken from *Useful Prescriptions* (1935) by Cloyce Wilson, M.D describes the use of Cannabis for Chronic Cystitis as follows:

Rx Sp. Med. Cannabis 3ss.
   Sp. Med. Fragrant Sumach 3iij.
   Sp. Med. Saw Palmetto 3ij.
   Elix. Simplex q.s. oz. iv. M.
   Sig: A teaspoonful every three hours.

Another formula, Dysmenine Compound, was produced by Keysall Pharmacy in Kansas City, MO, circa 1905. The label indicates that it was a uterine tonic and anti-spasmodic to be used for "Dysmenorrhea, Menstrual Colic and Cramps, Ovarian Neuralgia, and Nervous Hysterical conditions arising therefrom." The ingredients are listed as fluid extracts of Acetanilid, *Cannabis, Cyprepedium,* Skullcap, *Pulsatilla, Viburnum prunifolium,* Caullophylin, *Viburnum opulus,* and *Capsicum.*

In 1942, though it had been dropped from the National Formulary, *Cannabis* was described in the *Journal of the American Medical Association,* by its editor, as recommended for the treatment of catemenial headache (Russo)

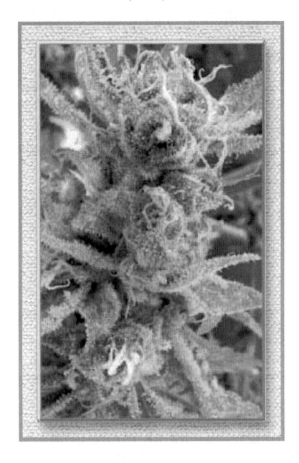

Herbalist Maude Grieve suggested the use of *Cannabis* tincture for menorrhagia, chronic cystitis, gonorrhea, and uterine prolapse (Russo).

Cannabis and Obstetrics Historically

The precedent for using *Cannabis* as a medicine in obstetrics is ancient and persists throughout the history of modern medicine, into the 20th century. The *Ebers Papyrus,* dating from somewhere between 3000 and 1534 BCE, references its use in difficult childbirth. The first Persian materia medica, written in the 9th century, discusses the use of *Cannabis* to "calm uterine pains, prevent miscarriage, and preserve fetuses in their mothers' abdomens" (Russo). An ancient Chinese medical text (*Bencao Gang Mu,* 1596), discusses the use of the seeds for postpartum difficulty, and the juice specifically for retained placenta and postpartum hemorrhage.

The use of *Cannabis* in childbirth is also common in folk medicine globally. In Cambodia and Vietnam it has been used to promote well-being in the new mother and to promote breast milk production when taken as a tea of flowering tops. In modern China it is still used to facilitate birth and improve lactation.

In the 1850s its use in childbirth was officially recognized in England and Ireland, and was endorsed in the medical literature (Christison, 1851; Grigor, 1852; Willis, 1859), for its efficacy in expediting protracted labors and improving the force of contractions via its oxytocic effects, relieving rigid *os uteri,* reducing pain in labor as well as the duration of pain, and was even reported to be useful in resolving "puerperal convulsions" (presumably eclampsia). It was popular in France around the same time for similar obstetric applications (Racime, 1876). It was favorably compared and often used preferentially to ergot, which was the most widely used oxytocic at the time.

In the early 1900s Eclectic physicians/pharmacists Felter and Lloyd reported *Cannabis*' ability to increase the strength or uterine contractions during childbirth, stating that it compared favorably to ergot without the side effects of that drug. Mentions in the obstetric literature in the 1920s cite its usefulness in treating impending abortion, postpartum hemorrhage, and improvement of sluggish labor when combined with ergot (Sajous and Sajous, 1924; Solis-Cohen, Githens, 1928).

There are some interesting topical uses of *Cannabis* in the treatment of painful breasts and nipples in postpartum women. For example, Czechoslovakian research in the 1960s found that an alcohol and glycerine extract applied to the nipples of breastfeeding mothers prevented mastitis from staphylococcal infections.

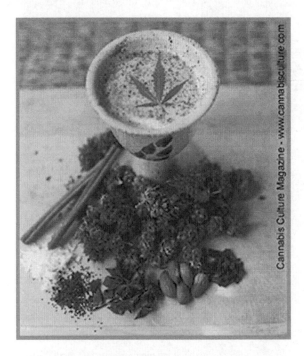

Cannabis and Obstetrics: Contemporary Use

Cannabis is not currently prescribed nor endorsed by most medical professionals for use during pregnancy and childbirth as it an illegal drug, and indications for medically approved use do not typically apply to childbearing women. Contemporary self-medication with *Cannabis* by pregnant, birthing, or postpartum women in US is not widely described or reported in the literature, likely largely due to its illegal status. The stigmas surrounding its use lead to underreporting of personal use. As author Lin-Curry (2002) states in her chapter "*Hyperemesis Gravidrarum* and Clinical *Cannabis*: To Eat or Not to Eat" in <u>Women and Cannabis: Medicine, Science, and Sociology:</u>
Most view the use of illicit drugs, especially during pregnancy, to be deviant, threatening, and something to avoid at all costs (Boyd 1999). Murphy and Rosenbaum (1999, p. 1) state, "In modern society the use of illegal drugs during pregnancy is commonly defined as the antithesis of responsible behavior and good health. The two statuses, pregnant woman and drug user, simply do not go together.

The reality is that a woman found to have a positive urine drug screen for *Cannabis* while pregnant, nursing, or raising small children may potentially face serious social and legal consequences. Thus, most women avoid its use in the childbearing year, and those who do choose to use it medicinally will often not disclose use.

While as many as 60% or more of pregnant women experiment with some form of complementary and alternative therapy during pregnancy, including herbal medicines, most women are also unlikely to be aware of the potential medicinal uses and benefits of *Cannabis* during pregnancy, so the thought of using it would not cross their minds. While a number of studies have explored the impact of maternal use on adverse outcomes in the child, there is a paucity of studies on intentional medicinal use in pregnancy and childbirth. As clinicians we must rely primarily on anecdotal and historical evidence of use, tempered by safety data from a limited number of contemporary safety studies.

Excellent support exists for the efficacy of *Cannabis* for the treatment of nausea and vomiting, and thus it has natural applications for nausea and vomiting of pregnancy (NVP). It can be particularly helpful in the treatment of the more severe form of NVP called *Hyperemsis gravidarum* (HG). However, symptoms of NVP and HG are experienced daily by the sufferer, and over a prolonged period of time, generally weeks to months. Treatment might require daily, regular use and smoking is not advised due to potential long-term impacts on the child (see *Safety*). The safety of daily tincture use in pregnancy has not been assessed.

While no comparative studies exist on the safety and efficacy of anti-nausea medications versus *Cannabis*, for many women, Ondansetron, the typically prescribed medication, is often cost-prohibitive for women -- at least several hundred dollars per month -- and considerably more expensive than an equivalent treatment supply of *Cannabis*.

A paper by Westphal et al. examined the use of *Cannabis* for the treatment of NVP, along with general use patterns amongst a cohort of 84 female users of medicinal cannabis. Of the seventy-nine respondents who had experienced pregnancy, 51 (65%) reported using cannabis during their pregnancies. While 59 (77%) of the respondents who had been pregnant had experienced nausea and/or vomiting of pregnancy, 40 (68%) had used cannabis to treat the condition, and of these respondents, 37 (over 92%) rated cannabis as 'extremely effective' or 'effective' (Westfall, Janssen, Lucas, & Capler, 2006)

Some women have reported a reduction in insomnia, a common pregnancy complaint particularly in the second and third pregnancy trimesters, after smoking a very small amount of marijuana. It is also sometimes used instead of Tylenol by women who experience chronic tension headaches or migraines in pregnancy.

Beneficial effects have been observed by midwives and reported by women giving birth at home who have used *Cannabis* to mitigate pain and to facilitate a protracted labor. Its combined actions of stimulating uterine contractions, its analgesic effects, and ability to promote a relaxed state, create the synergy that facilitates these outcomes. No contemporary studies have evaluated effects on postpartum hemorrhage and it is not recommended for this purpose.

The form in which marijuana is used has a definite impact on its effects. Tincture tends to impart anodyne and analgesic effects without the high; it can also be useful in the reduction of nausea and vomiting — it is the most advisable form for optimal outcome with minimal side-effects of "high." A typical dose is 1-3 mL, and it may be repeated up to every 30 minutes for acute management of pain, less frequently for other symptoms. Smoking is highly effective for sleep promotion and the relief of nausea and vomiting, but imparts more psychotropic effects. The high is dose dependent and follows a generally predictable response; with symptom relief lasting for a couple of hours, typically followed by increased appetite and sleepiness. Edible products are not recommended. They are generally prepared by cooking the *Cannabis* in an oil base, i.e. coconut oil) which is then added to the remaining ingredients, yielding significant amounts of highly lipohilic THC into the final product. Such products lead to a substantial "high" with an unpredictable response time that is commonly experienced as uncomfortable, and is followed by significant tiredness. Vaporizers are an optional alternative to smoking. Pharmaceutical marijuana products have not been studied in pregnancy at all and are not recommended. They also require physician prescription.

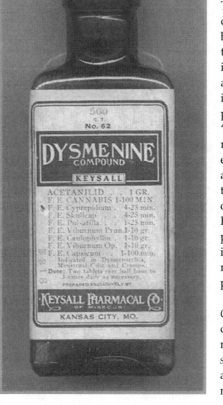

Cannabis indica is the most commonly recommended medicinal species; *Cannabis sativa* is often somewhat milder and may also be used medicinally.

Safety Concerns

The safety of most botanicals in pregnancy, including *Cannabis*, has not been thoroughly investigated, so safety is not fully understood. Further, the safety of *Cannabis* use as a therapeutic agent in pregnancy has never been studied (Westphal et al., 2006). However, *Cannabis* is reported to be the most widely used recreational drug in pregnancy and, as such, its effects are relatively well studied. (Park, McPartland, & Glass, 2004: Wang, Dow-Edwards, Anderson, Minkoff, & Hurd, 2004)

The widespread use of *Cannabis* amongst pregnant women, and the very low numbers of reported adverse effects, suggests that a general level of overall safety rare or occasional use can be expected. All of the studies that I have identified involve smoked marijuana products. A multi-site study of 7470 women in the US at low risk for adverse perinatal outcomes in whom the use of cannabis was assessed by interview and serum assay, reported no correlation between *Cannabis* use and prematurity, low birth weight, or *abruptio placentae* after adjustment for tobacco use (Shiono, Klebanoff, Nugent, Cotch, Wilkins, Rollins, Carey, Behrman, 1995). A study of perinatal deaths in Jamaica, involving 9919 singleton births, found no correlation between maternal cannabis use and rates of perinatal mortality or morbidity (Greenwood & McCaw, 1994).

newborns. The results were adjusted for cigarette smoking. In seven studies, information on *Cannabis* use was collected prenatally. Five studies reported results for differences in mean birth weight associated with maternal *Cannabis* use. 32,483 women giving birth to live-born infants were included. Three analyses of the studies on mean birth weight were conducted to avoid double-counting women from one study. The largest reduction in mean birth weight for any *Cannabis* use during pregnancy was 48 g. Mean birth weight was increased by 62 g (among infrequent users (< or = weekly) whereas *Cannabis* use at least four times per week had a 131 g reduction in mean birth weight. Based on these studies there is inadequate evidence that *Cannabis*, at the amount typically consumed by pregnant women, causes low birth weight (English, Hulse, Milne, Holman, & Bower, 1997).

Abortifacient activity is not expected with rare use, but the plant does have reported oxytocic activity, so caution is absolutely advised. Studies suggest that *Cannabis* does not affect plasma levels of follicle-stimulating hormone or luteinizing hormone in men or women nor does it usually human prolactin levels in women or plasma levels of thyroid hormones or glucocorticosteroids (Block, Farinpour, & Schlechte, 1991; Erdolu, Saglam, & Harmankaya, 1985; Kolodny, Masters, Kolodner, & Toro, 1974; Kolodny, Webster, Tullman, & Dornbush, 1979).

Two major areas of concern regarding maternal marijuana use in pregnancy have to do with the potential for low birth weight in the infants, and neurocognitive or developmental problems. A meta-analysis of 10 studies evaluated the role of marijuana smoking on low-birth weight in

Based on several studies looking specifically at neurocognitive development in infants and toddlers up to age 3 whose mothers have smoked marijuana during pregnancy, there appears to be little effect upon the cognitive development of these children. However, starting at age 3 and extending through adolescence, several studies suggest that some aspects of executive functioning may be affected in children whose mothers ingested marijuana in pregnancy. Specifically affected may be problem solving abilities that rely on complex visual perception integration and attention and impulsivity. However, the authors concluded that the long-term consequences of prenatal exposure to cannabis, if any, are subtle (Fride, 2002; O'Connell & Fried, 1991). The mothers in the studies often smoked marijuana heavily and regularly for up to several years prior to pregnancy, and may have smoked regularly and often during the pregnancy, thus it is impossible to extrapolate these findings to women who are otherwise not regular marijuana smokers who then use marijuana only infrequently for medicinal use, or in forms other than smoking, i.e. in the form of tincture. Also, other confounding factors might contribute to behavioral outcomes; for example, analysis of one studies demonstrated the way in which home environment conditions, particularly high levels of aggression, could magnify effects of prenatal exposure to *Cannabis* on postnatal outcomes (Day, Richardson, Goldschmidt, Robles, Taylor, Stoffer, Cornelius, & D Geva, 1994).

Marijuana use is not recommended for any woman who has not tried it before; some women will experience anxiety or paranoia as a result of intoxication. Anyone who has previously had an unpleasant experience while smoking marijuana is advised not to use it in labor, which is already an emotionally heightened time.

Clearly a great deal remains unknown about the safety of use of marijuana in pregnancy, particularly on the offspring. Available studies analyze use in regular smokers, not in those who use *Cannabis* rarely, medically, in small amounts only, and in other forms than smoking, i.e., tincture. *Cannabis* is a valuable medicinal plant. Whether it is appropriate for use in pregnancy has not been scientifically established. However neither has the safety of most pharmaceutical drugs prescribed medicinally during pregnancy by physicians. Each woman will need to weigh not only the available known risks and benefits of using marijuana for medical conditions that might arise in pregnancy for which it might have efficacy, but also the political and legal ramifications of use.

To answer more of these questions, herbalist Roy Upton and I, along with Ethan Russo, MD, one of the world's leading medical *Cannabis* researchers, are co-editing monograph on *Cannabis* spp. for the American Herbal Pharmacopoeia. Publication is expected sometime in the next 18 months. I also highly recommend the book Women and Cannabis.

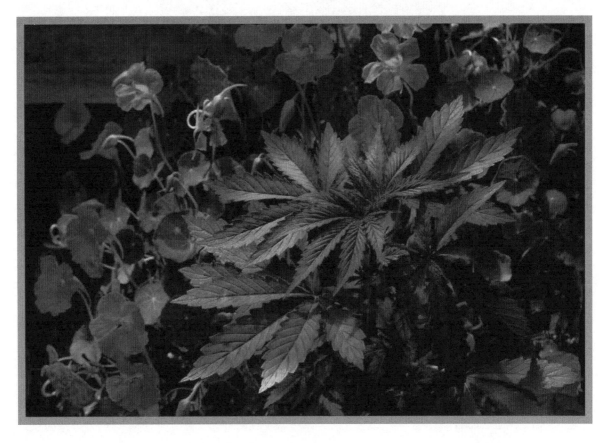

References

Block RI, Farinpour R, and JA Schlechte. 1991. Effects of chronic marijuana use on testosterone, luteinizing hormone, follicle stimulating hormone, prolactin and cortisol in men and women. *Drug Alcohol Dependence* 28: 121–28.

Christison, A. 1851. On the natural history, action, and uses of Indian hemp. *Monthly J of Medical Science of Edinburgh, Scotland* 13:26-45, 117-21.

Day NL, Richardson GA, Goldschmidt L, Robles N, Taylor PM, Stoffer DS, Cornelius MD, and D Geva. 1994. Effect of prenatal marijuana exposure on the cognitive development of offspring at age three. *Neurotoxicol Teratol* 16:169-75.

Dreher MC, Nugent K, and Hudgins R. 1994. Prenatal Marijuana Exposure and Neonatal Outcomes in Jamaica: An Ethnographic Study *Pediatrics*; 93:254.

English DR, Hulse GK, Milne E, Holman CD, and Bower. 1997. Maternal cannabis use and birth weight: a meta-analysis. *Addiction* 92:1553-60.

Erdolu, C., Saglam, R. and C Harmankaya. 1985. The effects of marihuana and tranquilizers on male sexual functions. *Bull Gulhane Mil Med Acad* 27: 77–82.

Fishbein, M. 1942. Migraine Associated with Menstruation. *J Amer Med Assoc* 237:326.

Fride, E. 2002. Cannabinoids and feeding: The Role of the Endogenous Cannabinoid System as a Trigger for Newborn Suckling. In Russo E, Dreher M, and Mathre ML (eds), *Women and Cannabis: Medicine, Science, and Society*. New York: Haworth.

Greenwood R and B McCaw. 1994. Does maternal behaviour influence the risk of perinatal death in Jamaica? *Paediatric Perinatal Epidemiol* 8(Suppl 1):54–65.

Grieve, M. 1971. *A Modern Herbal*. New York: Dover Publications.

Grigor, J. 1852. Indian hemp as an oxytocic. *Monthly J of Medical Sciences* 14:124.

Kolodny RC, Webster SK, Tullman GD, and RI Dornbush. 1979. Chronic marihuana use by women: menstrual cycle and endocrine findings. Presented at the New York Postgraduate Medical School 2nd Annual Conference on Marihuana: Biomedical Effects and Social Implications, June 28–29, 1979, per Abel, E.L. 1981. Marihuana and sex: a critical survey. *Drug Alcohol Dependence* 8:1–22.

Kolodny RC, Masters WH, Kolodner RM and G Toro. 1974. Depression of plasma testosterone levels after chronic intensive marihuana use. *New Eng. J. Med* 290:872–74.

Lin Curry, W-N. 2002. *Hyperemesis Gravidarum* and Clinical Cannabis: To Eat or Not to Eat? In Russo E, Dreher M, and Mathre ML (eds), *Women and Cannabis: Medicine, Science, and Society*. New York: Haworth.

O'Connell CM and PA Fried. 1991. Prenatal exposure to cannabis: a preliminary report of postnatal consequences in school-age children. *Neurotoxicol Teratol* 13:631-9.

Park B, McPartland JM, and M Glass. 2004. Cannabis, cannabinoids and reproduction. *Prostaglandins, Leukot Essent Fatty Acids* 70(2):189–97.

Racime, H. 1876. Le Haschisch ou chanvre indien. *Montpelier Medical* 36:432-49.

Russo, E. Cannabis Treatments in Obstetrics and Gynecology: A Historial Review. In Russo E, Dreher M, and Mathre ML (eds), *Women and Cannabis: Medicine, Science, and Society*. New York: Haworth.

Sajous, C., and M. Sajous. 1924. Cannabis indica (Indian hemp: hashish). In *Sajous's Analytic Cyclopedia of Practical Medicine*. Philadelphia: Davis.

Shiono PH, Klebanoff MA, Nugent RP, Cotch MF, Wilkins DG, Rollins DE, Carey JC, Behrman RE. 1995. The impact of cocaine and marijuana use on low birth weight and preterm birth: a multicenter study. *Am J Obstet Gynecol* 172:19–27.

Solis-Cohen, S., and TS. Githens. 1928. *Pharmacotherapeutics, Materia Medica and Drug Action*. New York: D. Appleton.

Wang XY, Dow-Edwards D, Anderson V, Minkoff H, Hurd YL. 2004. In utero marijuana exposure associated with abnormal amygdale dopamine D-2 gene expression in the human fetus. *Biol Psychiatry* 56(12):909–15.

Westfall RE, Janssen PA, Lucas P, and R Capler. 2006. Survey of medicinal cannabis use among childbearing women: Patterns of its use in pregnancy and retroactive self-assessment of its efficacy against 'morning sickness' *Complementary Therapies in Clinical Practice* 12, 27–33.

Willis, I.P. 1859. *Cannabis indica. Boston Med Surg J* 61:173-8.

Wilson, C. 1935. *Useful Prescriptions*. Cincinnati: Lloyd Brother, Pharmacists.

205

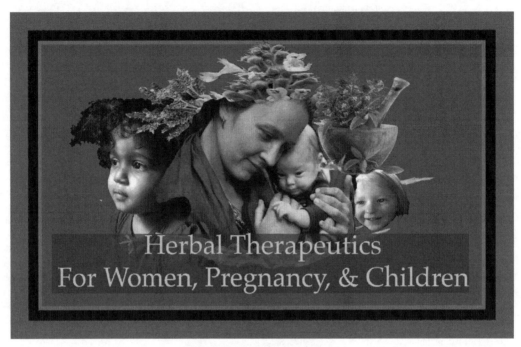

Herbal Therapeutics
For Women, Pregnancy, & Children

BIRTH TRAUMA

Healing with Herbs

by Juliette Abigail Carr

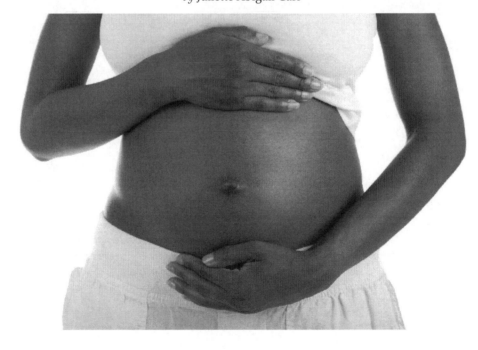

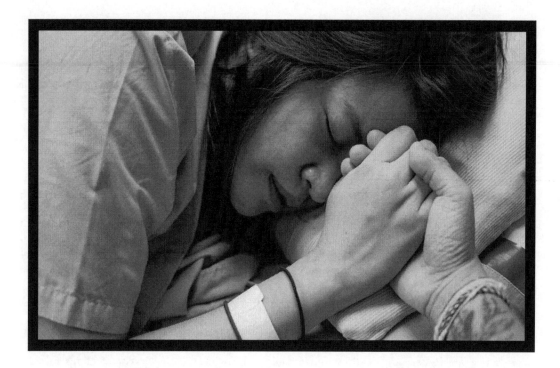

Birth trauma is incredibly prevalent: mention the phrase "traumatic birth" in any group of parents and prepare to be immersed in stories of fear, pain, and loss of autonomy. Regardless of whether the birth involved an unarguably scary sequence of events, a bad injury, or a personal perception that others may not share, trauma can be indelibly wrapped up in the birth experience and stored in the body's memory. This is true for the whole family: it is not simply the birthing parent who can experience and store trauma, but everyone who is close to the birth. Everyone touched by birth trauma should be supported to move through trauma into self-empowerment.

The ideal time to start trauma healing is during the natural postpartum healing process. This can help prevent a true trauma response with internalization and triggers, turning it into a memory instead of imbuing it with power as it lies in wait to strike. However, many of us walk through our lives with deeply internalized trauma, and processing it is important work that happens when the time is right—a major life transition, moments of clarity and self-reflection, and very often in a subsequent birth. Supporting the harder, longer process of healing from old trauma is often part of the birth process and postpartum healing.

Herbs are extremely useful for processing birth trauma, along with adjunct therapies and therapeutic communication techniques. While we cannot take away an experience, we can help others integrate the experience into their life story in a way that is empowering instead of traumatic.

The ultimate goal is to help people step into their deepest power, which is only revealed through transformative hardship: the odyssey shapes the hero.

Types of Birth Trauma

Birth is an unpredictable mystery that can be incredibly jarring for people, upsetting their sense of autonomy and bodily control, even with a good outcome. It is important to respect that a person may experience trauma in a situation that other people wouldn't; they are the authority on their experience, and it is not on us (or anyone else) to try to explain how their birth was fine/normal/expected/etc.

Physical Trauma

There are many possibilities for physical trauma to the birthing parent, including a bad tear, episiotomy, prolapse, hemorrhage, infection, vacuum assisted delivery, and surgical birth (caesarian section). For the new baby, physical trauma can include a wide variety of events both in utero and during the birth process, including problems with the fetal heart rate, difficult fetal positioning, maternal or fetal bleeding, infection, problems with the placenta, umbilical cord issues, vacuum assisted delivery, and difficulty fitting. Families that experience these types of events may feel fine about them, or they may experience emotional trauma as well as tissue injury.

Emotional Trauma

Often, emotional trauma surrounding birth includes feelings of the loss or theft of autonomy or control; lack of trust in self, support people, or providers; loss of self-efficacy or self-esteem; and fear of irreparable harm or death of self, infant, or beloved. These types of feelings may be expressed after a normal birth as well as a physically difficult one.

Somatic Trauma Processing

Somatic trauma, physical or emotional trauma stored in the body itself, is particularly common in the realm of birth trauma, as our bodies go through a tremendous upheaval. The healing and integration process following a physiologically and emotionally healthy birth is not a return to the prepregnancy normal, but instead develops a new normal in a body that is transformed by parenthood. When that postpartum healing process is accompanied by the need to heal from trauma, it is extremely common for the physical symptoms, feelings, memories, and subsequent triggers to become healed into the body during the healing process—think of the formation of scar tissue, both physically and metaphorically, holding an old injury in place and supporting healing around it, allowing the body and mind to function around an old area of weakness through the development of strong but inflexible tissue.

It is very common to see birthing people process old somatic trauma during birth as the physical transformation takes place, whether that be from a previous difficult birth experience, miscarriage, car accident (especially affecting pelvis or lower back), body dysphoria, sexual assault, long-standing eating disorders or other conditions involving self-deprivation and body image, emotional abuse, and chronically internalizing negative feelings about oneself. This sudden processing of internalized somatic trauma can be frightening if the birthing person is not prepared for it, so a discussion ahead of time can be helpful in cases of a known history. Birth workers can assist in supporting this process as it happens with drop doses of heart openers and stimulating dispersants as described below, to help them look at the experience without fear and let go of it.

Reactivation of Past Trauma

It is extraordinarily common to see a reactivation of past trauma, as everything comes out in the birth process, from body fluids to old scars to eventually a brand new person. Managed well, this breaking up of trauma scar tissue can be an acute healing crisis as the person processes deeply internalized trauma during the birth transformation, as discussed above. However, sometimes the past trauma can be reactivated and compounded by a traumatic birth, in which case speedy intervention in the postpartum period is absolutely essential.

Family Trauma

It is essential to remember that the partner, other children, parents, and other loved ones can experience trauma too, especially if the birthing person is the central pillar or force around whom the rest of the family organizes their sense of selves. It can be earth-shattering to think that your beloved might die right now, or your mama, or your child, and yet the family is often forgotten in the shuffle of supporting the most visibly affected person. Witnesses and close family usually benefit from a therapeutic herbal regimen as well.

Useful Herbs for Birth Trauma:

Physical Healing

Vulneraries are an essential class of herbs for supporting physical healing. Combine them with **astringents** and **antimicrobials** for tears, episiotomies, hemorrhoids, and other tissue injuries. I like to blend Yarrow, Calendula, Plantain, Witch Hazel, and sea salt, provided warm in the squirt bottle with every pad change, or as a sitz blend in the bath tub, or soaked onto pads before freezing to make herbal ice packs.

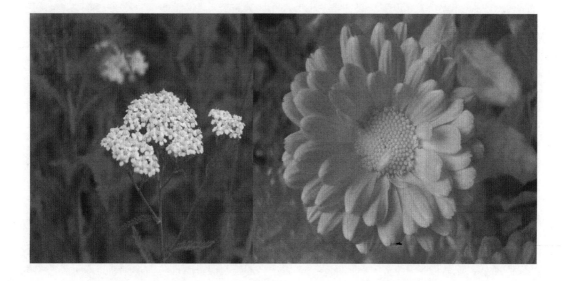

For people who have hemorrhaged, it is essential to support the regeneration of their blood count. These people should drink as much water and tea as possible and sleep as much as their body will allow, and their support people need to be cognizant of that plan. Mineral-rich tea can speed up the process, as well as helping prevent milk supply issues following hemorrhage (which are unfortunately common in those who do not rest, hydrate, and eat appropriately following a major blood loss, as their body simply does not have the extra it needs for lactogenesis). Nettles, Oatstraw, Alfalfa, Yarrow flowers and Raspberry make a nice base,

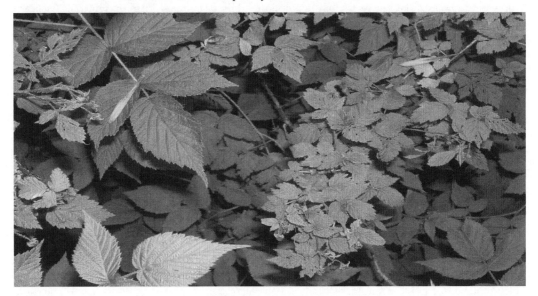

Tinctures of Yarrow flower and Lady's Mantle are wonderful allies to help tighten lax uterine tissues and speed the healing process following hemorrhage; this is also true of uterine prolapse.

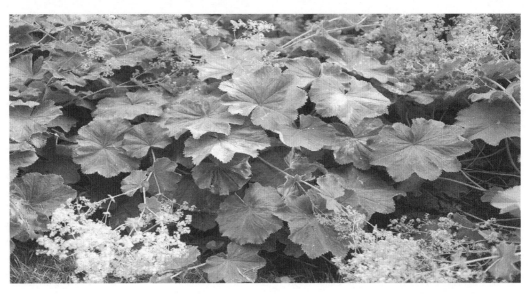

For those who have an infection now, had one in labor, or are at a risk of developing one postpartum, **antimicrobials** and **immune stimulants** are warranted. Echinacea is safe internally for breastfeeding parents, as are Elder and Spilanthes.

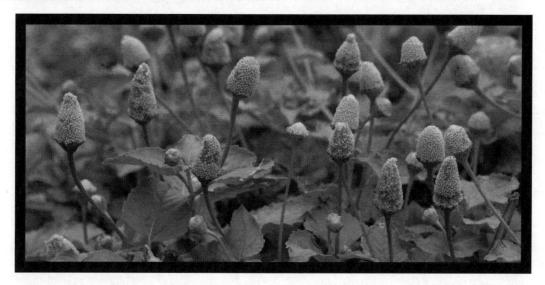

Tinctures can be added to squirt bottles for direct perineal application, or taken internally as usual. It is important to realize that the immune system may not be functioning at its utmost capacity following birth due to exhaustion, depletion of nutrients, and blood loss, so provide support early and often.

Muscle pain is extremely common and can be supported with any of your usual **anti-inflammatory** and **analgesic** liniments, massage oils, and salves, as well as baths and resting on a heating pad or hot water bottle. Muscle pain that persists past the first 2 or 3 days may be indicative of an actual injury, such as a muscle or ligament torn in the birth process. In these cases, rest, massage, and more aggressive musculoskeletal support may be warranted (Arnica massage oil, Solomon's Seal, etc.). Abdominal binders are very helpful for postpartum back or pelvic pain that appears musculoskeletal in origin, as supporting the musculature helps tissues heal in the right places without straining or over-stretching, in the absence of abdominal muscles.

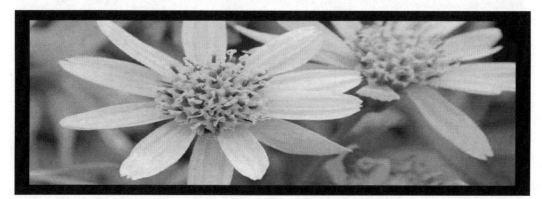

Emotional Healing

To support emotional healing in the wake of a traumatic birth, we prioritize uplifting mood, supporting the development of circadian rhythm and an appropriate sleep routine, managing healthy lactation, and preventing postpartum depression.

Non-drowsy uplifting **nervines** are essential for this type of healing. Milky Oats tincture is one of my absolute favorites, as it works quickly when you need it and has an increasing effect with regular use, and gives an overall feeling of rejuvenation that is so essential for the chrysalis-shedding of the healing process. It helps prevent postpartum depression, a major risk following traumatic birth (especially if someone has a history of depression), combined with Mimosa flowers for great effect. Lemon Balm is another nervine perfect for this type of healing as it can help with feelings of exhaustion and depletion as well, especially in warm weather; it can be added to a daily tea or taken as a tincture or oxymel. Small doses of Skullcap tincture are appropriate for anxiety or bouts of fury, especially with drop doses of heart openers as discussed below.

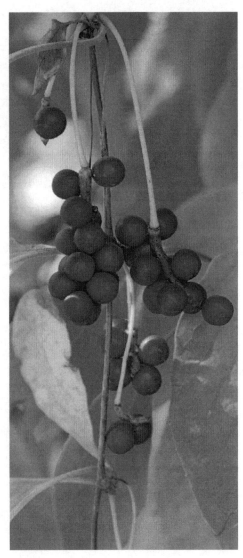

Adaptogens also have an important place in supporting healing from emotional trauma, but they should be chosen based on the specific presentation instead of one-size-fits-all (…like always). If the person seems especially run down, in particular after hemorrhage, infection requiring antibiotics, multi-day induction, or other long drawn-out saga, Ashwaganda is an excellent anabolic ally to rebuild deep strength. I turn to Shatavari if there is a major circadian rhythm disruption that their hormones would normally have regulated (like they aren't able to rouse to nurse, or aren't able to nap), and if there is a true milk supply issue, which is actually much less common than people think—often what is called "milk supply" is actually a latch issue, engorgement, or dehydration, so it is essential to be sure there is actually a milk supply issue before telling their body to make more milk; galactagogues are often not the answer. For circadian rhythm disruptions together with depression, anxiety, or fury, Schisandra is a perfect ally, especially as a honey.

Spiritual Healing: Heart Openers & Stimulating Dispersants

If the person is dissociating, distancing from their family, reports postpartum depression, the emotional trauma is deeply rooted in a forest of pre-existing traumas, or the birth was not recent, supporting spiritual healing is appropriate as well. The goals here are to help them reintegrate their experiences and sense of self, and to help the family find tangible means of love and support, to help hold the person through an important grief and healing process.

The term "Heart Openers" has become so overused as to become almost generic, with some practitioners using it to mean almost any herb that makes them feel calm, happy, or physically present. I'm using the term in a specific sense, to mean herbs that help us access experiences and feelings that we otherwise wall off inside ourselves as a coping mechanism. Accessing those experiences, taking them out and looking at them, allows us to process them appropriately following a difficult event, which can help prevent us from internalizing the trauma and thus creating a deep-seated, long term trauma point that can affect us for years to come.

In these situations, we combine **stimulating dispersants** with **heart openers** specific for grief and trauma that are uplifting and improving to motivation. Doses range from drop doses up to 1/8 teaspoon. This helps the person take out the memory, look at it without fear, and let go. Guided visualization or meditation can be helpful with this, as they breath it out or blow it away or watch it flow out of their fingertips or whatever works for them. These formulas should always be combined with an appropriate **nervine** to support emotional well-being simultaneously: **do not cover them with the raw meat of their memories and leave them to the wolves**.

One of my favorite formulas is a honey made from Hawthorn, Rose, and Prickly Ash, with the Hawthorn and Rose working as uplifting trauma-specific heart openers that improve motivation, the Prickly Ash as a stimulating dispersant, and the sweetness of the honey sending the medicine deep in the body to help loosen stored memories.

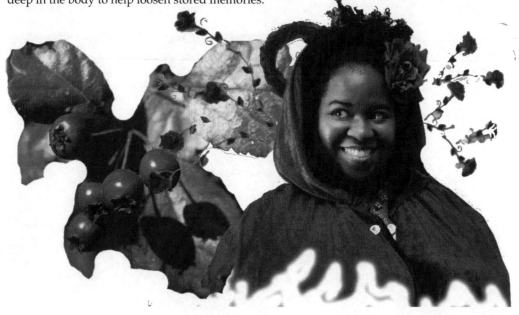

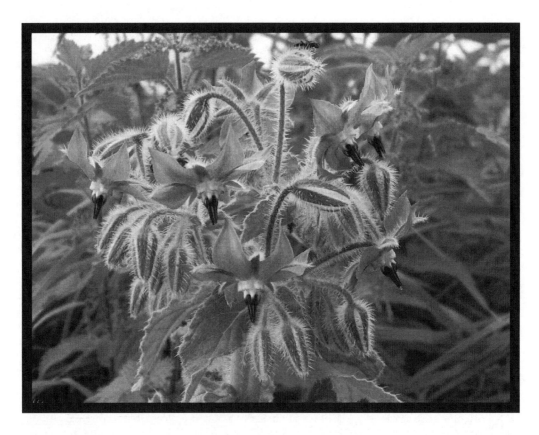

I also love Borage, for its mood-uplifting nature and how it helps us stand firm in the face of adversity, which can be really helpful for staring down bad memories, especially for assault survivors. I use drop doses of Borage generally, but they can take larger doses if they are not nursing and after miscarriage, especially as an oxymel with Lemon Balm and Ginger.

If grounding is needed, burdock or elecampane can be useful allies depending on the person's constitution.

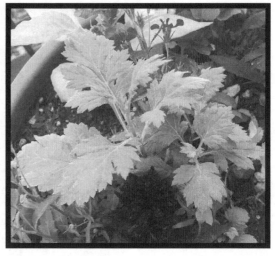

Other stimulating dispersants useful in this application include Ginger, Elecampane, Pine, Artemisia, Juniper, Wormwood, and Mugwort, depending on the person's constitution and how the trauma is manifesting itself (i.e. during dreams, Mugwort).

Additional Techniques

Nutrition

Nutrition provides the foundation for healing. Rest, hydration, and a healing diet high in quality protein, fat, minerals, and vitamins is essential for tissue repair, regeneration of blood cells, healthy nervous system and immune function, and milk supply development. Diets must provide ample iron, calcium, fat, and protein, with vitamin C and vitamin D to improve absorption. We give our cells every advantage when we build them from a strong foundation: grounding, nourishing, warming foods support physical and emotional healing. Foods like bone broth, stews, seaweed, live cultures, high quality meat, leafy greens, eggs, fish, avocados, and sweet fruit are ideal. Balance healthy food with comfort food: the warming stick-to-your-ribs nourishment of our families is often an essential expression of love, and should not be thrown out with the bathwater. Instead, encourage the family to integrate healthy foods into their diet in creative ways, or have the lasagna/tamales/fried chicken/macaroni and cheese for dinner and bone broth miso soup for lunch.

Therapeutic Language

The words you use when speaking about someone's birth experience matter. Ask for their impressions instead of making assumptions. As each person is the authority on their own health and body, it is inappropriate to engage in downplaying or ranking traumas, as in the common practice of informing birthing people that an experience perceived as terrifying is actually normal or common, or that they didn't have it that bad, etc.

Asking for their birth story and using limbic resonance to really be there with them is extremely therapeutic, whether it was traumatic or not: "Tell me about your birth, how was it?" is a great opener. In the days after birth a family is integrating the experience and talking about it in

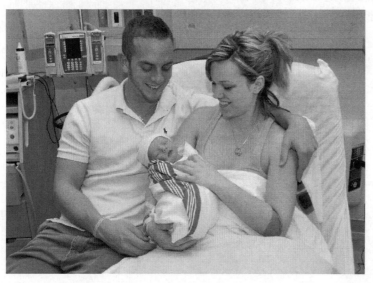

detail can help prevent it from becoming traumatizing if it was scary, and regardless help it become a source of power for both parents. Use their words back to them; if the partner says "She was like a fertility goddess, I still can't believe it," referring to her goddessness a few minutes later reinforces the importance of the partner's perceptions and communicates to the partner that their role is central to the narrative.

215

Partners are often ignored, especially in emergencies; this can be hard even in normal birth, but especially when things get scary. This is also true of other children. Eliciting their impressions, feelings, and stories with gravity can help them integrate the experience and be able to step into a caregiving role more fully.

One of the most common pieces of sadness that people carry in their hearts for decades is the idea that they didn't "really" give birth if they gave birth surgically via caesarian section, which is ableist garbage. Unfortunately, this idea is reinforced by our natural health community's narrative that the "right" way to birth is unmedicated, at home, ideally in a tub; while this is a very nice birth it's certainly not the only way, and the narrative is racist, classist, ableist, and completely tone deaf to the complex multifactorial influences on health outcomes that dictate how our bodies are able to birth safely, especially those related to socioeconomic status and race. It is a backlash against the overmedicalization of birth and the destruction of a home birth as old as time, powered by the glorious resurgence that we've seen in the last 2 decades. It's an understandable narrative trying to normalize natural birth; however, it is very untherapeutic for our many friends and loved ones 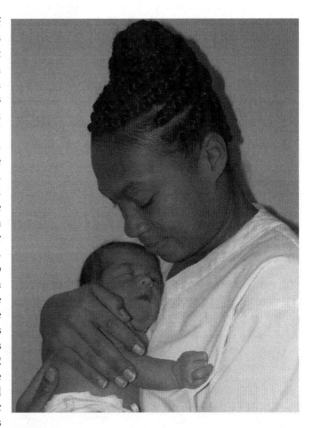 who need to birth differently. Instead of surgery or c-section, referring to "surgical birth" is an important distinction, and peppering the conversation with phrases like "when you gave birth," "your birth," "giving birth," etc. is an essential act, as it can help them reframe the experience and ameliorate feelings of insufficiency, making space for self-empowerment.

Never assume that a train wreck was traumatic; likewise, don't assume that a good outcome was not. I've worked with innumerable families who experienced trauma when births veered off their planned path but were still routine, like a long induction or a baby with jaundice therapy, as well as families who had a very challenging experience and emerged without feeling traumatized (i.e. emergency surgery, baby needing resuscitation or medications, someone being flown to a bigger hospital in a helicopter). It is possible to go through these things and feel okay about it, like "that was really scary, I'm glad it's over, thank goodness we're all okay," integrating the experience as a hard day in the past.

Integrating The Experience

As parents, we often don't allow ourselves the luxury of time and space to grieve, as there are so many demands on every moment of our lives. It is appropriate for many people to grieve after a traumatic experience: maybe they grieve for the birth they hoped to have, maybe for the person they were before, maybe for what they learned about themselves in the process...allowing time to grieve improves the chances of a solid integration. This is most effective right away, during the postpartum healing process.

Validate their feelings and encourage them to claim their power. Using therapeutic language combined with limbic resonance and reflecting feelings is helpful, while trying to help them reframe the experience with themselves as the protagonist, as opposed to someone powerless that has things done to them. Help them identify sources of power and claim them over and over until it sticks. Phrases like, "you never knew exactly how strong you were before, and no one can ever take that knowledge from you" can be helpful. Look to your heart openers and nervines, as discussed throughout.

Adjunct Therapies

Numerous other modalities can be extremely helpful as adjuncts. Limbic resonance is always a helpful tool when speaking to people about personal topics, and in particular when dealing with trauma. Some people may benefit from talk therapy, EMDR, or other trauma-specific therapy modalities, especially those experiencing reactivation or compounding of past trauma. Mindfulness meditation can be helpful for people who have experienced numerous traumatic events in their life.

Massage, acupuncture, and yoga can help release somatic trauma, especially combined with heart openers and visualization. Massage can make use of herbal infused oils to increase efficacy. Gentle massage can also be very helpful for newborns after a difficult birth. In yoga, hip opening poses are especially helpful. Moxibustion can be a powerful acupuncture tool to send the medicine deep. I have had great results in my practice with using these tools concurrently with herbs to release stored trauma; however, it is possible for the person to experience a healing crisis when memories are initially triggered, so it is essential that it happen on their timeframe, when they feel strong, and that they are provided with a rescue formula for anxiety, fury, or panic if relevant. Craniosacral therapy can be wonderful for somatic trauma stored in the pelvis or lower back, as well as postpartum back pain. However, my absolute favorite use of craniosacral therapy is for newborns who had a rough delivery. Often, these kids may not be nursing well because they don't feel good, which is a set up for further problems like jaundice, latch problems, or mastitis. They might not be sleeping comfortably because one side of their head or shoulder hurts. Craniosacral can work wonders in this situation.

Final Thoughts

Although birth trauma is extremely common, it is by no means universal. All birthing families should receive the gift of love and caring from their community, as life transformations are challenging. Holding a family up as they shed the chrysalis of their old structure is a mitzvah that builds our energy as well as theirs. Using herbs and adjunct therapies together with the language of birth self-empowerment helps them step through trauma and into their power, as only transformative hardship can do.

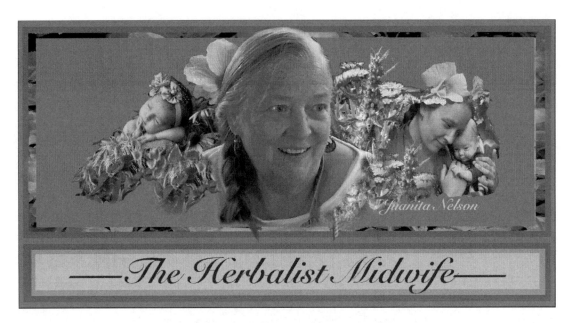

HERBS IN BREASTFEEDING

by Jaunita Nelson

Juanita is an amazing S.W. midwife and plant healer, whose periodic articles will add much to the Quarterly, and who's classes at the <u>Good Medicine Confluence</u> are much treasured.

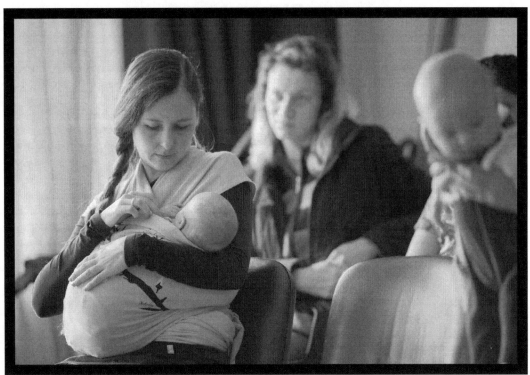

206

With this article, my goal is to give you some basics about the mechanics of how various substances go from being taken or ingested by the mother. their transformation into breast milk, their delivery to the baby via breastfeeding, and eventually the effect on the nursing baby. We'll talk about how that knowledge can inform you, as an herbalist, in the way you prescribe, how those herbs might affect both mother and baby, what to be cautious about, how to apply your knowledge within the context of recent research. I want to give you some tips on prescribing based on who you're trying to treat (mom or baby) and info for issues specific to breastfeeding. Once we get a basic feel of the issues, I hope to enter into a discussion about the specific concerns about cannabis use while nursing and the legal ramifications of continuing to breastfeed here in Colorado.

I want to start this discussion with some commentary about the difference between the scientific view of how and what substances enter into the breast milk and the traditional, historical view. There has been an explosion of information recently about both the physiology of milk production, the pharmacology of drugs and herbs, and most exciting-the amazing transformative ability of the body to sense specific environmental stimuli that then alters the chemical make-up of breast milk in direct response to the baby's needs. This is mind-blowing information that has to change the way we view both the mother/baby dyad and the way we treat and prescribe herbs.

While research is coming in fast and furious now, studying how drugs/herbs effect the baby it has not historically been a major focus of study. There are a few reasons for this. First, nursing has not been particularly valued by the medical community, not because the effect on baby wasn't a concern but that the importance of breastfeeding itself was not taken into consideration. If there were maternal health concerns that required medical interventions most recommendations were to temporarily or permanently stop breastfeeding because there was no in depth understanding(much less research) of how treatment might affect the baby.

The focus was on the mother's needs and how cessation of nursing might affect both partners was irrelevant. Because formula has become a mainstay in our culture and easily available it became the standard response to addressing maternal issues rather that finding a way to keep mom and baby together during treatment and maintaining breastfeeding. For many years, rather than increasing research, the standard was to categorize both pharmaceuticals and botanicals as potentially harmful to the baby so the options were to not treat or if the situation was concerning enough to recommend not nursing. Hopefully, some of that is changing but there is still a long way to go. Case in point, the CDC recently recommended that breastfeeding mother's with the flu either stop caring for their baby and/or stop nursing implying that the risk of the baby contracting the flu was worse than the benefits of continuing to breastfeed. The ramification of that statement were widely criticized for not taking into considerations the relationship between the nursing mother and baby and the profound impact of separating them. Consumer response is changing the way things are viewed.

Second, there has never been a strong incentive to study breastfeeding because there was no demonstrable, financial incentive by the pharmaceutical companies who fund most of the research. The side effects to the baby of a particular drug prescribed to the mother was always downplayed because there were alternatives available. Formula companies and pharmaceutical companies were happily partnered. Proving the benefits of formula over breastfeeding was for many years the incentive of the formula makers as a way to market their product-downplaying and disregarding breastfeeding and discouraging research into the profound health benefits thereby affecting generations of babies in all parts of the world.

Third, the misunderstanding of the difference of the physiology of pregnancy with that of the nursing mother was poorly understood. They tend to get lumped together in treatment considerations. The statement "If pregnant or nursing consult your provider before using" is

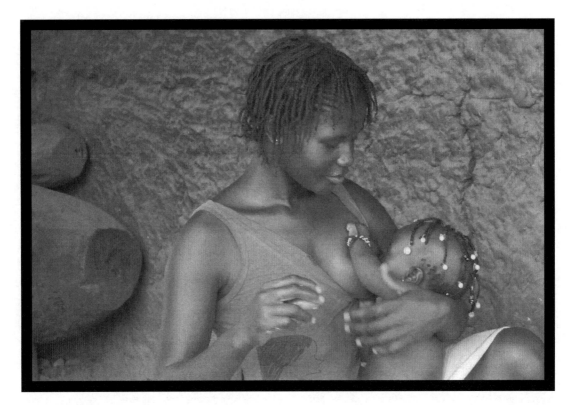

still a common finding and few people make a distinction between the two. The concerns we have for the impact of herbs during pregnancy have very little correlation during the nursing period and the herbalist can play a role in understanding the difference.

Empirically, how we address issues for the breastfeeding pair has been somewhat different than the scientific model. Herbalist, midwives, and folks caring for new moms and babies have always recognized the essential value and importance of the breastfeeding couple. Financial incentives have rarely played much of a part in providing care. However, the one area we have been somewhat lax is the treatment of maternal health issues during the breastfeeding period. So much of the time we back off of any significant treatment for fear of negatively affecting the baby. While important, I think we need to re-evaluate how herbs cross into the milk supply and re-think our treatment protocols. The way we do this is to understand both the physiology of milk production and the pharmacology of the herbs we want to use.

So how do herbs enter into the milk supply? It is a fairly straight-forward process defined by a few specific factors. Substances enter into the milk supply after being ingested by the mother, processed by her body, and delivered into her blood supply. As the maternal blood passes by the alveolar cells lining the milk buds within the milk sacs, substances are diffused across the cell membranes. Herbs, or their components, must pass through both lipid membranes to enter into the milk supply. The degree that substances pass is affected initially by the gaps between the alveolar cells. During the first 3-4 days postpartum the gaps are larger and allow for greater diffusion of herbs, immunoglobulins, and maternal proteins. Once prolactin, a hormone produced in the pituitary gland, begins to enlarge the size and number of the alveolar cells, the gaps between the cells is dramatically decreased and the exchange of substances transferring from the maternal blood supply is reduced. Once milk production is established the amount of any substance entering into the milk supply is relatively small. The standard, with some exceptions, is that 1% of the drug/herb ingested by the mother, ie. maternal dose, makes it's way into the milk supply and ultimately into the baby. There are some substance that will cross more readily or accumulate in the milk up to 10% but the 1%-10% standard defines that substance as "safe." [1]

There are a few factors that will influence how well a substance will enter into the milk supply. The most important of these is the mother's plasma levels. Remember that whatever herb/ drug the mother ingests must traverse through her own metabolic process in order to be active. If the substance does not easily enter into the maternal plasma it will be greatly reduced in the milk supply, thus the bio- availability of the substance is reduced.. As the level of the herb increases in the mother's plasma it will increase in the milk supply. It enters into the milk supply as a process of diffusion as the body seeks equilibrium between fluids. As the plasma levels decrease they will automatically decrease in the milk. There are exceptions to this: a few substances may actually concentrate in the milk supply because of a change in pH or affecting an active pumping system in the alveolar wall preventing them from traversing back across the membranes from the milk supply into the maternal plasma. Iodine and alkaloids do this and therefore can be in higher concentrations in the milk supply compared to other substances.
Other factors that influence the degree at which a substance enters the milk supply are lipid solubility, protein binding, the half-life of the substance in the maternal plasma, and the molecular size and weight. If a substance is highly lipid soluble in the maternal circulation then it will enter into the milk supply in higher quantities.

Cannabis, because of it's fat soluble qualities is an example here-although the actual effects of that higher concentration is under debate. It has generally been understood that .8% of the maternal plasma levels is found in the milk supply-however, even that number has recently come under question. Protein binding in the maternal circulation greatly affects the way a substance accumulates in the milk supply. The higher the percentage of protein binding, the less

the substance will cross the membranes into the milk supply. [1]

When considering whether or not an herb is relatively safe during breastfeeding there are a few things to consider. This is true whether you are the herbal provider prescribing specific herbs for a particular condition or a breastfeeding mother trying to treat a cold. Knowing the age and weight of the child is significant. A 3 day old infant is much more at risk for having a stronger reaction because of the degree which substances can cross the plasma/milk barrier than a 6 month old baby whose metabolism has matured and organs have developed. The amount of milk consumed is significant. An older baby may consume more milk but will also weigh more and be able to process substances differently as their metabolism matures. A premature or low-birth weight baby is more at risk for adverse reactions.

There is a Lactation Risk Category that can prove helpful in deciding on a specific substance. It ranges from L1-safest to L5-contraindicated. The problem with these categories is there are almost no extensive lists that define specific risk levels for herbs. Pharmaceuticals have had a much more rigorous scientific exploration in terms of their affects on breastfeeding-whether baby, mom, or the affect on nursing itself. However, even here there is very little in-depth information and many new drugs often have no studies done. Interestingly enough, the lack of studies has not deterred the basic blanket statement that most drugs (and by referral most herbs) are considered safe to use during nursing. There are almost no studies that track the use of drugs or herbs across the full spectrum of nursing gauging bio-availability, maternal and newborn serum levels, protein binding, or half-life at different times in the relationship at differing degrees of nursing. [1]

The American Herbal Products Association's Botanical Safety Handbook has created it's own set of safety classes. Class 1 is herbs that can be safely consumed when used appropriately and Class 2 as herbs for which the following use restrictions apply, unless otherwise directed by an expert qualified in the use of the described substance.

Class 2a: For external use only
Class 2b: Not to be used during pregnancy
Class 2c: Not to be used during lactation.
Class 2d: Other specific use restrictions as noted
Class 3 includes herbs to be used under the supervision of a qualified expert. Specific labeling is recommended for Class 3 herbs. [2]

While, in general, most herbs are going to be safe for mom and baby there are a few categories of herbs that I do try to avoid during breastfeeding.

Here is a basic list:

1. Known toxic herbs
2. Herbs containing PA's unless they're being used strictly topically
3. Herbs that have the potential of reducing Mom's prolactin levels 4. Strong laxatives
4. Herbs containing high levels of caffeine

One of the concerns about the few studies that are done on herbs and lactation is the relatively small range of the 1. length of time that the study was conducted and 2. the number of people studied. The gold standard of a double-blind, placebo controlled study that assesses a large number of breastfeeding pairs over a long period of time have not been done. What we are left with are small, often poorly designed studies that investigated a small number of breastfeeding pairs and then applied results onto the larger population.

So where does that leave us as herbalists trying to navigate the information available and help the moms and babies seeking our help? In general, I think we can be pretty happy about what we do know while always striving to increase our knowledge base. One thing we can access is the empirical knowledge that has been passed down for generations about how plants can provide specific actions on either mom, baby, or both. Over thousands of years of observation, the traditional healers witnessed the results of their prescriptions and treatment and some of that knowledge is available to us even now.

When we can plant our feet in both worlds and take the improving scientific information that is exploding right now and balance it with our deep intuitive knowledge about plant use we can meld the two together to create a comprehensive way of caring for moms and babies as they journey through their breastfeeding time.

There are a few things I take into consideration when I'm working with breastfeeding moms and babies. I try to break it down into a few categories to help myself determine the best route of care. First, determine who (what) I'm treating. Is this a breastfeeding issue? Is it straight mechanics: sore nipples, engorgement, clogged ducts, full-blown mastitis, weaning? Sometimes increasing or decreasing the milk supply is a simple mechanical issue and sometimes it's a more involved hormonal issue. Is there a medical issue happening and mom happens to be nursing as well? How significant is the issue? Does she have a cold or is she dealing with something more serious? Is this something that was present prior to pregnancy, birth, and postpartum or is this something new. Was it being treated before and in what way? Herbs, pharmaceuticals? What worked historically?

Am I trying to treat the baby through mom's milk? While we now understand that only a small percentage of herbs make it into the milk supply, yet empirically I have seen baby's respond to treatment by treating the mother. It's possible that there is something else going on here that has nothing to do with the chemical substance transferred into the milk supply. The more we learn about the adaptability of the chemical composition of milk on a day to day basis, and its ability to directly respond to the needs of the baby, the more I think that there is a mechanism for treating baby here. Certainly if there is a cold circulating within the family it is possible to boost the mother's immune system with both herbs and vitamins. A portion of those substance will get into the milk supply but so will the mother's increased antibodies thereby decreasing the chance that baby will get sick.

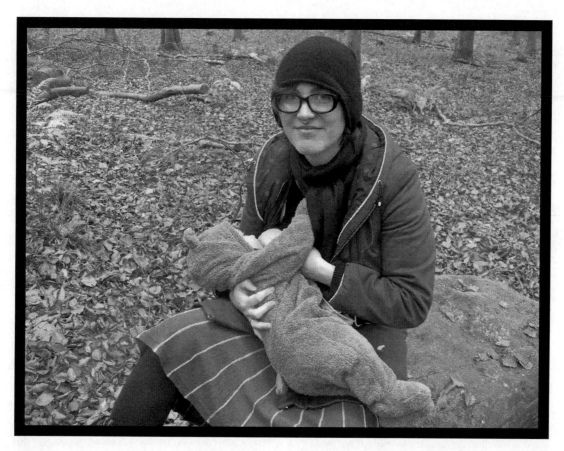

There is some controversy about whether or not foods ingested by the mother will adversely affect the newborn. The scientific analysis of breast milk after eating strong substance like onions, broccoli, or chocolate will tell us that there is very little chemical presence of those foods transferred into the milk. But tell that to the mother whose child has spent the night awake crying and it becomes clear that there is something else at work here. I've seen babies with chronic issues resolve seemingly overnight by simply removing certain foods from the mother's diet. I usually recommend that new mothers start our with restricting a few basic foods until we know how this particular baby responds. Early postpartum can be challenging enough without adding in a fussy baby due to mom ingesting certain foods.

Here is the list of foods I recommend being careful with:

1. Cruciferous vegetables, Broccoli, Cabbage, Cauliflower, Brussel Sprouts, Kale
2. Stimulants containing caffeine
3. Onions, Tarlic, Curry, Chili
4. Very acidic foods like Tomatoes (sauce), Pineapple, Citrus
5. Foods that the mother is sensitive to. If the mother is truly gluten sensitive then not eating food high in gluten will make everybody happier.
6. Foods know to be specific for increasing specific issues: for example dairy and reflux disease

I want to talk a minute here about looking at the bigger picture when working with breastfeeding folks. Taking into consideration the overall situation with this pair will guide you in your recommendations. It is really easy to want to prescribe an herb, for example, a galactagogue to increase milk supply. I would encourage you to take a step back and really investigate what might be creating that need. Understanding some basic physiology and it's timing can make a huge difference. Here's an example of what I'm talking about.

You receive a phone call from a new mother who is concerned because she doesn't think she is producing enough milk and she wants your recommendation for a tea that will increase her milk supply. She is in day 3 postpartum. She had a normal, vaginal delivery and her baby weighed 9 # at birth but has dropped to 8# 8 oz. She nurses every 3 hours around the clock usually. There is nothing wrong here! While colostrum is produced early and provides the perfect food it is not produced in quantity. At three days postpartum, the milk may not be "in" and you have a baby who is big, hungry, and maybe not nursing frequently enough to trigger prolactin production-yet. A certain amount of weight loss in the first few days is normal and not unusual and in this case is not excessive. You want to encourage maternal hydration and ensure she is receiving adequate protein and calorie intake, but the best advice you can give her is to nurse, eat, and rest. Three to four days postpartum is often when the reality of caring for this newborn is starting to settle in, hormones are starting to shift, and mom needs encouragement. She may need to evaluate how well baby is latching with someone who is well trained in lactation support. If you give her something to increase her milk supply right now then you may make the days following this one more difficult rather than less so. Engorgement happens in differing degrees for different moms but when the milk does come in she often will have more than she knows what to do with. Baby will get satisfied soon. Eventually, there is a regulation of production that happens. This is how it's designed. When you increase the volume at that time you make it much harder for baby to latch well and run the risk of creating a clogged duct or worse mastitis.

Now, let's compare that to another scenario. A mother and her 6 month old baby come to see you about herbal support for nursing. You spend some time with her and start to understand some of her history. This is her third child and there is a three year old and a 6 year old at home. Her baby is exclusively breastfed and nurses during the day every 2 hours for around 10 minutes. At night the baby is sleeping through the night. At a recent well-baby check the baby has started to plateau in weight gain and length. Mom is pretty proud of the fact that she weighs a few pounds less than she did before she got pregnant. She has had a couple of bouts of mastitis. She is concerned about her milk supply and wants to know what she can take to increase it. Before you pull our the galacatagogues, take some time to look at the bigger picture here.

There are a lot of reasons for a decrease in milk volume. The two at the top of the list are mostly mechanical. If this mom did not establish good habits early in the breastfeeding relationship, she may have not created a good latching pattern with the baby and while baby still gets some milk, it's not the fat-rich milk that is triggered with a relaxed prolonged nursing session. If the mother is not focused on high quality protein and calorie intake, she made not be producing enough milk. The body will sacrifice milk production before it sacrifices maternal tissue and or function. While sleeping through the night might have been a well-meaning goal for this mother, it is not necessarily an appropriate one. Babies need to nurse frequently enough and long enough to maintain high prolactin levels. Prescribing a galactogogue may be really helpful here (Fenugreek is my favorite) but supporting this mom to spend more time at each feeding with an actively sucking baby until the fat milk descends, go back to nursing at night, and increasing her protein and caloric intake will do wonders. There are "breastfeeding lifestyle" issues that need to be addressed or the Fenugreek tea will have only limited success.

The take away here is that expanding your knowledge about why something might be occurring through expanding your history-taking, clinical skills will only improve the success you have as an herbalist treating breastfeeding couples. Breastfeeding is a mechanical, hormonal, emotional, social, and culturally influenced activity that can be enhanced through providing a wide-range of community support. Mom's need a full spectrum of support during this time that goes beyond herbal teas.

So, lets talk about some specific breastfeeding issues that can be treated with herbs. I want to re-iterate the importance of knowing where the mother and baby are in their nursing journey. How you address a newborn/new mother's concerns will be very different from treating a mother with a nursing toddler. Before I recommend anything to the new mom I want to know a few things. How was the birth itself? Long? Super fast? Were there any pharmaceuticals used in labor? How soon after the birth did baby latch on and nurse? How long has it been since the birth? How often has baby nursed since then? How long will the baby nurse during each session? Has the milk come in yet? How often is baby pooping?

It seems like a lot of questions to ask but getting a sense of how both mom and baby are adapting to breast feeding will go a long ways towards helping you know how to support both the Mom and baby.

Cracked, Sore Nipples

Going from occasionally having someone interested in your breast to having a baby attached 24/7 can be a huge transition for a lot of women. In the beginning, most women find that some soreness is par for the course as the sensitive skin gets used to being sucked on. If the baby's position and latch have been well evaluated and corrected if necessary, treating the skin becomes the focus. If the nipples have cracked and are bleeding, it becomes the challenge of wound care. Mom should be encouraged to continue nursing and changing up the baby's position for each feeding. That provides a slightly different point of pressure and can give the sorest areas a chance to heal. Air drying off the breast before putting it away can reduce the risk of fungal infections. Once the baby has finished with the nursing session, I like putting a vulnerary rich salve on the nipple. My favorite is a combination plantain leaf and comfrey leaf made into an olive oil/beeswax salve. I know there are people concerned about comfrey and the PA's but when used for a few days I believe it to be safe. Calendula salve is also a wonderful choice. Any residual can be gently wiped off before the start of the next nursing session. I do not recommend straight or even diluted essential oils as I find them to be more more problematic- inflammation of the sensitive nipple tissue as a result of their being too strong or having an allergic reaction in mom or baby is an unnecessary result. It is important to remind mom that practicing good hygiene is important here. Changing a diaper and then grabbing the breast to nurse without washing her hands (and yes, we've all done it) can lead to all kinds of contamination and infection.

Thrush

Thrush, a fungal infection, can be transferred from baby's mouth to the mother's breasts and can cause extremely sore nipples as well as pain in the baby's mouth. This can usually be differentiated from normal sore nipples because it often happens after the initial soreness of new nursing has worn off. My first line of defense is not specifically herbs but rather treating it as an imbalance rather than an infection. Probiotics given to the mother and infant probiotics given to the baby by letting them suck it off mom's finger 3-4 times a day will often times be enough. In really stubborn cases I will have the mother wash her nipple with Yerba Manza decoction after each feeding. That along with eliminating obvious sugar intake will usually kick it.

Clogged Ducts/Mastitis

When you look at the anatomy of the breast you have alveolar milk sacs that channel down into the ducts that then carry the milk out through the nipple. When these ducts don't get drained completely they can plug up and cause a painful lump. This is differentiated from mastitis in that the former is uncomfortable where as the latter causes increased inflammation, fever, and the potential for going systemic. A clogged duct can easily lead to mastitis if left untreated but is often much easier to resolve. When a mother calls me complaining of a sore spot on her breast

225

that is hard and painful unless she's running a fever, I will treat it as a clogged duct. The most important piece here is to release the plug and get the milk to flow again. Baby is the most efficient at this so encouraging nursing from that affected side is essential. (Caution the mom to not neglect the other side but to not shy away from the sore side because of pain.) If baby is not nursing every 1 1/2 to 2 hours around the clock then I have mothers use a breast pump. Standing in the shower and letting hot water flow over the breast, using hot water compresses, and massaging the breast with downward and outward strokes can help release the clog. Grated potatoes or bruised cabbage leaves applied to the sore area covered with a warm washcloth helps to soften and draw out the clog. This alternating with massage, nursing/pumping and repeating until the pain has eased will usually release it.

If there is fever and red inflammation visible from the outside then we've crossed a line into true mastitis. It feels like you've been hit by a truck and can come on very fast. All of the above recommendations are still suggested but to reduce the inflammation I will have them alternate hot compresses with cold packs. I have them take 250 mg of Vt. C, 60 gtts of Echinacea tincture every 2 hours around the clock. I like Calendula and Chamomile tea to help ease and relax. It's important to let folks know that this will not resolve in a few hours and they will need to commit to stopping everything else and take care of themselves. I see these women describe their lives as overwhelming. They are trying to care for their baby, their partner and family, often a job or other responsibilities and life is stressful and chaotic. When asked they often describe dealing with increased life stress, lack of sleep, forgetting to hydrate, not eating well, and underwire bras. Moms with other children at home sometimes forget to take the time to fully empty their breasts by letting baby nurse longer or more frequently feeling the pressure to be up and doing. Supporting these moms with infusions of lemon balm, motherwort, and nettles is both nutritive and calming and helps remind them to slow down and take care of themselves.

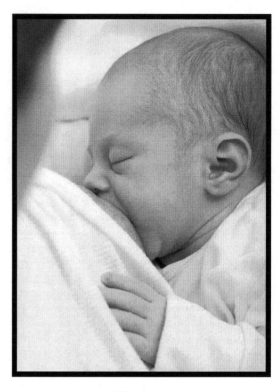

Milk Supply

The concern about whether or not a mom feels like she has enough milk is a universal theme. Because the actual amount of milk transferred to baby via breastfeeding is invisible it can make the question come up over and over. Knowing where they are in their breastfeeding journey like we talked about before is important. Habits that are created early postpartum can continue for a long time. It's often not until the baby is a few months old that milk supply, or a decrease in it, becomes more apparent. When a mom calls or comes in to see me it becomes pretty obvious quickly that her biggest concern is milk supply. Often this is because she has taken her baby to a doctor and they have indicated that the baby is not gaining enough weight. A typical scenario starts to be revealed. She describes baby as "fussy", he/she is sleeping through the night, there is often three hours between feedings inter-mixed with periods of cluster feeding when she can't put the baby down, pooping has decreased to once a day or every few days. Mom has lost all her pregnancy weight and struggles to find time to eat during the day. Her menstrual cycle may have returned. Not everybody has all these but everybody will have some of them. Before I look at hormonal issues that might be affecting supply, I look at this as a mechanical issue. There is so much information available to folks about proper feeding schedules, and the importance of babies sleeping through the night, and the extreme pressure that moms feel to be "functional." It's not a surprise that a simple supply and demand cycle gets thrown off.

There are some basic elements that need to be present to both avoid a lack of supply or to bring it back. These things are:

1. Nursing frequently enough and for long enough to trigger the regular, consistent production of milk.

This means baby is nursing at least a couple of times throughout the night as well as often enough during the day to maintain supply. When baby nurses long enough they trigger a second let- down reflex that will bring milk down from the rear milk sacs. This milk is higher in fat content and will sustain baby and encourage growth. The milk that is released in the beginning of each session is higher in sugar content and is designed to stimulate and waken baby for continued nursing. If that is the only milk they receive then eventually they will get hungry, fussy, grow less, and the milk supply will decrease.

2. Ensuring a good latch.

This is a hot topic these days. Unless the latch has been evaluated and there is a clear indication of a problem, I encourage Moms to not assume the worse. Tongue tie is the issue dujour but I have seen latching problems with no tongue tie and dramatic tongue tie that does not affect latching in the least. Getting the nipple far enough back in the baby's mouth up against the palate triggers the release of milk and is the whole point of a good latch

3. Making sure that mom is consuming enough protein and calories and water to make the milk.

4. This seems obvious but so many times the need to lose weight and/or a busy life style with influence how much mom is eating. The other thing I see is that so many people are so focused on what they can't or shouldn't eat they forget that **they just need to eat.**

The best way I have ever found to increase a milk supply that has dwindled is to send mom and baby to bed naked. They are instructed to let baby touch, taste, smell, and handle the breasts as much as possible. Let baby nurse as much as they want. They literally just get to hang out together and nurse. Make sure that mom has plenty of food and water and all other pursuits of the day are put aside. The idea here is to re-set the hormonal triggers that support good milk production. I suggest doing that for 24 hours and watch what happens. Occasionally, it might need to be 48 or 72 hours but almost without fail the supply will be back and everyone happy again.
In support of this process, adding herbs into the mix can be very beneficial. Fenugreek is my favorite tea to increase the supply. I have moms drink 3-4 cups a day. Here is where good evaluation skills come into play. If the mom has described being anxious or stressed out then adding plants that will help her relax and enjoy each nursing session can be included into your mix. Lemon balm with nettles added to the Fenugreek, combined with an hourly dose of motherwort tincture can help her overcome some of that daily anxiety. If mom is describing depression then adding St. John's Wort to the mix is helpful. Creating support systems so that this mother has multiple people/avenues to decrease isolation becomes essential.

Cannabis & Breast Milk

Now, let's talk about the use of Cannabis during breastfeeding. As you know, recreational Marijuana use in adults was legalized a few years back in Colorado (and more recently in California.) THC, both recreational and medicinal, is still considered a Schedule 1 drug under both federal and Colorado law. Schedule 1 drugs are defined as 1. The drug or other substance has a high potential for abuse. 2. The drug or other substance has no currently accepted medical use in treatment in the United States. 3. There is a lack of accepted safety for use of the drug or other substance under medical supervision.

Based on that definition alone it's easy to see that there is discrepancy in how Marijuana is classified. With the current administration, the chances of Marijuana being removed from the Schedule 1 list and re-classified are slim.

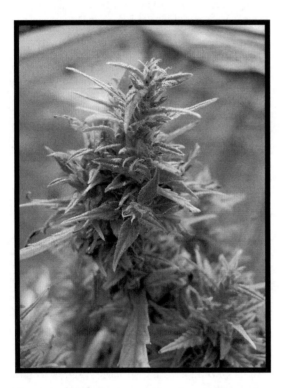

Current Colorado law states that if a women voluntarily reports Marijuana use to their health care provider and/or have a positive drug test during a prenatal visit that information can not be used in a criminal investigation. However, once she has been flagged, she has implicitly given her permission to test her baby after the birth for THC. If baby tests positive at birth for a Schedule 1 substance, Colorado law defines that as an instance of child neglect which automatically requires a report to social services. Social services is required to follow up by doing interviews, home visits, and blood testing to ensure that there is no ongoing exposure. If a

mother is breastfeeding her baby and has been identified as a Marijuana user or baby tested positive for any amount of THC after the birth she is required to stop breastfeeding. If she declines or baby is re-tested and tests positive for THC then Social Services has the right to begin legal proceedings to remove the baby from the mother's care and the home. [7]

ACOG, the American College of Obstetricians and Gynecologists, came out with a position statement titled "Marijuana Use During Pregnancy and Lactation in October," 2017. While it goes into detail about the concerns about Marijuana use during pregnancy, it's policy on breastfeeding is considerably more limited. It states that "There are insufficient data to evaluate the effects of Marijuana use on infants during lactation and breastfeeding, and in the absence of such data, Marijuana use is discouraged. Breastfeeding women should be informed that the potential risks of exposure to Marijuana metabolites are unknown and should be encouraged to discontinue Marijuana use." It also went on to list the supposed social impact of Marijuana use as creating dysfunctional mothers who would neglect their babies and/or that Marijuana use was hand in hand with cocaine, heroin, and pharmaceutical abuse. [5]

Currently, the status of research concerning 1. the amount of THC that is crossing into the mother's milk and 2. it's affect both short and long term on baby is extremely limited. The studies that have been done have been irregularly if not poorly designed. Many of the studies have included the simultaneous use of tobacco and/or other drugs. Most studies are done on animals with the results applied to humans as proven fact (studies done are rats are especially misleading as there is a 1:1 or 100% transfer of substances in maternal plasma into the milk supply compared to humans which is commonly 1%.) Some of the studies have started with a defined negative bias. Some of the studies have extrapolated information on a statistically small number of participants and applied that information to the general public. One study that has been used to define policy had a total of two participants. With other herbs, individual case studies have been introduced into the literature and helped define risks of use and exposure, but in *no other case has the widespread release of poorly done research so dramatically defined policy or so impacted families.*

There is an independent study currently being implemented by Dr. Thomas Hale out of the University of Texas that is being done in Colorado using specific cannabis strains and amounts and then testing breast milk for quantity of THC. [7] I don't believe that study is also testing any short or long term effects on babies who are ingesting the milk. Previous studies done on the amount of THC transferred to baby in the milk are contradictory. They state that anywhere between <1% to >10% of the maternal dose gets into baby's circulation. Maternal dose is the biggest factor but the wide range of products and the wide range of THC in those products is not taken into consideration.

Clearly, there is a huge gap in our knowledge of how maternal Marijuana use affects babies that are breastfed. Here's what we think we know.

1. THC rapidly distributes to the baby from the milk supply into both brains and adipose tissue
2. THC is easily stored in fat tissues for up to a few months.
3. Cannabinoids easily bind with human endocannabinoid receptors and can either act as an agonist or antagonist to the action of that receptor. [6]

How the presence of THC in brain tissue affects neural development and cognitive function is the crux of the matter. Some studies have indicated that using Marijuana during breastfeeding in the newborn period decreases motor function when tested at 1 year of age. Except those studies where not done on humans but rather baby rats. Other studies have indicated that there is no change in expected cognitive or motor development at one year of age but the number of participants was very small. Another study indicated that using Marijuana at three months postpartum seemed to have no side effects on baby.

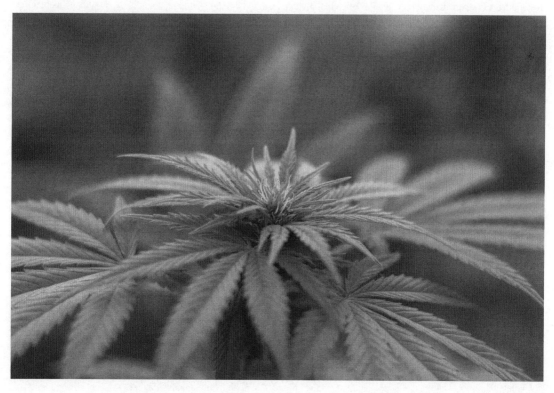

The other factor that has been studied is the effect on cannabinoids (specifically THC) on maternal prolactin levels. Animal studies suggest that Marijuana could inhibit lactation by inhibiting prolactin production and possibly by a direct action on the mammary glands. There have been no human studies to date to either prove or disprove this assumption.

So how do you take all this information and make suggestions to your clients when they ask for recommendations on using Marijuana and breastfeeding? We know that folks are going to use it and some of those folks are going to be breastfeeding. As an herbalist, your job is to gather information about the bigger picture in this mother's life. Asking about the way she has, is, or wants to use Marijuana can help. Is she using it recreationally or is there a medical reason? Does she smoke a joint to help herself relax due to high stress in her life? Is she smoking or ingesting flowers or is she taking something more concentrated? What is the legal status of Marijuana use in your state? Is there a precedent for alerting social services and are they actively pursuing women who continue breastfeeding? Are they actively prosecuting women for child endangerment or abuse and removing children from the home? As an herbalist, can you provide herbal alternatives that can help produce similar actions for the mother without the legal or potential physical ramifications?

Here is how I've begun talking to folks.

1. There may be some long term affects on cognitive and motor function in baby but the research is mixed. Until good quality studies are done that prove cause and affect it's probably better to avoid it if possible especially in the first couple of months postpartum.
2. There may be some effect on actual milk production. If there has been a problem with maintaining milk production/prolactin levels in the past it may be best to avoid it. If there is no sign of reduced milk supply or decrease or lack

of baby's growth it's good, however those things may or may not be apparent immediately.
3. Know your legal rights. Just because a substance is legal for adults does not mean that the state, county, hospital, or provider wont pursue legal action if your baby tests positive for THC and you are continuing to breastfeed.
4. Encourage parents to push for scientific studies that will clarify the actual effects on baby and breastfeeding and support legislation that is reflective of that research.

What you can do as the herb specialist in your community is to understand your clients needs and support them accordingly. Teaching a new mother how to make a cup of tea and what to use gives her a process for daily ceremony. When you encourage her to take the time everyday to make her medicine and even share it with others you empower her to make healthy choices. Acknowledging that what she does is valuable and essential to her child's well-being reminds her that she is doing sacred work.

References

1. Hale, Thomas. Medications and Mother's Milk, Ninth Edition 2000: 5-22. Pharmasoft Publishing
2. Gardner, Zoe, McGuffin, Michael. Botnical Safety Handbook, Second Edition, 2013: Appendix 4. 989-998. CRC Press
3. Romm MD, Aviva. Botanical Medicine For Women's Health. Second Edition 2018: 464-484, Elsevier
4. The American College of Obestricians and Gynecologists, Committee Opinion No. 722, October, 2017
5. Merritt, T. Allen, Wilkinson, B., Chervenak, C. Maternal Use of Marijuana During Pregnancy and Lactation: Implications for Infant and Child Development and Their Well-Being. November 4, 2016. Academic Journal of Pediatrics and Neonatology.
6. Simmons, Kate McKee. Breastfeeding and Cannabis: New Colorado Study Looking For Participants, Westword, March 7, 2017.
7. Colorado Department of Public Health and Environment, Marijuana Pregnancy Guidance For Colorado Health Care Providers. March, 2015

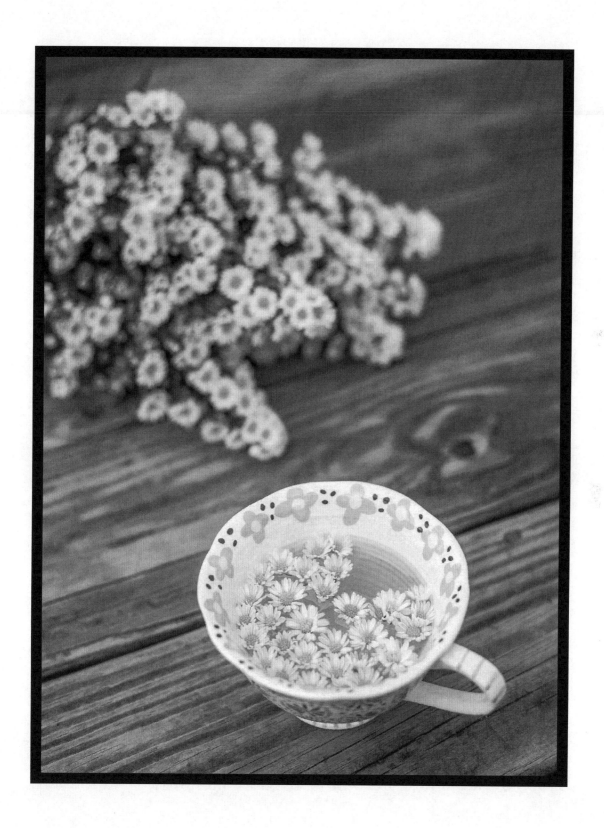

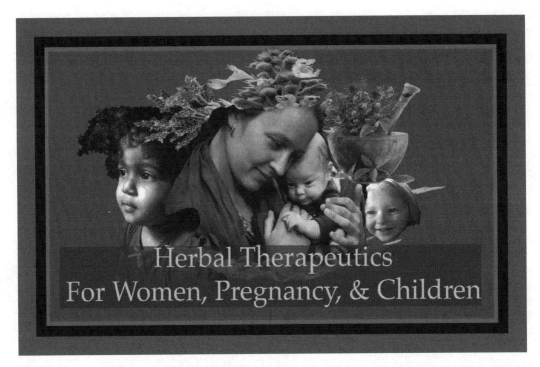

Herbal Therapeutics
For Women, Pregnancy, & Children

PHYTOESTROGENS DEMYSTIFIED

by Juliet Blankespoor

Estrogens are a group of steroid hormones, which function as the primary female reproductive messengers. Estrogen has its etymological roots in the Anglo-Saxon goddess of fertility Oestre, and can be broken down as follows; from *estrus* (period of fertility for female mammals) + *gen* (to generate).

There are three types of estrogens known:

- **Estradiol**- the most potent and abundant estrogen, produced primarily from the follicles and corpus luteum in the ovaries. Primary hormone involved in the development of secondary sex characteristics and the menstrual cycle.
- **Estrone** – least abundant estrogen; levels higher during menopause (think crone)
- **Estriol** – primarily produced in pregnancy by the placenta

Estrogens are primarily produced in the ovaries but some of the body's supply comes from the conversion of androgens (male reproductive hormones) by the aromatase enzyme. This conversion (aromatisation) takes place primarily in adipose tissue (fat) but also occurs in the brain, skin, muscle, and bones. This secondary source of estrogen is particularly important after menopause as it supplies most of the body's estrogen. During the reproductive years this process can account for a significant gain in circulating estrogen levels as evidenced by the experience of some women who have undergone surgical removal of their ovaries without menopausal symptoms. Excess aromatisation has been linked to breast, adrenal and prostate cancers.

Estrogen is responsible for the development of secondary sex characteristics during puberty and the growth of the endometrial lining during the menstrual cycle. Other affects seen in the presence of estrogen are strengthening bones, maintaining skin and blood vessel elasticity, increasing vaginal lubrication, increasing platelet adhesiveness (clotting), and increasing HDL cholesterol while lowering LDL cholesterol. In addition, estrogens can elicit cell proliferation in estrogen dependent tissue such as the breasts and endometrium.

Endogenous estrogens are produced within the human body, as opposed to the externally generated phytoestrogens and xenoestrogens. (Endo= within; gen=generated)

Endocrine disruptors, or hormone disruptors, are human-made chemicals in the environment that interfere with the development and function of body systems in animals, including humans. The endocrine system is the body's messenger service, integrating all other systems through hormones, which deliver the actual messages. Hormones regulate metabolism, sexual development and reproduction, mental processes, growth, and prenatal development.

Xenoestrogens are a subclass of endocrine disruptors which are able to bind to estrogen receptor sites and elicit an estrogenic affect.

Hormone disruptors interfere with the healthy functioning of the endocrine system by binding to hormone receptor sites, thus producing a number of unnatural responses. They may mimic the natural hormones in our bodies, such as estrogens. They may also block our natural hormones, such as androgens (male hormones), thyroid hormones and progesterone. Finally, they can alter the way in which natural hormones are produced, eliminated, or metabolized.

Since the 1940s, approximately 87,000 synthetic new chemicals have been produced in the United States alone. Only between 1.5 and 3 percent of synthetic chemicals have been tested for their cancer-causing properties, and even fewer have been tested for hormone disrupting properties.

These human-made chemicals are the building blocks or byproducts of pesticides, fuels, detergents, plastics, and many everyday household objects. They can be found anywhere from cheese and the plastic wrap that it is sold in, to children's toys and teething rings. Some common examples are dioxins (created when plastic is manufactured and burned), PCBs (previously used as electrical insulator, adhesive, and lubricant), and DDT (banned from use in this country but still manufactured domestically and sold abroad). These chemicals do not observe political boundaries and travel freely through air and water currents. For example, DDT sprayed in Peru to control mosquito populations can end up in the breast milk of an Aleutian mother in Alaska five years later.

Environmental chemicals enter our body through the food we ingest, the water we drink and bathe in, and the air we breathe. They evade our natural internal "checks and balances" and may persist in the body for decades or even a lifetime. Whether you live in remote Alaska or Calcutta, India, your fat cells are harboring a dozen to 500 chemicals in measurable quantities. Hormone-disrupting chemicals are found in the air, soil, water, plants, and in the bodies of animals, including humans, on every continent and in every body of water.

The process of bio-magnification is particularly concerning. As hormone disruptors move up the food chain, they become more concentrated. A herring gull eating a diet of trout from the Great Lakes stores a chemical in its tissue that is 25 million times more magnified than it was in the plankton where the chemical first entered the food chain. This process is often illustrated with the wolf as the predator on the top of the food chain. But in reality, it is the wolf pups that the mother nurses who are even higher.

Mammals, including humans, pass on the majority of their lifetime stores of fat-soluble chemicals when they nurse their first-born. Human infants are exposed to a higher concentration of fat-soluble chemicals, such as PCBs and DDT, during breast-feeding than at any other time in their lives. In the United States and Europe a six-month old baby is fed five times the allowable daily levels of PCBs set by international health standards for a 150-pound adult. They will also have already received the maximum recommended lifetime supply of dioxin via breast milk.

This said, breast milk is still vastly superior to formula in its nutritional, immunological, and developmental capacities. As a mother who breast-fed and breast-feeding advocate, I believe every mother considering breast-feeding should be empowered with this information so we can work towards a healthier planet and healthier babies.

Substances which have demonstrated estrogenic effects on animals (including humans)

- atrazine (weedkiller)
- 4-Methylbenzylidene camphor (4-MBC) (sunscreen lotions)
- butylated hydroxyanisole / BHA (food preservative)
- bisphenol A (monomer for polycarbonate plastic and epoxy resin; antioxidant in plasticizers)
- dichlorodiphenyldichloroethylene (one of the breakdown products of DDT)
- dieldrin (insecticide)
- DDT (insecticide)
- erythrosine / FD&C Red No. 3
- ethinylestradiol (combined oral contraceptive pill) (released into the environment as a xenoestrogen)
- heptachlor (insecticide)
- lindane / hexachlorocyclohexane (insecticide)

1. Go Organic and eat wild food! Growing your own organic food and supporting local organic farmers affects not only your health, but also the integrity and future of the entire planet. Eating organic whole foods is the number one way to avoid endocrine disruptors.

Ninety percent of our exposure to PCBs and dioxins comes from the food we ingest, especially conventionally grown (non-organic) meat and dairy products and processed foods. Non-organic meat and dairy products contain the highest levels of environmental contaminants for a number of reasons. Conventional animals are fed the most heavily sprayed crops and often contain rendered fat laced with melted plastics. In addition, they are often given synthetic growth enhancers such as Bovine Growth Hormone (BGH), which has been implicated in the increased risk of breast cancer. Finally, toxins such as pesticides and pharmaceutical residues concentrate and persist in fat cells. According to the EPA, 90–95 percent of pesticide residues are ingested through conventionally produced meat and dairy products.

2. Purify the water you drink and bathe in (unless you are fortunate enough to have clean spring or well water).

3. Avoid letting plastic touch your food and water. Bisphenol A (BPA), a component of plastic, is one of the top fifty chemicals currently being produced. According to laboratory studies it exerts an estrogenic effect in the human body. BPA can be found in invisible linings of metal food cans, in dental composite fillings, and in polycarbonate plastic containers used for some types of baby bottles, and the hard, clear water containers sold in stores to refill purified water. It is also used in the manufacturing of water bottles used in sports or camping. Use glass or stainless steel water and food containers instead. Avoid using cling-wrap next to food and don't microwave food in plastic containers.

4. Live simply for the health of all beings. Avoid dry-cleaning clothing and synthetic body-care and housecleaning products.

How can we remove endocrine disruptors from our bodies?

We can limit our exposure to environmental contaminants, but we cannot completely avoid them. Minimizing toxins stored in the body is beneficial for all people, but especially important for the woman considering pregnancy and breast-feeding. Detoxification is an intense and rewarding process, but should not be undertaken during pregnancy or nursing as toxins being flushed from fat cells may enter the bloodstream and reach the fetus or breast milk. Remember that your body is sacred and amazingly powerful at protecting itself from foreign substances with which it has not evolved. Visualize fasting and cleansing as augmenting the light and beauty you already possess!

Phytoestrogens are a diverse group of compounds found in plants which have the ability to bind to estrogen receptor sites and elicit an estrogenic effect (*phyto*=plant, *estrogen* = estrus (period of fertility for female mammals) + *gen* = to generate). They are found in many commonly eaten seeds, grains, and beans and are present in many medicinal herbs used to treat female reproductive disorders. Their effects are the subject of thousands of studies and it can be quite complex to unravel the seemingly contradictory findings.

It appears that phytoestrogens exert a weaker estrogenic effect on cells than endogenous estrogens or xenoestrogens. Different substances may bind to the same receptor site and the change they bring about can vary depending on the exact fit. Phytoestrogens exert an anti-estrogenic effect premenopausally by competitive inhibition of hormone receptor sites. If the receptor sites are occupied with the less estrogenic phytoestrogens, than there are less sites available for the more potent endogenous estrogens or xenoestrogens. Thus eating a whole foods diet rich in naturally occurring phytoestrogens is one of the ways we can protect ourselves from the harmful effects of environmental xenoestrogens. In menopausal and post-menopausal women there is a net reduction in estrogen as the ovaries begin to rest. In this case the phytoestrogens can increase the positive effects of estrogen by increasing the estrogenic effect on the body. Although they are less estrogenic than endogenous estrogens they still increase the net estrogenic effect. This is evidenced by epidemiological studies demonstrating fewer menopausal symptoms, greater bone density, and lower breast cancer in populations of women who regularly consume phytoestrogens as part of their diet.

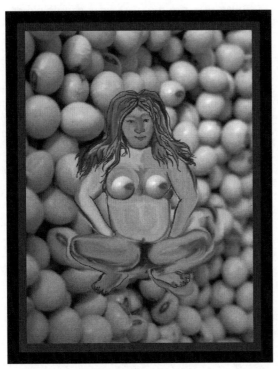

Isoflavones (genistein, daidzein, formononetin, and biochanin A) are produced primarily in the bean or legume family (Fabaceae) and are some of the most potent and studied phytoestrogens. Isoflavones are anti-oxidant compounds and have demonstrated activity against breast and prostate cancer.

The best dietary sources of isoflavones are produced from soy beans (*Glycine max*). Soy foods, listed in order of isoflavone content, include miso, tempeh, soy milk, tofu, and edamame. Other beans and peanuts contain some isoflavones, but to a much lesser extent.

Isoflavone absorption is greatly enhanced by healthy populations of intestinal flora. Many studies have been conducted utilizing isolated isoflavones in isolated cell lines *in vitro* (petri dish), many of which have fueled the soy debate. Some in vitro studies conducted with genistein as an isolate have demonstrated promotion of breast cancer cell lines but the majority of studies have demonstrated positive health effects such as increased bone density and lower LDL cholesterol levels. It appears that soy consumption via breast feeding (with mothers who consume soy foods) and in youth reduces breast and prostate cancer later in life. Early consumption of soy is also linked to a reduced amount of menopausal symptoms in population studies.

Herbal sources of isoflavones such as Red clover (*Trifolium pratense, Fabaceae*) and Alfalfa (*Medicago sativa, Fabaceae*) may not be readily water soluble as tea and may be poorer choices for isoflavones ingestion than dietary sources.

Lignans are the most widely consumed phytoestrogen precursors found in the western diet and are found in high concentrations in flax and sesame seeds and to a lesser extent in other seeds, whole grains, fruits, vegetables and beans. Intestinal flora act upon the lignans to convert them to their active forms; enterodiol and enterolactone. Enterolactone has been shown to inhibit the proliferation of prostate cancer *in vitro*. These phytoestrogens metabolites generally have a weaker estrogenic effect compared to the isoflavones. Note the importance of intestinal flora health in phytoestrogen metabolism. The repeated use of antibiotics and subsequent damage to intestinal bacteria has been linked to breast cancer risk, perhaps in part due to the lowered production of active phytoestrogen metabolites. As would be expected, increased dietary intake enhances enterolactone production.

Coumestrol is a phytoestrogen found in high concentrations in sprouted soy and red clover, and to a lesser extent in non-sprouted beans and peas.

Flavanoids are known for their potent anti-oxidant and anti-inflammatory effect but most also demonstrate a weak phytoestrogenic affect. Most yellow, red, purple and black fruits contain ample flavanoids.

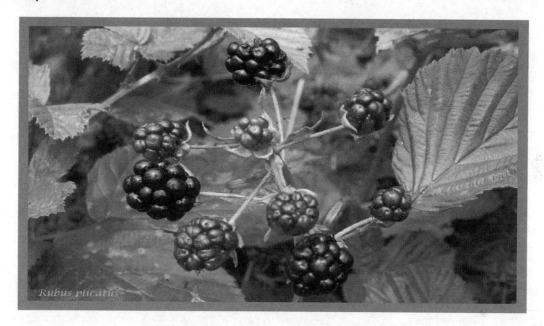

Rubus plicatus

Resources/bibliography

Women, Hormones and the Menstrual Cycle – Ruth Trickey
In depth coverage of the disease process, and dietary, lifestyle and herbal remedies for most of the female reproductive disorders encountered. Advanced and somewhat technical – geared towards health practitioners.

Botanical Medicine for Women's Health. Aviva Romm

Hormone Deception. D. Lindsey Berkson.

Our Stolen Future: Are we Threatening our Fertility, Intelligence and Survival? A Scientific Detective Story. Theo Colborn, Dianne Dumankoski and John Peterson Myers.

Herbal Constituents: Foundations of Phytochemistry. Lisa Ganora

Having Faith: An Ecologist's Journey to Motherhood. Sandra Steingraber

Hormonal Enzyme Systems and Botanical Agents. Jillian Stansbury, ND. P134-137. Medicines from the Earth. Offical Proceedings. June 4-7, 2010.

Gene Expression and Reproductive Health. Jillian Stansbury, ND. P138-142. See above.

237

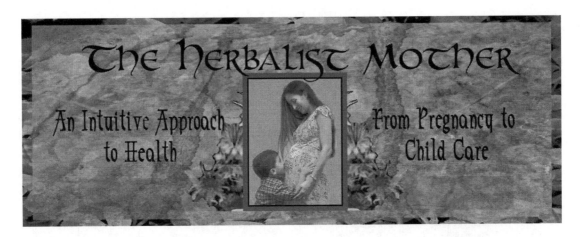

DEEPENING OUR CONNECTION WITH OURSELVES DURING PREGNANCY, BIRTH, & POSTPARTUM

by Sabrina Lutes

Each pregnancy is unique in that every woman and baby is unique. Each mother brings the culmination of her life experiences to her pregnancy and later birth. There are moments off elation, dread, happiness, terrifying revelations, love and every other emotion we humans hold within our framework. Sometimes these boil over and make it hard to connect to a child during pregnancy even when that child is deeply loved and desired. When we begin to work on these feelings, we can use the natural world to help circumvent, soothe or meaningfully mark these moments. There will also be times when a mother must choose other paths to help her in dealing with things that are making her pregnancy more difficult and it is

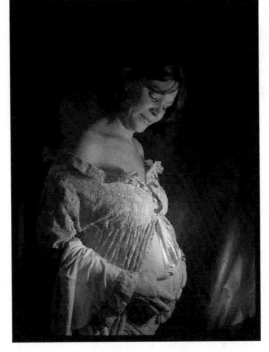

always a good thing to seek out help and understanding. Even in these moments, our trusted plants can be carried with us.

Connection comes in so many ways. Pregnancy is a time of losing some part of ourselves to allow the life another part to emerge. The new mother! She is both powerful and delicate and sometimes ambivalent. It's hard to give up who we were. To grapple with the idea that we will soon be responsible for a being that will depend completely on us. It can cause some turmoil within us. This can feel so disorientating and we can feel caught up in the burgeoning drive of life that is growing a baby. Many find it exciting, some will be fearful, others will be ambivalent.

Testing the waters and going slow and deliberate can help our minds catch up to the moment. Choosing a particular plant to carry with us, one or possibly a bundle of plants in a small sachet that reminds you of the work you are doing. These may be gathered from the plants that grow near you, or ordered from herbalists that gather with ceremony and care. A story can be attached to each plant, so that as you handle your bag, the smells that come from within or the way a root feels under your fingers, can remind you of what you may have forgotten or become a signal you to relax and stay focused. I learned this from a woman at a Renaissance faire, of all places. I call them story pouches and the contents are stitched up within fabric. You simply pull them out and feel for the items within. It is a sensing exercise. I have carried them with me to births and they contain small figurines, herbs, and stones that help remind me to stay calm and focused at each birth. This is something easily done and when created with thoughtfulness can become something really special. This is your story bag. It can be whatever you choose, simple or elaborate. Some examples: Artemesia for dreams, Comfrey root for tenacity and healing, chamomile and lavender for relaxation.

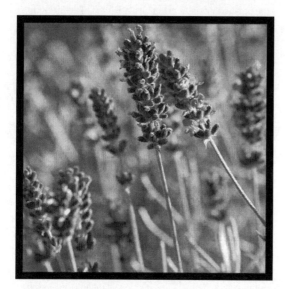

It's very important, especially for pregnant women, to really listen to how information feels. Pregnancy is such a soft and open time and things can get into our heads and cause all sorts of worries that weren't there to begin with. I have learned it best to just say no to advice or

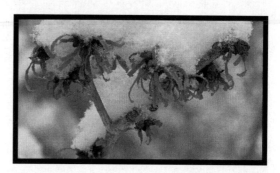

stories that feel like they might ruminate inside of me. I'm always amazed at how pregnant women are targets to every sort of advice under the sun and every wild horror story about birth and pregnancy that people can think of. Only listen if you want to, otherwise feel ok about the word "no".

Pregnancy Garden

If you are able to start a garden, pregnancy is such a wonderful time for this. The movements required to tend plants: squatting, stretching, carrying water meet many of the physical needs of the pregnant body. Caring for plants helps to shift our minds to something task oriented. It's an outward expression of all the internal work that is occurring in our bodies. There are also wonderful plants to begin growing that will serve your pregnancy and birth and beyond. Lavender (*Lavendula angustifolia*), Rosemary (*Rosmarinus officinalis*), Oatstraw (*Avena sativa*), Calendula (*Calendula officinalis*), Violet (*Viola* spp.), Red Raspberry(*Rubus idaeus*), Nettles (*Urtica dioica*) are all wonderful additions to a pregnancy and birth herb garden. If a garden is too much, try potted plants. Tending things keeps our minds from wandering too much. Planting a special plant for your baby is a beautiful gesture as well. Some women choose to plant a tree or special perennial, with the baby's placenta. If this is something that calls to you, perhaps you could begin that plant by seed, early in your pregnancy, so that it is ready when your baby is. These activities are similar to baby quilts that some mothers sew for their children. Taking our tears, our joys, our worries into the garden can be very therapeutic. Fussing over seeds, and practicing the art of puttering, really prepares you for having small children around. If you already have children, being out in the sunshine, doing work they can help you with creates strong family bonds.

Birth & Pregnancy Recipes

The act of collecting supplies for our baby's birth can certainly help funnel some of the flyaway thoughts we can have in pregnancy. It helps to hone our awareness on tangible things we can do to get ready. Being prepared just plain feels good. Filling jars with sitz bath herbs, creating herbal oils for tender breasts and stretched skin, as well as creating herbal infusions to help our bodies recover nutrients lost during gestation.

Belly Oil

1 part Elderflower (*Sambucus nigra*)
1 party Pink Rose petals (I really love damask Rose petals for their subtle, sweet scent they impart into this oil)
1 part Violet leaf
½ part cut and sifted Marshmallow root (*Althaea officinalis*)
1/8 part Vanilla bean cut into small pieces (*Vanilla planifolia*)
Grapeseed oil enough to cover herbs

Fill a clean, very dry jar to the top with herb material (or as close as possible) using the parts listed above. One way to do this is to divide the jar into the appropriate parts. Cover with grapeseed oil, cover and set in a warm place. A sunny window is lovely for this oil as it really brings out the vanilla. If it is warm enough, the oil will be ready in 3-4 days. Otherwise give it 6 weeks. Using dried herbs and a container that is absolutely dry, drastically reduces the risk of mold contamination. I enjoy grapeseed oil because it is drier and less greasy and mostly odorless, but you could substitute another oil of your choosing. This oil has a beautiful and subtle smell that could be overpowered by the oil you use.

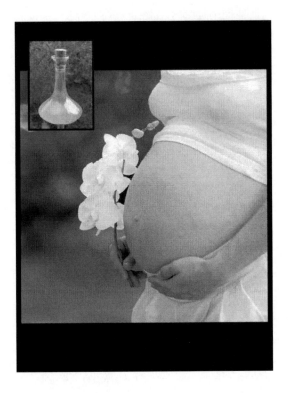

Sitz Bath Herbs

A sitz bath can be done in a few different ways. You can be sure that your tub is impeccably clean and follow the directions listed below. You could make a strong infusion and place in a Peri-bottle (a soft squishy bottle made to easily apply cleansing water to the perineal area, your health care provider or a drug store should be able to supply these). The third way is to use a specifically designed sitz bath contraption that fits into the toilet seat and allows the perineum to come into contact with the fluid.

Calendula blossoms, Blackberry leaf (*Rubus fruticosus*), Witch Hazel bark (*Hamamelis virginiana*), Lavender buds, Rose petals blended with salt are all wonderful additions for a sitz bath. Leaning heavily on the astringent and antimicrobial as well as skin soothing qualities of these herbs they can be very beneficial to the aches, nicks and tears as well as hemorrhoids after birth. You could choose one or a combination of all of these herbs to aid in healing. A basic recipe is:

240

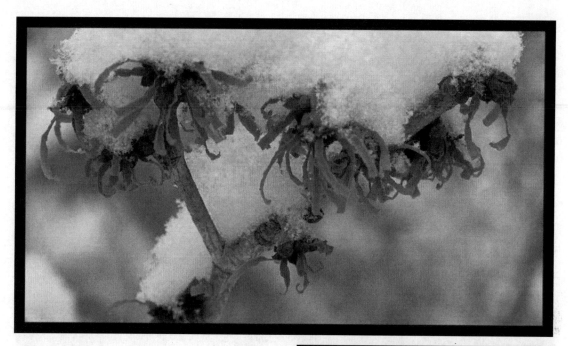

1 part Witch Hazel bark
1 part Calendula blossoms
½ part Lavender buds
½ part salt (the crushed, larger salt crystals are better than the fine)
Boil a gallon of water, remove from heat and add 1 cup of herbal blend, let steep for an hour and pour this mixture into a bath.

Perineal Compresses

As a midwife assistant, I would help the midwife in creating compresses. These were made using sanitary pads and a strong infusion of herbs. The plants would typically contain skin healing and soothing qualities like calendula and rose, sometimes comfrey leaf if there was bruising but no tearing, witch hazel bark and plantain to be placed on hemorrhoids. We would then pour the fluid onto the pads, and freeze them individually in baggies, so that they remained very clean and ready for use this is such a treat for a sore and bruised bottom. It is always a good idea to discuss with your health care provider your plans to do this or sitz bath herbs. They may have reasons for limiting soaking due to the extent of injury. You also want to be sure that the herbs have been boiled to kill any microbes. If there were any vaginal or perineal tears you do not want to introduce bacteria.

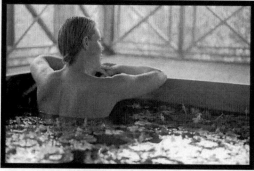

Warm Herbal Baths & Foot Soaks

Nothing can soothe an aching, tight body like a warm bath or foot soak. It is such a beautiful moment of bliss, one where we can literally sink into an embrace and be held and supported by the water around us. As things grow and shift inside of us, our buoyancy in water can be a welcome sensation. Add to this a sweet herbal concoction that you created and you have a beautiful ceremony for yourself and your little one.   A milk and honey foot bath with rose water drizzled in, is a divine way to spend an evening. Set aside an evening that you can have the house to yourself especially if you have little ones already. Have towels and warm socks close by and ready for when you finish, and just crawl into bed afterwards.

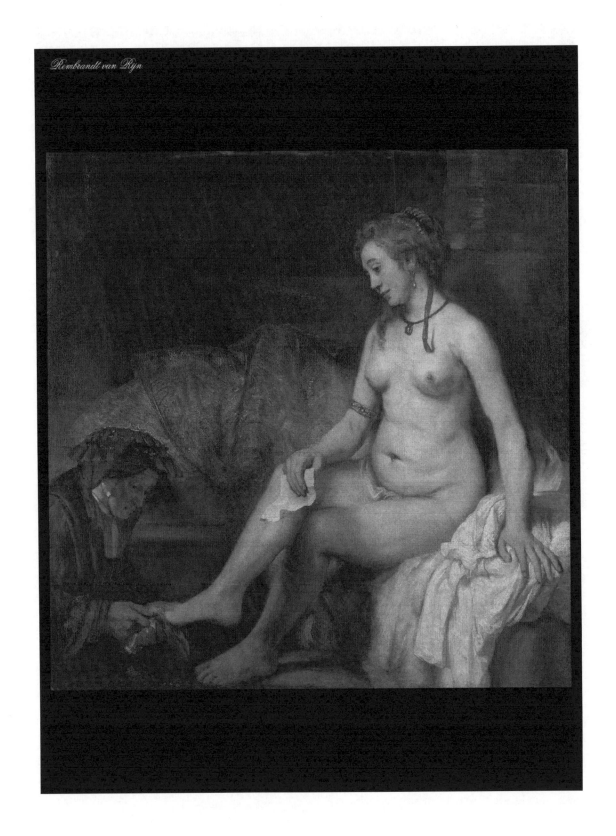

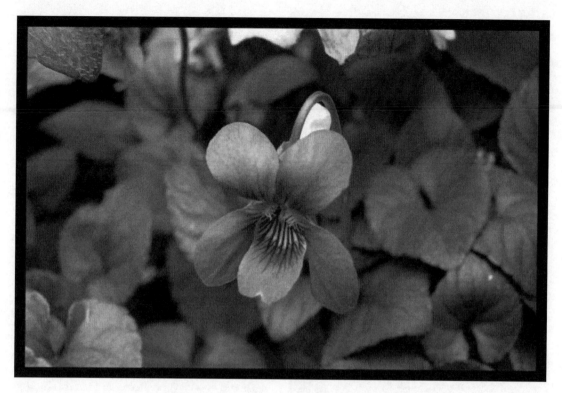

Tuck a lavender and rose sachet under your pillow. Have a mug of warm Red Raspberry leaf tea. Think about the baby you're carrying and your feelings about your pregnancy in that moment. Staying in the moment, as cliché as that can sound can help foster more connection, particularly if you are feeling tender. Some ideas for your bath: (take any combination of these herbs that feels right and smells good and add them to a muslin bag the size of your hand. You then tuck them into the bath with you and even use them to rub on your skin) Rose (pink and red), Oat tops, Rolled Oats, Calendula petals, Lavender, Marshmallow root, Elderflower, Plantain (Plantago spp.), Violet leaf.

The above are a few suggestions to make something beautiful and possibly helpful for yourself during a time when self-care may not be as easy. These herbs may not work for everybody, situation or pregnancy. Take some time to research each herb you may consider using for pregnancy and birth. We must discover for ourselves what is best. Our bodies know how to create a baby as well as prepare for labor. Herbs can be adjuncts to this when needed. Seek out a knowledgeable midwife or herbalist if you feel you need to take herbs for specific complaints. Anytime you put a new substance or herb on your body, check in for sensitivities by doing a spot test.

Preparation

Taking the time in pregnancy to create nutritious frozen meals can seriously reduce stress levels. Some families are able to continue on with life relatively seamlessly, but others cannot. As a doula and a mother, I don't suggest trying to live up to some impossible standard. Postpartum is a time for healing and snuggling a new baby, and adapting to a new rhythm both for the parent(s) and/or siblings.

Asking others to cook a meal for your freezer or to bring one over on a specific day after baby arrives is another wonderful way to put well-meaning offers of help to good use. Generally after a baby is born, people want to come hold your infant. This can be a welcome event or a source of stress. If you have a plan in place beforehand and a meal train set up, people can focus on helping in ways that are beneficial to the new family. Clarity and boundaries about what you need is immensely important during this time. This planning is such a sweet way to gift yourself and your family. It can also be a time when you have friends over, pour some herbal tea, and cook together! It allows a sense of autonomy and control at a time where we are working hard on surrendering. When we give ourselves the permission to prepare in concrete ways, that will be welcome after any scenario, it feels very empowering and can deepen our connection to our baby and ourselves. It allows us to really ask that our needs be met in a very concrete way. To think about how the interplay of others will be received during your transition into first time motherhood or with subsequent pregnancies, may never be fully clear before it actually happens. It can change day to day even, yet having a strong network of basic care, ready and waiting, goes so very far.

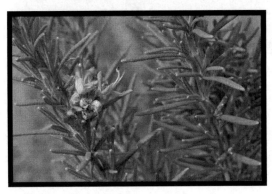

Reading lovely books about herbs and pregnancy and birth can also help us find connection. They can paint pictures for us that we have not yet begun for ourselves. The author can help guide us in lyrical ways. Books that I have found helpful are *The Natural Pregnancy Book* by Aviva Romm, *Herbal Healing for Women*, and Rosemary Gladstar's *Family Herbal*.

The plants can help ground us and even help us to become lucid and soothed when that is necessary. Allowing our minds to experience a bit of magic in pregnancy is so very wonderful. Being amongst beautiful roses, dripping with petals and wonderful smells, can carry us when we are unable to carry ourselves. When things get too heavy and need to be lightened, the vibrant fragrance of lavender may be just what is needed. When we need a grounding presence, keen observation and focus, breaking a twig of rosemary can direct that for us. If you can, go into the woods to sit and listen or to hike. I loved exploring the same trail over and over again as my belly swelled, feeling the changes so much more acutely because the trail was familiar. I could feel imbalances as I became more awkward in my movements. It forced me to tune inward and notice when I could push myself or when I needed to slow down and let my structure catch up to loosening ligaments and increased fluids. Visiting this same area throughout the months also heightened my senses to the changing seasons. It would be a long while before I could pay so much attention to the world around me. After my son was born, my focus became so intensely aware of his needs that the world around me became unfocused.

I have found that pregnancy can be so amazing for some, and so hard for others. I think that each and every experience is valid and should be honored. When we honor something for what it is, instead of immediately trying to change it, we can find so much about ourselves. These are just merely a reminder of ways that we can connect into a time in our lives that is so very fleeting. If tuning in is something that we as mothers have consciously chosen to do then it will be easier to work towards that goal. If it feel s like one more thing to complete, then my suggestion is to leave it be. There is nothing that says we must do or act a specific way in pregnancy. There is so much out there telling women how to feel and what to do that it adds even more separation. As I mentioned before, learning how to filter information and allowing "no" into our vocabulary, either out loud or silently to ourselves, it is its own form of tuning inward.

This path of pregnancy is different for each of us. When we move into our sensing selves, we find our own unique way. This may include a network of women, a wise midwife, a kind obstetrician. It may include using plants intently for remedies and specific ailments, or it may just be listening to the winds or watching the sunrise as our labor begins and our baby emerges.

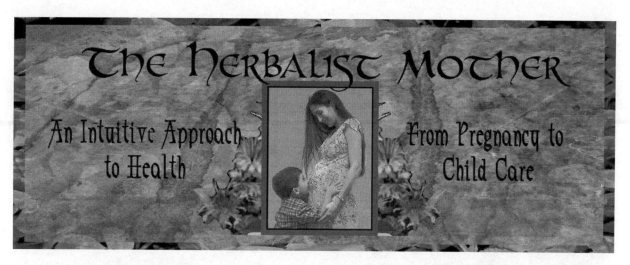

THE HERBALIST MOTHER

An Intuitive Approach to Health

From Pregnancy to Child Care

"The moment a child is born, the mother is also born. She never existed before. The woman existed, but the mother, never. A mother is something absolutely new."
–Bhagwan Shree Rajneesh

Herbal Rituals For New Mothers

by Sabrina Lutes

Mothering in those first few moments, days and weeks can feel otherworldly. As if the mother is between worlds. Some women may feel elated and at ease in their new role, others may struggle. This is how it goes with birth. Transitions are awe-inspiring, oftentimes messy, and for us humans they come with all sorts of cultural and self-appointed issues to live up to and within. It's no wonder after a baby's birth a new mother may find herself feeling a little lost. Lost in her newborn's gaze, lost in the emotions of vulnerability and helplessness, lost in her own power.

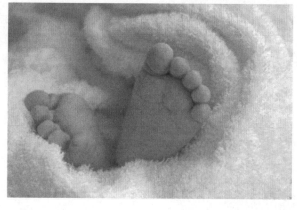

In my work as a doula and midwife assistant I have witnessed many births. In doing so I have learned that my presence and the presence of others, if undertaken in a humble and reverent way can go far in helping a woman come into her new role of mother. I love using the plants and a touch of ceremony to do this. The herbs and plants can be very grounding, soothing and healing to both the physical body and the ethereal body. The ceremony speaks to us on an ancestral level. It taps into our limbic system and calms the fight or flight response. I feel that when done with reverence, ceremony crosses cultural and religious barriers. It also connects us as healers to the women and families we serve. I invite you, if you are involved in birth in any way to use these simple and profound ways to be present for the mother/child dyad.

My particular way of helping mothers after birth is to sit quietly with them. I like to listen deeply to them before I "do" anything. Mothers know what support they need to help them find their way. For me, my ceremony is simple. Before I go to a mother I will hold her in my heart and say a small prayer. Sometimes I will light a candle or burn some incense, thinking specifically of the work I am about to engage in. When I arrive at her house, which is typically where I do my work, I assess what is going on; take a peek at the dishes, maybe the trash, where she is resting or maybe not resting and whether she has something to eat and drink etc. This gives me an idea of how things are going and how I can be most helpful. Then I hold the space for her so that I can let her tell me what she needs. A guideline that I follow in my practice with mothers and really young babies are not to use essential oils with them. A baby is learning the sweet scent of his mother's milk, of her skin, and the others around him. When we use powerful scents I feel this can confuse infants. I will bring herbal infused oils of Lavender, Rose, Calendula and others. Motherhood beckons me to choose more of the floral medicines and some of the traditional resinous herbs like Frankincense and Amber. I also

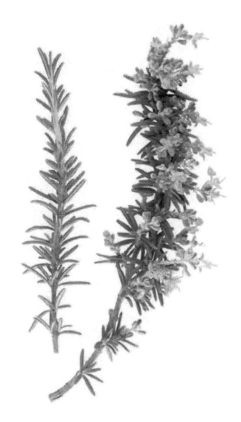

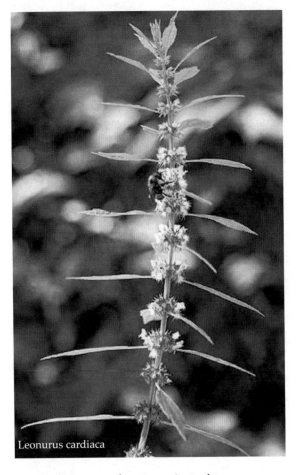

Leonurus cardiaca

use fresh flowers when I can obtain them.

If a woman had a particularly long and exhausting birth, maybe a surgical birth or the birth just didn't unfold as she had hoped I would use Rosemary infused oil to massage her body. Dim the lights and make her warm. Wrap her in warm blankets. Gather a warm water bottle to place at her feet. Keep her baby close to her if at all possible.

Rosemary (Rosmarinus officinalis) is strengthening to the system. I may also bring a fresh Rosemary twig for her to crush in her hand. Speak warmly to this mother. Allow her to tell me her story. I would also brew her some Oatstraw (Avena sativa) infusion. She may be grieving her experience and Oatstraw is very healing and strengthening to the spirit.

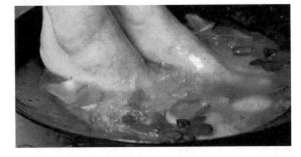

If a woman is having trouble breastfeeding, my first offering to her is a foot bath. Something warm and soothing to help her relax and get her milk flowing. When a mother relaxes, her baby will also. To this I might add some red Rose petals (Rosa centifolia), honey, and fresh milk. I find that massaging a

246

mother's feet and sitting below her in reverence and respect for her present self and who she is becoming can be very helpful. I also ask that she holds her baby close, skin to skin and allow the baby to suckle while we work together. Dimming the lights and warming the room is also nice. I enjoy lighting a beeswax candle for her to gaze at as well. For breastfeeding issues at any point, just taking a mother's mind off the immediacy and urgency she is experiencing with nourishing her baby may just be the trick she needs to let it happen on its own. I would also brew a cup of delicious tea with red Raspberry leaf (Rubus idaeus) and Oatstraw or other nourishing herbs. I generally hold off on specific galactagogues until I know if the mother has a true low milk supply. Sometimes we can interfere too much and then more milk becomes another problem in itself. There may be other factors involved, and as long as the baby is not in any immediate medical need, a few moments of peace can be a first gift to this new mother. If things do not improve then other measures should be employed, including providing the mother with a reference to a good lactation consultant.

For the mother that is feeling out of sorts and anxious, perhaps feeling a little down or depressed. I offer her warm teas and tinctures of Lemon Balm (Melissa officinalis), Motherwort (Leonurus cardiac), Lemongrass (Cymbopogon Citratus), and Oatstraw. For these mothers, it's important to be sure she is just experiencing normal postpartum blues and not the more serious postpartum depression (PPD). You can still be of service to a mother suffering from PPD but it is prudent to be sure she is under the care of someone who specializes in this. I often inquire if the woman has a good network of support. Bringing fresh flowers can bring joy to women feeling a little low. Checking in about her nutrition is also important. If a mother has too much on her plate and is not caring for herself she can begin having low days. You can use infusions of Nettles (Urtica dioica) to help her build her blood and give her body a boost of nutrient dense nutrition. Drawing a warm bath with Lavender (Lavendula spp.) buds tied in a sachet can bring calm and foster pleasant thoughts. Frankincense (Boswellia Thurifera) infused in a light oil can foster clarity and strength. These mothers also need an open heart and lots of deep listening.

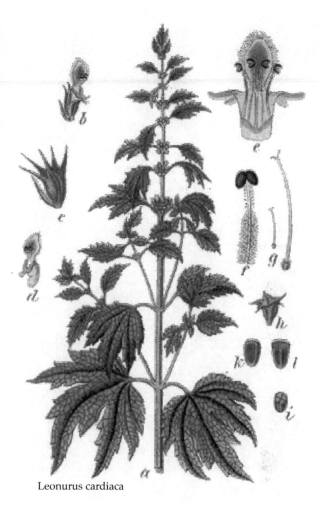

Leonurus cardiaca

These are just a few of the scenarios we may come across as birth practitioners, partners, friends and family when working with new mothers. My hope is that it gives a sense of deep reverence and simple acts of caring that we can bring to mothers and their babies. When mothers are listened to, cared for, and nourished both in body and soul they can continue giving more and more of themselves to their families and to the world beyond. Using the healing herbs in this work can also bring us as practitioners to a deeper understanding of the great transition and transformation women go through to become mothers. By using gentle medicines that not only heal physically because of their chemical constituents but also from the energies they radiate we can see the magic of nature work we can have a greater trust for the ebb and flow of motherhood.

Recipes and instructions

Rosemary Infused oil:

Fresh Rosemary, if flowering include them
1 Quart jar
Lightly scented oil, grapeseed is a nice one

Pack the jar loosely with Rosemary (chopping it helps release more of the aromatics), pour oil over the plant, poking with a chopstick to get rid of air bubbles. Cover and place in a cool place. In 24 hours check that all the plant material is still covered, if it is not add oil all the way to the top. Leave for 2-6 weeks, checking frequently to be sure no mold is forming. Strain and store in bottles.

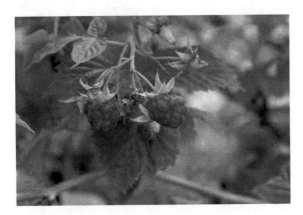

Foot bath:

Rose petals (any aromatic variety will do), enough to fill a muslin bag
½ cup of milk, coconut would work nicely but I use cow's milk
A tablespoon of honey

Warm enough water to fill your container half way. Go a little warmer than you'd think because it will cool as you get it prepared. Leave some heating on the stove so you can reheat the bath. Transfer your water to a container. I use a large turkey roasting pan for foot baths. It seems to be just the right size and depth. Add your bag of Rose petals (you can also brew a strong infusion of Roses and reheat this for your water). Check temperature and when it feels warm but not burning, add your honey and milk and stir with your hands. If you will be massaging her feet and legs adding a tablespoon of grape seed oil to the bath makes things smoother. Have towels under the basin and nearby to dry her feet when you are done. Have some warm socks for the woman to wear after you are done as well.

Simple Nourishing Brew:

1 Part Oatstraw
1 Part Red Raspberry leaf

Add 1 ounce to a quart jar, fill to top with boiling water. Let steep for 4 hours or longer. Strain and add honey to taste.

Bright Days Tea:

1 Part Lemon Balm
1 Part Oatstraw
¼ Part Lemon grass

This is fine as an infusion or strong tea. She can take 20 drops of Motherwort tincture if she is feeling especially fragile. Take this in water separately as it can be a bit bitter.

Frankincense infused oil:

1 Tablespoon Ground Frankincense
1 Pint of grape seed oil

I have had good luck grinding (taking a large wooden pestle and beating it) the resin and then infusing in the sun to warm it. I leave it a couple of days. You can also place the jar in a crock pot set to "keep warm", filled with just enough water to come within a finger's space beneath the lid of the jar. Do this for 12 hours or so, keeping an eye on it so it doesn't get too warm. Strain and bottle.

Resources:

Postpartum Depression- http://www.postpartum.net/
Lactation Consultants- http://www.ilca.org/i4a/pages/index.cfm?pageid=1

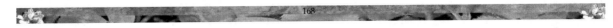

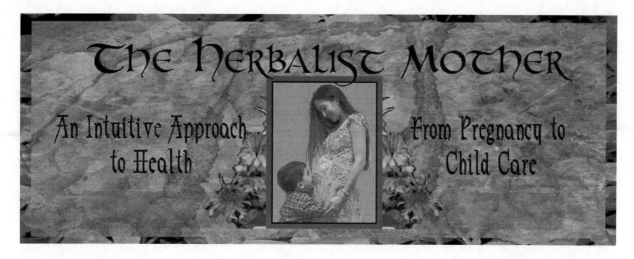

Life must continue as normal, the show must go on, push through it and get over it. Our lives and illnesses are one big rush to get onto the next activity. As a mother I have honed the art of convalescing. Seeing the rewards it gives is never disappointing. Yet failing to honor it, surely brings minor discomforts in the least, and major secondary issues in the worst. I have tried to push the edges a bit, to get back to my regularly scheduled programming as quickly as I think it's alright to do so, only to have it back fire. It is always in everyone's best interest to stay the course and artfully as I like to call it, convalesce.

I feel that this is one of the larger missing pieces in caring for our own. It's super tough to be confined at home with little kids. My hopes are that some of the things I have learned and am sharing with you will help to bring this practice to the

The Art of Recovering

Holding & Making Space for Healing to Continue

by Sabrina Lutes

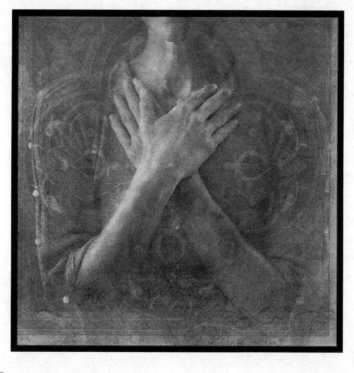

forefront of the healing we do in our families. When I sit with and feel the power in this time period, after the acute illness has subsided yet everyone is still tired and cranky and waking back up to the world, I see that this is the one part that I can play in an illness to bring things around just a bit and nurture the experience for my little one. This is where I can nourish deeply, and with greater ease than when my mind is worrying over my child's illness. My little one is also more receptive to the healing soups, foods, playtime and herbal medicines than during the acute stage, since that is the time his body is working overtime to bring itself back into balance and has often had its fill of lighter meals or no food at all, simple liquids, herbal popsicles, and dose upon dose of tinctures. I feel there are a few key areas to focus on when helping a child or anyone recover from an illness and come out of it a bit stronger. The first nutrition and herbs, the second the environment (home space), third physical activity and getting back out in the world.

Nutrition and Herbals

During the convalescence period it is a good idea to slowly introduce more substantial, wholesome meals. Children normally have no problem letting you know that they are hungry after illness, and are willing to jump in ravenously. With this in mind I choose foods accordingly. Leafy green veggies and herbs chopped finely along with small amounts of protein added to broth to which I've simmered mushrooms (such as Reishi, *Ganoderma lucidum*), maitake, *Grifola frondosa*) and herbs to help strengthen immunity (such as astragalus, *Astragalus membranaceus*). I will leave a pot of this warming on the stove to have a warm meal ready when my little one asks. If the illness didn't involve vomiting or diarrhea I like to add healthy fats in as soon as

tolerated. Grass fed butter, ghee, coconut oil if tolerated, high fat red meat, and fatty fish. Very small amounts are all that is necessary while the child heals. Seaweeds are also a wonderful way to revitalize mineral depletion in the body that happens during fever, and dehydration. For recovery I would simmer these in broth and serve in a soup rather than dry, which will cause the body to require even more liquids. Yogurt is also remarkably healing to a gut that has been dealing with gastritis.

Normally I would use full fat yogurts, but in times of gastric upset, I will go low fat, stirring raw, local honey into it with a dash of warming herbs such ginger or cinnamon. Convalescence is a great time to make a large batch of infused herbs and offer this to the child instead of water. Some of my favorites are Hibiscus (*Hibiscus rosa-sinensis*), Spearmint (*Mentha spicata*), Oat Straw (*Avena sativa*), and Nettles (*Urtica dioica*). These can be sweetened with a bit of Licorice (*Glycyrrhiza glabra*) or Stevia (*Stevia rebaudiana*) depending on preference or energetics of the illness.

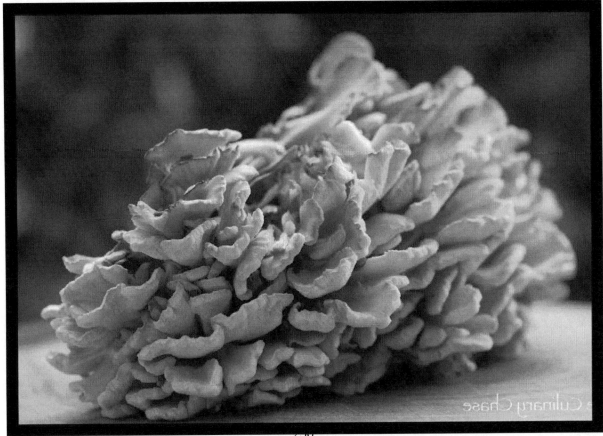

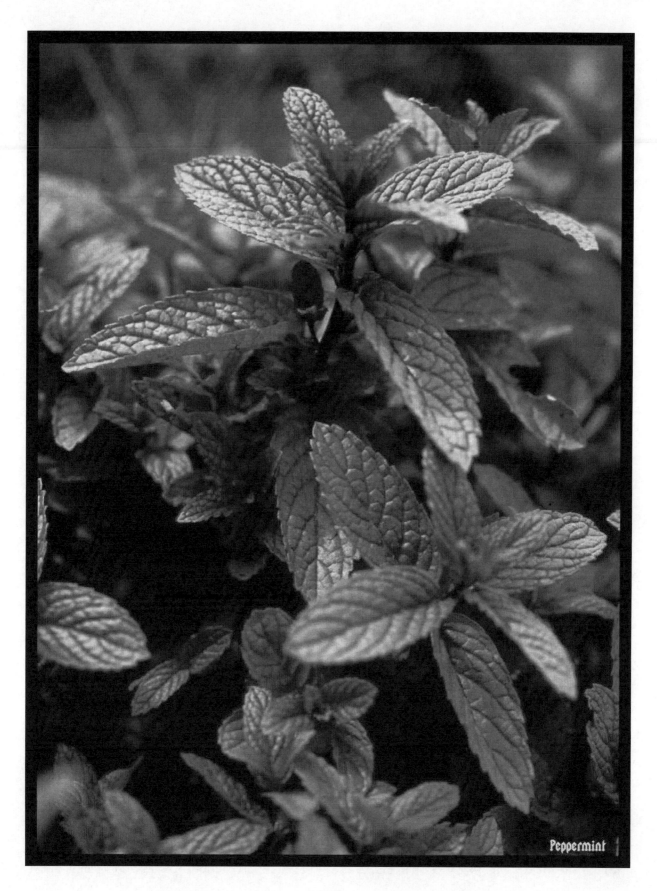

Peppermint

251

Environment

When preparing your home during and after illness, I like to think of the energy of the illness. Just as we do for internal remedies. Is it hot/dry, damp/cold? An example is acute gastritis, which is hot/dry consisting of high fever, and vomiting but very dry. I like to add peppermint to the environment by putting a drop in the toilet or vomit receptacle. It clears the air, is cooling, and decreases smells which is unpleasant for both the person who is sick as well as the caregiver. I continue this in a vaporizer while the child recovers or until the illness changes. I also make cooling/moistening infusions to drink, with marshmallow, licorice, fennel. These can be continued until the child feels well and the GI tract appears healed. After this type of illness I like to give my house a thorough scrubbing. It makes everyone feel better! Fresh linens, lavender spritzed into the room to moisten and calm everyone, a wipe down with diluted thyme tincture and lavender blended with citrus infused vinegar. I also enjoy bringing favorite things into the recovering persons view and senses. Fresh flowers or greenery from out of doors, embroidered herbal hot packs, and beautiful tea cups filled with steaming or chilled drinks.

By tailoring my cleaning products, room sprays, compresses, simmering herbs and smudging herbs to what is happening in the person's body, I can bring healing to the larger environment and it just feels good. These are the things that will continue into the convalescence period. Once the acute herbal remedies and round the clock care have helped where they needed to help, the care of the environment sets the stage for healing and strength to continue. Your children will remember how the house smelled and appeared during their illness. Is it in disarray or is it neat and inviting? Do the things around the child who is healing, help or hinder their process? These things may seem a little bit 1950's housewife, and indeed I fought it long and hard. Yet now that I have my own child and I see how effected he is by his greater environment, I feel it is a very important piece in healing to place our focus as parents and caregivers. The herbs and plants make this so easy to do. Their effects are immediate, their beauty effortless.

Another piece is modeling good care practices ourselves. This can be difficult at times for us as parents if we are concerned over an illness, wary after days of constant care or nights of frequent waking. Are we as parents helping our child stay grounded and still while they are healing? Are we rushing around while we are ill or are we practicing healthy recovery skills; eating well, getting to bed early, drinking plenty of nourishing liquids? How is our energy around illness and recovery? Are we telling ourselves to just get over it and get back to work? Do we appear frantic and worried? This also can have a big impact on our child's energy and ultimately how they view disease and illness. Can we pass on a redeemed paradigm of convalescing? I try my best to make myself a daily or three cups of hot tea, filled with immune boosting roots and lovely smelling herbs. This re-centers me and refills my self-care cup. What do you require for self-care when your routine is disrupted to care for a little one? The more you can do, the more you will have to give to your child when they need it most. It may also keep you from falling ill as well.

Physical Activity/Venturing Out

I enjoy getting my little one outside as soon as humanly possible. Even if I he is carried on shoulders until he asks to return inside. Ours first ventures outside will be very brief, particularly after an exhausting bout with illness. If the weather is beautiful, I will coax my little one out by asking him to come gather some flowers for the house, or to sunbathe in a warm location. He understands that the sun is healing and will generally comply (not always!).

Knowing when to take your child out into public depends on the disease. There is a general time frame when the illness is contagious, and I try to follow this as much as I can. It can be difficult if your child is begging for play time with friends as you wipe a thick, gooey nose. I like to err on the side of cautious because not only am I exposing others to my little ones illness, I am also taking my child out, still ill and not fully recovered, which could lead to another illness to deal with right away. This is why convalescing is so important and healthy. It gives our bodies time to fully recover *and* strengthen before going out in the world. My rule of thumb is no symptoms plus 24 hours and a full day of eating really good food. This works in our home, and I urge you to come up with your own way of handling the recovery period. If I were dealing with a more serious illness, I would extend the recovery time. I've learned that the more I honor this, the happier and healthier everyone is.

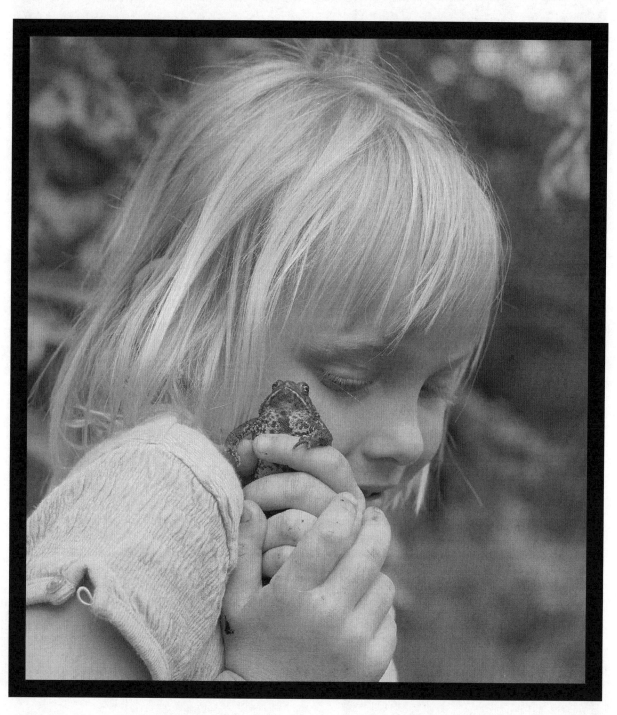

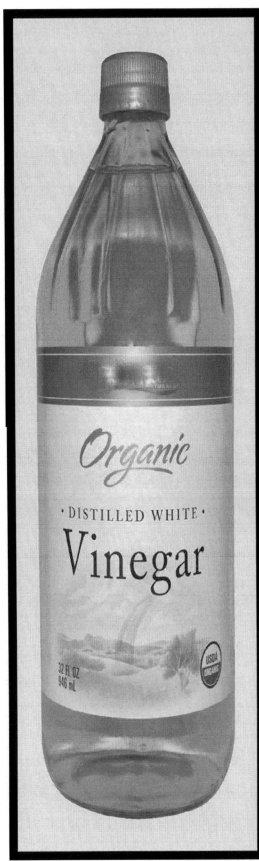

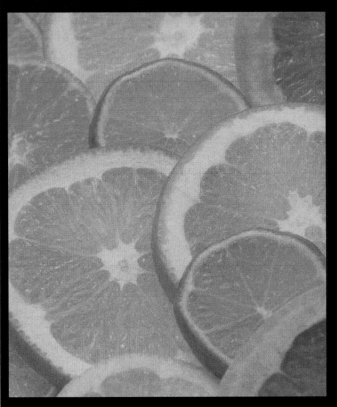

Recipes

Citrus Vinegar

I try to save citrus peels wherever I am! I love this simple household cleanser. I didn't create it, it's all over the internet, but I suggest to everyone I meet to have some handy.

Citrus peels/ or halves enough to fill whatever glass container you have
White vinegar to fill to above peels
Cap with a plastic lid (metal will disintegrate from vinegar)
Let this sit until ready to use. I will be the old lady with jars of this stashed everywhere, I love it so and make it so often. It is a great base to create your own cleaning sprays.
Cleaning spray
1 part thyme tincture or 2 parts strong infusion
1 part lavender tincture or 2 parts strong infusion
1 part citrus vinegar
10 parts water

Place in spray bottle, shake and cap. If you are using infusions instead of tinctures this will not keep and will also decrease germicidal activity. You can store in refrigerator a few days.

Do a test before using this on furniture or appliances you may need to dilute with more water. This is what works for my household.

Simmering Herbs

I will use a pot of herbs simmering on my stove (watch very closely or use a crockpot with the lid off) turned down as low as possible, during an illness and all through recovery. The scents cleanse the space; add moisture, and healing to both the caregiver and the child. I generally just throw a handful or two into a big pot of water and let them steam away. With children in the home it's a good idea to place it on a back burner.

• Vomiting and diarrhea:

Ginger (Zingiber officinale), peppermint (Mentha piperita), lavender (Lavendula)

• Colds/Sinus congestion:

Eucalyptus (Eucalyptus globulus), peppermint, lavender, thyme (Thymus vulgaris)

• Flu:

Ginger, garlic, lavender, thyme

Smudging: I enjoy smudging our home after an illness. I feel that it resets the space, clears out any funk and brings a sense of order. My little one will follow me all over the place with a little broom helping to get the smoke everywhere. I have used lavender as well as sage when I smudge.

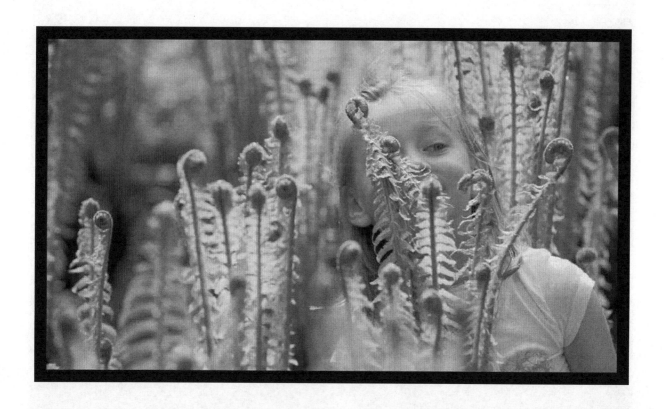

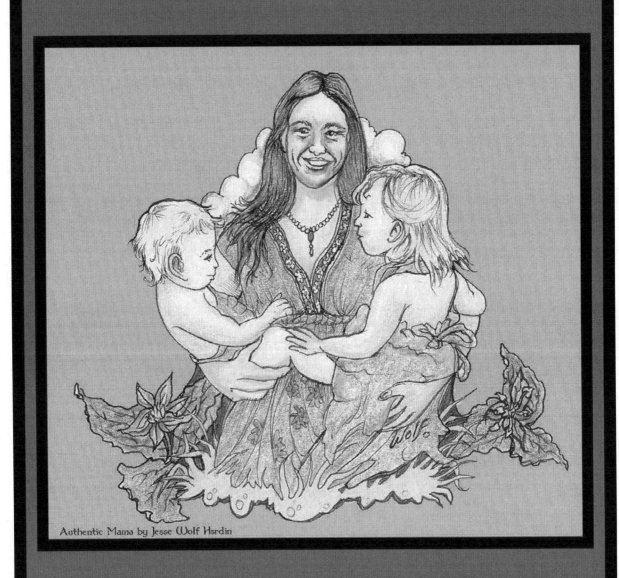

Authentic Mama by Jesse Wolf Hardin

To be the best Mama that you can be,
take the time to sweetly mother your own needing self
-Jesse Wolf Hardin

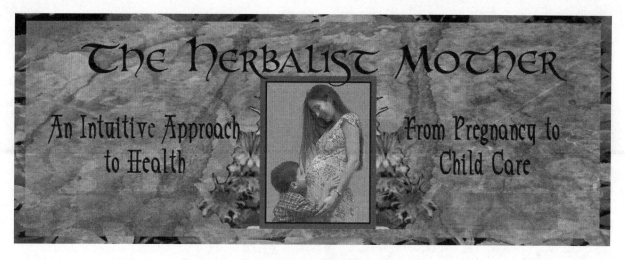

SELF-CARE FOR DOULAS:

Herbals and Common Sense Wisdom

by Sabrina Lutes

A doula is someone who serves women while they are birthing their babies. An ancient form of caregiving that requires a deepening sense of self and stamina, a doula is the container for a woman to find her edges in birth. She is there to comfort, offer support, and care for the birthing woman's needs. Many times this includes physically holding a woman's entire weight as she is draped around your neck while she pushes, supporting a leg when needed, or burying your knuckles into the sacrum of a hurting back due to a posterior baby's head. It will include hours or days of sleeplessness. Being on call and having to drop everything to make it to a woman's side. It will entail tears of joy, pain and sadness, witnessing triumphs and despair. Whispering in a mother's ear that she can do what needs to be done to give birth to her child.

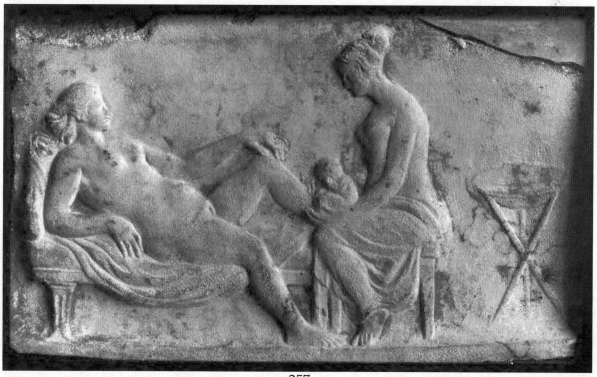

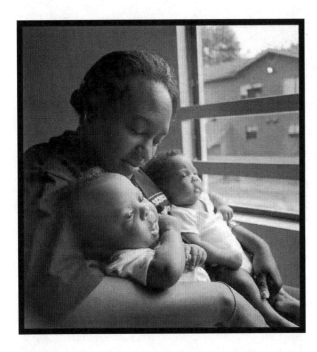

So much of this work requires a calmness and tenacity of spirit. A grounded-ness that comes mostly when we are well taken care of ourselves! When I began my practice many years ago and many babies later, I realized that doing a few key things really helped me continue my work joyfully. The new to doula-ing me, would pack a huge birth bag. Just about everything in my rolling cart was for the comfort of the birthing mother. Herbal rice socks, aromatherapy, massagers, music, and on and on. I fussed over my bag and worried over the contents always wanting to be ever more prepared. As I became more seasoned in my work, I slowly began to carry less and less that was mother specific and began to carry things that would help me be ever more present and comfortable. I also learned what I needed to be well cared for nutritionally to help prepare for and recover from the rigors of supporting laboring moms. This job is not for the faint of heart. You must be physically strong and able to put in long hours, and depending on your client load some of those hours are back to back births. Your mind must also be capable of staying in tune with the laboring woman as well as able to get you home after a marathon birth.

Sleep is huge in birth work. You're either awoken from it at all hours or you aren't getting it because you are at a birth, or you are having trouble getting to sleep because you have just come home from a birth and are full of adrenaline. Making good choices helps this aspect of doula work so much. Many times this requires saying no to going out late, missing that late night caffeine laden dessert or drink, and just getting into a rhythm and routine that allows for an early bedtime. A warm herbal tea before bed that has Chamomile (*Matricaria chamomilla*) and Fennel seed (*Foeniculum vulgare*) is a wonderful night cap. Passionflower (*Passiflora* spp.) can be added for a jittery mind.

Keeping a sachet stuffed with Lavender and Roses under the pillow helps, particularly after hours of being in a hospital environment. I also got into a strict routine of bed making! If I wasn't called away, then I made sure that I made my bed up each morning, and spritzed the sheets with a Lavender (*Lavandula*) hydrosol or strong infusion of lavender blossoms with enough alcohol for preservation. The reason for this was to allow me ease and bring sleep quickly when arriving home.

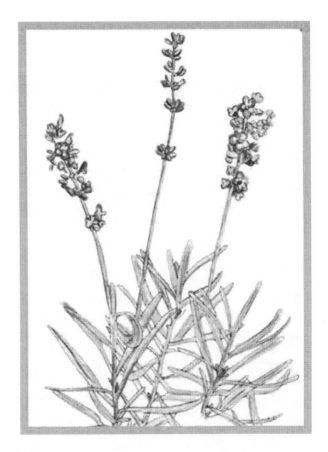

Many things about being a doula are apt to wear your immunity down. Long hours, irregular schedule, hospitals, many hours without eating, stress. It will only serve you and your clients if you can stay as healthy as possible. I love Elder (*Sambucus nigra*), berry and flowers so very much. It is delicious and I would take it throughout cold and flu season. I used the jam on my sandwiches and added syrup to mineral water. I also consumed large quantities of very garlicky chicken soup, filled with seaweed, veggies, and Shiitake (*Lentinula edodes*) or Maitake (*Grifola frondosa*) mushrooms.

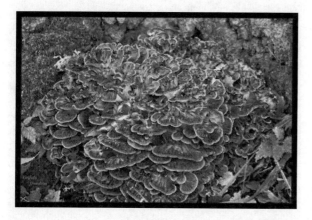

I would keep Echinacea throat spray in my bag just in case I felt exposed while working. Stress is best dealt with beforehand. Tulsi (*Ocimum tenuiflorum*) is a beautiful adaptogen to keep on hand. It has served me in so many ways! Keep ready-made tea bags with you while you work. Since adaptogens work better when taken over a period of time, find one that works well for you. There is so much written about them, and with some trial and error you can tease out one suited for your own constitution and needs. Time in nature is paramount for someone who works with birthing moms. Exercise will keep you physically strong and boost immunity as well as ward off fatigue. Eating nourishing foods several times throughout the day regularly, keeps us capable. All these may seem common sense, but when most people can skip a meal and it won't affect them, whereas doulas' we skip some part of self-care it may be days before we can right that indiscretion.

Staying hydrated is another key aspect to this work. Depending on the level of care you are giving a mom, as some labors you may be there just as quiet support, and others you are spending hours within physical contact, you may forget to drink. I tried to keep a water bottle in my line of sight as much as I could. I also kept things such as Oatstraw (*Avena sativa*) infusion, lemon and honey water, or Hibiscus (*Hibiscus sabdariffa*, Roselle) in it. If your practice takes you to lots of hospital births, including a few moistening herbs is really helpful. One of my favorites is Oatstraw and Linden (*Tilia Americana*), these herbs are nervines first but with use I have discovered their moistening qualities. Since they are so effective for soothing frazzled nerves, they create a great combo.

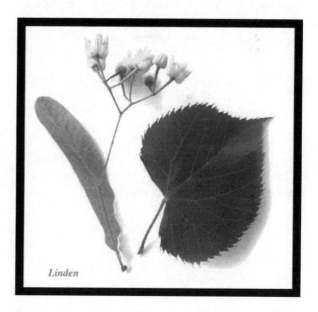

Linden

A little jar of honey kept in your bag goes a long way to help quell a dry throat and adds a boost of energy when needed. Midwives I worked with would also give it to a laboring woman if she was particularly tired and needed some energy. An herbal adaptogen infused honey would be marvelous for this. I enjoy Tulsi and Schisandra (*Schisandra chinensis*).

Oh sweet doula, your body will ache after birth. The blinding exhaustion that hits after a three day labor, you will feel it in your bones. Those deep tissue massage maneuvers you performed because a mother's pain threshold is so high and she's begging you to press harder, you'll feel those also. Your adrenaline is high enough that you agree. The clock at a birth stands still for everyone. You think you are holding a position for moments, when in reality it may be hours. You will be bruised. Of course not every birth is like this, but most likely some will be. If I could get a hot bath before I crashed, that was best; Epsom salts mixed with herbs that help dull the ache and push the buildup of tension out of my muscles. Bodywork from a sensitive caregiver is so extremely important. This can soothe the nerves as well after particularly intense births. It also serves as a way to process without having to talk about it, which is great because your client information is confidential.

Doula work is a calling that is really heart centered work. You must be open and giving and gentle. Your work is a gift and the gifts you receive are found in first breaths and beads of sweat as a mother claims herself no matter the outcome. I hope this inspires you to take good care of yourself as you walk the path of birth doula. A lovely herbal creation to carry with you is a heart centered elixir. Keep it in a lovely bag with rose quartz and other birth talismans. This can be used before and after births, or during if you just need to re-center yourself and remember why you are doing the work you do.

A Doula's Self-Care Bag:
Things to Bring
To a Birth

•A small jar of honey (herbal infused is really nice, if you happen to give some to laboring mother, be sure the herbs you used are safe during pregnancy).
•Tea bags with herbal blends (Mountain Rose Herbs sell press and seal bags that work great) Hibiscus, Tulsi, Spearmint are excellent choices).
•A muslin bag with Rosemary (*Rosmarinus officinalis*) and Lavender (fresh scents can help refresh and rejuvenate during a long birth. As I developed my practice I moved away from essential oils and began using whole plants. The scent is easier to control. Essential oils may not be the safest around brand new babies. Once essential oil is used, it is hard to remove it should a mother grow tired of it.)

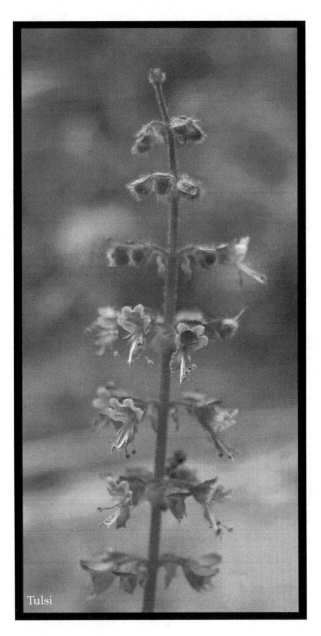

Tulsi

•Echinacea throat spray- you can make your own, but I really love Herb Pharm's Soothing Throat spray.
•A bag of nuts
•A water bottle (one that can handle hot liquids so you can make tea in it)
•An herbal infused oil like Calendula (*Calendula officinalis*), Saint John's wort (*Hypericum perforatum*), arnica(*Arnica montana*). If you make St John's Wort or Arnica these can help with the muscle aches that occur with the work)
•A small first aid kit
•A good quality salt like Himalayan to add to water to help hydrate

260

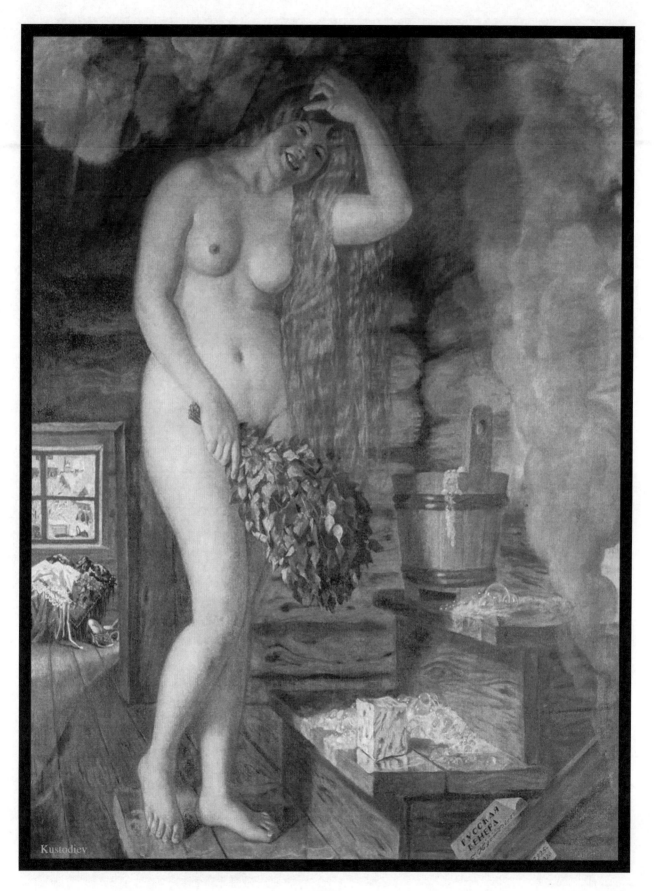

Kustodiev

261

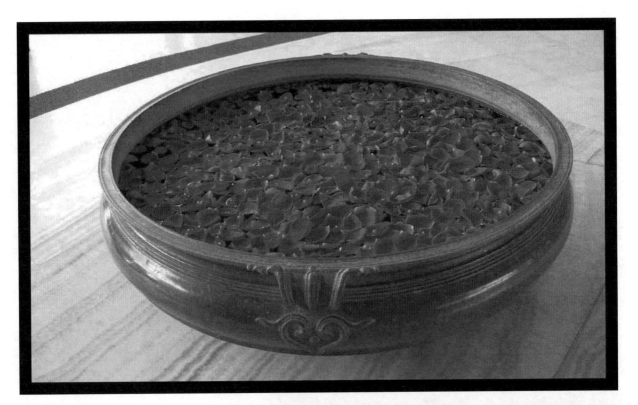

Herbal Bath:

You can create your bath herbs all at once and keep them stored tightly in a glass jar. Scoop out 1 Cup of herbs and place in a muslin bag. Run the bath and toss the herbs in. Add the Epsom salts directly. I usually use 1-2 cups. These herbs can be used singly or you can create your own mixture. If I were blending them, I might choose one aromatic (rose, lavender, Pine (*Pinus strobus*), Rosemary and add the other herbs to that, although Rosemary and Lavender together are sublime.

Ideas- Epsom salts, Rose petals, Willow Bark (*Salix alba*), Rosemary, Comfrey (*Symphytum uplandica* x), Pine, Lavender, Calendula

Moistening Infusion:

2 parts Oatstraw
1 Part Linden

Add one ounce to French press, fill with one quart boiled water. Let steep for a

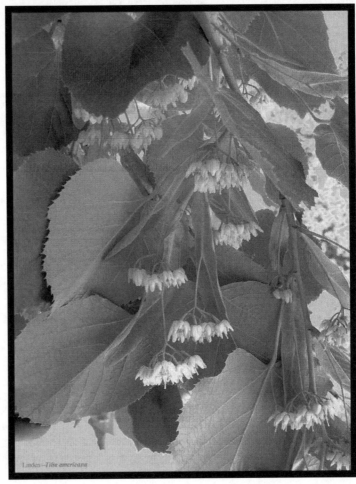

Linden—*Tilia americana*

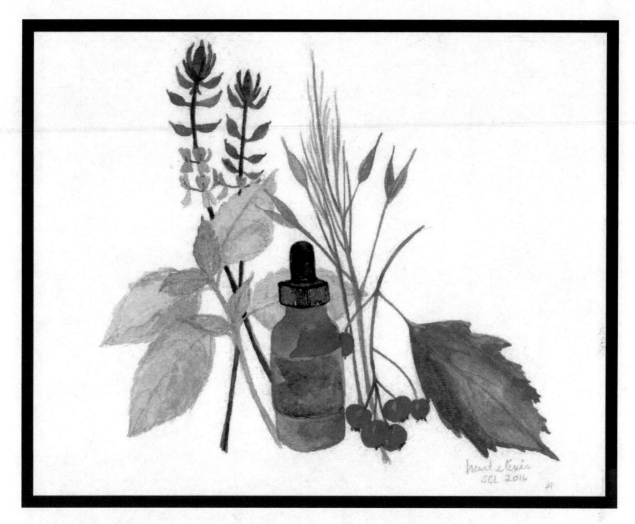

few hours. Drink warm with a dash of Cinnamon, or chilled with honey or without.

Lavender room spray:

1 Cup of lavender blossom
2 cups water

Bring water to a boil, turn off heat and add blossoms. Let sit until cool. Strain and add enough clear alcohol such as ever-clear or high proof vodka to make a 20% alcohol solution. The ratio will be different depending on the alcohol and amount of liquid you have. Place in a spritzer bottle and use when needed.

Heart Centered Elixir:

1 Part Hawthorn (*Cratageus* spp.) tincture
1 Part Tulsi tincture
1 Part Oatstraw tincture
½ part honey

Blend tinctures and honey in a dropper bottle. Label and use a few drops at a time.

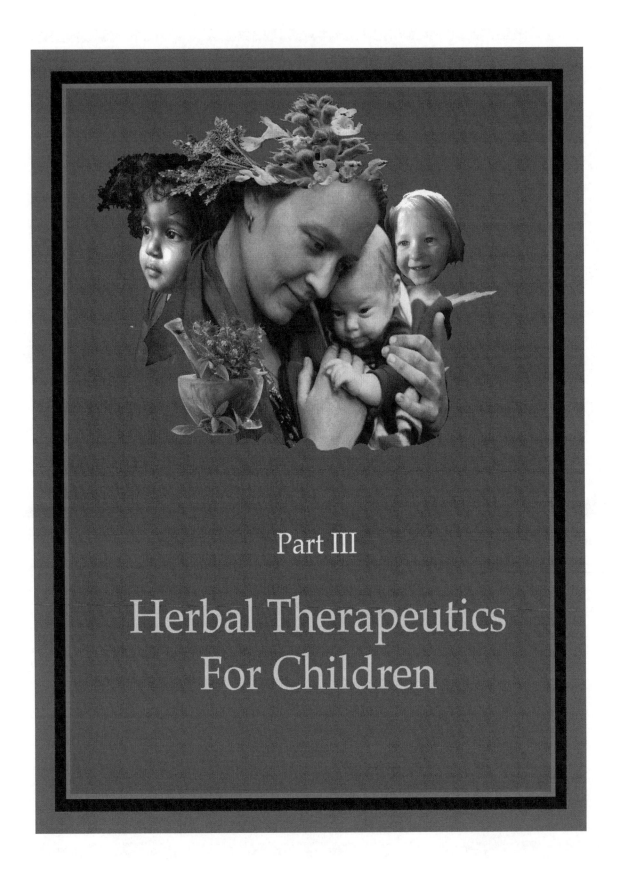

Part III

Herbal Therapeutics For Children

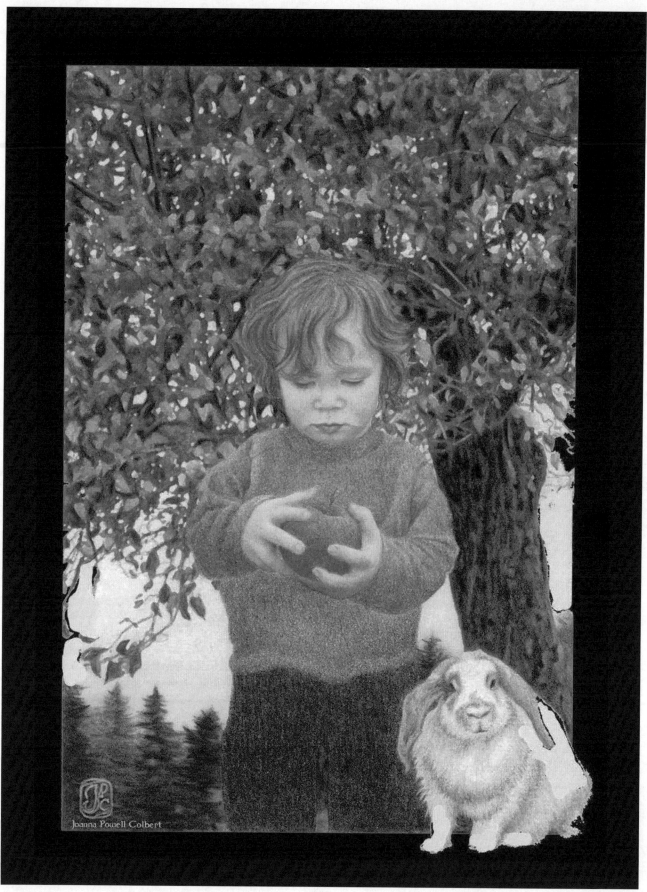

Joanna Powell Colbert

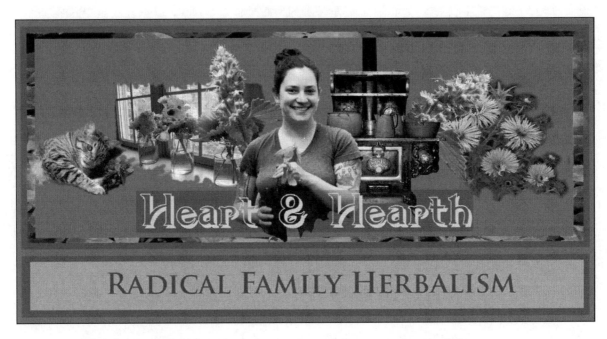

HERBS FOR THE POSTPARTUM YEAR

Birthing Parent's Toolkit

by Juliette Abigail Carr

Home herbalism is who we are and how our families work, healing practiced around the kitchen table around the world and across the centuries. Thank the Good Green Earth that home herbalism happens as a reflex, intuition built on a foundation of herbal fluency that allows us to live as herbalists in every moment.

Childbirth and caring for a newborn are some of the most common inspirations for families to turn to herbs, but not enough attention is paid to the postpartum period itself. This year *Heart & Hearth* is focusing on creating useful toolkits to support a family throughout the postpartum year, including herbal toolkits for parents, newborns, and nursing.

Leading up to childbirth, much of the emphasis is placed on the birth itself, as a grand finale of the pregnancy—and the importance of the period after the baby is born is minimized to our great detriment. This is a deep failing in the dominant culture, as the postpartum period is absolutely essential to the physical and emotional well-being of every member of the family. Traditionally, childbearing parents are lovingly cared for by extended family, friends, and community members, allowing them time to recuperate and adjust. In many parts of the world this is still true, just as it is still true in communities that live by traditional values throughout the US.

Unfortunately, the isolation of most modern childbearing families in the US is deeply problematic and is associated with serious negative health outcomes for birthing parents. Often, birthing parents are too quick to get back on their feet due to the ceaseless demands of the free market: even if there is no rush to return to work, a lack of continuous postpartum support forces modern parents to care for themselves and their families instead of emphasizing rest and healing for the first few weeks, which increases the likelihood of postpartum preeclampsia, blood clots, hemorrhage, infection, pelvic floor injury, prolapse, diastasis recti, and pain related to structural misalignment, as well as the ever-present specter of postpartum depression.

266

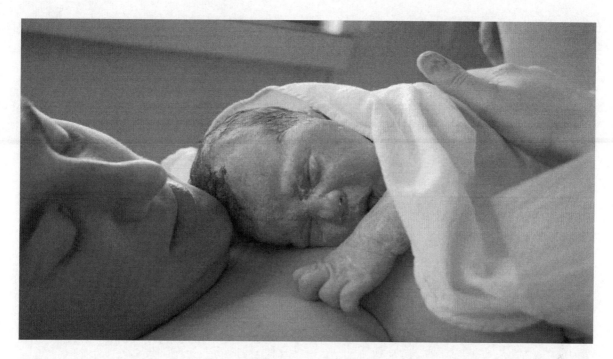

Postpartum connectedness is becoming more emphasized within local radical communities and natural health communities, which is absolutely essential to improving birth outcomes, especially among birthing people of color—particularly BIPOC—who suffer birth morbidity and mortality rates exponentially more severe than their white counterparts. Building support networks into the childbearing era, both prenatally and postnatally, has a significant effect on the wellbeing of the whole family, as seen in the dramatic shifts in long-term health outcomes of Black and Indigenous mothers who receive culturally relevant doula care.

There is much that can be done to support our community members as they birth: bringing a meal, babysitting older children, doing the dishes or laundry, and providing a nonjudgemental listening (adult!) ear all go a long way towards helping families rest and heal from the chrysalis-shedding of birth. As herbalists, bringing trustworthy remedies into a home is an incredibly helpful gift: not only are we preparing the medicine itself, but we've removed the burdens of problem identification, safety research, and logistics from the family. Providing an herbal toolkit as a prenatal or postpartum gift means that all they have to do is ask a visitor to make them a cup of tea or hand them a tincture bottle, no mental or physical effort required. It also gives us a chance to check in again, every contact an opportunity to ensure that postpartum depression, nursing problems, and other difficulties are not being missed, and that they have enough emotional and physical support.

Peri Tea

To support healing of tears, episiotomies, hemorrhoids, and other pains in the bottom, combine vulneraries, demulcents, astringents, and antimicrobials. My favorite formula for this is 2 parts each of Yarrow, Calendula, Violet, Plantain, and 1 part each finely shredded Witch Hazel and epsom salt. This formula drastically speeds the healing of injured tissue, helps prevent infection, and decreases pain as a moistening anti-inflammatory. Someone who loves the birthing person (not the person themself) brews this tea as needed, using several handfuls in a big jar so it's nice and strong, and storing it in the fridge. With each pad change, mix 50/50 with hot tap water so it is warm in the squirt bottle and use it in the squirt bottle.

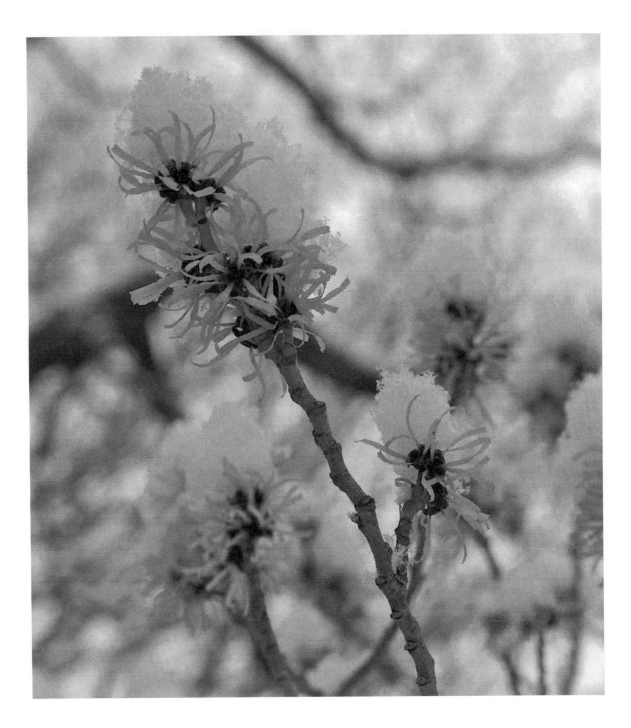

Witch Hazel Ice Pads

These anti-inflammatory, astringent ice packs are just the best, whether there is a tear, hemorrhoid, or just a normally swollen bottom after giving birth. Do this for everyone you love! Fill a bowl with witch hazel, either homemade or store bought. Dip 40-50 cotton makeup remover pads or 20-30 panty liners, then freeze on a cookie sheet (so they don't stick together). When frozen, store in a jar, bag, or container in the freezer. Use 1 panty liner or 1-2 makeup pads on top of the pad at every pad change for the first 3 or 4 days.

Cramps Tincture

This is an easy-to-make formula for one of the most common postpartum complaints. Combine equal parts of Cramp Bark, Black Haw, Lady's Mantle, and Motherwort tinctures. Give 15 to 30 drops, diluted in water or tea, as needed for postpartum cramps.

Massage Oil

Muscle pain is extremely common after the hard work of creating life and the transformation of parenthood, especially in the first two days or so postpartum. Herbal infused oils containing anti-inflammatory and pain relieving herbs are helpful to support soothing touch. Including aromatics and circulatory stimulants in the formula can assist integration into tissue. I no longer use any essential oils due to their serious ecological impact, but I have found that making infused oils of aromatics and antimicrobials (Eucalyptus, Thyme, Rosemary, Lavender, etc.) fills the gap seamlessly in my practice. For sore muscles, I like Willow, Meadowsweet, Black Birch, Lavender, and Mint, infused into a blend of olive and almond oil and used to massage the back, neck, upper arms, and feet. If the legs are to be massaged, wait until the person is regularly walking around and massage toward the feet, due to the potential for blood clots, which are rare but pose a serious threat postpartum. Oils can also be added to bath water (ideally after the person has gotten in to avoid a slippery tub), or mixed in with epsom salts. Abdominal binders are useful in the early days as well, especially for back or pelvic pain, as they help support posture while the body heals.

NORMAL-T(ea)

This is an easy-to-source tea base that covers the most common postpartum concerns, based on the commonly used NORA tea. The name is an acronym: **N**ettles leaf, **O**atstraw, **R**aspberry leaf, **M**otherwort aboveground parts, **A**lfalfa, **L**emon balm aboveground parts, and **T**ulsi aboveground parts. NORMAL-T is a mineral-rich anabolic trophorestorative, promoting endocrine function, nervous system stability, red blood cell regeneration, and water/electrolyte balance. These actions promote appropriate physiological responses postpartum, engaging the parasympathetic nervous system to allow for cell and hormone generation, supporting lactogenesis II and ongoing milk supply, HPA-axis function, neurotransmission, establishment of appropriate postpartum circadian rhythm, healing of damaged tissues, uterine toning, and emotional coping in the face of significant hormone shifts and physical challenges, making it one of the single most useful interventions to help promote a healthy postpartum adjustment and prevent postpartum depression. Herbs can be added to this base as appropriate for a person's specific needs: consider yarrow and lady's mantle tinctures following prolapse or hemorrhage, rose for birth trauma, etc.

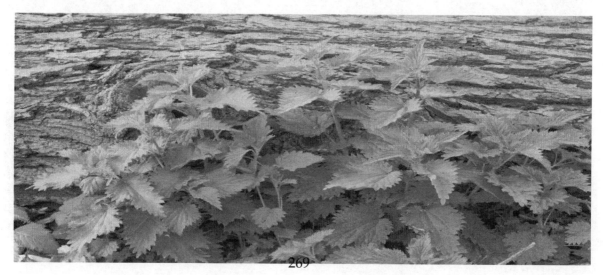

Sleep Tincture

The development of an appropriate postpartum circadian rhythm is absolutely essential for physical and mental health, from rebuilding blood supply and having sufficient milk to avoiding postpartum depression. A nursing parent needs to be able to rouse from a deep sleep easily, nurse, and go back to sleep, adapting to the baby's sleep cycle. Instead of simply turning off the lights with a hypnotic —which is dangerous for cosleeping families in particular— support the development of circadian rhythm using nervines & adaptogens, to help the nervous and endocrine systems function the way they should postpartum. Adaptogens also support lactation & help prevent postpartum depression via hormone balance. NORMAL-T is a strong starting place and delivers enough balance for most of us, but if a birthing person needs more support than that, blend equal parts of Milky Oats tincture and Ashwagandha tincture. Milky Oats is a trophorestorative nervine that imparts an overall feeling of rejuvenation and helps us helps shed the chrysalis to step fully into our transformed family. Ashwagandha is a powerful anabolic adaptogen to rebuild deep strength when especially run down, working on the endocrine system to affect the sleep-wake cycle. Schisandra is also a great addition, when circadian rhythm dysfunction is accompanied by depression, anxiety, fury, or unusually labile mood, and when an autoimmune disorder is present. I will also occasionally use Shatavari, but only in the rare instance of a true milk supply issue (more on this in the upcoming Nursing Toolkit).

Herbs for Emotional Wellbeing

Emotional healing is just as universal of a priority in the postpartum period as physical healing. We often don't consider it except in clear cases of postpartum depression, which misses an important opportunity to fully support our community, and leads to invisible cases of postpartum depression, postpartum anxiety, and birth trauma.

Family Nervine Formula: All members of the family, including the birthing parent, benefit from a basic nervine formula in the early days. Birth is a major transformation for everyone, and it can take the gut-brain and limbic system time to adapt to the new family structure. Combine Lemon Balm and Milky Oats, and add something else if circumstances indicate.

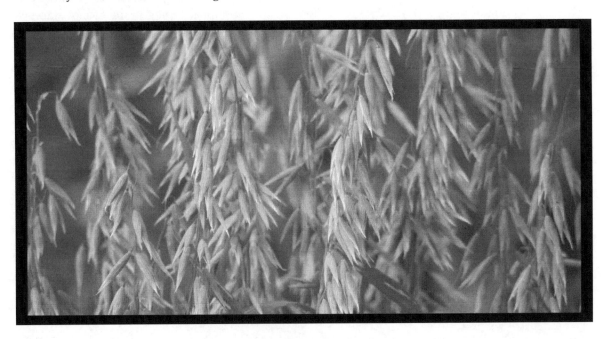

Postpartum Depression, Anxiety, or Rage: Parents who experience physical trauma may be fine otherwise, or they may experience emotional trauma too. Physical injury, especially long-lasting issues like diastasis recti, painful sex (dyspareunia), incontinence, and chronic back pain, is a serious risk factor for both birth trauma and postpartum depression later in the postpartum period; screening people with these risk factors is essential to catching it early. Other risk factors include previous history of depression, survivorship, recent grief, circadian rhythm dysfunction, and milk supply issues. Remember that fully 1/4 of birthing people will experience some measure of postpartum depression, anxiety, or rage during their childbearing years: that is a crazy statistic, and one that has deeply felt ramifications for the rest of the family as well.

Basic PPD Formula: Milky oats, Mimosa, Tulsi, and St John's Wort or Blue Vervain (depending on constitution) is a nice general formula that can be adjusted based on the individual person.

Consider adding one of the following herbs as appropriate:

•Schisandra: labile mood or rage, plus circadian rhythm disruption or autoimmunity; especially as a honey

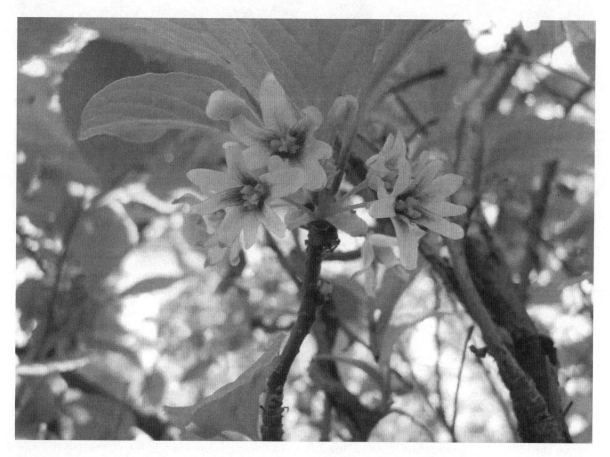

•Black Cohosh: role upheaval anxiety (esp. gender-related or self-efficacy) or with backache or headache
•Linden: labile mood, hypervigilance activities, and difficulty sleeping
•Catnip: anxiety-related stomach aches or nightmares and hypervigilance activities

271

• Peach blossom: grief, deep sadness, needing patience and hope
• Lilac: fear, sadness, needing to feel safe

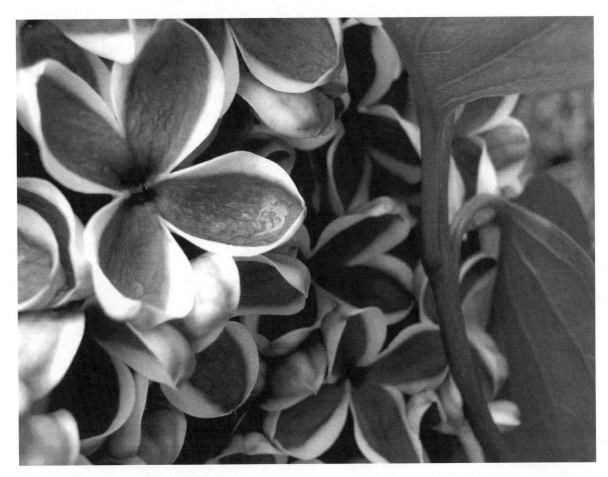

Family PPD Formula: If the birthing parent is struggling with any flavor of postpartum depression, supporting the rest of the family is appropriate. Add an adaptogen like Tulsi to the Family Nervine formula, to help them cope and support each other and the birthing parent.

Family Trauma Formula: Fearing for the life of your beloved/child/mother/parent is earth-shakingly terrifying, and yet witnesses are often ignored after a potentially traumatic birth experience. If there is the potential for trauma in the partner or other children, add a trauma-specific heart opener to the above Family Nervine formula like Motherwort, Lilac, or Rose-Hawthorn, to help them cope with those feelings and effectively move through them. Children in particular benefit from lilac to help them feel safe in the family again.

Providing pre-made herbal formulas for the most common postpartum complaints is an act of loving compassion for our community members as they go through the childbearing transformation. It is a thoughtful, useful gift, but more importantly it sends the nonverbal message that we see them and understand what they're going through, both positive and negative. Empathetic connection is one of the single most powerful gifts we can give each other in this era of isolation: the more connected we each are, the stronger we all are.

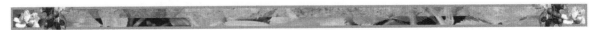

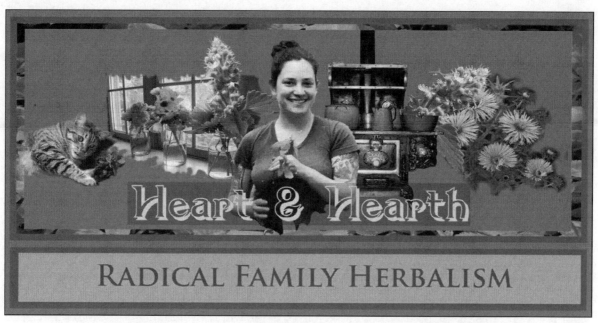

HERBS FOR THE POSTPARTUM YEAR

Newborn Toolkit

by Juliette Abigail Carr

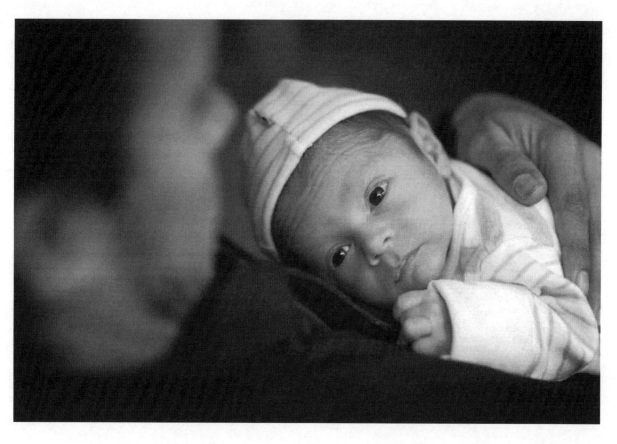

Home herbalism is who we are and how our families work, healing practiced around the kitchen table around the world and across the centuries. Thank the Good Green Earth that home herbalism happens as a reflex, intuition built on a foundation of herbal fluency that allows us to live as herbalists in every moment.

Childbirth and caring for a newborn are some of the most common inspirations for families to turn to herbs, but it can be very difficult to create remedies out of whole cloth during the postpartum period, a time characterized by an extreme learning curve in difficult circumstances.

This year *Heart & Hearth* is focusing on creating useful toolkits to support a family throughout the postpartum year. Previous articles this year have presented herbal toolkits for immediately postpartum parents and for nursing couplets. Here, we create a toolkit of the most versatile newborn-friendly herbs. It can be customized in the moment if needed, avoiding a sleep-deprived frenzy of researching and cooking up remedies when they are needed most. This toolkit contains some of the most-used herbs in my practice.

Baby Basics

Babies are considered "newborns" for the first three months, then they to transition into "infants" for the rest of their babyhood, as they awaken fully to the world around them. The older they get, the more problems arise: teething, starting solids and its attendant gas and constipation, overstimulation, catching colds from playmates, etc.

Generally, newborns should not need much herbal support, if any at all. Nursing provides for all their nutritional needs; plenty of microbiome support for immune, digestive, blood, and nervous system development; comfort, attachment, and safety; stability of body temperature, respiratory function, and blood sugar; and much of their important developmental tasks related to connectedness and interpersonal communication.

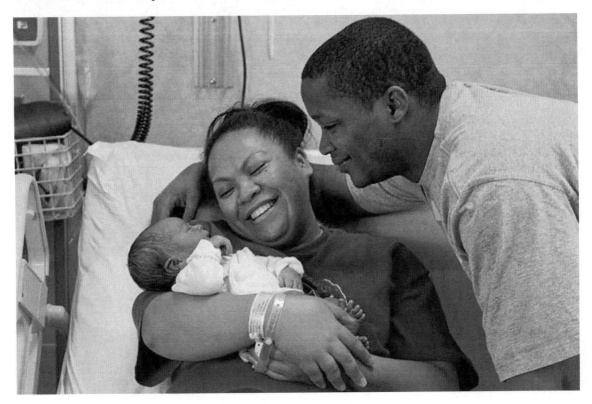

Newborn Microbiome

If a baby was exposed to antibiotics during or following birth, skin-to-skin contact is doubly important to allow for speedy microbiome colonization. If the parent took antibiotics, a diet rich in fermented foods, soluble fiber, fat, vitamins, minerals, and antioxidants is key to recolonizing healthfully; that sounds like a lot, but a breakfast of oatmeal, whole milk yogurt, berries, and nuts checks those boxes.

Dietary improvements are a much more effective means of microbiome colonization and maintenance than supplementation, but in the immediate postpartum period it is appropriate to consider parental supplementation to hedge your bets. Choose a probiotic that contains bacteria associated with vaginas and babies, especially *Lactobacillus rhamnosus, L. reuteri,* and *Bifidobacterium adolescentis, B. bifidum, B. breve,* and *B. longum.* There are products marketed for yeast infections that contain these strains.

Newborn probiotic supplementation is not indicated: the baby's body is made to work with milk and snuggles, so we should be careful about attempting long-term changes to something as pivotal and as poorly understood as the microbiome. There is no tradition of giving live foods to babies before they're eating solids, and their systems did not evolve to introduce microbiota that way. The most recent research indicates questionable benefits to newborn supplementation, and even a potential increase in childhood infections, although the science is far from settled. Regardless of the iffy science, giving newborns probiotics isn't called for, as babies will be effectively colonized with their parents' microbiome through skin-to-skin contact and nursing as nature intended. Instead, concerned parents can supplement and improve their diets.

Milk Transfer of Herbs

When babies have uncomfortable symptoms, our first line of defense is always nursing (or giving a bottle), snuggling, skin-to-skin, and other comforting routines. If that is insufficient to soothe the baby, a nursing parent may take newborn-safe herbs. This is especially true for things like colds, where you really want their immune system to learn how to work, but you also might want to ease their symptoms if they're super uncomfortable.

The timing for tea is about an hour on an empty stomach before nursing, or two hours on a full stomach before nursing; for tinctures, about an hour and a half on an empty stomach before nursing, or three hours on a full stomach before nursing. Most of the medicine will not transfer into the milk, as the digestive system, liver, and lactation system will filter out most of it; but as the body builds custom milk for every feed, a small percentage does transfer to the baby.

We do not have good data on exactly how much of each herb transfers to the baby (due to a paucity of research), and milk transfer of herbs is also affected by diet, hydration, metabolism, and nursing frequency. The research on pharmaceuticals during lactation is somewhat better (although still lacking) and indicates that small percentages of bioactive compounds pass into the milk. Generally, most herbs that have been studied have been found to transfer in smaller amounts than the pharmaceuticals that are considered safe during lactation, such as antidepressants. Fat soluble molecules are larger and tend to concentrate in milk, delivering a larger-than-intended dose to the baby, so herbs like cannabis that contain a high proportion of bioactive fat-soluble molecules should not be used in this way. Alcohol builds up and is cleared from milk at the same rate as it does in blood, which is why nursing parents are no longer instructed to "pump and dump." The rule now is "if you can drive, you can nurse," which can apply to baby-safe herbs in tincture form as well.

This toolkit is meant to be useful for common baby discomforts that often benefit from a little extra support beyond nursing and parental supplementation. All of the newborn remedies here can carry over into the infant period, as well, making them particularly useful to have on hand throughout the whole first year. There are many other herbs that can be used instead, but I have prioritized easy-to-find herbs that have very versatile applications and an endlessly long, multicultural tradition of use for babies.

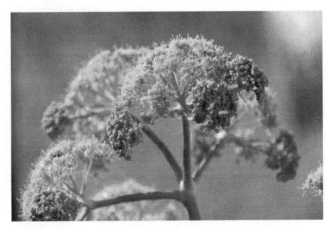

Fennel is a perennially reliable digestive aid for babies (and through childhood, really). It is unparalleled for colic, and the first thing I reach for with reflux/infant GERD. As infants start to eat solids and gas and constipation become an issue, fennel continues to be the perfect key for that

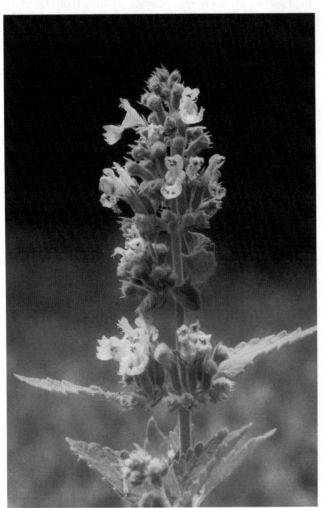

lock. It has additional nice uses in toddlerhood and childhood, but digestion is my favorite application in babies for this workhouse of an ally.

Note: If a baby is gassy, painfully refluxes, and spits up a lot, see a lactation consultant to assess the latch and rule out a tongue tie. Sometimes ongoing digestive upset happens because the baby is gulping air while nursing. Believe it or not, adjusting the latch and doing tongue-tie exercises can go a long way. Craniosacral can also be helpful, especially if the birth was traumatic or very fast, as this can leave some residual jacked-ness to their posture that can affect latching.

Catnip is another just flat-out indispensable herb in my practice. It is a lovely, soothing nervine with an affinity for digestion. I use it for inconsolable fussiness, overstimulation, stress, angst, and emotional overwhelm, especially when those feelings, pain, and digestive upset occur together. I always combine it with fennel when colic or gas is an issue at night, or occur together with those difficult feelings. It is wonderful for teething pain in particular.

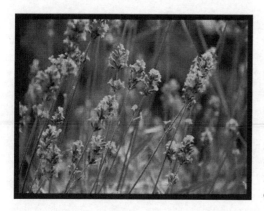

Lavender is basically good for everything. No baby-friendly apothecary is complete without it. It is a gentling, soothing friend in times of general fussiness, overstimulation, and broken-routine exhaustion. It soothes pain and fussiness related to teething, as well as the lumps, bumps, and bruises that come along with learning how to move your body in a world with gravity and hard objects. It is a soothing antimicrobial astringent useful for skin issues and hot, red, irritated rashes. I also like it as a digestive aid for gas and colic, especially if the baby seems emotionally distraught.

Chamomile is a well-played fiddle of a childhood remedy, but that's for a reason (thank you, Mrs. Josephine Rabbit, and many thousands of generations of mothers before her). Chamomile, like lavender, is something of a panacea. It is a useful ally for gas, colic, and general indigestion. Chamomile combines well with lavender for general fussiness and pain, especially for teething. It is also very helpful for rashes and boo-boos, especially itchy ones.

Calendula flower and **Marshmallow** flower (or leaf, if you want it stronger) is a magical combination for skin issues of all types. Boo-boos, rashes, dry skin…you name it, the moistening antimicrobial vulnerary power of these common, easy-to-grow flowers turns a skin ailment right around.

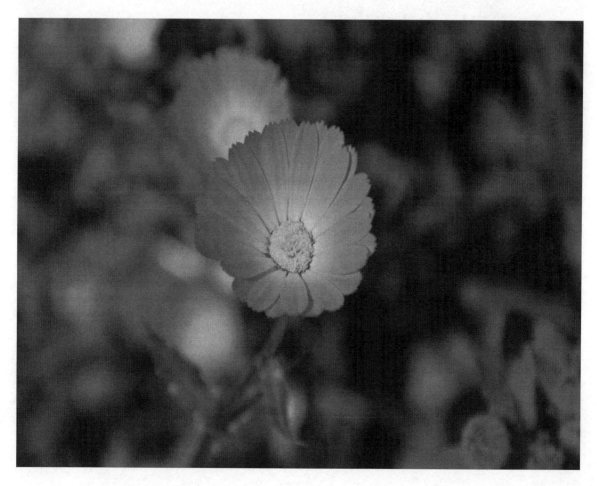

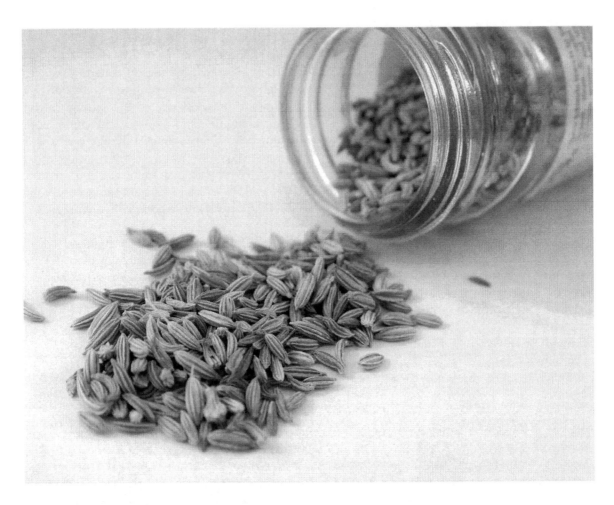

Basic Useful Formulas to Keep On Hand

Massage Oil

Combine equal parts Lavender, Catnip, Chamomile, and Fennel in a double boiler at a 1:3 ratio with olive oil and almond oil. Cover and heat slowly, keeping oil at 100 degrees or body temperature to avoid oxidizing the oil, for at least 4 hours. Store in a jar in a dark place for 1 month, then strain and put into a pretty glass bottle. (detailed infused oil-making instructions available on my website, oldwaysherbal.com)

For gas and constipation, gentle massage the baby's tummy using a circular motion. Alternate tummy massage with "bicycle legs," moving their legs like they're pedaling help release trapped gas. After a couple of repetitions, put them on their tummy (prone) to help release trapped gas; you can also massage their lower back in this position. Watch their posture: arching is usually reflux or painful gas, whereas rigid legs often signifies constipation or gas that is ready to pass—sometimes babies respond to that feeling of something about to come out by squeezing against it.

If you have a difficult sleeper, a stress-prone baby, or a baby with ongoing nighttime digestive upset, a nightly massage after bath as part of your routine can be helpful to settle down. It can also help for occasional stress, like from traveling or a disrupted routine. Add calendula oil and you can skip moisturizing!

278

Teething & Pain Tincture

Tincture equal parts Chamomile, Lavender, and Catnip in brandy at 1:2 fresh or 1:4 dried. Clove makes a nice addition here, too.

Generally, one hopes the baby doesn't experience pain, but things do happen as we learn how to move, especially in a world with gravity and siblings. Some babies don't start to teeth until they're well into the infant period, but others start earlier, and honestly it can come up very suddenly so it's nice to have something on hand. This is also helpful for pain related to vaccination. Simply put one drop on your finger and let the baby suck it off or massage it into their ouchy gums, then immediately nurse the baby or give a pacifier or bottle (depending on how you feed your baby). Sucking is a primary source of pain relief, so this step is actually really important.

For ongoing pain like a broken bone, make a sugar-based syrup with this tincture and give it every 3-4 hours—it's easier to stay ahead of pain than it is to play catch-up later. The research is clear that sucrose has a significant pain-reducing capacity in babies. Avoid honey due to the risk of infant botulism.

Diaper Cream

Make a salve using infused oils of Lavender, Calendula, Chamomile, and Marshmallow leaf, in a base of olive oil and sweet almond oil. Go heavy on the oil and light on the wax for a looser, easier-to-apply texture. Avoid essential oils, as they are not safe for babies' skin or for the environment.

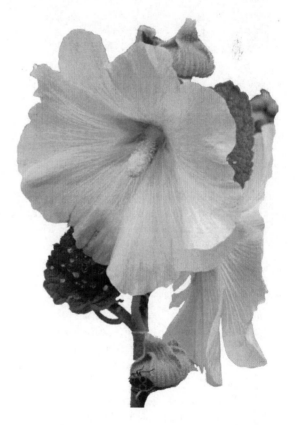

Salve is safe for cloth diapers and easy to make in advance. These vulnerary, anti-fungal, anti-bacterial herbs moisten and soothe skin to promote healing and prevent ongoing infection. It's also nice for dry, chapped skin, which is a big issue here in my wintery climate, and perhaps in yours as well.

These basic formulas build a basic general apothecary that is useful to have on hand throughout babyhood and beyond, as newborns grow into infants and then into toddlers. The older babies get, the more likely they are to benefit from herbal support in acute situations. There are many other herbs that can be substituted for reasons of bioregional availability, just be sure to emphasize both versatility of applications and a long tradition of use in babies, as well as environmental stewardship: there is no reason to use an at-risk herb when a weedy ally works just as well.

Note: For more information on choosing safe herbs for babies and children, please refer to Heart & Hearth #5, "Choosing Safe, Effective Herbal Remedies for Toddlers & Young Children," in *Plant Healer Quarterly* Summer 2019, Vol. 9 Issue 3_. For Materia Medica specific for the next era of toddlerhood, please refer to Heart & Hearth #7, "Essential Materia Medica for Toddlers & Young Children," in *Plant Healer Quarterly* Fall 2019, Vol. 9 Issue 4

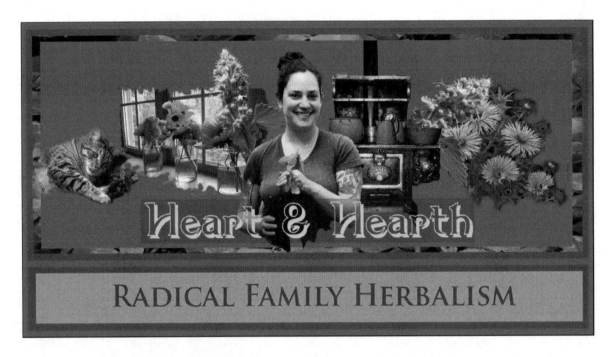

HERBS FOR THE POSTPARTUM YEAR:

The Nursing Parent's Toolkit

by Juliette Abigail Carr
Old Ways Herbal School of Plant Medicine

Home herbalism is who we are and how our families work, healing practiced around the kitchen table around the world and across the centuries. Thank the Good Green Earth that home herbalism happens as a reflex, intuition built on a foundation of herbal fluency that allows us to live as herbalists in every moment.

Childbirth and caring for a newborn are some of the most common inspirations for families to turn to herbs, but not enough attention is paid to the postpartum period itself. This year *Heart & Hearth* is focusing on creating useful toolkits to support a family throughout the postpartum year. This article presents my practice's most-used remedies related to nursing. Last time we talked about an herbal toolkit for birthing parents in the immediate postpartum period, and the next installment covers remedies to have on hand for newborns.

I find lactation to be completely magical. Nursing parents respond to subliminal messages from their baby to provide perfectly customized milk: pheromones, skin temperature, and germs on their skin all influence the makeup of our milk, from fat/sugar balance to immune cells. Newborns' breathing and blood sugar are stabilized by contact with our skin, and our skin temperature increases or decreases based on the temperature of our baby's skin. Milk is usually higher in sugar in the morning to be all rise-and-shiny, and higher in fat at night to promote longer sleep periods. There are twin studies where each twin is nursed exclusively on one side, and the milk produced on one side is completely different from what the other twin gets, based on their individual metabolic and immune needs. Come on, that's amazing!

280

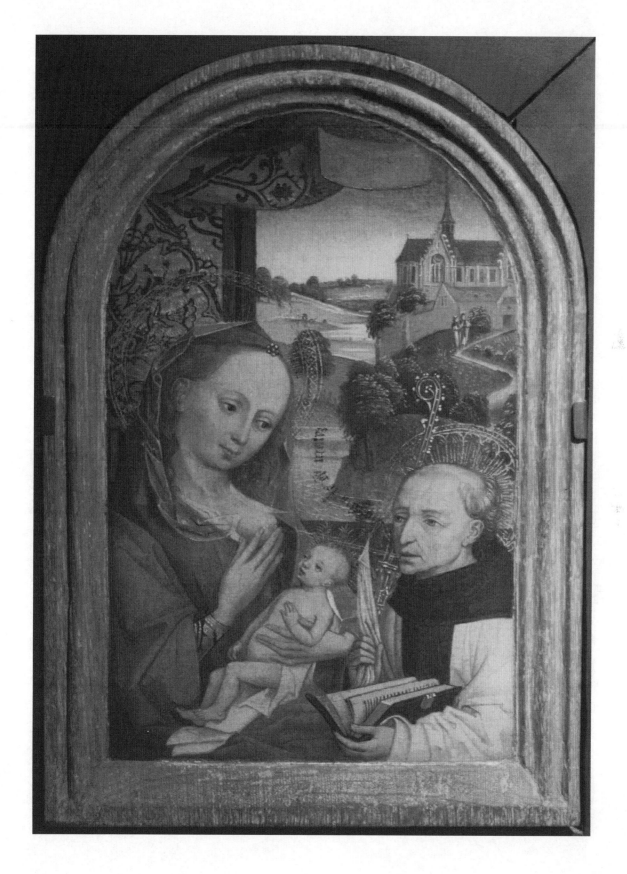

Lactation is a supply-and-demand operation run by feedback. If the breasts are completely empty, it signals to the body that more milk is needed, especially if sucking or pumping continues. If the breasts are a little engorged, it tells the body that too much milk was made last time, which down-regulates tomorrow's supply. For this reason, paying attention to breast emptying and engorgement is an important part of analyzing lactation on an ongoing basis.

It is also important to pay attention to the baby's behavior during and after nursing. A baby who appears calm and satisfied, falls asleep after nursing, fills diapers, and gains weight is getting plenty of milk. A baby who seems frustrated, angry, fussy at the breast, or otherwise uncomfortable should be checked out.

NORMAL-T(ea)

This is an easy-to-source tea base that covers the most common postpartum concerns, based on the widely used NORA tea. The ingredients are inexpensive and easy to find at the food co-op— and bulk herbs can even be bought with food stamps/SNAP benefits, making easy-to-source tea one of the most accessible ways to offer herbal medicine.

The name is an acronym: **N**ettles leaf, **O**atstraw, **R**aspberry leaf, **M**otherwort aboveground parts, **A**lfalfa, **L**emon balm aboveground parts, and **T**ulsi aboveground parts. The herbs in this formula are often thought of as allies for nursing and/or blood building, but they are much more than that.

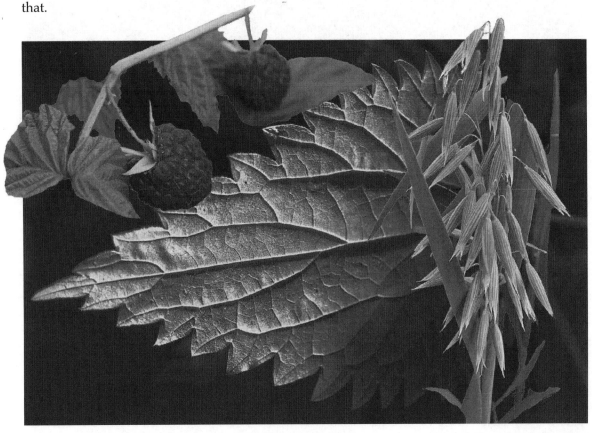

NORMAL-T is a mineral-rich anabolic trophorestorative that improves endocrine function, nervous system stability, red blood cell regeneration, and water/electrolyte balance. These actions promote appropriate physiological responses postpartum, engaging the parasympathetic nervous system to allow for cell and hormone generation, supporting lactogenesis II and ongoing milk supply, HPA-axis function, neurotransmission, establishment of appropriate postpartum circadian rhythm, healing of damaged tissues, uterine toning, and emotional coping in the face of significant hormone shifts and physical challenges, making it one of the single most useful interventions to help promote a healthy postpartum adjustment and prevent postpartum depression.

NORMAL-T is appropriate for almost everyone who nurses, unless one of the herbs is directly contraindicated or there is a drug interaction. Motherwort, Nettles, and Raspberry are gentle, replenishing, hormone-balancing galactagogues, rich in minerals. Gentle galactagogues are less likely to cause issues like oversupply, plugged ducts, mastitis, hormone surges, and dehydration than their stronger counterparts, and are gentle enough for daily use when nursing is going as expected. Tulsi is an adaptogen that supports lactation through emotional and physical calm, endocrine balance, and circadian rhythm regulation—which in turn help prevent postpartum depression. NORMAL-T is a daily tea for health maximization, but additional problem-focused herbs can be added to this base as appropriate; consider yarrow and lady's mantle tinctures following prolapse or hemorrhage, rose for birth trauma, etc.

Sore Nipples

Sore nipples are a huge deal in the first week or so of nursing. I actually don't use an herbal nipple cream/butter/salve because I've never found one that I thought worked as well as **lanolin**, which is cheap, plentiful, and natural, as well as fine for babies to ingest. If you have a nipple cream that you think is as good as or better than lanolin, I'd love to see it, please get in touch!

As well as lanolin, I really like refrigerated Aloe, although it is not appropriate for babies to eat. Cut an aloe leaf off and put it in the fridge, then put the goopy insides on a cotton nursing pad and wear it after nursing. Gently wash the nipple before nursing next time.

Too Little Milk

Insufficient milk supply is often wrongly blamed for nursing difficulties. It seems like a simple answer as to why a baby may be unsatisfied, losing weight, struggling with jaundice, or extra fussy—but it is rarely in fact the culprit (prior to about 3-4 months when the hormone drivers of lactation drop). This is made worse by a very aggressive marketing campaign run secretively by formula companies called "fed is best," which attempts to sow doubt in the minds of new parents about their own abilities to promote formula sales. "Fed is best" has been debunked and called out by the scientific community and every major maternal-child health organization, including the World Health Organization, as fear-based marketing propaganda and nothing more. If someone in your sphere starts in with statements like "there's just no way to tell if the baby is getting enough," they are probably the unwitting victims of this campaign (there are lots of ways to tell, see the beginning of this Plant Healer article).

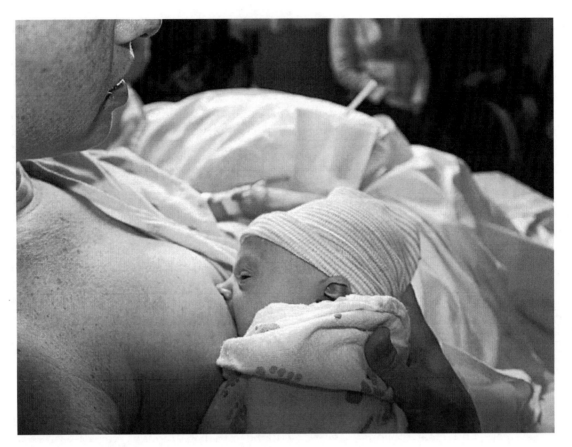

It is much more likely that a nursing problem is one of these, which are far more common than a flat-out inability to make enough milk:

• Shallow latch
• Disorganized suck/swallow (often related to prematurity or substance exposure)
• Anatomy of the infant's mouth, like tongue or lip ties
• Anatomy of the nipple or breast, like decreased glandular tissue or breast reduction surgery
• Parental dehydration, lack of nutrition, or lack of sleep
• Birth trauma to parent or child
• Reactivation of survivor trauma for the parent

Over-diagnosis of insufficient milk supply causes significant harm to the nursing couplet, in that helpful interventions are often bypassed—i.e. craniosacral therapy for newborn discomfort after a difficult birth, or EMDR for reactivation of past trauma in the parent—in favor of stimulating more and more milk to be produced. When milk is produced without being effectively removed from the milk ducts, problems arise that can have long-term impacts on the nursing couplet. Impacts of stimulating supply without ensuring adequate milk transfer include plugged ducts, mastitis, and down-regulation of supply, at which point the parent really might not make enough milk going forward. Continued ineffective nursing can lead to jaundice, serious newborn nutritional impacts, and significant emotional ramifications for the nursing parent—including an increase in the likelihood of postpartum depression and compounding birth trauma.

Refer to a lactation consultant before settling on milk supply as the root of the problem, to avoid compounding the issue. Also consider referring the baby to craniosacral therapy if there is an issue with the latch or birth trauma, and trauma-targeted therapies can be helpful for parents as appropriate.

If there's really a milk supply issue, a **galactagogue tincture** of Shatavari, Fennel, Fenugreek, Nettles, and Blessed Thistle is magical, taken 3-4 times per day in water or tea, ideally during or immediately after nursing if possible.

A **nervine-adaptogen formula** is also called for, as nursing difficulties are exhausting, stressful, and one of the most common precipitating factors of postpartum depression; a simple formula like Milky Oats, Lemon Balm, and Ashwagandha has a big impact. It's appropriate for the other parent to take nervines, also, and age-appropriate nervines may be helpful to older siblings (more about this in the previous installment in this column).

The nursing parent should drink 1-2 quarts per day of NORMAL-T and 1-2 quarts per day of water, for a total of 3-4 quarts of non-caffeinated, non-sugary hydration. The nursing parent absolutely must sleep, regardless of other obligations: I tell my clients that I'm "prescribing" nap time, since you just.can't.make.milk.if.you.don't.sleep. Period. This is a great opportunity for loved ones to step in to help out: instead of buying newborn clothes, they can make put the baby in a ring sling and vacuum the house while the parents sleep.

Protein, fat, iron, calcium, magnesium, vitamin C, vitamin D, water, and sleep are all essential for lactation. Nourishing, warming foods support both physical and emotional healing, and provide a strong foundation for cells; things like bone broth, clean meats, seaweed, fermented foods, nuts, leafy greens, eggs, fish, avocados, and sweet fruit are great choices.

That said, it is important to balance healthy food with comfort food: the warming stick-to-your-ribs nourishment of our families is an essential expression of love, and it's important for birthing families to feel nurtured by their larger family and community, especially if things are difficult. Try to work healthy ingredients into comfort foods and into every meal, to ensure adequate nutrition for lactation.

Manual breast massage immediately prior to nursing or pumping is very helpful to promote let-down for everyone who nurses. Pumping during waking hours is great to increase stimulation, especially when the issue is anatomical, but it must be balanced with sleep and self-care or it increases the likelihood of postpartum depression; sometimes clients report that they're pumping every two hours by alarm clock all night in addition to nursing. If that's not a recipe for a postpartum mood disorder, I don't know what is.

A clinical assessment of hormone balance and autoimmunity is warranted. If the birthing parent is found to have a condition that affects hormones of lactation or the development of glandular tissue, such as polycystic ovarian syndrome, supporting realistic goal-setting is an important intervention to help prevent postpartum depression.

Too Much Milk

At the other end of the spectrum of nursing discomforts is engorgement, oversupply, and plugged ducts. Engorgement happens to most people when their milk first comes in and can usually be managed well by nursing the baby, as well as cold packs to decrease swelling. If more help is needed, my favorite topical remedy is to take two leaves of green cabbage, ideally out of the fridge so they're very cold, and place one leaf inside each bra cup for 10 minutes. It works wonders on the swelling and feels fantastic, although you don't want to leave them on too long or you can overly down-regulate supply. Willow tincture is helpful if engorgement is painful, although it is slow to kick in, so take it before you need it.

Oversupply is also pretty common, especially with tongue-tied newborns—perhaps this is an attempt to compensate for decreased vacuum when sucking. Many people with oversupply simply pump once or twice a day and freeze the excess, but for some people oversupply is extreme enough to lead to plugged ducts and mastitis.

The cabbage leaf trick above is useful for oversupply. If it's done immediately following a feed, it will signal the body to down-regulate supply. Sage infused oil is very helpful as a gentle massage, avoiding the nipple and areola. Be sure not to massage firmly, as vigorous breast massage increases milk supply.

It can be helpful to pump to comfort so that the parent isn't in pain, without fully emptying the breast so that the supply will still be down-regulated by incomplete emptying of the breast. There are nursing techniques to decrease supply including block feeding and single-side feeding, which are appropriate to explore.

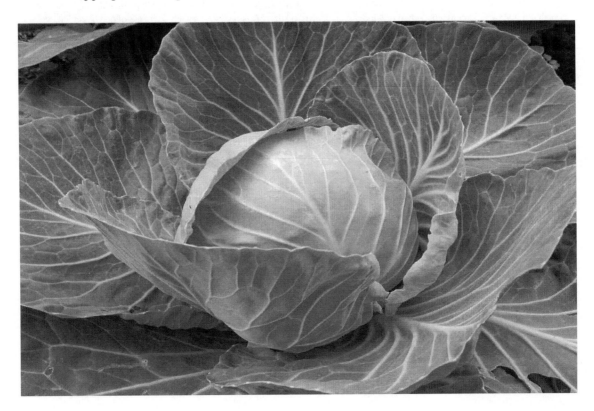

It can be helpful to pump to comfort so that the parent isn't in pain, without fully emptying the breast so that the supply will still be down-regulated by incomplete emptying of the breast. There are nursing techniques to decrease supply including block feeding and single-side feeding, which are appropriate to explore.

If a plugged duct does develop, apply a compress made from very hot red clover tea with salt immediately before nursing; I use a newborn cloth diaper, as they're the perfect size and very absorbent. Compress the sore spot during nursing, and apply sage oil as described above following the feed. It is also a good idea to take garlic, elderberry, and echinacea tincture internally to stave off mastitis, since a plugged duct can quickly progress to mastitis. Avoid echinacea products containing goldenseal, as they are unsafe for the newborn liver (…and goldenseal is endangered, so please stop using it unless you're cultivating it yourself—Japanese barberry works just as well and is an aggressive invasive in goldenseal's biome). Be sure to keep nursing on the affected side.

A Word on Referrals

Whether it's your lactation experience, a friend or loved one's, or even a client, it is important to request the help you need: refer early and often. Childbirth and child-rearing is weird in that everyone thinks they're an expert, and they want to lecture you about how you could do it better from their vast experience as a parent. of two, or whatever. It's a manifestation of patriarchy: no one would walk up to a strange man in line at the grocery store, put their hands on his belly, and lecture him—and then be deeply offended if he politely asks them not to touch him, or refuses their advice about epidurals/discipline/whatever. Can you imagine?

So yes, everyone's an expert and they're all up in your armpits and most of them have no idea what they're talking about. Let us take each other's experiences with a grain of salt, recognizing that they were true for someone and they might be helpful for us, or not—and let us ask for help from people who do in fact know what they're doing, early and often. It is so easy for things to be missed if you don't know what to look for, which can cause problems later—things like tongue ties and oversupply, which may not seem like a big deal when the parent's body is compensating, until the hormone drivers of lactation drop off around 3 or 4 months and suddenly the milk supply is gone because it's just demand-based and the baby's mouth can't form a good vacuum. It's always better to have too many people checking in than too few; community connectedness is a primary prevention again postpartum depression.

Not to say that nursing isn't the most normal, natural thing in the world, or that we aren't equipped to care for each other as a community without professional intervention at every turn, but that it's okay for us to acknowledge our limits as support people and professionals. When my oldest was a newborn and I struggled with getting a deep latch due to oversupply, a colleague of my midwife got frustrated and instructed me to just wait the baby out, that eventually she would get hungry enough to latch on her own. This is hands-down the worst nursing advice I have ever heard from a professional. Luckily I knew it was bad advice, but how many people wouldn't have known enough to question it, leading inevitably to worsening engorgement and all its attendant problems—continued inability to latch, plugged ducts, mastitis, decreased supply, etc. I advocated for myself by requesting lactation support elsewhere, but a referral would have been a good idea for her to offer when she hit the limit of her knowledge.

Preparing for nursing before the baby is born is a sensible choice for childbearing families. Providing pre-made herbal formulas for the most common nursing complaints is an act of loving compassion for our community members as they go through the childbearing transformation. It is a thoughtful, useful gift, but more importantly it sends the nonverbal message that we see them and understand what they're going through, both positive and negative. Lactation support is a great opportunity to surround a family with love: checking in regularly is one of the best measures against postpartum depression, which affects 1 in 4 families. Empathetic connection is one of the single most powerful gifts we can give each other in this era of isolation: the more connected we each are, the stronger we all are.

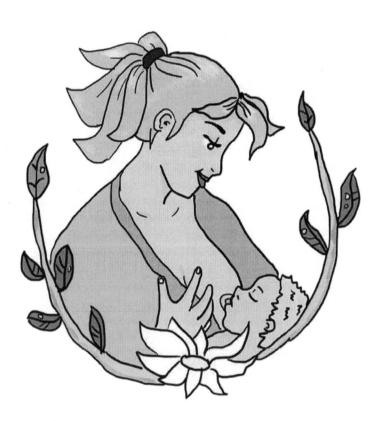

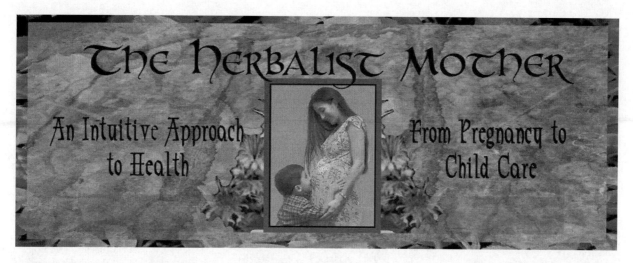

THE HERBALIST MOTHER

An Intuitive Approach to Health

From Pregnancy to Child Care

When a baby emerges from the womb, he is primed for living on the earth. Squeezed and pushed by the woman's body, fluid is expelled from his lungs. Beneficial microbes gifted from his mother, colonize his body. When he takes his first suckle from the breast his body is nourished and his immune system stimulated by the golden liquid colostrum. It is an amazing orchestra of events that happen between mother and infant to facilitate his life and functioning.

 When we step back and realize that most, if not all of the processes that occur in birth are for very specific reasons, the less we wish to interfere. And so it was when my son was born. In my initial imaginings, while pregnant, I saw myself using all sorts of herbal concoctions with him, only to give birth to him, seeing first hand just how amazing the mother and child dyad work together, I found that simple really can be more.

It's a powerful thing to use beautiful, tried and true remedies in a very simple way. It's also very empowering to use these remedies knowing that there is a very subtle shift that happens and they do not overpower the mother's own mechanisms of protection and healing offered to her infant. No strong scents, subtle nudges of healing, gentleness are what these herbs can offer. I laugh at myself now, because I narrowed my healer's basket to these very few plants in that first year, especially when I

Mother's Healing Basket:
1st Year

by Sabrina Lutes

think of the sheer number of remedies I had dreamed up. When I talk to mothers and clients now, I continue to feel that these plants are precious to me for use with little babies. They made many of my son's transitions much easier, as well as my transition as a mother. My hope is to introduce you to some different ways to use herbals for that first year and of course beyond.

There is no right or wrong way to approach this, as long as the herbs are safe to use with babies, pick ways to use them that feel good to you. These were my tried and true plants, ones that I would return to over and over again. These became my plant allies in mothering. Their energy worked well with my son and almost all ills and discomforts were eased by them. As you work with each of the herbs, and I suggest, like many wise mentors before me, to pick one herb at a time to work with, that your basket will grow to match the needs of your family.

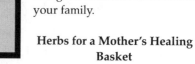

Herbs for a Mother's Healing Basket

German Chamomile (*Matricaria recutita*)
 Uses: soothing and calming to nervous system, fever reducing, stomach discomfort and gas, teething pain
My method of preparation: dried whole blossoms, tincture, infused oil, strong tea in ice cube trays in the freezer

289

Catnip (*Nepeta cataria*)
Uses: fevers, fussiness, teething pain
My method of preparation: dried herb, tincture, strong tea in ice cube trays in freezer

Elderberry (*Sambucus canadensis*, my native Florida plant but they grow all over so with proper ID you probably have your own native Elder growing near you)
Uses: viral infections; infusions, syrup, elixir for mom to take while nursing for babies not yet taking solids, added to other less pleasant tasting herbs for popsicles etc.
My methods of preparation: dried berries, frozen berries, syrup, elixir, infusion frozen in ice cube trays

Linden (*Tillia spp*)
dried herb
Uses: fevers, colds, fussiness
My method of preparation: infusions, and infusions frozen in ice trays

Lavender (*Lavandula spp*)
Uses: over-tiredness, fussiness, transitions, skin irritations, diaper rash
My method of preparation: dried buds, infused oil, buds in a muslin sachet, strong infusion poured into baths, tea

Rose(*Rosa damascene and spp*)
Uses: skin infections and wounds, massage, herbal baths for relaxation
My method of preparation: strong infusions in baths, stuffed into muslin bags, infused in oil

Olive oil or other suitable oil (grapeseed, jojoba)
Uses: massage, skin dryness or irritation (not Staph type infections since it may seal in infection)
Method of preparation: kept plain, or herbs infused into it

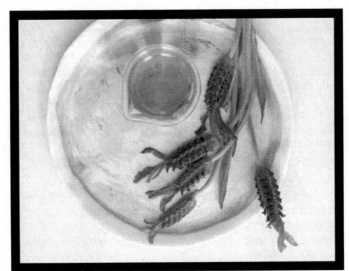

Bentonite clay (internal use quality)
Uses: dry powder to dust skin for diaper rash, wet (plain water or mixed with an herbal infusion such as chamomile, lavender or rose) for diaper rash spots, bug bites
My method of preparation: dry, mixed with a little lavender or chamomile infusion

Herbal Therapeutics

Teething:

Oh teething! I remember feeling like this was some mysterious thing that happened to babies. All of us first time mothers talked about it, we knew it was going to happen, just not exactly when or how. Every little crankiness or fussiness, little fevers, or runny noses all got blamed on teething. Normally after the fact, our child would seem off for a few days and then, a tooth would appear, and we all would sigh and say, he/she was just teething! Phew! I tried all the remedies, sometimes they didn't work, sometimes they would all work. Oh, I was just mesmerized by it (and a little exasperated by it). My little one's favorite remedy for this was when I would crush up herbal infused ice cubes and tie them in a muslin cloth (leave a long tail, and watch your baby so that they don't end up trying to swallow the cloth). It was like an herbal Popsicle! Chamomile and catnip for the pain and fussiness, elderberry and linden if I thought there may have been a virus involved, lavender for over tiredness or lack of sleep from sore gums.

Sleep/Relaxation

My son's first direct tactile experience of herbs was with lavender. At about 3 weeks of age, I filled his bath with beautiful blue water, colored by the flower buds of lavender. I remember my mother sense coming alive and I felt so happy being able to bathe my baby in this lovely floral water. It was a simple, sweet ritual we continued that first year. I'd fill a cloth bag with the buds and allow the warm water to run over it as I gently squeezed. The scent and color helped to calm my mood and relax my babe.

Massage with herbal infused oils is a lovely way to relax both yourself and baby. When we offer loving touch to our children, it boosts their immune function, decreases perception of pain and increases their parasympathetic nervous system response (the opposite of fight or flight), it is also a powerful bonding tool and has many more benefits. Lavender, rose and chamomile infused oils are wonderful to use on your baby's sweet skin. I always suggest waiting a few months before introducing any massage oil with a scent, even if it is just infused oil. Unlike a bath, where the scent is momentary, the oil stays on and little bitty babes are still learning their mother's sweet smell. I don't like interfering with that. Unless there is a specific reason, as in treating a skin issue and the herb's healing properties are needed.

Diaper Rash

Diaper rashes can have many different causes. Chemical sensitivity (detergents in wash if your using cloth diapers, if you use disposables there are chemicals in the diaper from scents to gel fluid absorbers and other things), irritation from friction

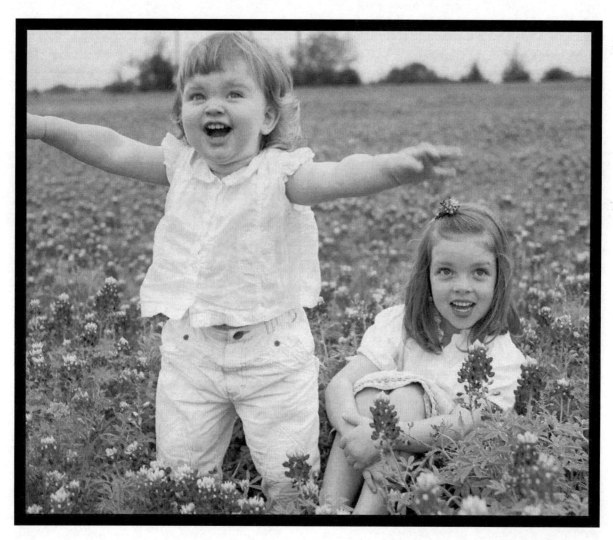

which can lead to secondary issues of bacteria and yeast if not caught. For the most part my little one was diaper less, and we rinsed him in plain water. Yet, sometimes he managed to get a diaper rash. I treated it with bentonite clay, either sprinkled on or mixed with a little infusion (lavender, chamomile, linden) and placed directly on the sores. It's always a good idea to know what type of rash you are dealing with, since that changes the treatment. If you have tried simple home remedies and it is getting worse, or not improving, I encourage you to check in with a midwife or doctor for a diagnosis. Once you know what's causing it, you can tailor your treatment better. If I felt my son's bottom was a little infected, I'd soak him in rose and lavender infusion every chance I got and allowed his bottom plenty of sunshine. This worked well for us. Yet some babies may get more severe rashes and you may need different herbs than what is covered in this article.

Easing Transitions

Another wonderful use of herbs I discovered in my mothering was for car rides! My son hated the car. Needless to say, I didn't get out much that first year! Yet there were days when I needed to leave the house or just not have a gut wrenching scream fest while we drove to our destination. Desperate to find help, and not finding answers that fit within the parameters in which I wished to raise my little guy, I stuffed a muslin bag with every soothing herb I had on hand! Lavender buds, chamomile flowers, cardamom pods (why the hell not? They smelled really lovely), vanilla. I laid it next to his nose while he was placed in his car seat, rubbed a little Bach's rescue remedy on his toes, and low and behold quiet! He even slept. This didn't work every time mind you, but it got us through some really tough moments. I continued to use these little muslin bags, filled with herbs, tucked in my bags for travel, under our pillows and in the car, just to help ease our day to day transitions.

Fevers and Illness

Once you have ruled out any serious causes of fever, it's best to support the baby in clearing the infection and getting well. I loved giving my baby warm baths in chamomile infusion for this. When he was old enough to eat I offered sips of linden infusion, chamomile, catnip and elderberry. I would either pull some ice cubes out of the freezer or allow him to suck on them (using the same method for teething and tying them in cloth), I would gently warm the ice cubes on the stove, or I would create a fresh batch of infusion. Most of these herbs children will love. All these herbs have antimicrobial, antiviral, and fever reducing qualities. I found that for my son, mixing them up throughout the day helped with compliance. I would also continue the herbs for as long as I remembered to after the illness was on its way out. This way the immune system continues to be supported. And, of course your own breast milk is full of beneficial help for your sick child. Nurse them for as long as you are willing. Older babies and children still benefit from your nourishment particularly when sick.

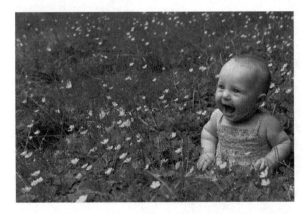

As a new mother, I really enjoyed assembling a beautiful basket of healing remedies for my child. Those that needed to be frozen, I kept in a special place in the freezer. I loved carefully labeling the bottles and decorating them with images that made me think of my son's special energy. This made the medicine more powerful in my mind. My love and intention for my little boy went into the contents as well as my love of the Earth and the plants for the healing they provided. I suggest you try this while assembling your own Mother's Healing basket. I treasure an old, empty tincture bottle I have recently found with my son's name on it, labeled Respiratory blend. The label was tattered and stained, because of frequent refills as the tincture was used up. That was a tough illness, yet instead of feeling sadness in seeing that bottle, I felt much empowered by it.

Some things to think about when working with very young babies:

•Fevers in babies 3 months or younger should always be taken seriously and let a skilled practitioner or pediatrician take a look.
•Fevers in babies 4 months to a year, best to get counsel from a pediatrician.
•It's good to ally yourself with a pediatrician that is aware of natural and herbal remedies or at least into working with you in using them.
•When a baby is very new, the first 6 weeks or so, I typically treat through the mother. Infusions and tinctures get through the breast milk in very small amounts, thus helping the baby in that regard. You could also bathe the baby in a strong herbal infusion.
•If you are going to use something on a baby's skin, even though it's natural, always test first! It's better to deal with a small amount of irritation, than an all-over contact dermatitis.
•Do your own research in a few different sources. Make sure that you can cross reference the information. This will help you, not only in herbal healing but in other matters of medicine as well.

Know whether an herb you wish to use has been used for many generations on infants. Even things written by so called experts can have in correct information. Trust your gut and listen to your baby. My little guy was very helpful in helping me figure out what he needed.

References:

Infant massage benefits: http://www.infantmassageusa.org/learn-to-massage-your-baby/benefits-of-infant-massage/
Diaper rash: http://www.askdrsears.com/topics/skin-care/diaper-rash
Fevers in babies: http://www.parenting.com/health-guide/fever/when-call-doctor
Books:
Naturally Healthy Babies and Children, Aviva Romm

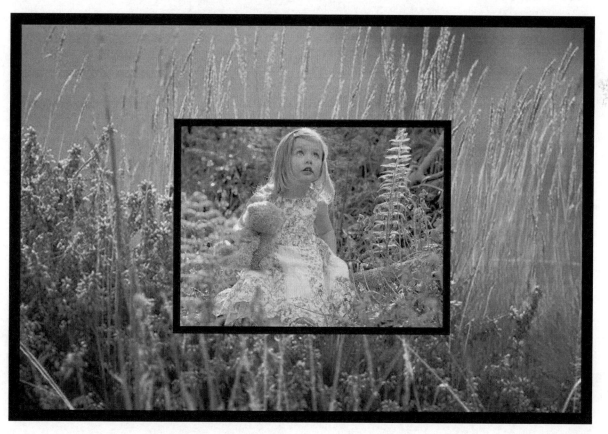

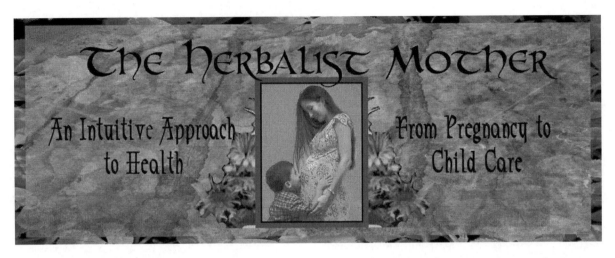

THE HERBALIST MOTHER

An Intuitive Approach to Health

From Pregnancy to Child Care

You've held your baby close, kept him warm and safe within your arms. Now is his time to begin pulling away and exploring more than what's just within your (or their caregiver's) arm's reach. He will begin walking and running, eating a variety of different foods, fully engaging with the environment

A Mother's Healing Basket:
Beyond the First Year

By Sabrina Lutes

around him. He will get bumped and bruised, cut and scraped, and deal with more and more organisms for his immune system to sort out. It's certainly time for your basket to have more herbs for these occurrences! In Part 1 of this article we discussed some gentle herbs for the first year of a child's life. Continue to use what has worked for you and learn the gifts of those plants, and just like your child is broadening their exploration of the world, you can broaden your exploration of the plants and their help in bringing health to your family.

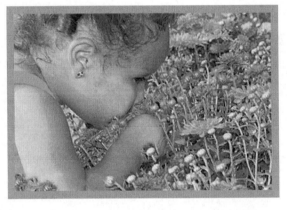

As my son began his journey into the bigger world, I decided that I needed a few more things to aid that journey. He also knows these herbs well, now that he is older, and asks for them when they are needed. I suggest allowing these older children to help you prepare your herbal remedies. . Much like you would bake cookies with them! They will delight in the colors and smells and learn this beautiful

healing art that you are passing down to them. You can also take your children into the woods with you or plant a garden. Many of these plants are found growing wild around you, most are easy to grow in your own garden or in pots. Teach them the Latin names of the plants as well as the common names. I find that this keeps them fresh in my mind and allows my son to know the importance of a universal language for safety's sake and for keeping the knowledge alive.

Herbs:

Hibiscus *Hibiscus sabdariffa* (dried petals): cooling, high in vitamin C
Uses: fevers, hydration

My method of preparation: popsicles, herbal jello, infusions (hot and cold)

Ginger root *Zingiber officinalis* (dried and fresh): warming
Uses: colds and flu, warming the body, easing muscle aches, belly aches
My method of preparation: tea, infusion poured into bath, infused oil

Thyme *Thymus vulgaris*: antimicrobial

Uses: colds and flus, congestion, cuts and scrapes

My method of preparation: Tincture, infusion

Plantain *Plantago lanceolata, Plantago major* (fresh leaf): cooling, antiinflammatory

Uses: Bruises, wounds, bug bites

My method of preparation: fresh plant poultice, infusion, tincture

Spearmint *Mentha spicata* (dried and fresh): muscle aches, cooling

Uses: growing pains, flavoring

My method of preparation: infused oil, added to water based infusions for flavoring.

Cinnamon (powder): warming, antimicrobial

Uses: colds and flu, fevers, sore throat, warming a chilled body

My method of preparation: mixed in honey, sprinkled in warmed milk and over toast

Honey (raw, unfiltered): (please only give internally to babies older than 1 year) antimicrobial

Uses: wounds, sore throat

My method of preparation: placed directly on wound, taken by spoon, mixed with herbs

Nettles (*Urtica dioica*): mineral rich, antihistamine
Uses: a nutritional boost

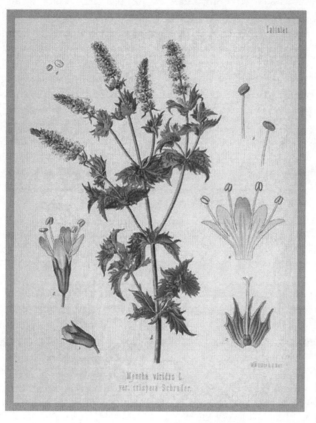

Mentha viridis L.
var. crispata Schrader.

My method of preparation: freshly cooked (must be cooked because of the stinging hairs) in soups or as a steamed green, infusion

Growing pains: These are heart wrenching in our house. Waking us in the middle of the night, being begged to be rubbed and warmed. We keep a special bottle of oil just for this purpose. My son is comforted by its smell and calls it his growing pain oil. In the case of growing pains, and my own research, if your child is waking up with severe pain, please have someone take a look and be sure more is not going on. Once we felt confident that we were dealing with stretching muscles and grumbly tendons we offer love and support and lots of massage until my little one falls back to sleep. You can rub oil into the sore places being sure to cover the whole area. Squeezing and kneading the muscle and gently pressing into the stiffer tendons. After I have massaged his legs, sometimes my son will fall asleep, or he will ask for a warm bath or a hot water bottle. You can tuck the water bottle into a towel and wrap the body part in that. Hot flax socks are great for this as well (just be sure they are evenly heated, as the oils in the seeds can get extremely hot in some places, and may burn the skin). To these socks you can add soothing herbs like lavender (*Lavandula spp*), chamomile(*Matricaria recutita)*, or spearmint.

Cuts/Scrapes: I love using thyme and plantain infusion to rinse the wound. I also keep raw, unfiltered honey to place on my son's wounds. It helps ease pain and keeps it from getting infected and also keeps the bandage from sticking. For surface scrapes I use a thin layer of honey and as the wound heals and begins to scab over and itch I put a salve made of plantain and lavender onto it. These are for minor wounds. It is not within the scope of this article to discuss issues of vaccination for tetanus, please use your good judgment and discuss with a knowledgeable care provider any injury that may be at risk for tetanus.

Bug Bites: plantain poultice and infusions, as well as infused oils. Nettle infusion to help ease the histamine response. If you know your kid is prone to itchy, irritated bug bites allow them ample nettle infusion throughout bug season.

Illness (self-limiting viruses): I like to treat these at the first sign. That way I feel the illness can be shortened or at least kept from getting too extreme or drawn out. If I notice those glazed eyes, cranky and tender moods then off to a hot bath my little guy goes. I give him thyme tincture mixed with honey, about a dropperful every hour. Then into a warm bed for snuggles and quiet time. I also try to get him to eat lots of nutrient dense foods. Kale and salmon are our favorites, and I mix the kale cooking water with a bone broth for a beverage. This

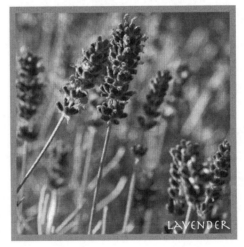
LAVENDER

way he gets lots of healthy food into his system so that when he does lose his appetite, I can feel comfortable with him listening to his body and eating sparingly. I also make popsicles, herbal jello or a warm tea of elderberry, depending on his symptoms. If it's a cold cold (chills, pallor) then a warm tea, if he's flushed and hot with a sore throat I'll allow him a popsicle or jello. I'll also use elderberry syrup, a teaspoon every hour. Ginger is also useful for colds that are cold in nature. I'll pour some infusion into a bath or add a small amount to a tea. Go easy though, since children are more sensitive to ginger's spiciness. I also love cinnamon for warming my son's body on chilled days and sprinkle it into milk, on toast or yogurt and infuse it into teas.

Sometimes it's hard to get remedies into kids (another reason I like to catch it early, when my son is more willing to cooperate with his mama). If they won't take something, don't force it. In those moments I just meditate on the strength of my child and his ability to get through this illness on his own terms. This seems more healthy and whole to me than forcing remedies down his throat. Go with your gut on this. In my household we have only dealt with self-limiting issues. I always take a watchful wait stance on my child's illnesses if I ever feel things are serious, I wouldn't hesitate to see our pediatrician. This is a great link to visit to help you decide if you need medical help for your child's illness: http://www.virtualpediatrichospital.org/patients/cqqa/callthedoctor.shtml. It's always a good idea to have a practitioner you know and who knows your child in case you have any questions.

Crankiness, Tantrums, & Moodiness: Here's the thing. I'm no expert on this and just when I think I have it figured out, my son throws a curve ball or I'm having a rough go of things and my son mirrors it right back. This is when your ability to love what is becomes so important. Go easy on yourself and your child. It also helps to remember that they have only been on this planet a short while. If adults haven't figured it out, why do we expect children to have done so? I do feel strongly that herbs can help either acutely, when feelings are strong and angry, or they can help soothe hurt and frazzled nerves. If things feel a bit out of control or out of the ordinary, look at diet. This is another area where I drag out the nutritional heavy hitters. I give my boy lots of deep green vegetables, cut out sugars except low sugar fruits, and am sure he is well hydrated. I love switching water for high mineral infusions like nettles and hibiscus. If things need some soothing energy, I love to use linden (Tillia spp) infusion. These are home days, where we pull our energy in and focus on loving each other and decreasing demands. These are the times to take your child in close and use the things that helped soothe them as tiny babies (refer to my previous article on easing transitions). Warm baths with chamomile and lavender infusions are so sweet and lovely for both you and your little one. Before bed, make warm milk (any milk will do) infused with honey and lavender or chamomile buds.

Recipes:

Herbal Jello:
4 packages of gelatin, I use Knox but there is a grass-fed brand, Great Lakes, you could try.
1 cup cold herbal infusion
3 cups of hot herbal infusion
Honey to taste

Sprinkle gelatin over cold infusion, stir this mixture into hot infusion allowing gelatin to dissolve. Add honey to taste, pour into mold, allow to set in the refrigerator. Cut into cubes. (herbs for this are Hibiscus, elderberry, linden or any other combination you like that tastes good)

Herbal Milk:
½ Cup of milk (whatever your child drinks)
1 teaspoon of lavender buds, chamomile buds or a combination of both.
1 teaspoon of honey

Brink milk to steaming (NOT boiling), I use this time to think about my relationship with my boy. When you see steam just beginning to rise, pour the milk into a favorite mug, stir in the herbs and honey and let steep a few minutes. I use one of those strainer balls for tea. I do this ritualistically. I use the same mug, do it in the same order. I feel that it allows me to come to a place of calm and centeredness before giving it to my child. It makes the medicine strong.

I'm Growing Oil Rub:
Oil of your choice (we love grapeseed, jojoba, and olive oils for oil infusions)
½ part Spearmint Leaf (dried)
1 part Sassafrass root(dried)
1 part White willow bark (dried)

Place the herbs into a crockpot that allows a "keep warm" setting, pour in oil until herbs are just covered and turn the crock pot on warm. I keep an eye on it until things are warm but not hot, like warm bath water. Allow to steep a few hours, turning crock on and off to keep temperature just right. Strain your herbs into jar and use as needed. You can add a few drops of essential oils that your child finds pleasing.

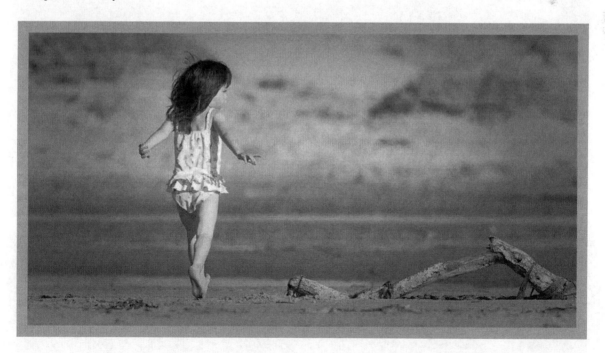

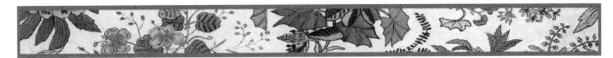

ASSESSING & TREATING THE YOUNG

Using Herbs & Other Natural Healing Modalities

by Briana Wiles (with Holly Torgerson)

As parents we want to do everything right for our children, so when they are sick we want them to get the best care possible. Sometimes that involves going to the doctor, but usually it's staying home and doing simple remedies that support the healing process. It's helpful to know what things we can do to make our children feel better and to have a good framework for knowing when it is perfectly ok to treat an illness at home. Most childhood illnesses will resolve on their own with a little love, at the same time the accompaniment of herbs or alternative practices can really help ease the discomforts of sickness. In the instances where an ailment seems to need the advice or help of a doctor, please do not hesitate to do so. Here we will address some of the most common childhood complaints and give you tools to assess when you need to stay home and rest and when you need outside help. Children catch many viruses and infections during the first 5 years of life, making this a valuable place to begin and focus on. From earaches, to coughs, fevers, vomiting and more, discover some useful tips and tricks from experienced mom herbalists.

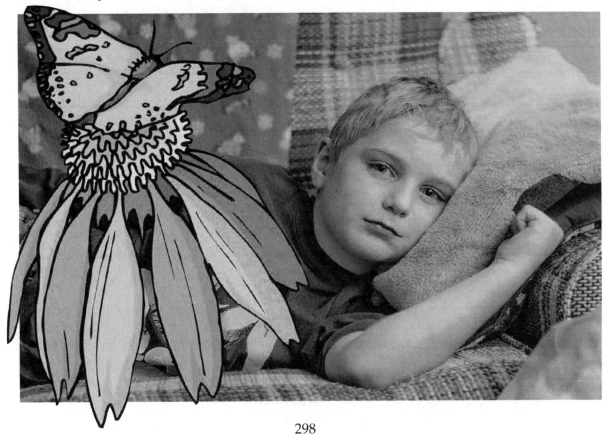

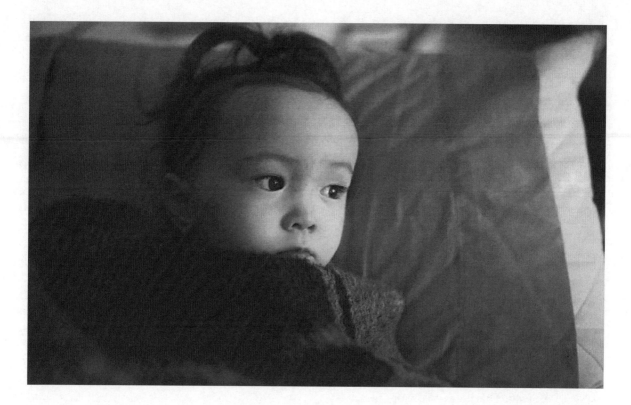

The joy of infants and children is that they are learning about the world in every single thing that they do. This is doubly true for the immune system. The immune system is constantly learning about the world and how to react appropriately. Early childhood is the window where the immune system learns the ropes. For better or for worse, this is the reason that so many vaccines are clustered in the early years. There are so many viruses out there that we are constantly exposed to, so it's no surprise that small children always seem to be sporting a runny nose. That's just the reality of the immune system contending with innumerable viruses for the first time. Fever, mucus, and cough are all important ways the immune system protects and defends the body so they should be encouraged within reason. Secretions are the first line of protection for the body. Then comes the immune response with fever. For the most part kids just roll with it but some kids really feel it. Sometimes you see a child with a 102°F fever who is still happily playing and is not apparently sick. Some kids run hot. Some kids are miserable with the slightest elevation of temperature. This is why it's important to watch the child and not the thermometer. Check in and do a full assessment. Many people run to urgent care or to their pediatrician at any hint of fever. I see them post on social media and if their co-pays are what my co-pays are they are spending hundreds of dollars a year on fever panic. It's really not necessary to know exactly what a child is fighting and how to help treat it.

Children are unreliable in telling you what is going on with their bodies and pediatricians tend to err on the side of caution with treatment. But I want to tell you that you know you child. *You know your child*. Full stop. If you feel like something is wrong then you know. If you feel scared, honor that feeling. Be honest with yourself. Going to the doctor for their opinion doesn't lock you into a treatment modality, but it can give you valuable information you do not have. Your pediatrician is intimately aware of the illnesses circulating in your community and they have information more valuable than a google search. At the same time a pediatrician's office is a hotbed of disease so avoiding it when a child has a mild illness can help prevent bringing something more unpleasant home.

Physical assessment is an important part of caring for children. Infants are unable to tell us what is wrong so they cry and may be very upset. As they get older they will point and fuss, hold their ears or heads, scratch their skin, or hold their tummies. A 3-5 year old will start telling you verbally what's bothering them. Because children's bodies aren't yet mature, they're susceptible to diseases affecting their lungs, immune system and digestive system.

- Temperature is the primary at home assessment people are comfortable performing. In babies any temperature over 102°F is cause for concern, but older children can reach higher temperatures up to 104°F so long as they don't have any other concerning symptoms and it is not sustained. 5 days is usually the cutoff for a sustained fever.
- Skin and lymph. Look for rashes, color changes, bruising, lumps. Viral illness often produces a rash on the skin so it is wise to regularly look at the skin when an infant or toddler is beginning to act sick or uncharacteristically fussy. You may see small red bumps show up on the trunk, red flushing on the cheeks, small fluid filled blisters on the palms of the hands or feet, blisters or sores in the mouth or on the tongue. You might have a child that is fussy for a few days and then is better but you find a sore in their mouth characteristic of hand foot and mouth disease. You might never know they were sick or potentially contagious if you didn't look in their mouth. Also check the eyes for redness. The lymph nodes might become swollen or sore. Feel the neck and armpits. Some kids hold their armpits when they are sick.
- You can look for signs of dehydration by noticing wet diapers or trips to the bathroom, lack of tears, in infants you can feel the fontanel to see if feels sunken in (bulging is another issue), or press the nails to see how quickly they pink back up.
- Bowels. Diarrhea or constipation.
- Look in the ears for redness or signs of drainage or rupture. Ear pulling and crying or pain when lying down.
- Lung sounds. Listen for wheezing or gasping. Croup sounds like a barking seal and the cough is quieted by cold air or steam. If you see the child's rib cage or the area above the breastbone sucking in when they breathe, then they are struggling to get enough air. It could be severe croup or pneumonia. Doubly concerning is if the lips or fingers have a bluish tinge.
- Respiratory rate. Observe for a minute. Infants have periodic breathing so observe for longer than than a few seconds.
- Heart rate. In acute illness the heart rate can be rapid especially if there is fever.
- Tension or laxity. Tone of the body. Both flaccidity and rigidity are signs that something is not right.
- The tongue can also give you information. A white coated tongue shows mucus and dampness. A healthy kid tongue have a very light to minimal coat, a healthy pink color that isn't red, smooth with few to no bumps *papillae*. Redness, bumps, and yellowness point to heat and to something irritating the body and immune system. A white coated tongue that then peels (strawberry tongue) is a sign of strep scarlet fever and is a red flag symptom.
- Mood is another big thing to pay attention to. A child who has a mild illness will definitely feel sick, but it's concerning when they are downright miserable, don't want to play, listen to stories, or watch a movie. They might be in too much pain or discomfort, might be too dehydrated to focus, or lethargic to do anything and this is concerning. Dehydration is far too common an issue. It makes it much harder for the body to respond to an illness and it can put major stress on the internal organs like the kidneys. This past flu season saw a lot of complications, many of which might have been prevented by proper hydration. Not just water, but electrolytes too. Recovery takes longer too if electrolytes are off.

I am sure this all sounds like a lot. Having a sick kid can be nerve wracking, but being able to confidently assess the situation goes a long way to calming some of the panic that goes with it.

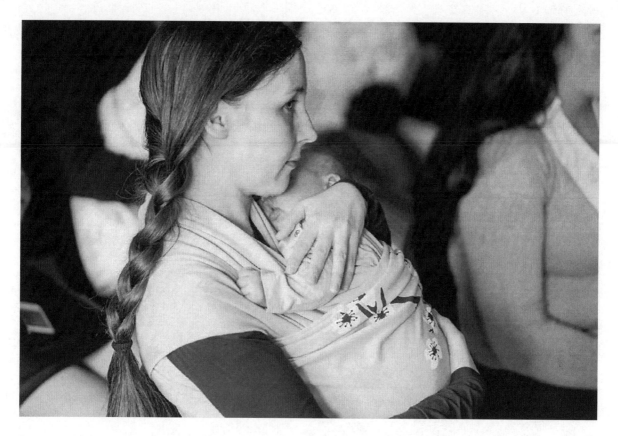

Just a quick note on vaccines, whether you do or don't, there is a big misconception that bothers me. When you have immunity to a disease it doesn't mean you have a magical shield where a virus just bounces off you. If you have immunity and are exposed you will actually be infected but have an effective immune response that shuts it down. You can still spread disease. So be mindful of this as there are a lot of people out there who might be susceptible.

Herbal allies can be formed at young ages with the proper guidance and administration. With proper selection you can help your child grow to love herbs just as much as you do. But, you can also turn your child off to herbs even quicker with the wrong taste, feel, reaction, or preparation. The consistency and application of homemade remedies is really important for the compliance of our little ones. Ways to make topical oils, teas, steams, soaks, tinctures, glycerin, alcohol, honey, vinegar, poultices and infused honey's will be shared.

It is extremely beneficial to know the energetics of the herbs your are using, especially with children, who are much more sensitive to what we put in them, on them, and around them. For this reason essential oils can both be useful, and harmful. Young infants should not be exposed to the strong principles and dilutions of essential oils. Especially really strong essential oils such as, eucalyptus, and camphor. Even using small amounts in oil blends or in diffusers can cause problems if the infant is highly sensitive or exposed to this during long periods of time. Energetics of herbs are the way herbs interact with us, which is different for each of us depending on constitution and temperament. Every herb has its own array of uses, therapeutics and energetic offerings, such as being aromatic, diaphoretic, demulcent, nervine, lymphatic, alterative, decongestant, anti-microbial, and so forth. Becoming familiar with which herbs are drying, warming, cooling or moistening is important in gauging which herb to use for your little one. For example, colds can be exacerbated by the use of too dry an herb, leaving the mucus membranes feeling dry and worse than better. Kids and babies are mucousy, and the demulcent love of marshmallow tea will never go unappreciated.

301

Finding and choosing alternative practitioners to take your children to can be overwhelming and hard, although sometimes it is an easy referral from the community of parents. Get acquainted with what is offered in your area with naturopathy, herbalism, osteopathy, bodyworkers, chiropractic, and energy work. Things like recurring ear aches should be checked out by someone who manipulates bones or soft tissue, such as a chiropractor or osteopath, before administering dose after dose of antibiotics or resorting to tubes.

Little people can turn the world upside down when unhappy and ill. Make sure to stay alert and read your child's behavior first and foremost when observing a sick kid. Never hesitate to seek medical attention, especially when symptoms are progressively getting worse. Herbs and alternative medicine have a lot to offer, but do not negate the fact that modern medicine can also serve our health and safety.

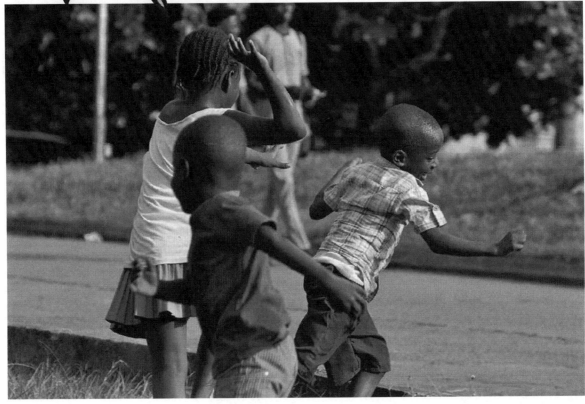

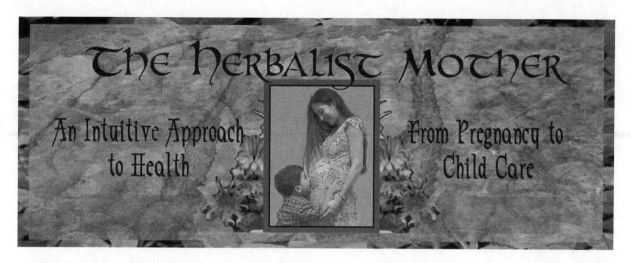

THE HERBALIST MOTHER

An Intuitive Approach to Health · From Pregnancy to Child Care

I began my journey with herbal medicine at the same time that I began my journey of motherhood. Birthwork come closely on the heels of parenting and herbal work. I gratefully remember every tidbit of information specific to treating babies and children that I learned from my early teachers of herbalism and for the writings of herbalist like Aviva Romm and Anne McIntyre

Working With Children & Herbs:

Approaches, Diagnostics, Therapeutics, & Materia Medica

by Erin Poirier

who wrote fine books on these topics. When I began expanding my herbalism outside of the small circle of my family and close friends, the first class I taught was Herbs for Children's Health, a class I still offer periodically. Like most herbalists I know, who make a living practicing herbalism, I was trained and practice as a generalist. I will see just about anyone and am

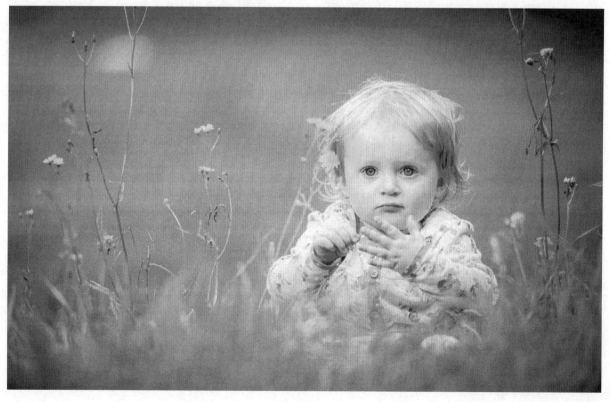

willing to talk about just about any problem, but as a homebirth midwife and traditional Western Herbalist I have carved out a little niche for myself working with babies and children and teaching parents, herbal students and other practitioners about the unique health needs of babies and children and how to use herbs for and with them. I estimate that about one-quarter of my clients are little ones and in this article I will share with you some little tidbits I hope are helpful in preparing for and working with little ones and their parents in your herbal practice.

Get Ready, Get Set: Crawlers, Roamers, Explorers, Toys and Tantrums (And Maybe Snacks)

If you don't have children yourself or you don't see many children in your practice, having toddlers and little children around can throw you out of your groove and feel a little disruptive. It is true that working with little ones requires some flexibility on your part.

I schedule shorter appointments for individual children. By virtue of not having lived as long, their stories are typically shorter we don't need the same amount of time for intake. In my practice it is most often the mother who brings in her child. She may also bring her other children with her. I typically spend the initial minutes of the consultation talking with the mother about what's going on with her child. When you practice Traditional Western Herbalism and you are used to getting lots and lots of information from your client about what it is like to live in their bodies, it is challenging to look at a little child, say 2 or 3, who has some significant health issues but can't verbally explain to you what he or she is feeling. You have to rely on the mother's observations. Mama will tell you why she's brought her little one to see you, but I always make sure that by the time we have finished talking I have asked her about sleep, mood and temperament, energy level, any history of accidents or infectious illnesses, the skin, allergies, digestion, elimination (both bowel movements and urination as she observes it), respiratory health, how often her child gets sick and what that is typically like I ask follow up

questions whenever necessary. I usually ask the mother her if she feels that her child is hot or cold, how her child sweats, what color or how concentrated the child's urine is and if she has commonly noticed (or been told by a physician) that her child has swollen glands or tonsils? I find those particular questions to yield very helpful bits of information in assessing the child's constitution or energetic pattern. These questions get me thinking about hot and cold, damp and dry, a periphery that may need to be opened and relaxed or astringed, whether or not lymphagogues may be in order. Mom may not have the answer to all of those questions and that's ok. She will probably think about them going forward and have an answer for you next time. It's also a wonderful starting point for a conversation with her that illuminates your truly holistic (not just natural) approach to health care. If your client is a little bit older, you may try asking them questions directly. With older children I gauge their interest level in talking with me and adjust accordingly. Remember that maturity level can vary greatly. There are some seven year olds who will gladly sit and answer your questions and others would much rather play with toys. For older children and teens (or any child who shows interest in the interview) gear your questions directly to them and not to their mother. Honor their personhood. Sometimes when I know a woman is bringing in an older child I may ask her to email me any information that may be potentially embarrassing or discomfiting to the older child. I also speak communicate directly to older children how normal and common certain problems and affirm the young person's health and wholeness whenever I can. I believe that a young person, or any person for that matter, should not leave a consultation with me feeling that they are broken and maybe I will fix them.

During this interview time hopefully our little friend is playing with the toys I keep in my consultation space. It is very helpful to prepare a basket or bin with toys for your young clients. If you are fortunate enough to have a large consultation space or clinic, consider having a corner or area devoted to children's toys for different ages. This is really worth your small

304

investment in money and space. The toys feel welcoming to the child, it also usually buys you and the mom a little time and space to talk without a bored and/or apprehensive kid doing what bored and apprehensive kids do, (which is usually bug their mothers in ways characteristic to their ages and personalities). Some kids are not interested in your lovely toy basket (sorry!). Some very little people have just learned to walk and crawl and they would like to walk and crawl all around your office or home and maybe rip the pages out of a magazine or pulls some books off the shelf. Bold, curious, confident children of all ages have no qualms about checking out the rest of the house. These young extraverts may also have a lot of questions about your space. Little kids also graze all day. That's just what they do. Moms are usually prepared for this and may have brought snacks. These snacks may end up on your floor. Sometimes mom doesn't bring snacks and it's almost lunch time. Sometimes junior has already toured your kitchen and has spotted the bananas on the counter, or opened the cupboard. If it's ok with mom, let him have a snack. Diapers may need to be changed mid consultation. Babies may need to nurse. If all this sounds like kind of a pain in the butt, think of it this way: being a parent is hard, your hospitable gestures to this family is your gift as a person who serves, being generous of spirit will make you feel good and I promise it will not go unnoticed. Moms talk to other moms—a lot— and if going to the herbalist is a fun and pleasant experience you will get referrals. I sometimes serve whole groups of moms where all the friends in the group see me, or lots of families from the same neighborhood, homeschool co-op or church. At the end of the day, it's good for business.

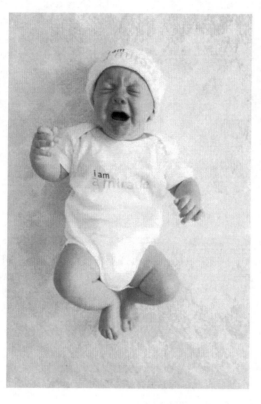

Tongue Assessment and Small People

After the intake interview I usually observe and assess the tongue. Many Western herbalists use tongue assessment. This is just as valuable with little ones as with adults. Virtually every child fours old and older will show you his tongue when asked. Most three year olds will as well. With children under three this can be hit or miss. If the toddler is apprehensive or timid, try lightening the mood and make yourself as non-threatening as possible. Get down on the floor. Act silly. Stick out your own tongue. Get a mirror and offer to show the child his or her tongue in the mirror. Have mom stick out her tongue. Smile a lot with sincerity. If the toddler doesn't respond to your overtures and seems determined not to stick out her tongue, don't push it. Respect her boundaries. You will simply have to work without this information, relying more on your knowledge of the materia medica. Remember that you can also gather some useful information about a child's energetic patterns or constitution with the type of careful questioning and observations described in the previous section. You can visualize the redness and inflammation, duskiness in the complexion, pallor. You can ask to touch the child's hand and feel for yourself the moisture level in the skin.

Be aware that babies one year of age and younger most often exhibit the tissue state described by Matthew Wood as damp/relaxed. The whole system seems relaxed and prone to discharge. They are soft and doughy. The tongue is very wet with copious saliva. They most often have dilute, copious urine (some moms using cloth diapers change them up to twelve times daily). They drool, spit up, have loose stools, pee all the time. I have come to view this as not pathological dampness but normal human baby physiological dampness. I don't know what purpose it serves and would be very interested in the theories of others herbalists, but I am quite confident that it is normal. Of much greater concern to me is the less typical baby with a dry tongue.

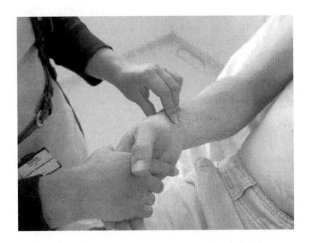

Pulse Testing & the Younger Crowd

I utilize pulse testing as a final aid in my attempts to match an herb or herbs with an individual. This is a non-diagnostic practice taught to me by Lise Wolff and Matthew Wood, where I attempt to let the client's body lead the way, revealing what it likes, what it would prefer to work on, what feels good, restores the flow, and what has the potential to transform. I pulse test babies and young toddlers in their mother's arms. I view the mother-babe as an energetic unit. Sometimes I test the child's pulse directly while being held by the mother. Sometimes if the child is fearful or rejects the touch of a stranger or is simply too squirmy, I test the mother while she holds the child or even while she breastfeeds the child. In my mind there is no clear cut-off moment at which time a child becomes separate from the mother, although it is very fascinating to consider those boundaries and how they may affect pulse testing. I sometimes wonder if a remedy is really a remedy that is more for the mother. The bold, confident and brave child announces his own energetic independence by his own choice to simply hop up on the chair to

be tested. If the child is reticent or hesitant, I acknowledge his preference to remain connected to his mother during this process. Again, you may need to remain flexible during this time. Be prepared to get down on the floor if you have to. Have some toys or books that the caregiver can show the child to distract them. Be very selective in your remedies. You may only have a minute or two. Your little client may not have the patience to wait for you to test 30 different remedies in many combinations. Be decisive. Give your gut instincts free reign. Some little children feel very compelled to put their fingers in the drops of tincture. Try giving the child the tissue and letting her wipe off the drops. Some young children are very sensitive, just as some adults are very sensitive. Some children are able to articulate their feelings about certain herbs. The child may tell you that a particular herb feels good or feels bad. Listen to this as you would listen to it with an adult. With older children and teens you can usually proceed with pulse testing just as you would with an adult.

Acute Care

In my practice I provide a lot of acute care to babies and children including care during fever, coughs, colds, sore throats, upper respiratory infections of all sorts, earaches/ear infections, thrush and other fungal infections, boils, pinkeye and the like. I enjoy providing acute care. It's fun and gratifying. Acute conditions require a little bit less of a precise determination of constitution and energetics and we have so many choices of various regional herbs and types of preparations.

The challenge is that in your capacity as a trusted advisor you will be called upon to help make the determination of when to go to the doctor. Because one of my primary goals is empowerment of the client, I try not to allow the mother to hand authority over to me. It can give you a boost to your ego to have someone else give you the mantle of expert and decision-maker, but ultimately it doesn't help this mother become a more confident and competent steward of her child's health. I encourage you to explicitly put the decision back in her hands.

Answer questions, provide information, share your experience but listen for the feelings behind her questions. Help her tease out what she really wants to do. Sometimes women consult the herbalist or another natural health care practitioner really looking for someone to give them a permission slip to go the doctor. She is afraid for her child's well-being but is conflicted about taking the child to the doctor because this makes her feel she is giving up on her natural health ideals. Mother guilt and pressure to be an ideal parent is rampant in our culture and this is especially true in idealistic natural parenting communities. If you sense that she wants a permission slip from you, don't be a jerk and try to talk her out of it. Give the woman not only permission to go to the doctor with her sick little child but also give her your support and affirmation. Tell her she should always trust her intuition. Tell her that when she feels out of her depth, there is no shame in getting help. Help her realize her choice is not a failure and that by walking through the door of the clinic she is not failing, nor does she have to wholeheartedly accept the physician's view on things. Going to a clinic to rule out something serious is a totally reasonable option. Help her formulate the questions she can ask her physician. Remind her that she does not need to have an uncomfortable conflict with her physician. She can take the prescription for antibiotics and choose not to fill it. Herbal medicine and conventional medication for acute illness are rarely incompatible. Help her make a plan to combine natural treatments and conventional treatments. She can utilize your consultation services and your products in addition to conventional care to create a individualized approach to health for her child.

If you do provide acute care or find yourself in the role of trusted advisor it is important that you are familiar with signs and symptoms that really ought to be checked out by a physician. While this is not a comprehensive list, I would include: an infant whose fever and lethargy makes them unwilling to feed potentially resulting in serious dehydration, labored or rapid respirations that could be a sign of pneumonia, rash accompanied by fever. A fever and a rash could be a simple as a self-limiting case of hand, foot and mouth disease or fifths disease or something more serious like measles

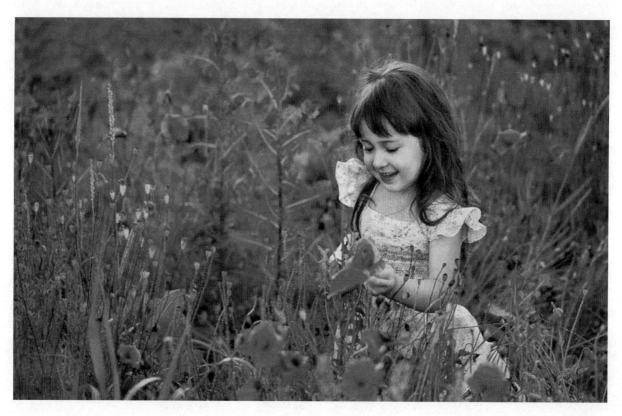

or meningitis. My rule of thumb is rash+fever= the doc should check it out! Other symptoms that should be assessed are seizures or convulsions in a child who does not have a history of seizures and blood in the stool that is not from an evident hemorrhoid. There is no magic number on the thermometer at which a parent must take their kid to the clinic. Nor is there a magic number of days of coughing after which someone must go to the doctor. The overall impression of wellness or illness shown by a child is more important than the number on the thermometer or the number of day the child has been ill.

Educating about Normal and Teaching Acceptance

Not everything in life needs an herb. This can be hard for herbalists to face sometimes, but it is true. Not everything can or needs to be fixed and this is sometimes hard for the contemporary natural Mama to understand. Some things are just kind of normal, no matter how annoying it is, or how much it stresses out mom and dad. Babies wake a lot in the night in spite of our cultural obsession with sleeping through the night. Babies are sometimes fussy, just like grown-ups babies sometimes feel crabby and pissed off. They are not always allergic to something that mom ate. A four year old boy who wets the bed, probably doesn't have a problem, especially if his dad wet the bed too as a child. They grow out of it. Everybody gets sick a couple times a year. Eight year old boys have a *lot* of energy.

What does the herbalist do when faced with the possibility that the most issue is really the mom's anxiety or unrealistic expectations? I keep three key concepts in mind when dealing with these types of situations: empathy for the mother's struggles, affirming the child's wholeness, and common sense. Let the mom know that you know it's really hard when her baby wakes often to feed or whatever the issues is. If the child seems really healthy, well and normal to you, convey this kindly and repeatedly if necessary and offer common sense advice and non-

overwhelming steps she can take make everyone in the family feel better. Many times has a consultation for a baby or child in my practice been expanded to include a quickie consult for mom. Some nervines like Motherwort, Blue Vervain, or many others can take the edge off the anxiety and tension caused by the struggles of mothering and make the whole situation a lot more manageable.

Forms of Herbal Medicine for Babies and Children

I primarily work with tinctures, even with babies and kids. I love tinctures for their potency, convenience, ease of storage and administration for the client. I give tinctures to just about everyone over the age of one. I feel that precision that comes from a constitutional and energetic approach with tongue assessment, pulse testing and specific indications allows me to use sublingual drop doses most of the time. I really don't worry about the tiny bit of alcohol, even when I use doses more in the range of .5 to 1 ml. For acute illness, there are many more possibilities including yummy sage tea with honey, elderberry syrup, blossoms in the bathtub to treat a fever, an aromatic chest rub made with essential oils, drops for earaches. Tiny infants are meant to be exclusively breastfed. Avoid exposing babies to any unnecessary foods, herbs or drugs during the first six months of life. Their little guts and little livers and little immune systems are just starting to get warmed up. When herbs are necessary begin with the gentlest preparations and the lowest possible dose. Start with weak teas. Tea should be cooled to lukewarm and given to baby in doses from 1-3 teaspoons. In situations like colic, coughs, digestive upset, use small doses every 1-3 hours. Herbal baths can be an effective alternative to internal use of remedies. Baths are especially beneficial for fever or for any problem characterized by tension or emotional upset. Move to higher doses or stronger preparations when necessary for instance, I will use tinctures such as diluted Black Walnut for thrush or one or two drops of Yellow Dock for reflux.

Working with babies, children and their caregivers can be fun, gratifying and profitable for you as an herbalist although it does present some challenges. Educate yourself on breastfeeding, normal infant behaviors, acute infections of all sorts including warning signs requiring physician consultation and chronic health issues childhood such as eczema, ADHD asthma etc. Be flexible and open in your manner and approach. Good luck!

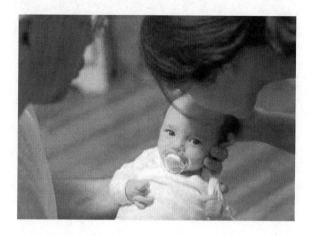

A Non-Comprehensive Off-the-Cuff Materia Medica for Babies and Children
(based on the practice of just one herbalist Who sees a lot of kids)

• Agrimony (*Agrimonia eupatorium*) sometimes this rose family astringent nervine is the just the ticket for bedwetting in the older child.

• Black Walnut (*Juglans nigra*) This powerful remedy is simultaneously gentle enough to give to infants. I recommend diluting the tincture in water and using for a rinse/wash for cases of oral thrush. It's also a good topical agent for ringworm. Useful for constipation, skin problems of the dry type, eczema, atopic illness, worms/parasites. Cold, dry or stagnant. Black Walnut treats them all!

• Blue Vervain (*Verbena hastata*) Even little ones can be tense! This nervine/antispasmodic is great for little teeth grinders and the kids who even as babies give off a tense vibe.

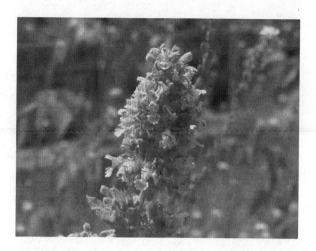

• Catnip (*Nepeta cataria*) A classic children's herb for colic, teething, fussiness and fevers. More sedating than many herbs, catnip can be dispensed in larger doses before long car trips or plane rides (it works!). Catnip and Chamomile (see below) are used for similar conditions. Catnip is specifically useful when the child's crabbiness involves anger, irritation, muscular tension. You know the type of baby. They flex their bodies angrily, arch their backs and try to launch out of your arms, resisting your attempts to snuggle them into a less crabby mood. (indebted to indications from Matthew Alfs).

• Chamomile (Roman, German, Pineapple Weed, I use them interchangeably). Not only a classic children's herb but a widely useful totally underutilized herb in general. I recommend Chamomile as an eyewash for conjunctivitis or pink eye. It is great orally for seasonal allergies in children and adults and it's good for a mild tummy ache or as a slight enhancer of digestion. Like Catnip, it's used for teething, fussiness and colic but these babies are fretful, whiny and clingy, not so angry, more like the type that doesn't want you to put them down for the entire duration of their discomfort or illness. (some indications from Matthew Wood).

• Chickeweed (*Stellaria media* and other *Stellaria* species) awesome topical for eczema and really anything that itches, burns or is swollen.

• Cinquefoil (*Potentilla* spp.) Another Rose family nervine for bedwetting in the older kids.

309

• Cleavers (*Gallium aparine* and other *Gallium* species) This moistening lymphagogue is one of my favorite remedies for childhood eczema, and children with chronic upper respiratory infections, or chronic strep, especially when the tonsils and other lymph nodes are frequently swollen.

• Elder Blossoms (*Sambucus nigra* or *S. Canadensis*) Elder: the undisputed queen of herbs for the youngsters. Elder is a reliable diaphoretic and an aid in decongesting upper respiratory conditions and earaches. Elder is also a transformative medicine for children with eczema and atopic illness, ADHD and hyperactive behavior, frequent infections and a combination of pallor and bright, red, dry harsh inflamed cheeks. This is the remedy for kids who don't sweat. They are dry and harsh on the exterior and some combination of hot and cold.

• Elderberry (*Sambucus nigra*) Almost all children love the syrup or elixir which is a good anti-viral and shorten the duration of illnesses. Try making elderberry gummies—it's fun and kids and adults love them!

• Elecampane (*Inula helenium*) drop doses for upper respiratory tract infections especially with green infected mucus (indication from Matthew Wood).

• Goldenrod (*Solidago canadensis* and other species) Another favorite. This herb is great for eczema, allergies and sometimes kidney/urinary symptoms or poor digestion. The tongue coating is almost always thick, creamy or greasy.

• Ground Ivy or Creeping Charley (*Glechoma hederacea*) This little mint is useful for the common cold and upper respiratory infections, as well as earaches and ringing in the ears. Ground Ivy has a history of use for lead poisoning.

• Hawthorn (*Cratageus* spp.) I use the berry for ADHD and hyperactivity in hot, sanguine types.

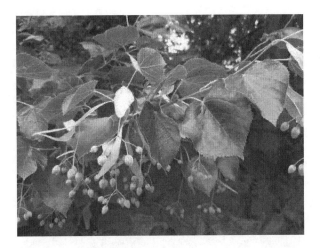

• Linden (*Tilia* spp.) The blossoms are another classic children's herb, particularly useful for fever and upper respiratory infection. Linden is also a nervine and promotes restful sleep in very active or anxious children and is also a choice herb for ADHD in children with hot, inflamed patterns.

• Mullein (*Verbascum thapsus*) The leaf will moisten dry coughs and is particularly useful when a child coughs until gagging or vomiting, bronchitis, croup, whooping cough, as well as more run of the mill dry coughs. The blossoms are for ear oil, of course. I cold infuse mine with garlic and add some Lavender essential oil.

• Oregon Grape Root (*Mahonia* species)— Excellent for those dry little ones, constipation, eczema, chronic swollen glands.

• Plantain (*Plantago majus*) allergies, common, non-serious upper respiratory infections, sinus infections, post nasal drip, cough, clear mucus. Topical for rashes.

• Poke (*Phytolacca americanum*) Just a tiny bit can be great in a formula for eczema, allergies, chronic swollen tonsils especially when the tongue shows signs of lymphatic imbalance.

• Red Clover (*Trifolium pratense*) another moistening lymphagogue in the kit to help those youngsters with eczema. Also good for general upper respiratory infections, coughs, mucus, head cold.

• Sage (*Salvia officinalis*) no better tea for sore throats, including strep. I recommend a strong tea with fresh herb (available year round even at the most conventional of grocery stores) with raw honey and lemon. Sage also makes an awesome infused honey.

• Wood Betony (*Stachys betonica*) thin intellectual, ungrounded, spacy style ADD, headaches and stomaches when nervous or worried (indications from Matthew Wood).

• Yellow Dock (*Rumex crispus*) Yellow Dock is the best remedy for GERD even in babies. The downward energy of this plant is amazing. Wonderful for constipation in larger doses without the discomfort associated with senna preparations.

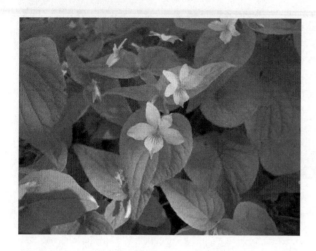

• Violet (*Viola* spp.) A very cooling lymphagogue. Great for high fevers. Sore throat, swollen gland, eczema.

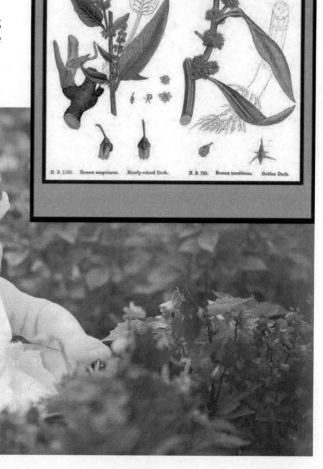

HERBAL HEALING FOR WEE FOLKS

by Debra Swanson

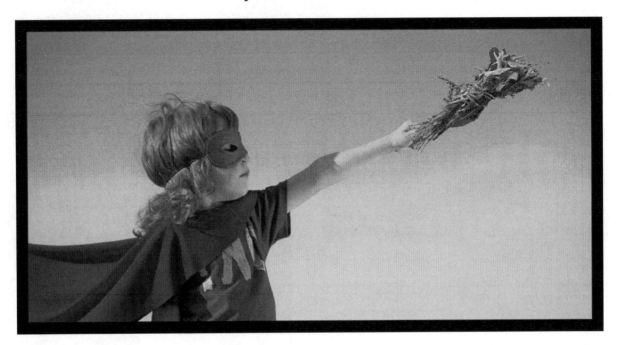

No one likes for their child to be sick or in pain! We naturally want to spring into action and fix the problem, but perhaps we aren't always 100% sure what the proper course of action is. I hope to share with you some simple and time tested solutions for the most common of childhood ailments, but first relax and know deep down that the resiliency of children is remarkable. Most childhood illnesses are a very natural part of growing and living and are no cause for alarm or panic. They are natural reactions to the act of living and usually can be treated at home with a good dose of common sense, and nurturing. As a society, we have lost touch with our ability to heal.

We need not look further than the pantry, refrigerator, kitchen cabinets, or what is growing outside the back door for medicine to treat common colds, flus, fevers and common ailments. It is my wish to demystify this. It is not magic, or "silly" folk medicine but practical wisdom with sturdy roots that have held strong over time. This is the brilliance, wonder and perfection of how how life used to be. Our mothers, grannies and great grannies looked no further than themselves, home and neighbors to treat so many of the common ailments of childhood. Unfortunately, we have turned away from that model to one based on pharmaceutical solutions for every bump or pain. Let's explore why and how we can return to a more natural healing path with confidence!

In our modern world, where time moves at an exponentially fast pace, we have forgotten such simple things. We have demonized what is natural and have put blind faith into over-the-counter medications or medications that are made in a lab. The new holy robes are in the form of a white jacket. Everything is so medicalized and sophisticated these days and many parents are left feeling helpless and disempowered because they have little faith in their innate ability to nurture and heal. We have been conditioned to think that taking our child to the doctor is the best and prudent choice for any condition that is out of the ordinary, when in truth, a nurturing response coupled with time to heal and some simple natural remedies would be far more beneficial than a trip to the doctor and the resulting prescription that might follow. When I was growing up and got sick my grandmother would come over. We would pull out a deck of cards and she would brew up a big pot of hot lemonade with ginger and honey. She would wrap my blankets around me tightly, and I was so comforted by that simple act. In fact, I almost looked forward to being sick and to those moments when she came over and and we could spend
that special time together.

Our connection to nature has been short circuited and we have lost touch with many ancient, time honored means of healing that have worked for thousands of years. For a host of reasons, we have put our faith in big pharmacy and diagnostics based on hierarchal authority. So many common childhood illnesses do not constitute going to the doctor and were once easily treated at home. The wisdom of generations has been thrown out the window in search of a quick fix that may come at a cost to both parent and child. The quick medical fix does not take into account a child's emerging immune system, nor the fact that a quick fix is rarely the best answer. Most childhood ailments are easily treated, we simply need to slow down and embrace the nurturing aspect of parenting that should include healing the bumps and basic illnesses of childhood.

We are now seeing side effects of over prescribed and mis-prescribed drugs and the loss of the big picture when it comes to childhood ailments. Let's take eczema for example. A typical visit to the doctors office for the treatment of eczema, which is a common ailment, will most likely end with a prescription for cortisone. This powerful drug is effective, but no consideration is given to the root cause, not to mention, the long term effect of such a strong drug. The skin is a membrane that is permeable. All medications are absorbed and go into general circulation. Cortisone suppresses the immune system and we are seeing a relationship between suppressed immunity and asthma. A child that has been given cortisone is likely, later in life to develop problems related to suppressed immunity. Looking at the child as a whole and not jumping to a fast draw and easy solutions is critical. In treating anyone, it is important to know that time is valuable, that slow is not bad, that nature has it's way and rhythm and when we use herbs to heal naturally we are getting in sync with a more natural pattern. By using natural ways to heal that support our system, rather than undermining it for the short term goal with quick fixes and powerful drugs, we are healing naturally and aligning our health with a natural pattern that we have stepped away from in this fast paced world.

Many parents don't have the time that is needed to wait out a cold or the flu. We feel such urgency to get back to work and back to earning that our natural inclination to nurture and support in times of need is undermined. For some people, fear comes into play. No one wants to see their child in pain or discomfort. But of course, discomfort and pain are vital parts of growing on so many levels, and to short circuit this is to undermine your child and to create a person that has no ability to persevere through adversity. No one likes fever or discomfort, but perhaps if we reassess our fears we can see them as an opportunity to dig deeper into nurturing. Let's look at fever in particular, as it is scary for many. Fevers are a natural function of the immune process.Fever is what the body does to stimulate the immune system. It's how we grow strong children. The natural responses might take time, but are a bridge to a pattern of health that is life long.

Another example that I see often is the very common childhood ear infection. Many parents come to the herb shop with complaints of ear infections, and wanting the quick fix, they have gone to the doctor for antibiotics. That worked briefly, but then they are at the herb shop a week or month later, with the same complaints, this time hoping to heal the underlying problem that was the root cause in the first place. After a protocol of time tested remedies, the problem is usually fixed. When we find the time to bond and establish patterns of health, natural healing can be our go-to for all the common illnesses of childhood.
Below you will find some traditional herbal remedies that
are time tested for some of childhoods most common maladies.

Fevers

For fevers I recommend:

Relaxing Diaphoretics:

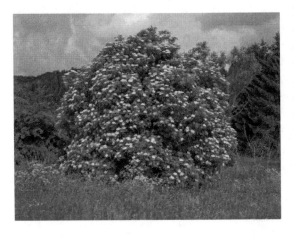

Elder Flowers (*Sambucus nigra*): Used as a relaxing diaphoretic. It opens the pores when a fever rises and allows the body to sweat. This allows the tension in the muscles and nervous system to relax and allows for blood to flow from the core to the surface.This has a soothing and relaxing effect. Great for restless agitated fevers that are hot, dry, painful and possibly with irritability.

Catnip (*Nepeta cataria*)gentle relaxant helps to relieve the pain of fever, allowing for rest and repair. improves circulation so that vital energy flows through to he body.

Boneset (*Eupatorium perfoliatum*) : Relaxing. Allows the vital force to flow. Very specific for the feeling of bone breaking fever that alternates between cold chills and hot fever. This is a very bitter tea, but nothing quite
relieves pain like this.

Stimulatiing Diaphoretics:

Brings blood from the core to the periphery by using herbs that are warming. This is helpful for the child who is cold, listless and in the initial stages of fever where it is making you feel cold and clammy. They may be sweating, but they feel cold. Many of your kitchen spices can be helpful.

Ginger for fever with nausea. Cinnamon is warming and good for diarrhea, mucilaginous and helps to coat the mucus membranes, Cayenne to really get the blood moving and increase peripheral circulation.

Colds, Flu, & Congestion

Colds, flu and congestion will benefit from this simple hydrotherapy technique.

The Cold Sock Treatment is a simple hydrotherapy technique that is especially effective for relieving nasal congestion in bed at night (frequently better than medications and without the side effects). It also helps to stimulate the immune system in the upper respiratory tract and is relaxing for aches and chills, and helps bring on a more restful night's sleep when sick. We find it helpful in such conditions as colds, "flu" (not the "stomach flu"), earaches, sore throats, and sinus infections. It is useful with people of any age from infants to the elderly. The Cold Sock Treatment is especially good to use with the nasal congestion of colds and influenza.

Preparations. In the evening before going to bed, prepare by having a pair of cotton socks and a pair of wool socks. They must be at least 90% cotton and 90% wool, respectively. Most sporting goods stores and some department stores carry wool socks. For small children you can use safety-pins to hold a wool sock on that is too large, or rap wool cloth around each foot.

Step 1. Soak the foot part of the cotton socks in cold tap water and wring them out thoroughly. Place the socks close to the basin or bathtub used in the next step. Note: If your feet are already warm (e.g., you have already been in bed) you can skip to Step 3.

Step 2. Put your feet into a basin or bathtub of hot water to warm up your feet. Soak them for a few minutes until they are hot and pink.

Step 3. Remove your feet from the hot water and quickly dry them off. Immediately put on the cold wet cotton
socks, and then over them, put on the dry wool socks.

Step 4. Go directly to bed and keep the feet covered through the night. The therapy does not work if you or your feet are uncovered, such as when walking around or sitting in a chair uncovered.

When the Cold Sock Treatment procedure is followed correctly the feet will start warming up within a few minutes of getting covered in bed. The congestion will usually start to be relieved within 30 minutes. It will often work better than a decongestant or antihistamine to relieve congestion during sleep. In addition, it is not uncommon to see a small child or infant fall immediately to sleep after they are put to bed with the Cold Sock Treatment. After approximately four hours the socks should be totally dry, the feet warm, and the symptoms will be much improved (if not gone).

If necessary the Cold Sock Treatment can be repeated through the night or used on consecutive nights. In repeating the treatment in the same night or if an illness starts during the night, it is not necessary to warm the feet in hot water since they will already be warm. Simply apply the wrung out cold wet socks and the dry wool socks and go back to bed. Similarly, a cool cotton cloth on the throat with a neck warmer on top activates the lymphatic system.

Cough & Respiratory Infections

In Colorado we are high and dry. Most folks in the SW are living between 6000-9000 and the air is thin and dry dry dry! The respiratory infections that I often see are different from the east or west coast where there is an abundance of humidity. My first premise when working with kids is to liquify and add humidify. A humidifier in the bedroom with some aromatic essential oils is soothing and healing. Disinfecting essential oils like eucalyptus, thyme, and rosemary are also wonderful.

A steam inhalation is one of the best home remedies for cold and coughs and is also an effective sinus infection home remedy. Steam inhalations can also to relieve sore throats and catarrh.

Inhalations are easy to do and can be made more effective by adding essential oils, especially oils with decongestant, antibacterial and antiviral properties. Some of the most useful oils are Eucalyptus, Pine, Lavender, Rosemary, Peppermint and Tea Tree.

How to Make a Steam Inhalation

Simply heat up water up to boiling point on a stove or in an electric kettle. Remove from heat and pour the water into a large bowl. Add 3-4 drops of essential oil, cover your head and the bowl with a large bath towel, place your face above the bowl but not so close that the steam will burn your face, and inhale the hot steam for several minutes. I do up to ten minutes or until the water cools down.

Make sure you don't burn yourself, and supervise kids closely with the steaming bowl. If you have a cold, a persistent cough or a sinus infection, steam inhalations can be done several times a day. This is not recommended for people with asthma.
Many of these readily available culinary herbs are highly anti microbial and loaded with volatile oils that will disperse into hot water for a simple steam inhalation. Just think spaghetti sauce!

For convenience, the following essential oils are great to
have on hand.Rosemary, Thyme, Oregano, and Marjoram

Essential Oils For Steam Inhalation

•Colds: Eucalyptus (*Eucalyptus globulus* or *radiata*) is one of the best oils for colds; it is antiviral, antibacterial and decongestant. Other useful oils are Lavender (*Lavandula angustifolia*) –antibacterial, antiviral, decongestant and relaxing, Pine (*Pinus sylvestris*) – a good decongestant, Tea Tree (*Melaleuca alternifolia*) – one of the best antiviral oils but not as good for clearing up the nasal passages as Eucalyptus. Peppermint (*Mentha piperita*) is an effective decongestant but it is quite strong and not everyone can take it.

•Coughs: Eucalyptus steam inhalation is one of the easiest home remedies for coughs. The oil relieves congestion and if there is an infection, it also fights the bacteria. For dry and irritating coughs, try Benzoin (*Styrax benzoin)* or Frankincense (*Boswellia carterii*).

•Sinus infection: a steam inhalation several times a day can relieve the pain, the congestion and the infection. Try Eucalyptus, Lavender, Peppermint, Pine, Thyme (*Thymus vulgaris*) or Tea Tree.

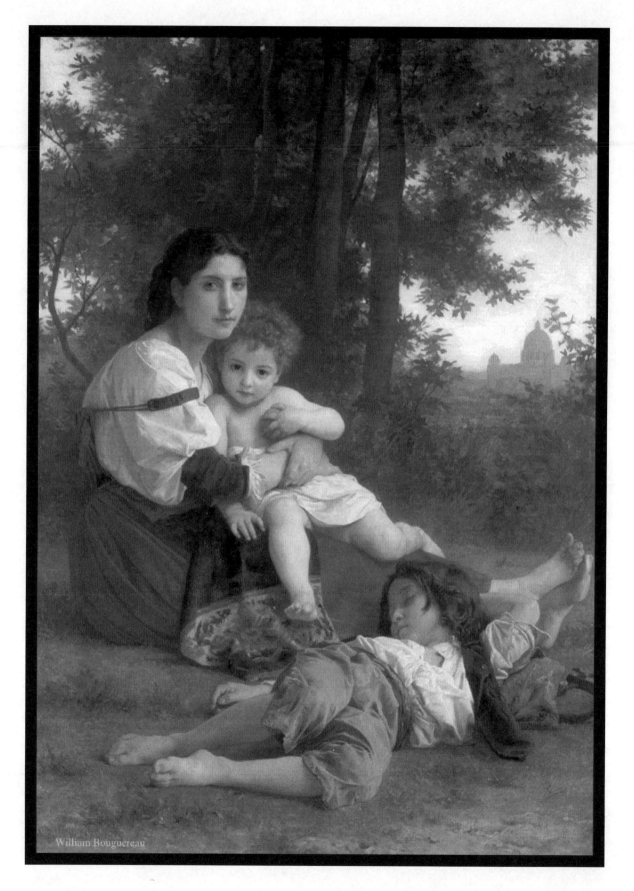

William Bouguereau

317

Sore throat: steam inhalations can ease irritation and soreness in the throat, whether it is caused by an infection or if you've just been talking too much. Benzoin, Lavender and Thyme are all good choices.

<h2 style="text-align:center">Ear Aches</h2>

A Mullein Garlic ear oil is an essential remedy to have on hand when ear aches strike in the middle of the night. When in a bind, one can simply crush and then strain one clove of Garlic into 2oz of olive oil.

To Use: Gently warm oil in a hot water bath to just warm on the wrist. Place 3 to 5 drops of infused oil in both ears and take a warm wash cloth and gently cradle each ear. The warmth is incredibly soothing and the oil will fight infection and reduce inflammation.

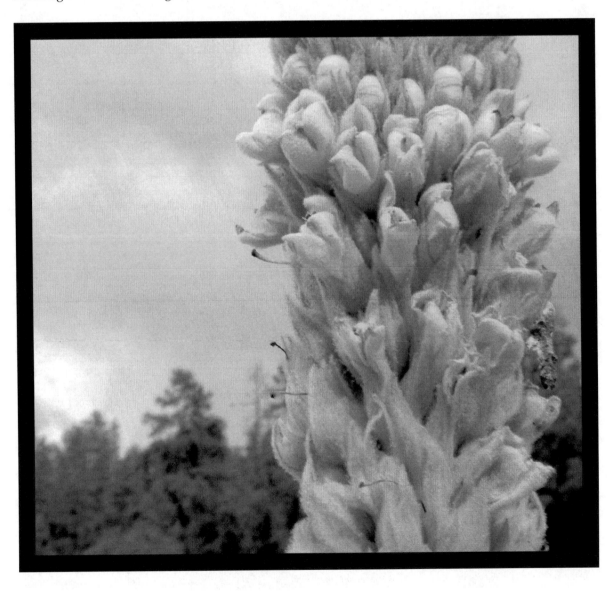

Here are some common facts about fever from Seattle Children's Hospital that we can all agree on!

Many parents have false beliefs myths about fever. They think fever will hurt their child. They worry and lose sleep when their child has a fever. In fact, fevers are harmless and often helpful. Let these facts help you better understand fever.

Myth*:* My child feels warm, so she has a fever.

Fact: Children can feel warm for a many reasons. Examples are playing hard, crying, getting out of a warm bed or hot weather. They are "giving off heat". Their skin temperature should return to normal in 10 to 20 minutes. About 80% of children who act sick and feel warm do have a fever. If you want to be sure, take the temperature. These are the cutoffs for fever using different types of thermometers:

•Rectal, ear or forehead temperature: 100.4° F (38.0° C) or higher
•Oral mouth temperature: 100° F (37.8° C) or higher
•Under the arm Armpit temperature: 99° F (37.2° C) or higher

Myth*:* All fevers are bad for children.

Fact: Fevers turn on the body's immune system. They help the body fight infection. Normal fevers between 100° and 104° F (37.8° - 40° C) are good for sick children.

Myth*:* Fevers above 104° F (40° C) are dangerous. They can cause brain damage.

Fact: Fevers with infections don't cause brain damage. Only temperatures above 108° F (42° C) can cause brain damage. It's very rare for the body temperature to climb this high. It only happens if the air temperature is very high. An example is a child left in a closed car during hot weather.

Myth*:* Anyone can have a seizure triggered by fever.

Fact: Only 4% of children can have a seizure with fever.

Myth*:* Seizures with fever are harmful.

Fact: These seizures are scary to watch, but they stop within 5 minutes. They don't cause any permanent harm. They don't increase the risk for speech delays, learning problems, or seizures without fever.

Myth*:* All fevers need to be treated with fever medicine.

Fact: Fevers only need to be treated if they cause discomfort. Most fevers don't cause discomfort until they go above 102° or 103° F (39° or 39.5° C).

Myth*:* Without treatment, fevers will keep going higher.

Fact: Wrong, because the brain has a thermostat. Most fevers from infection don't go above 103° or 104° F (39.5°- 40° C). They rarely go to 105° or 106° F (40.6° or 41.1° C). While these are "high" fevers, they also are harmless ones.

Myth: With treatment, fevers should come down to normal.

Fact: With treatment, most fevers come down 2° or 3° F (1° or 1.5° C).

Myth: If you can't "break the fever", the cause is serious.

Fact: Fevers that don't come down to normal can be caused by viruses or bacteria. The response to fever medicines tells us nothing about the cause of the infection.

Myth: Once the fever comes down with medicines, it should stay down.

Fact: It's normal for fevers with most viral infections to last for 2 or 3 days. When the fever medicine wears off, the fever will come back. It may need to be treated again. The fever will go away and not return once the body overpowers the virus. Most often, this is day 3 or 4. *MYTH.* If the fever is high, the cause is serious.

Fact: If the fever is high, the cause may or may not be serious. If your child looks very sick, the cause is more likely to be serious.

Myth: The exact number of the temperature is very important.

Fact: How your child looks is what's important. The exact temperature number is not.

Myth: Oral temperatures between 98.7° and 100° F (37.1° to 37.8° C) are low-grade fevers.

Fact: These temperatures are normal. The body's normal temperature changes throughout the day. It peaks in the late afternoon and evening. A true low- grade fever is 100° F to 102° F (37.8° - 39° C).

Summary: Keep in mind that fever is fighting off your child's infection. Fever is one of the good guys. We grow strong children to be open and receptive to life and its natural processes. We expose them to dirt and germs, and nature, because it is unnatural not to. We talk about love, we talk about sex, we talk about dying. We talk about things that scare us so they don't take hold in our subconscious. We can offer so many nurturing and effective home and herbal remedies that heal and support the common illnesses of childhood while growing our faith in the power of family, love and nature.

Sources:

Fevers Myth and Facts Seattle Children's Hospital via Jim McDonald

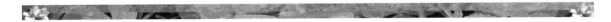

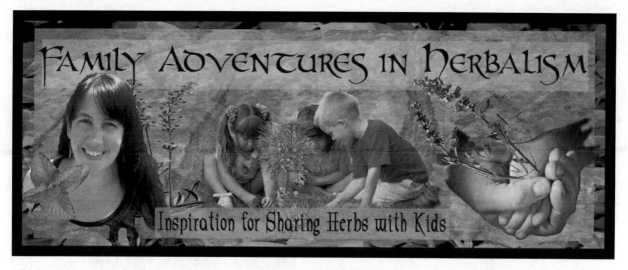

CHILDREN'S SLEEPYTIME SELF-CARE

by Angela Justis

Make bedtime fun and enjoyable for kids with the addition of lovely herbs to create a soothing bedtime ritual. Empower your child in their own self-care and help them create bedtime teas to sip, soothing baths to take, and foot rubs to enjoy! Friendly herbs can be used every night or just on occasion when sleep might be difficult. Bringing herbs into the everyday activities of life is a powerful way to share herbalism with children while enhancing the quality of life!

enjoy! Favorite herbs for children's bedtime blends in my home include lemon balm, chamomile, linden, and rose. We also enjoy small amounts of catnip, skullcap, passionflower, and California poppy on occasion often with some honey to sweeten things up and make the tea pleasant for kids. Warming carminatives also make their way into our after dinner evening tea mug to help gently stimulate digestion, making it easier to sleep deeply.

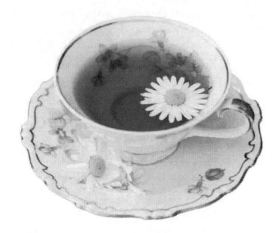

Say Goodnight with a Cup of Tea

Kids love to play in water and many herbs easily give their helpful constituents in this medium, making them readily available to the body. Many herbs make tasty bedtime teas that kids will

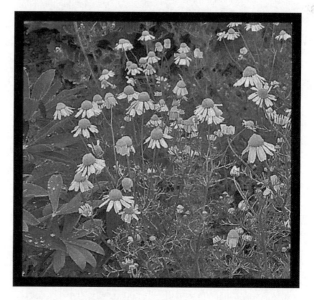

Chamomile (*Matricaria recutita*)

I like to think of chamomile as the "herbal mom" and with its wonderful calming action, a warm

321

cup of chamomile is like a comforting hug. This beloved nervine can gently nourish the nervous system, soothing away nervousness, irritability, anxiety, and insomnia. It is wonderful for settling a nervous stomach that is caused by emotional stress and strain. Herbalist Matthew Wood considers chamomile to be a remedy for babies, and not just actual babies but for the babyish behavior such as whining, fussiness, and tantrums that all of us are capable of exhibiting at one time or another. Call on chamomile to ease distress when someone in your family is fussy and cranky after a hard day.

Linden (*Tilla* species)

Children experience stress just like adults do and linden flower can help to ease some of that stress so the child can rest. Linden is especially useful when tension and anxiety manifest with physical discomfort such as muscle pains, headaches, and insomnia. It is wonderfully cooling and helps to calm overstimulation. Offer your child a cup of linden tea and a kind ear to talk to when they just can't calm down or are feeling anxious.

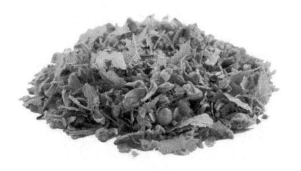

Lemon Balm (*Melissa officinalis*)

This delightful herb is particularly helpful for kids that are emotionally wound-up and over excited. As a lovely, happy herb, lemon balm is used to help lift the mood and dispel sadness while calming nervous stress and excitement. When I ask kids how lemon balm smells and tastes, I often get answers like "yummy, delicious, and happy!" It is great for grouchy children (and adults) who are so overtired and excited that they can't settle down.

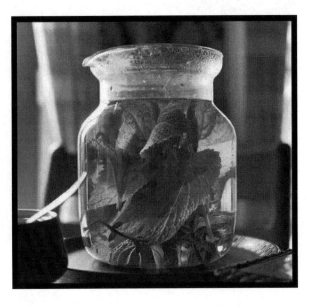

Rose petals (*Rosa* species)

Rose petals are useful for soothing nervousness especially if there is a sense of grief involved. Lovely and cooling, rose has long been used to comfort and calm the heart. Its gentle antidepressant and sedative properties can help uplift the emotions while providing a sense of ease.

A few simple things can make it more fun for your child to drink their tea. First get your child involved in making the tea! Use beautiful fragrant herbs and let your child hold, smell, and look at the herbs. Encourage your child choose the herbs for his or her tea from an appropriate selection of herbs. Start with simples so your child can get to know each herb separately and then encourage your child to try making their own blends. Brew up their tea in a little personal teapot or serve in a special mug that is just for your child. You can also serve the tea room temperature or cold with a straw if that is how they like to drink beverages most.

Kids are more sensitive than adults and respond strongly to mild herbs while stronger herbs may cause unwanted reactions in little bodies. Adjusting herb dosage for kids makes many herbs effective and safe for kids. Herbalist Rosemary Gladstar explains, "My experience has been that almost any herb that is safe for an adult is safe for a child as long as the size and weight of the child are accounted for and the dosage is adjusted accordingly" (Gladstar, 2001,

p. 163). She also says that these herbs should be used "in small amounts for short periods of time only, and in conjunction or formulated with milder herbs" (Gladstar, 2001, p. 163).

Using Clark's or Young's Rule is helpful for adjusting dosage size.
Clark's Rule based on the weight of the child and assumes that the adult dosage is for a 150 pound adult. To use Clark's Rule take the weight of your child and divide it by 150. For example, if your child weighs 38 pounds you would divide 38 by 150 (38/150 = .253 or ¼) so your child would take ¼ of the adult dosage (White et al., 1998).

Young's rule for figuring dosage is based on the child's age. To use, add 12 to the child's age and divide the child's age by this number. Here is an example for a 6 year old child: 6+12 = 18, then 6/18 = .3 from which you can calculate the fraction of the adult dosage to use. In this case 1/3 of the adult dosage (Gladstar, 2001).

Cozy Up in a Soothing Herbal Bath

A favorite herbal craft I have shared with many children is the fun art of making a sock bath. There is something special about a cuddly sock all stuffed with aromatic herbs that makes little ones smile! Children love stuffing the sock and giving it a good snuggle before using it to make a soothing bath - what could be better for bedtime?

Besides being fun to make, sock baths are easy to use and keep all the messiness of an herbal bath contained inside the sock while the goodness of the herbs soak right into the water! You and your child can make a supply of sock baths to have on hand or just create a special one using the herbs that call to your child that night. Your child can enjoy the tutorial in the recipe section for making their own sock bath!

Nourishing Bathtime Add-Ins

Beside herbs, there are other items that make a happy home in any sock bath! You probably have some of these useful add-ins in your kitchen right now.

Oatmeal – Perhaps one of the most delightful ingredients to include in any child's sock bath is oatmeal. It becomes slippery and slimy, releasing lots of lovely mucilage when soaked in water. Kids have great fun squeezing the sock and releasing the soothing slipperiness into the tub. They can then use the sock to gently scrub their skin. Beyond the breakfast bowl, oatmeal is

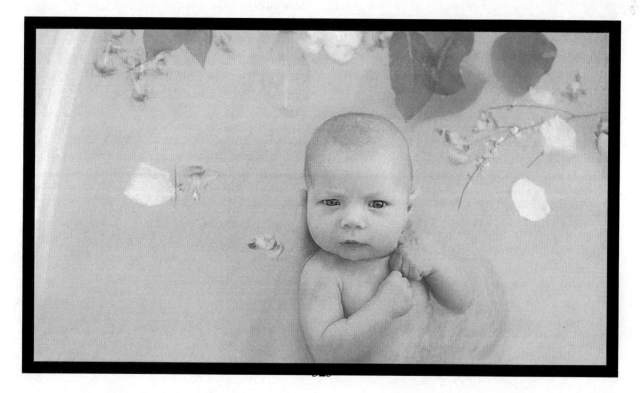

perhaps best known for its ability to soothe itchy skin. In the tub there really couldn't be anything better for those suffering from itchy rashes, dry skin, burns, and insect bites. The saponins in oatmeal also help to gently cleanse the skin, while oatmeal's emollient properties help to moisturize dry skin. When using oatmeal in the bath for a rash, use cool water as hot water may irritate and dry already sensitive skin.

Baking Soda – Baking soda is another wonderful addition to baths. Just like oatmeal, it is particularly good for soothing the itch of insect bites, poison ivy, and rashes. Plus, it adds a nice silky feel to the water!

Powdered Milk – Milk baths are so soft and silky. Milk in the bath helps to gently exfoliate and moisturize dry, rough skin. Plus it makes the water turn an interesting milky white.

Salts – Salts are used in the bath to help relax sore muscles. Salt baths also provide nourishing minerals to the body and can help to move lymph which is helpful during illness. My family's favorite salt to use in the tub is Epsom salt. Pretty pink Himalayan salt, sea salt, and Dead Sea salt are other great choices.

Finish Up With a Foot Rub!

A perfect time for a foot rub is after a nice warm relaxing bath. Oils infused with herbs are a great choice for a child's massage oil. Help your child learn the fine art of infusing oils and create their own infused oil for bedtime massage. Foot rubs and other types of massage invite us to slow down and relax. We can give tender care to our own bodies with a nice massage or share massages with loved ones as a lovely way to connect.

Herbs for Kids to Enjoy in Bedtime Baths & Infused Massage Oils

Herbal baths and massages with herb infused oils are wonderful for nourishing the skin and body with the beneficial properties of herbs by providing the opportunity for the herb to be soaked up by the skin. Here are some lovely herbs that make a happy home in any child's sock bath or infused massage oil.

Lavender Blossoms (*Lavandula* species) - The little blossoms have a delightful, sedating scent and also cleanse the skin, encourage wound healing, and ease muscle soreness.

Chamomile (*Matricaria recutita*) - These little apple-scented blossoms help to soothe inflammation and skin irritations, easing the pain of sore, tight muscles while calming and encouraging sleep.

Please Note: Chamomile is in the ragweed family and can cause reactions in susceptible individuals.

Linden (*Tillia* species) - The flowers and leaves are cooling and calming, help to ease muscle tension, and they smell wonderful!

Elder Flower (*Sambucus nigra*) - Delightful tiny cream-colored flowers soothe inflammation and rashes while promoting wound healing.

Roses (*Rosa* species) - These beautiful, fragrant flowers are anti-inflammatory, astringent, and heart opening!

Calendula (*Calendula officinalis*) -The pretty yellow-orange flowers help to happily heal irritated, injured skin, burns and bruises.

Lemon Balm (*Melissa officinalis*) - This herb smells delightful and makes a lovely, relaxing addition to the bath or as a infused oil for topical use.

Catnip (*Nepeta cataria*) - Even though catnip is exciting for kitties, it helps calm humans and can help to ease away pain. Put it in your bath and you may find that your kitty pays you a visit while you are in the tub!

Invite these gentle, calming herbs into your home! Please supervise young children on their herbal endeavors, offer guidance, and enjoy this special time together!

Hey Kids!

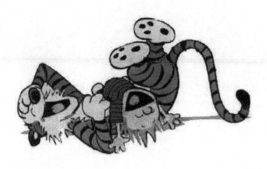

Do you want to make bedtime fun? You can invite our gentle herbal friends to help you make bedtime wonderful! Creating herbal preparations is a way to show gratitude for the herbs and the Earth from which the plants grew! Below are three different types of herbal preparations that you can make for a fun bedtime. Make all three to use or choose your favorites!

At my house we like to start getting ready for bed with a delicious cup of tea after dinner. We take time to read a book or color while sipping our tea. Then we follow up the tea with a soaky herbal bath and a foot rub before climbing into bed for the night! You can use these ideas to create your own lovely bedtime routine which will surely send you off to a dreamland!

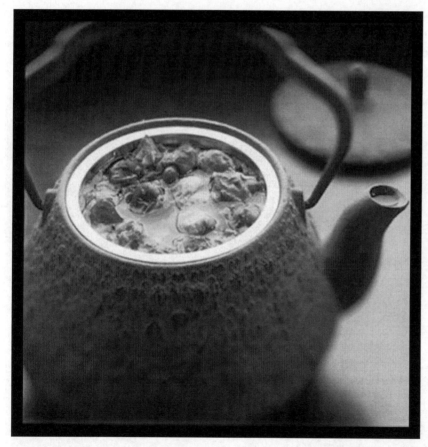

Brew Up Some Tea!

Sipping on a tasty warm cup of tea before bed is a great way to settle down from the excitement of the day and get ready to sleep. There are a lot of herbs to choose from! Some of my family's favorites to sip before bed include relaxing herbs that help calm us down. Good choices include chamomile, linden, rose, catnip, and lemon balm. Herbs that warm you up and help you digest your dinner also make tasty teas before bed. Try cinnamon, ginger, cardamom, anise seeds, and even mints - though mints can be more cooling than warming.

Teas are made by steeping 1 to 3 teaspoons of herb per cup of hot boiling water in a covered container for 4 to 30 minutes depending on the herb used. When making tea it is important to have your parent's permission before using the stove. Always ask for help if you need it so you don't get burned! Also be sure to cover your tea while it steeps. This helps to keep the lovely aromatic oils from the plants in your teacup, otherwise those oils will escape into the air with the steam.

325

Choose herbs to make your tea from the ideas above or try one of the recipes below!

A Few Tasty Tea Blends to Try

Sweet Dreams Kiddo Tea

My kids love this tea blend for soothing away nightmares. We enjoy drinking it as a family at the end of a stressful day or when things are just not settling right. The St. John's wort seems shine a little light into the dark of night giving some relief from nightmares and gentle chamomile relaxes away stress. Lavender blends well with the pepperiness of the St. John's wort and offers a little extra soothing relaxation to this blend!
Ingredients:
2 teaspoons St. John's wort (*Hypericum perforatum*)
2 teaspoons chamomile (*Matricaria chamomilla*)
Pinch of lavender (*Lavandula* spp.)
Honey to taste
2 cups of boiling hot water
Directions:
Combine the herbs and water and steep with a cover on top for around 4 minutes. Longer steeping time can make your tea bitter.
Add honey to taste and enjoy sipping!

Rosy Balm Tea

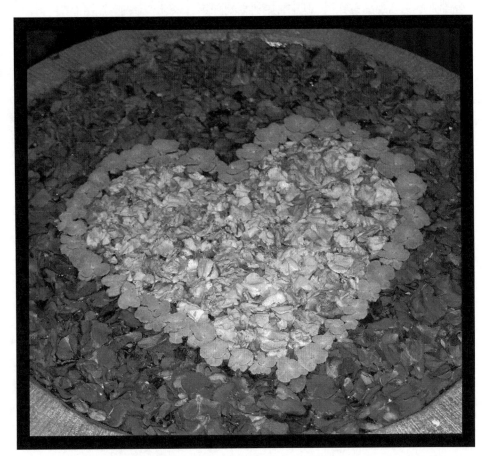

This tea is soothing and cooling making it a great tea for hot nights of summertime.

Ingredients:
2 teaspoons rose petals (*Rosa* spp.)
2 teaspoons lemon balm (*Melissa officinalis*)
1 teaspoon spearmint leaf (*Mentha spicata*)
Honey and lemon to taste
2 cups of boiling hot water
Directions:
Combine the herbs and water, cover and steep for 10 to 30 minutes.
Strain, add honey and lemon to taste, and enjoy hot or cold.

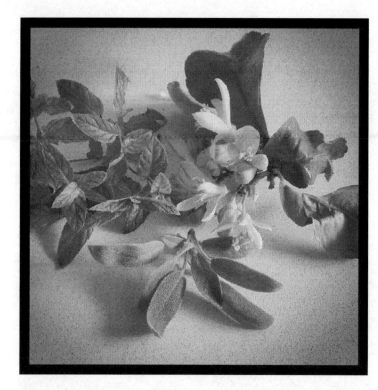

Calming Linden Tea

This recipe makes one big mug of tasty herbal tea, and is perfect to enjoy before bed or anytime a little calm is needed.
Ingredients:
2 teaspoons dried linden leaf and flower (*Tillia* spp.)
1 teaspoon dried spearmint (*Mentha spicata*)
1 teaspoon dried Calendula flowers (*Calendula officinalis*)
1 pinch catnip leaf (*Nepeta cataria*)
12 ounces boiling hot water
Directions:
Place all the herbs in a heatproof container and cover with boiling hot water.
Let steep for 15 to 30 minutes.
Strain and serve with honey if desired

Family Herbal Chai
Adapted many times from Yogi Bhajan

Warming and delicious, what could be better than a cup of herbal chai after dinner? Enjoy this tasty tea together as a family!

Ingredients:
6 cups water
10 cloves (*Syzygium aromaticum*)
14 whole black peppercorns (*Piper nigrum*)
14 green cardamom pods (*Elettaria cardamomum*)
2 to 4 cinnamon sticks (*Cinnamomum cassia*)
2 to 3 slices ginger root (*Zingiber officinale*)
½ to 1 teaspoon fennel seeds, optional (*Foeniculum vulgare*)
2 tablespoon rooibos, optional (*Aspalathus linearis*)
Up to 2 tablespoons total of other optional herbs, such as Astragalus (*Astragalus membranaceous*), turmeric (*Curcuma longa*), rose hips and petals (*Rosa* spp.), lycium berries (*Lycium barbarum*), Calendula flowers (*Calendula officinalis*), Echinacea (*Echinacea* spp.), or holy basil (*Ocimum tenuiflorum*)
1 to 2 cups of milk or milk alternative
Honey to taste

Directions:
Count the cardamon pods, cloves, peppercorns, and fennel seeds into a mortar. The is especially fun for young kiddos.

Have fun crushing the herbs with the pestle!!
Then place the all of the crushed herbs, ginger slices, and cinnamon sticks in a covered pot along with the water, covering the pot only half way.

Simmer the herbs in the water for 15 to 20 minutes being careful not to boil your tea.

Remove from the heat and add the rooibos. Steep for another 5 minutes.

Strain the herbs out of the tea, rinse out your pot and put the tea back into the pot.

Add the milk and honey to taste.

Gently warm until steamy hot.

Pour into mugs and enjoy!

Keep leftovers refrigerated and enjoy within a few days. This herbal chai is also delicious cooled and served over ice!

Make a Sock Bath

A warm bath before bedtime is just the thing for a restful sleep. Sock baths are kind of silly (who ever thought of bathing with a sock?) and fun to make! The sock gets stuffed with lovely herbs and other interesting things like oatmeal, then you toss it in the tub. The sock is kind of like a big tea bag and while it soaks in the hot water your bathtub becomes like a big cup of tea to soak in! Here is how to make your own sock bath.

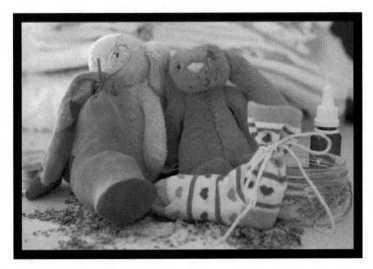

Ingredients:

A big clean, adult size sock

Herbs to choose from (see "Herbs for Kids to Enjoy in Bedtime Baths & Infused Massage Oils" for ideas)

Any of the following: oatmeal, powdered milk, baking soda, salts

A big plastic cup (a good choice because it won't break).

A big spoon

Instructions:

Gather all of your supplies and lay them out on a work surface such as a table.

Pick which ingredients you would like in your bath. Smell, touch and look at the herbs and other ingredients and pick your favorites!

Put a handful or big spoonful of each ingredient into the cup. This is the mixture that will go into the sock. You want to have around 1 to 2 cups of bath mixture in the cup when you are done.

Using the big spoon, mix the herbs and other ingredients inside the cup.

Stretch the opening of the sock over the top of the cup and then turn the cup over so that the contents fall into the sock.

Tie the top of the sock into a knot. If your sock is not long enough to tie, use a rubber band or piece of string to secure it shut.

Squeeze and smell the sock. This will release the good smells of the herbs inside! Give your sock a good cuddle and get ready to take a bath!

Ask your parent to help you get your bath ready and enjoy!

How To Take A Sock Bath

Here is our favorite way to take a sock bath:

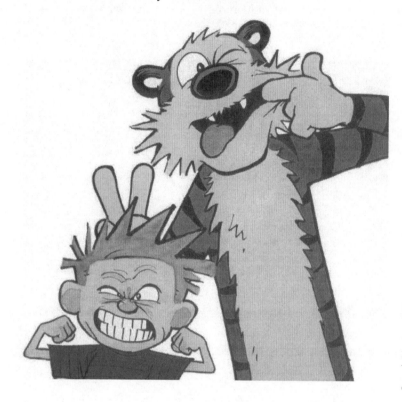

First, fill the tub with the hottest water you can get from your spout. You will need to ask for help from an adult to ensure that you don't get burned by the hot water.

Add the sock and then let it steep in the tub while the water cools down to bathing temperature. As it soaks, your sock becomes like a big tea bag and your tub like a big tea cup!

Ask an adult to help you check that the water is cool enough bathe in and then get into the tub.

Swish the sock around in the tub and squeeze it. All kinds of fun, lovely smelling herbal goodness will be released from the sock as you play! You can also use the sock to gently clean your skin if you want!

Enjoy a Foot Rub with Special Herbal Oil

Infused oils are an herbal preparation that herbalists love! When herbs are soaked in an oil, the goodness of the herbs moves from the herbs into the oil. Then you take the herbs out of the oil and are left with a lovely oil to massage on your body! You can also use your new herbal oil to make things like lip balms and salves - pretty cool uh?

There are a few different ways to make an infused oil. Here is a simple and easy way to make your own infused oils.

Materials:
Dried herb of your choice (see "Herbs for Kids to Enjoy in Bedtime Baths & Infused Massage Oils" for some great suggestions!)
Olive oil
Clean, sterile and dry jar with a tight fitting lid
Paper bag, optional
Cheesecloth

Instructions:

First, make sure your jar is sterile by either placing it in hot, boiled water or sanitizing it in the dishwasher. Stay safe and don't get burned - get help from an adult if you need it! Be sure to let your jar dry all the way before making your infused oil because water can cause your oil to spoil!

Next, loosely fill your jar with your chosen herb. Then slowly pour olive oil over the herbs until they are completely covered with oil. Place your lid on top. After a few hours check back on your oil. The herbs may have absorbed some of the oil. If that happens, add more oil until the herbs are covered again.

From here it is up to you!

You can set your jar in a cool, dark place or in a warm, sunny window to infuse. Some herbalists feel like it is important to keep their infusing oils cool, while others like to use heat to assist the oil in getting all of the goodies out of the herbs. If you chose to place your infusing oil in a warm, sunny window, you can place it in a paper bag for extra protection from light if you wish. You can even set your oil out at night to soak up the magic of the moon. My favorite? I like to infuse my oils right in the sun!

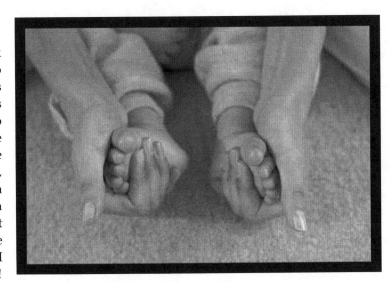

Be sure to label your oil! Include the plant you used, the part of the plant (such as flowers or leaves), and the date.

Shake the oil each day for 7 to 10 days if you are using the sun or for at least 2 weeks if you are keeping your oil cool.

Then strain the herbs out of the oil by pouring it through cheesecloth into a bowl or jar.
Place your herbal oil in a clean, dry jar and cap tightly. To keep it fresh, store your oil in a cool, dark place or in the fridge.

Now it is time for a bedtime foot rub! Take a little bit of oil and spread it on your hands. Then rub your feet, one foot at a time. Your feet carry you throughout your day - this is a great time to say thank you and appreciate all those adventures your feet have taken you on! Finish up by putting a cozy pair of sock on your feet. You can also ask a parent to give you a little massage and even trade massages if you wish! This is a great way to enjoy time with a loved one while settling down for the day.

Sweet Dreams!

Sources
Rosemary Gladstar's Family Herbal by Rosemary Gladstar
Kids, Herbs, & Health by Linda B. White, M.D. and Sunny Mavor
The View From Sunnyfield: Herbs To Treat Anger by Matthew Wood

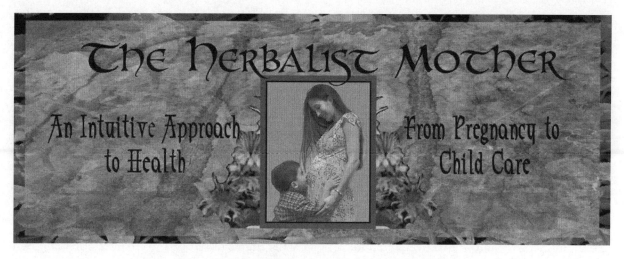

HERBS FOR CHILDHOOD FEAR

by Sabrina Lutes

Fear. It can be pretty alarming when your young one digs their heels into the earth and refuses to participate because they are afraid of something that may occur, or may even be a fabrication of their minds and we just don't understand all of what is going on for them. Real or imagined, their brains are reeling with thoughts of danger. Their bodies are pumped full of cortisol and adrenaline and they are looking to you for comfort and are understandably so, wildly unsure what to do with themselves. Their world view has become hyper focused and no amount of cajoling words or actions from you seem to help. As a parent who has experienced this and as an adult who once was that child experiencing these feelings, I fully appreciate the emotions of "oh fuck, now what do I do??".

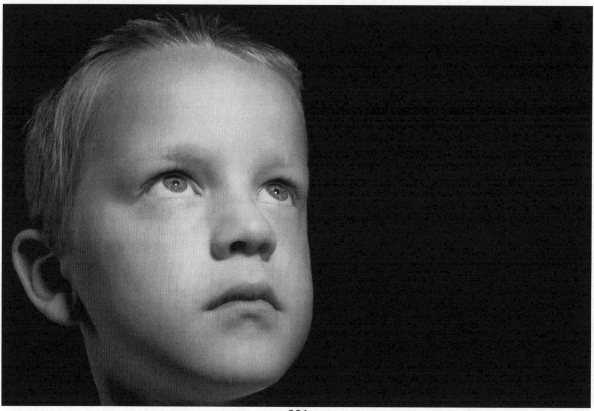

It's a tough road to navigate. So many childhood fears are developmental, completely normal, and certainly life preserving. We don't want them to simply go away. There are very real times when these skills are useful to us. Thunderstorms, natural disasters, fire, heights, dogs…all very real dangers. And unfortunately, many times these will interfere with everyday life. Learning to cope with what is a normal development for your child is paramount as well as being present for your child so that they may learn their own coping skills to either completely grow out of this fear, or have healthy strategies to work around it as they grow older. This may mean that we seek professional help and certainly remain loving throughout.

A child clings to her mother in the night, frightened with tears welling up in her eyes and lips quivering. Lightening streaks across the sky, the night air is filled with ozone and crackling molecules as a deafening BOOM shakes the windows. The young mother begins slowly telling a tale of the gods playing games in the sky, and sprays the air with the scent of Lavender and Chamomile. Slowly but surely the child calms and falls asleep after nervously asking that the story be repeated.

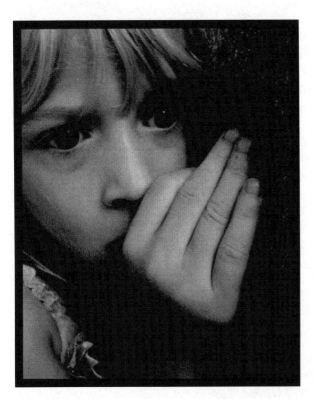

As parents and caregivers, we must seek to understand and help. Sometimes we mettle and things become worse, and sometimes we have breakthroughs and the child is able to come through the incident with a sense of accomplishment. The fear may not be gone, but with each experience it eases. Only by listening and paying close attention to our children, will we find some clues as to how to handle each situation.

Some things that have helped our family, and what I have observed in watching other children and families work through these occurrences, is to acknowledge the child's feelings, make a plan (be sure that everyone is on the same page if possible), don't force any action when the child is afraid unless it is something that is absolutely necessary, revisit what is causing the fear, if child is old enough and developmentally capable to understand you can try education (explain what happens in a storm), creating a story is immensely helpful. Use herbal remedies such as teas, balms, pastilles, aromatherapy, charms, and seek professional help from a caring counselor when things seem more than just developmental.

After a scary event, a little boy is begging his parents to not participate in an activity that he usually loves so much. For him, at this time, the world feels hard to be in and the class feels far away and hard to control what will happen. His mother packs small herbal pastilles made of vanilla and herbs and honey. On the box she has placed a word or symbol that the boy has learned means calm. Whenever he begins to feel afraid he can use them to sooth his mind and still the butterflies in his stomach. He uses them throughout the day, and while he is still afraid, they do bring some relief.

I use herbs and diet to help soothe frayed nerves and calm the storm that is fear. By bolstering a child with good nutrition and supportive herbs they are more capable of dealing with situations with more vigor. In my experience herbal remedies do not stop the emotion of fear from occurring. They are however a beautiful tool, and incredible ally when the world around us is feeling rocked by the chemical messengers within us, screaming at us to run for cover. It is my feeling that by placating these sensations, after the danger has passed or before a child must face an event that frightens them…soothe a stomach full of butterflies and cool the fire that consumes reason, then the child's brain that directs executive functioning can come back online and help redirect.

In observing fear within myself and others as well as my little one, I have found that it certainly presents in different physical ways. There is angry fear (the fight response), there is fear that leaves us cold and clammy and needing to be protected, there is a fear that forces us to run and since running is not an acceptable way of handling these situations in our society it often makes the child hysterical.

In angry fear there may be red cheeks, sour stomach, clenched fists, stamping feet. A child will refuse to do what is asked of them or tantrum before an event that they find frightening. They may appear anxious and pacing. Herbs that I have found useful for this are Lavender, Chamomile, Lemon Balm and Hibiscus. This is a great time to offer these herbs cold, in popsicle or jello form. My child feels very cared for when these treats are presented

and they help to cool the fire and calm the fears. A change in scenery may also help, go for a swim, give them a bath (with Chamomile bath tea of course!)

A child gets home from classes and is just not able to settle down. She is combative and mad. When asked how her day was, she stomps around the house, and later breaks down in huge hot sobs. She's sad and angry, and doesn't want to go back to school the next day. She is afraid that she will have to perform in front of the whole class. Instead of trying to allay her fears with words, her father gives her a hibiscus popsicle and draws a warm bath. He has stuffed a muslin bag with lavender, rose, and chamomile and allowed the warm water to draw out its sweetness. After the child is calmed and comforted they sit down and talk about an action plan that the child feels she can handle.

In what I call, cold fear, the child is pale, sullen, maybe shaking and feeling sick to their stomach. They may be withdrawn and quiet. For these moments I like to use warming herbs and herbs that help digestion. Chamomile, Fennel, Ginger, Marshmallow, Slippery Elm. This is a wonderful time to make warm teas, give pastilles, and use infused oil for massage.

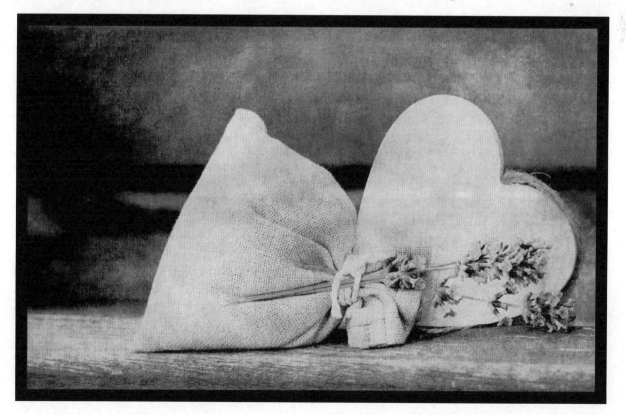

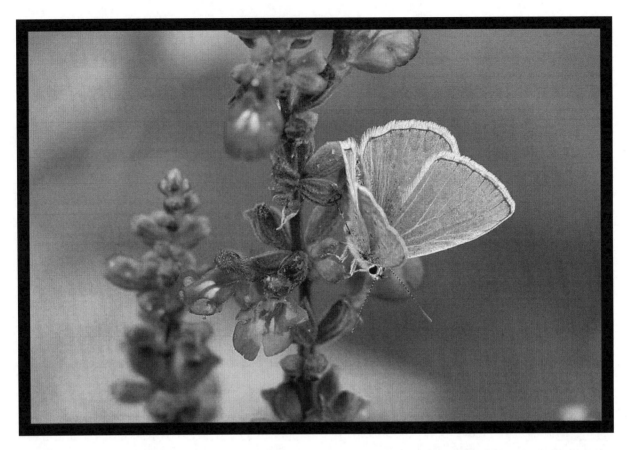

A child knew that a new program was about to begin, that new children would be there and new teachers. For days he worried and felt frightened about what it would be like, how it would feel. He wasn't sure he wanted to be away from home for so long. He became clingy and sad. He would hide behind his parents wherever they went, because he wasn't quite sure when things would start. His parents assured him that he would be told when his class would begin, but his young mind did not have a strong sense of time yet. So the days leading up to his new adventure his parents gave him warm teas of Chamomile, Oatstraw, and Fennel. They marked a calendar so that the little boy could get a sense of when things would indeed happen. They also spent plenty of time together as a family, doing special things to help anchor him in the new and upcoming routine. They discovered children books where the characters were experiencing similar situations. They also made it a point of getting to bed on time and eating well was also emphasized.

Nervines that help strengthen our nervous systems are truly a boon. Going into a situation already frazzled can make the physical responses even more overwhelming. When our nerves are nourished by healthy habits such as eating whole foods, getting enough sleep, plenty of outdoor activity, and balancing day to day requirements such as school and extracurricular activity blended with lots of down time.

Hysterical fear, in my experience, takes a different approach. It is my opinion that bringing a child to where they feel safe is a great way to handle this. I know that there are so many differing ideas out there, but my reasoning is that when a child, or anyone is in such a heightened state, requiring them to stay where they are scared will not help anyone. As a mother, my job is to help my little one feel safe. We can always return and either show them that the situation was indeed safe or we can agree with them that it was not and talk about it with them if they are old enough to process the information. Cuddles and soothing words or songs are such a wonderful way to help children through this as well as yourself. These moments can feel so wild and out of control!

I also believe that when we as caregivers are helping our little ones through these times that we can benefit from soothing nervines and taking care of our own needs. I discovered that my son experienced many fears that I had growing up and still do. When he was having moments of fright, my instinct was to feel it with him. It made it hard for me to be present in his experience without reliving some of my own. What helped me immensely was to remind myself that his physiology and perception, while seemingly similar, were actually his own! His brain was forming its own neural pathways in response to whatever it was that was scaring him. If I could just take care of myself, while helping him feel validated and safe then it would work out in the end. It meant giving myself lots of reminders, lots of warm tub soaks, and warm tea.

Mythology can also be utilized to help guide our young ones through their fears and can also help alleviate our adult need to fix things for our children. Knowing how to trust their process while supporting them through their journey is empowering to everyone involved. Much like Enki in Inanna's story of descent to the underworld (not a children's story), we can pick the dirt from our fingernails (experience) to create the creatures that would bring the food of life and water of life (our herbal allies, long sweet hugs, staying balanced and solid even as our child rides the waves of fear) so that they may be sent as aid to our children that they may be bolstered in a way that is strengthening. Stories can also create a sense of commonality of human experience for our children. They now have an animal hero, or a human heroine to attach their own desires to as they can, safely from your lap or by your side, experience feelings of fear and triumph as the story is told and retold. By choosing old fables and folk tales where the protagonist is experiencing a similar situation, a child can see that they are not alone, and it is a great teaching for us as adults as well, realizing that humans have experienced and overcome all throughout our history.

In closing, helping a child through childhood fear can feel daunting and lonely. It can be so very helpful to speak with trusted friends and allies when walking this labyrinth. Those that have gone before may have some helpful advice,

and those that are in it can sigh and say they get it. If your child is really suffering from fear, and things are just not letting up for them, it is so important to seek help from someone qualified and keenly aware of fear and anxiety issues for children.

Below is a list of the herbs and foods that I feel have supported us the most through our moments of fright and mother anxiety caused by them.

Oatstraw (*Avena sativa*): infusion is an old ally of mine. For those that can enjoy oats, a warm bowl of oatmeal can fill a nervous stomach up and give it something to stay busy with.

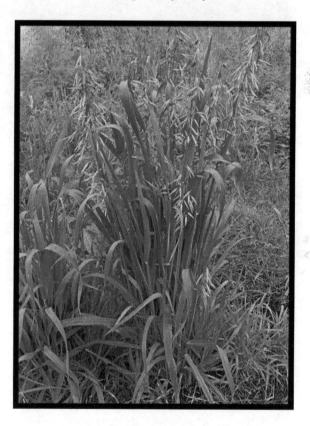

Lavender (*Lavendula spp.*): used in teas, bath sachet, room sprays. Massage oils
Lemon Balm (*Melissa officinalis*): tea, popsicles, jell-o
Rose: pastilles, popsicles, bath sachet, tea. Massage oil
Chamomile (*Matricaria chamomilla*): tea, bath sachet, room spray (calming, soothes stomach jitters)

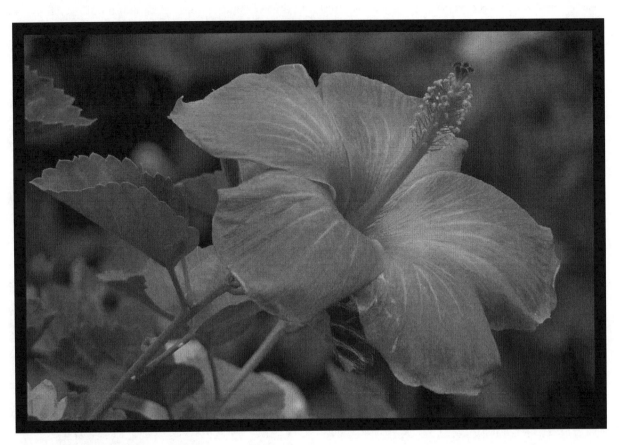

Ginger (*Zingiber officinale*): tea, pastilles (warming, settles nervous stomach)

Fennel (*Foeniculum vulgare*): tea

Marshmallow (*Althea officinalis*): pastilles, tea (soothing to stomach mucosa)

Slippery Elm (*Ulmus rubra*): pastilles (soothing to stomach mucosa, nourishing)

Vanilla (*Vanilla planifolia*): pastilles, tea, massage oil (calming, sweet)

Hibiscus flowers (*Hibiscus sabdariffa* L): cooling, very tasty

Healthy fats (avocado, fish, nuts, seeds, dairy, and grass-fed or wild animal meats): adds strength and resiliency to the myelin sheath that surrounds nerve cells and feeds the brain.

Recipes

Vanilla Honey Pastilles
1-part Slippery Elm powder
½ part Marshmallow root powder
Seeds scraped from 1 vanilla pod
1/16th part Ginger root powder
1/8th part of Rose infused brandy

Enough honey (infused honey makes a wonderful addition, chamomile or lavender honey would be great here) to create a paste

Mix all ingredients together until a stiff dough is formed that is easily rolled. Roll into a long coil and cut into peanut sized pieces or roll individually. Place in a warm oven on very low heat and allow to dry, or use dehydrator. Store in an air tight container (if left out in air the honey's natural tendency to attract water will make them go bad)

Calming Sleep Room Spray
1-part Chamomile flowers
1-part Lavender flowers

Blend and store in an airtight container.
Boil 1 cup of water, pour over 4 tablespoons of herbs and cap tightly. Allow to steep for 30 minutes. You want a strong smelling infusion! Add ¼ cup of ever clear to the infusion and pour into a spray bottle. Keeps refrigerated for about 2 weeks.

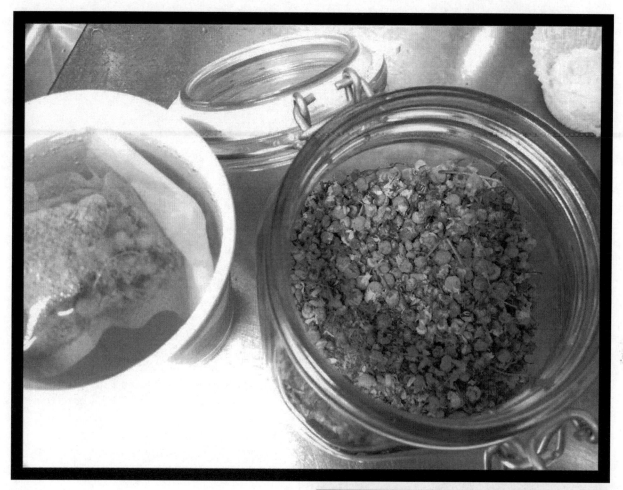

Infused Honey

Making infused honey is easy and also a lovely way to add herbs to children's preparations (as long as child is older than 1 year)

In whatever size jar you choose, fill up ¼ full with dried roots or berries, or ½ full for delicate plant parts like dried flowers or leaves. Fill the remaining with honey. Cover and let sit for two weeks.

Place jar in a double boiler and gently heat just until honey is thin enough to strain. Strain into a clean jar. Be careful not to get any water into your honey, or you will end up with fermentation.

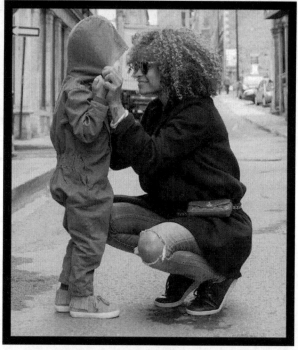

Natural Remedies for Children with Special Needs

by Elaine Sheff

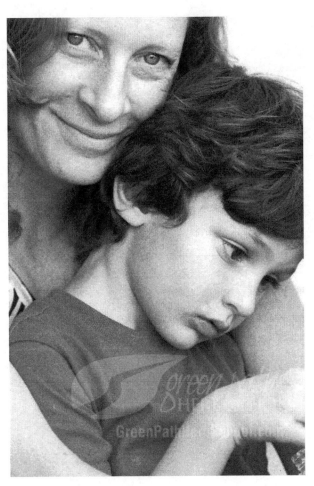

Elaine and her son Zane.

As both an herbalist and a mother of a special needs son, I have had many opportunities to apply the information I discuss in this article. I have had lots of occasions to try things and carefully watch outcomes. As my son Zane has grown and changed, so have the remedies and protocols that I use. My family's journey has been beautiful, exhausting, heart touching, filled with elation and tinged with deep pain. I would not change it for anything. We have had lots of help along the way. Teaching these classes is one of the ways I give back. If you have a special needs child, I hope this information is helpful for you and your loved ones. I am honored to share some of these natural and supportive tools with you.

Starting with a look at changelings and continuing on to statistics on children with special needs, this paper details six basic ways for children and their care-givers to stay healthy. It contains many herbs and recipes for the sensory challenged child. Relaxing and stimulating essential oils and flower essences are also discussed.

Changelings: A History of Special Needs Children

A changeling is typically described as a baby fairy, troll or elf that was secretly substituted for a human child. This idea was common among medieval folklore from diverse cultures such as Cornwall, Ireland, Scotland, England, Scandinavia, Spain, Whales, Nigeria, and the Philippines ("Changeling").

The concept of a changeling was used as a way to explain babies and children with unexplained diseases, deformities, or developmental challenges. The greater likelihood for boys to have birth defects correlates to the belief that male infants were more likely to be substituted.

It was believed that the changeling would initially resemble the human it substituted, but gradually they would grow "uglier" in appearance and behavior: "ill-featured, malformed, ill-tempered, given to screaming and biting." ("Kirkpatrick").

Historically, people believed that by treating the changeling cruelly, parents could force the return of their child. Methods used were quite abusive and included whipping, holding the child in a shovel over a fire, submerging the baby in water, or putting the child in a hot oven ("Changeling"). Changelings would often be left to die from exposure, or might even be murdered. Belief in changelings continued in parts of Ireland until as late as 1895, with the infamous killing of Bridget Cleary by her husband, who believed that she was a changeling. ("Kirkpatrick").

Many herbs and plants were used to ward off magical folk or to retrieve human children. Bathing the changeling it in a tea of toxic foxglove was thought to send it back to its true parents and retrieve the human child. A rowan tree could be planted near the threshold of the house to deter fairies. Other fairy deterrents included gorse, rosemary, dill, and St. Johnswort. A ritual of lighting a piece of fir-wood and carrying it three times around the bed of the mother and baby was thought to prevent child swaping. ("Kirkpatrick").

Today, some autistic people associate themselves with changelings. They cite their own feelings of being in a world where they feel they do not belong, or even wondering if they are the same species as the "neurotypical" people around them ("The").

I wonder if we might develop a new concept of a changeling. Many animals will kill and sometimes eat their young if they are sick or deformed ("Morell"). We have seen that the human species obviously has that instinct as well. But humans also have higher thinking processes and so can see a bigger picture. Certainly, we have an opportunity to open our minds to expand the ideas of what is valuable about the human condition. I suggest that "changelings" have several things to offer us, as a species and as individuals. We can learn a lot from people with special needs. Zane, for instance, sees the world in a unique way, from a different perspective. I think he will grow to be an amazing problem solver who can think outside the box. I know several parents of children with Downs Syndrome who say that their children have taught them how to open their hearts and love more deeply.

I offer that changelings, or special needs children are part of our evolutionary process as a species. Not all genetic mutations work out (and not all special needs children have genetic mutations), but those mutations that do work can help a species adapt to new environmental changes and pressures. Might this be another value of those humans that are different?

Most of the parents of special needs children that I know wouldn't change their beloved kids. I think most people who are considered special needs like who they are as well. Personally, it has been a hugely enriching experience for me to get to know more people of diverse abilities.

Zane with one of his creations that he calls "machines".

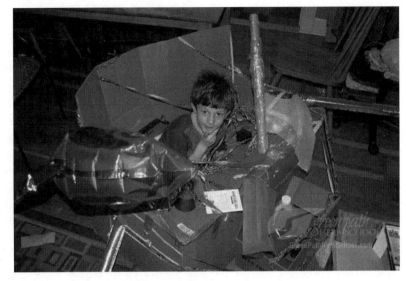

Children with Special Needs:

According to the Department of Health and Human Services, the definition of a special needs child is one who has or is at increased risk for a chronic physical, development, behavioral, or emotional condition and who also requires health and related services of a type or amount beyond that required by children generally.

Statistics on Special Needs Children and their Families:

• Childhood disability is on the rise. Emotional, behavioral, and neurological disabilities are now more prevalent than physical impairments ("U.S.").
• Approximately 10.2 million children in the US, which represents 15 percent of all US children, have special health care needs ("U.S.").
• More than a fifth of US households with children have at least one child with special needs ("U.S.").
• In 2009, it is estimated that 1,194,258 special needs children in the U.S. used at least one type of alternative health care or treatment ("Survey").

For caregivers and families, the statistics are similarly disturbing.
• 40 to 70 percent of parents and family caregivers have clinically significant symptoms of depression. About a quarter to half of these caregivers meet the diagnostic criteria for major depression ("Women").
• Caregivers who are often under extreme stress have been shown to age faster than their counterparts of the same age. This level of stress can take as much as 10 years off a family caregiver's life ("Elpel").
• The divorce rate among parents of kids with ADHD or Autism is nearly twice that of couples in the general population ("Robbers").
• Women who are family caregivers are 2.5 times more likely than non-caregivers to live in poverty and five times more likely to receive Supplemental Security Income (SSI). (Study conducted by researchers at Rice University and data compiled from the Health and Retirement Study funded by the National Institute of Aging and conducted by the University of Michigan, 1992-2004.)

An article by the author about the extreme challenges, and grace, of mothering her child with special needs: http://lalaland.mamalode.com/blog/2012/10/23/rising/

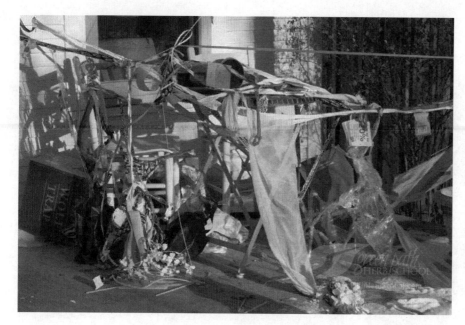

Zane's porch "machine".

As this machine grew over several months, we started to wonder if it might ensnure the mail carrier. It is impossible to see the true of intricacy of Zane's machines. There are literally layers upon layers of special little details taped into his work.

Helpful Fundamentals for Children, Parents, and Caregivers
(Or, how to stay healthy when things get hard.)

Six Basics for Keeping Our Kids (and Ourselves!) Healthy:

1) Drink more water.

Did you know that a normal adult is 60 to 70 percent water? Next to air, water is the most necessary element for human survival. All of our organs need water in order to function properly and eliminate wastes. The *minimum* amount of water for a healthy adult (150 pounds) is 8 to 10 eight-ounce glasses a day. Make sure to drink more if you exercise, sweat more or live in a hot climate.

Note: Dr. Paul Winchester, M.D., led a study reporting that birth defect rates in the U.S. were highest for women who conceived in the spring and summer months. This period of increased risk correlates with higher levels of chemicals and pesticides in surface water throughout the country. Experts suggested installing a reverse osmosis water system for drinking and cooking needs ("Clean").

2) Take a daily multivitamin.

The nutritional content of America's vegetables and fruits has declined during the past 50 years -- in some cases dramatically. Multivitamins assure that you get all the nutrients you need, even if there are gaps in your diet. Researchers are finding that some important vitamins (D and E particularly) and minerals are protective against disease in amounts that may be difficult to obtain through diet alone, no matter how conscientious you are. Supplements for children with special needs should include all the B vitamins, Vitamin C, Calcium, Magnesium, Omega 3's and vitamin D3. Probiotics are also extremely important. Choosing a high quality vitamin without fillers or binders will increase effectiveness. Capsules or liquids are easier to digest than tablets.

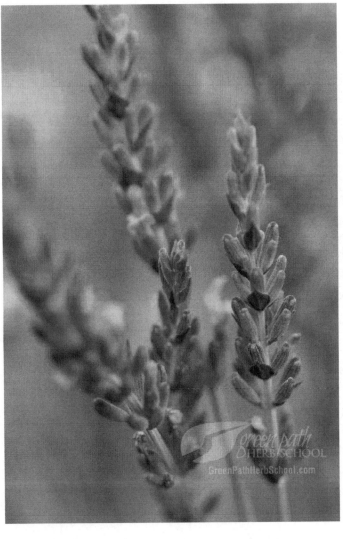

Lavandula angustifolia

3)Eat organic, whole foods.
Our organs, especially our digestive systems, have a hard time handling foods and chemicals that don't occur in nature. Whole foods are found in nature with all their parts intact. Fragmented foods include all foods that are missing original parts: they are modified by being refined, concentrated, fractionated, hydrogenated, preserved, colored or having additives. The Center for Science in the Public Interest reports that many common food dyes can increase risks for hyperactivity, cancer and allergies. Avoid ingredients such as artificial color, FD&C (Food, Drug and Cosmetic) Red #40, Yellow #6 and Blue #1. Common additives including BHA, BHT, TBHQ and MSG can also cause health problems. Headaches, hyperactivity and allergies can be common symptoms of exposure to food additives ("Clean").

Instead, focus on nutrient-dense, toxin-free, whole-foods including starchy & non-starchy vegetables, animal protein and fats, fermented foods, raw dairy (when tolerated) and fruit, nuts & seeds (in moderation). It is especially important to eat only organic animal products, as toxins accumulate the higher up you go in the food chain. No particular diet fits everyone.

Many special needs children have food allergies. I most often see reactions to gluten, casein, dairy eggs and sugar. Make sure to read labels carefully. To find out what works best for your family, consider keeping a health journal. Watch yourself and your child for symptoms of food reactions such as fatigue, anxiety, depression, insomnia, food cravings, ear infections, constipation, diarrhea, eczema, psoriasis, headaches or irritability. I often find an Elimination Diet (Elimination Diet PDF link) to be helpful.

Eliminate plastics including harmful chemicals such as BPA and phthalates, which can leach into your food or beverage from plastic packaging. BPA is also found in the linings of many canned goods. Use glass or stainless steel containers instead. When possible, choose fresh or frozen fruits and vegetables over canned ("Clean").

4) Get plenty of sleep.

Easier said than done, I know. Yet sleep rejuvenates our body and mind. It allows the brain to organize long-term memory and integrate new information, as well as giving our body a chance to repair and renew tissue, nerve cells and focus on parasympathetic body processes such as digestion and elimination. Getting enough sleep is especially important when you are sick or stressed. The average child needs 10-12 hours of sleep a night. Kids with special needs often need more, and can conversely have a harder time getting it.

5) Take a daily essential fatty acid supplement.

Essential fatty acids (EFA's) such as alpha linolenic acid (an omega 3 fatty acid) and linoleic acid (an omega 6 fatty acid) are called "essential" because our body can't make them - we need to eat them. They play a crucial role in brain function as well as normal growth and development: they make up the cell membrane for every cell in our body. EFA's help with heart health and can even improve insulin sensitivity to make our bodies better at using stored body fat for energy. They reduce joint pain, help with autoimmune diseases, reduce inflammation, and elevate mood. In the typical American diet, we get way more Omega 6 oils, so I recommend concentrating on the Omega 3's. Some of the food sources of essential fatty acids are fish, shellfish, flaxseed oil, hemp oil, chia seeds, pumpkin seeds, sunflower seeds, leafy green vegetables and walnuts.

6) Go green.

There is no doubt about it. There is a direct impact on our health and the health of our environment, from what we eat to what we breathe and the products we use. In July of 2011, a Stanford University study cited environmental factors as a cause of autism in 62% of the cases they found ("Digitale"). I recommend going through your home and reading your household labels, paying close attention to your home cleaning products, body care products, and the chemicals you use in and around your house. What you put on your skin is just as important as what you put into your body. Many household and personal care products also contain harmful chemicals that enter the body through direct contact with skin.

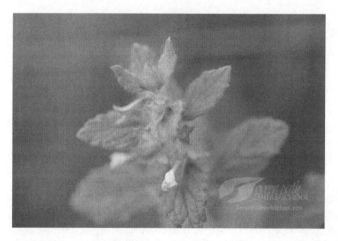

Melissa officinalis

Choose simple green replacements whenever you can. Look for products that are free of parabens, synthetic fragrances, petrochemicals, sulfates, lead (in some lipstick!), formaldehyde, phthalates, toluene, parabens and antimicrobial pesticides such as triclosan and triclocarban. Pay special attention to baby care items such as baby wipes, diaper creams and lotions. Avoid using artificial air fresheners, dryer sheets, fabric softeners, or other synthetic fragrances. Replace your vinyl shower curtain with one made of fabric, or install a glass shower door. ("Environmental"). Additional information regarding personal care product ingredients can be found on the Environmental Working Group's website at http://www.ewg.org ("Clean").

The Connection to the Nervous System:

The nervous system is the body's most rapid means of maintaining homeostasis. It has three main functions. The first is sensory. We sense changes in our body and the external environment. Next we interpret these changes – what do they mean? Lastly we integrate that information by responding with a muscular action or hormonal secretion.

Most special needs kids have issues with their central nervous systems. These challenges can be medical, emotional, or developmental. A few of the most common issues include ADD/ADHD, cerebral palsy, epilepsy, Down Syndrome, autism, learning problems, loss of a sense such as hearing, sight, or language, or having a diverse movement need such as a wheelchair or braces.

Sensory Processing Disorder:
I will focus here on sensory processing issues, as I consider them a common issue for most children with special needs. Sensory processing disorder is a condition in which the brain has trouble receiving and responding to information that comes in through the senses.

One of the main functions of the thalamus is to filter the sensory information coming to the brain such as noises, visual stimuli, sensations of touch, as well as information from our own muscles and organs. In this way, we can prioritize important information and eliminate the vast amount of incoming information we don't need. Imagine if that process didn't happen well. We have all had moments like these, but this is a common occurrence for people with sensory processing disorder, autism and schizophrenia. Sounds seem too loud, or not loud enough. Clothing, tags in particular, may feel uncomfortable and scratchy to the skin. Light pressure on the skin might feel uncomfortable or even painful.

Some children will only have a sensitivity in one area. Or they may be hypersensitive with one sense and under responsive with another. Their experience may also fluxuate so that sometimes that sense is over stimulated and sometimes it is under stimulated. An example of this would be a child that can generally not tolerate loud noises but at times makes lots of loud, repetitive noise themselves.

Let's consider each sense on its own.

Smell
Inside of our nasal cavities, we have specialized sensory cells, called olfactory sensory neurons. These cells connect directly to the brain ("How"). This means that smells can directly impact and influence the brain, changing mood and invoking memory. Smells can often be overwhelming to children with sensory processing disorder. This can lead the child to reject many foods or react strongly to overwhelming smells such as synthetic fragrances.

For a child that needs more olfactory input, pure essential oils are extremely useful. A few drops can be applied to a t-shirt or pillow, or added to an aromatherapy diffuser. For topical use, start with a 1% dilution such as 5 drops of essential oils mixed with 1 ounce of carrier (vegetable) oil. Be sure to research any essential oil before using it. Also let the child smell the oil prior to use. Choose oils that they are drawn to. If essential oils seem too overwhelming, they may be diluted more and/or applied to the feet. It is often helpful to rotate smells throughout the day, using more stimulating oils such as peppermint (*Menta piperita*), rosemary (*Rosmarinus officinalis*) or one of the citrus oils (*Citrus spp.*) in the daytime and more calming oils such as lavender (*Lavandula spp.*), ylang ylang (*Cananga odorata*) or Roman chamomile (*Chamaemelum nobile*) in the evening. See below for a more detailed list.

Menta piperita

Taste

We each have a unique perception and experience of the foods we taste.

Children affected by sensory processing issues can be very particular about food texture, color, smell and flavor. Some children, for instance, will only eat white foods. This can make it very challenging to provide a balanced, nutritious diet. Other
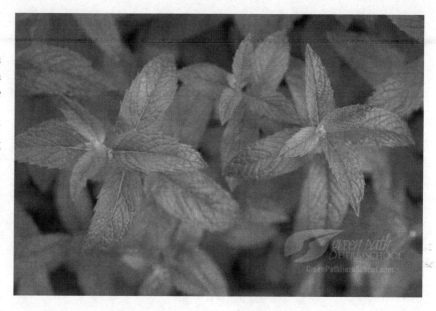
children may only be able to consume liquids through a feeding tube. To add extra nutrients to any diet, I recommend cooking with organic bone broth whenever possible.

Luckily, herbs can be taken in many different forms. Depending on the child, you might try a tea, syrup, tincture, hand made pill (powdered herbs incorporated into a sweet syrup such as honey or maple syrup and dried well) or herb infused honey (not for children under 1 year old). Applesauce, jelly, juice or food can also work well. In a pinch, I have even used ice cream.

Sight

I am always curious, when a child can see, what they are drawn to visually. For instance, in preschool my son used to gather and carry around ALL of the white crayons. When he was in kindergarten, he would only wear red shirts. Surrounding a child with colors that they are drawn to can be soothing and reassuring. Color therapy might be an interesting consideration for a child of this type. Sometimes, when in crowded environments with lots of visual stimulation or noise, my son preferred a blanket over his stroller. I have also seen children that are especially drawn to certain environments. Many children are soothed in nature and I find this an ideal and healing setting for most special needs children.

Touch

Touch provides many opportunities for healing or conversely for overstimulation. It is important to realize that some children can find even very light touch painful and overwhelming, where some children seek lots of tactile input. Sometimes even clothing such as seams, tags, waistbands, or rough textures can be intolerable. There are many tools for helping a child tolerate touch more easily or get the increased input they need. Yoga, massage and other forms of healing touch such as Reiki or cranial sacral therapy can be very healing.

Proprioception is the ability to sense stimuli within the body helping us know our body's position, motion, and equilibrium. For example, even if a person is blindfolded, he or she should know if they are standing up or lying down ("Proprioception"). If proprioception is hard for a child to evaluate, they often seek more physical input.

For children who need more physical input, there

sensory brushes, etc. Some schools are now using yoga balls or "T" shaped wooden chairs for their more fidgety students. Joint compression, a technique in which various joints are "pushed together" can help meet the need for deep pressure exhibited by many children with autism.

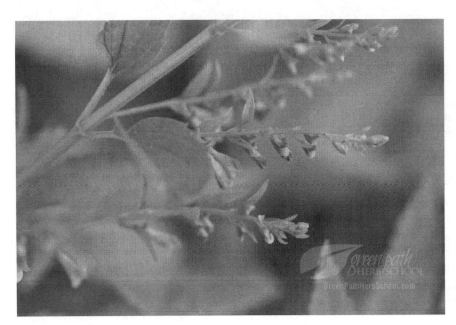

Scutellaria latifolia

Hearing
Noise has been the most challenging sense for my son. Zane's hearing is acute. When he was a baby, a sneeze would startle him to tears. I recall him standing at our living room window as a toddler and saying, "Train". I would hear nothing, but sure enough, a couple minutes later, I'd hear that train whistle. For more information about our family's auditory adventures read this: <u>http://mamalode.com/story/detail/the-sound-of-success</u>.

Depending on the child, you might try incorporating different types of music, starting at a very low volume. I have also tried small gongs and chimes. One of the best tools I have found for Zane is headphones used for noise reduction at shooting ranges. When he has had enough noise, he can put them on.

Sensory Diet:
Occupational Therapists can come up with a Sensory Diet for a child. This is a carefully designed, personalized activity plan that provides the sensory input they need to stay focused and organized throughout the day.

This is a helpful checklist that can help narrow down a child's sensitivities:
Sensory Checklist: <u>http://www.sensorysmartparent.com/sensory-checklist.pdf</u>

Herbs for the Nervous System:

In my experience, nervines (herbs that act on the nervous system) are quirky. A single nervine can have a very different effect on two different people. Let's use coffee (yes, it's an herb) as an example. Some people, such as myself, drink a small amount of coffee and feel jittery for hours. Others can drink a whole pot of coffee and then go right to sleep. I think it prudent to test nervines by using a single drop of tincture or a sip of tea. See how the child reacts and then decide if this particular plant will be beneficial to them. Similar to essential oils, timing is important. Generally, use stimulating nerviness earlier in the day and relaxing nervines in the afternoon or evening.

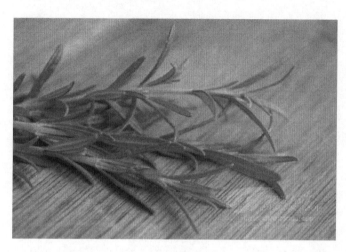

Rosmarinus officinalis

Stimulating Nervines for Boosting Energy:

Nervine Stimulants activate the nervous system. These herbs can be useful for those who are generally under-responsive. For certain other individuals, they can be used for an over-stimulated nervous system, much as the pharmaceutical stimulant Ritalin is used for hyperactive states. Many of these herbs contain caffeine, including coffee, guarana, kola, green and black tea, yerba mate and cocoa. Although it is tempting for people who are exhausted or burning the candle at both ends, I would caution that using caffeine will only increase fatigue and impair health in the long term. I recommend instead using adaptogens (see below). Interestingly, some herbs such as green tea, yerba mate, rosemary and cocoa are also high in antioxidants, which help stop the cascade effect of free radical damage in cells.

•Coffee (*Coffea arabica*): strongly stimulating to the nervous system. Many coffee beans on the grocery store shelf are rancid, so it is best to get locally roasted whole beans, store them in the freezer and grind them yourself.

•Guarana (*Paullinia cupana*): A powerful stimulant to the nervous system. Good for short term energy and memory.

•Kola (*Cola acuminata and Cola nitida*): a nervous system stimulatnt, kola nut is also a cardiac (heart) tonic.

•White, green or black tea (*Camellia sinensis*): white tea is the youngest leaf on the tea plant and has less caffeine. Green tea has more caffeine and fermented black teas have the highest caffeine content. Camellia is also an excellent source of antioxidants.

•Yerba mate (*Ilex paraguariensis*): can be highly stimulating for some people, and produce a subtle effect for others.

•Cocoa (*Theobroma cacao*): One of our favorite additions to sugar and milk, this bean is both stimulating and highly antioxidant.

•Rosemary (*Rosmarinus officinalis*): a good herb for memory and stimulating both to the mind and the senses, rosemary is an excellent antioxidant as well.

•Gotu kola (*Centella asiatica*): A rejuvenating nervine and adaptogen, gotu kola is especially good for the mind and memory. It is also good for adrenal fatigue and sluggish metabolism.

Adaptogens help the body, particularly the limbic system, adapt to stress and maintain balance. Some adaptogens are stimulating, especially if taken in excess. It is best to try an adaptogen in the morning and see how you react to it before incorporating it into a daily regime.

•American Ginseng (*Panax quinquefolius*): low dose and restorative providing energy and vitality.

•Eleuthro (*Eleutherococcus senticosus*): formerly called Siberian ginseng, eleuthero is a helpful adaptogen for overall stamina and hormone balance.

•Ashwaganda (*Withania somnifera*): a more relaxing herb, this is a wonderful plant for those that are over stimulated or having trouble sleeping.

•Gotu Kola (*Centella asiatica*): excellent for the mind and memory, this herb is useful for those that feel foggy or need extra brainpower.

•Licorice (*Glycyrrhiza glabra* and *G. uralensis*): this root is especially good for adrenal burnout. Contra-indications: high blood pressure. Using over longer periods of time (several weeks or months) can cause electrolyte imbalances. I like to use licorice in formulas with other herbs.

•Rhodiola (*Rhodiola rosea*): excellent for immune response and my favorite adaptogen for depression and deep fatigue.

•Holy Basil (*Ocimum spp.*): good for the immune system and for encouraging vital energy, holy basil decreases stress hormone levels, corticosterone in particular. It is also a powerful antioxidant and anti-inflammitory.

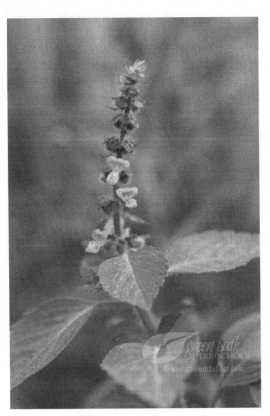

Ocimum sanctum

Stimulating Essential Oils:

A note on essential oils: essential oils are the scent molecules of plants. They are extremely potent and more is not better. Please research any oil before you use it, including its contra-indications. Some oils are not appropriate for children. Most oils should not be applied directly to the skin before first diluting them.

•Orange (*Citrus sinensis*): is refreshing, uplifting, and antidepressant. It is a wonderful, sunny fragrance that will brighten any environment.

•Atlas Cedar (*Cedrus atlanticus*): A circulatory stimulant, it is non-irritating and can be helpful for varicose veins. It is an excellent adrenals toner and is useful for emotional balancing and grounding.

•Peppermint (*Mentha piperita*): A cooling oil that is good for sluggishness, mild depression and headache, peppermint oil is also useful for the adrenal glands and digestive function.

•Rosemary (*Rosmarinus officinalis*) is helpful for mental fatigue. It is a tonic support for mind and memory. It is helpful to smell rosemary as you are learning something new and then smell it again when you want to recall that information. I often recommend this oil to students.

•Spruce (*Picea mariana*): Spruce helps tonify the adrenals and balance the emotions. It combines nicely with Atlas cedar and peppermint. It is expectorant and anti-bacterial for respiratory infections.

Supportive Nervines:
Nervine Tonics help one manage stress better by strengthening and supporting the nervous system. They combine nicely with adaptogens and relaxing nervines.
•Oat Seed, Fresh (*Avena fatua and A. sativa*): an incredible tonic and support for those under long-term stress.
•Lemon Balm (*Melissa officinalis*): a gentle and calming restorative to the nervous system, this herb makes an uplifting, nutritious and delicious tea.
•St. Johnswort (*Hypericum perforatum*): a deep nervous system tonic, it is useful for mild to moderate depression. St. Johnswort is calming and relaxing.

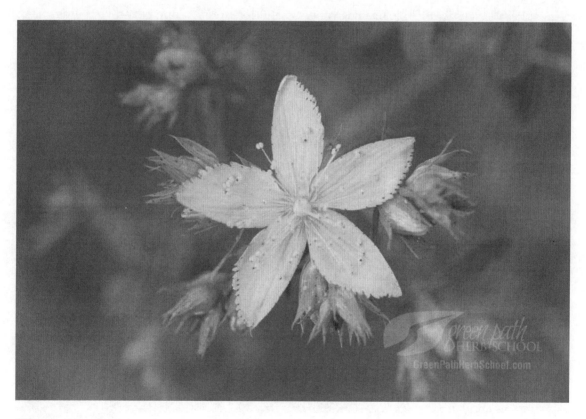

Hypericum perforatum

Relaxing Nervines to Encourage Calmness and Reduce Stress:
As they are calming but not sedating, these herbs can be taken throughout the day instead of just at night to lower the overall stress response in the body.
•Skullcap (*Scutellaria spp.*): a soothing nervine for overwhelment and stress. Skullcap is one of my favorite herbs for sensory processing issues, or as I call them "Skullcap Moments". http://sylvanbotanical.com/wp-content/uploads/2014/07/Volume-1-Issue-2-2014-final.pdf
•Passionflower (*Passiflora incarnata*): an relaxing and calming herb, passionflower is also good for heart palpitations and easing one into a natural sleep.

•Oat Seed, Fresh (*Avena fatua and A. sativa*): an incredible tonic and support for those under long-term stress with an over-worked brain.

•Motherwort (*Leonarus cardiaca*): a grounding and centering herb, this plant is useful for agitation and nervous energy. Motherwort is also one of my favorite herbs for menopausal distress and hot flashes.

•Lavender (*Lavandula spp.*): A gentle relaxer, this herb is an aromatic addition to a tea. It is useful for insomnia, nervous stomach, anxiety, and headache. For some people, a little can go a long way.

•Chamomile (*Matricaria recutita*): a gentle and soothing herb useful for both children and adults. The tea is soothing to the nerves and aids digestion. The fresh flower tincture is stronger and useful for insomnia.

•Linden flower (*Tilia spp.*): is an excellent remedy for calming and relaxing nervous tension and stress. A gentle antidepressant, it is an appropriate relaxing herb for both children and the elderly.

•Kava (*Piper methysticum*): This relaxing root is useful for stress, insomnia and pain. It is one of my favorite herbs for anxiety and panic attacks.

•Catnip (*Nepeta cataria*): is a very gentle relaxer appropriate for sensitive or small children and adults. It is a useful remedy for stomach upset and to aid digestion.

•Wood betony (*Stachys officinalis*): a good tonic for relaxation, stress and pain, including headaches.

Valeriana officinalis

Relaxing Essential Oils:

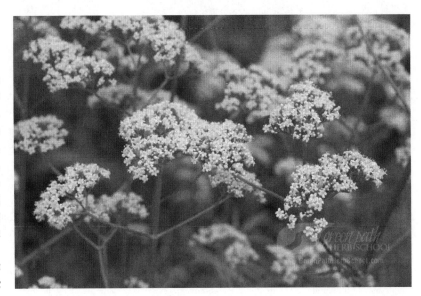

•Roman Chamomile (*Chamaemelum nobile*): is gently relaxing and calming for nervous tension and depression. It is anti-spasmodic, anti-inflammatory, emotionally balancing and safe for use during pregnancy and with small children.

•Lavender (*Lavandula spp.*): has an amphoteric action, meaning it can be relaxing or stimulating based on dilution. Use a small amount for calming and a large amount for stimulation. It is a wonderful first aid oil and can be used full strength on most people's skin for burns, infections, bug bites and skin inflammation and irritation (do a patch test first by applying a small amount to the skin and watching for redness or irritation). It is helpful for pain and headaches as well as being soothing for emotional upset.

•Marjoram (*Origanum marjorama*): is calming, relaxing, emotionally balancing and sedating. It is a useful anti-spasmodic for intestinal cramps, menstrual cramps or skeletal muscle cramping. It is helpful for countering long term stress.

•Mandarin (*Citrus reticulate*): This is an excellent oil for anxiety and hyperactivity in children or adults. It is a helpful sedative for chronic insomnia as well as being a good emotional balancer for dark moods or depression. Citrus oils may increase photo-sensitivity so be cautious applying this oil to the skin when you will be outside.

•Spikenard (*Nardostachys jatamansi*): smells just like valerian root and acts in a similar fashion as a strongly sedating nervine for insomnia and pain. It is also helpful for reducing anxiety.

•Ylang ylang (*Cananga odorata*): is antidepressant, and helpful for both stress and anxiety. It is extremely sedating.

Sedating Nervines to Encourage Sleep:

•Valerian (*Valeriana spp.*): is helpful for pain, tension, sleeplessness and smooth muscle cramps. For some children with ADD, hyperactivity or ADHD, it can help them with focus and attentiveness.

•Hops (*Humulus lupulus*): an exceptional remedy for encouraging sleep, hops is also used as a digestive bitter. Be warned: it is very bitter.

•Wild lettuce (*Lactuca virosa*): a helpful anodyne (pain reliever), wild lettuce has tranquilizing effect useful for insomnia and nervousness. It is sedative and antispasmodic.

•California poppy (*Eschscholzia californica*): an excellent herb for stress, helping to encourage sleep. California poppy is also pain relieving and soothing for agitation, nervousness or anxiety.

•Catnip (*Nepeta cataria*): is a very gentle relaxer appropriate for sensitive or small children and adults. It is a useful remedy for stomach upset and to aid digestion.

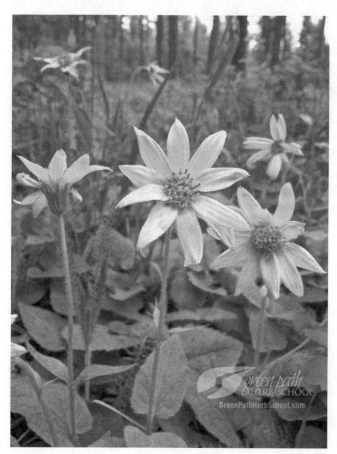

Arnica cordifolia

Flower Essences

Flower essences are gentle, yet profound. I find them very helpful for assisting movement and aiding resolution with the emotional and spiritual aspects of healing that often accompany physical health issues. They are safe to use with prescription medications and can be used either orally or externally on the skin. A dosage is around 3 drops.

•Rescue Remedy or Five Flower Formula: this formula contains five essences including Rock Rose, Impatiens, Clematis, Star of Bethlehem and Cherry Plum. It is useful for stress, anxiety, trauma and panic attacks. It is especially helpful in emergency situations.

•Chamomile (*Matricaria recutita*): encourages emotional balance. Chamomile is helpful for those who are moody, easily upset or irritable.

•Arnica (*Arnica mollis*): aids recovery from deep-seated strain, shock or

scarring from past traumas. I have used it for medical trauma.
•Pretty Face (*Triteleia ixioides*): helps one reconnect to their body after severe neurological injury. Encourages self-acceptance in relation to one's personal appearance.
•Cosmos (*Cosmos bipinnatus*): helps a child come into his/her body and out into the world. Encourages coherent speech and communication.
•Shooting Star (*Dodecatheon hendersonii*): useful for grounding, and helping ease feelings of profound alienation.
•Indian Paintbrush (*Castilleja miniata*): helps to integrate the body and the soul. Good for low vitality and exhaustion.
•Yarrow (*Achillea millefolium*): helpful for creating a protective shield when one feels vulnerable and easily depleted.

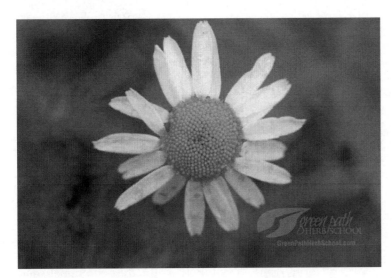

(*Chamaemelum nobile*)

Herbal Formulas:
I hope that parents and caregivers will use these recipes both for themselves and for their children. When taking care of a special needs child, it is extremely important to take breaks and practice self-care. Note: remember to use Freid's Rule or Clark's Rule when deciding the dosage for a child (see below). The tincture dosages below (and on most herbal product labels) are for adults.

Awake! Tincture
An herbal tincture is a liquid extraction of an herb that you can use internally, or topically as a liniment. This internal formula can be used to stimulate and enliven the senses and the mind. Although it is designed as a tincture formula, you can also make it as a capsule or a tea. Dosage: 30-60 drops up to 3 times a day, 2 "00" capsules 3 times a day, or 3 cups of tea a day.
•1 part Gotu Kola (*Centella asiatica*) tincture
•1 part Eleuthero (*Eleutherococcus senticosus*) tincture
•1 part Holy basil (*Ocimum spp.*) tincture
•½ part Rosemary (*Rosmarinus officinalis*) tincture
•½ part Peppermint (*Mentha piperita*) tincture

Relaxing Tea
This gentle tea is appropriate for both adults and children. It can be used as a daily nourishing tea and will give the body extra nutritive support during times of physical, emotional or mental stress. It can be drunk throughout the day and may be diluted if the flavor is too strong or made into ice cubes and added to water.
Use one part of each of the following: (by weight)

- Chamomile flowers (*Matricaria recutita*)
- Catnip herb (*Nepeta cataria*)
- Peppermint herb (*Mentha piperita*)
- Nettles herb (*Urtica spp.*)
- Horsetail herb (*Equisetum spp.*)

Mix herbs together. Use ¼ ounce of the blend per cup of water. Boil water and pour over the tea. Let steep for 30 minutes to 2 hours, strain and enjoy!

Equisetum hyemale

Stress Relief Bath Blend

After a long, difficult day, this bath is a wonderful treat to help relieve tension and encourage relaxation. If you know a caregiver of a special needs child, this bath salt makes a great gift!

- 2 cups unscented bath salts (you can use sea salt, Epsom salt, Celtic sea salts, Dead Sea salts, etc. Don't use table salt as it has anti-caking agents that are counterproductive to the healing process.)
- 30 drops Lavender (*Lavandula spp.*) essential oil
- 30 drops Mandarin (*Citrus reticulate*) essential oil
- 30 drops Rose geranium (*Pelargoneum spp.*) essential oil
- 10 drops Roman chamomile (*Chamaemelum nobile*) essential oil

Mix bath salts and essential oils well and store in an airtight glass jar. Unplug the phone and light a candle. Put on some relaxing music. Draw a hot bath and slip into it. Add 2 tablespoons Stress Relief Bath Blend, sit back and relax!

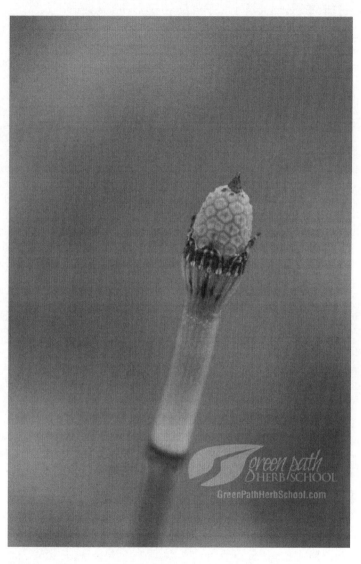

Nervine Tonic Tincture

This formula can be used as a daily support for stress, low energy and to encourage mental acuity. Take 60-90drops 3 x a day. Measure the tinctures by volume to create the formula.

- 3 parts Eleuthero (*Eleutherococcus senticosus*) tincture
- 2 parts Skullcap (*Scutellaria spp.*) tincture
- 2 parts St. Johnswort (*Hypericum perforatum*) tincture
- 1 part fresh Oat Seed (*Avena spp.*) tincture
- 1 part Vegetable Glycerine

Sweet Dreams Spray
•1 2/3 ounce Water
•1/3 ounce Brandy (to preserve your mixture)
•4 drops Hornbeam (*Carpinus betula*) flower essence
•4 drops White Chestnut (*Aesculus hippocastanum)* flower essence
•4 drops Oak (*Quercus robur*) flower essence
•10 drops Lavender (*Lavandula spp.*) essential oil
•5 drops Clary Sage (*Salvia sclarea*) essential oil
•3 drops Sandalwood (*Santalum Spicatum*) essential oil
Shake well. Spray on face, wrists, and pillow, or add a few sprays to your evening bath. Sweet dreams!

Insomnia Tincture
I like tinctures for sleep issues, because they work really fast. You can use the tincture when first going to bed, or take it if you wake in the middle of the night. If you are sensitive, try these herbs individually before making them into a formula. That way, you can exclude any that don't work. Make sure you try them on an evening when you don't have an important event scheduled the next day.
•1 part Skullcap (*Scutellaria spp.*) tincture
•1 part Passion Flower (*Passiflora incarnata*) tincture
•1/2 part Valerian (*Valeriana spp.*) tincture
•1/2 part fresh Chamomile (*Matricaria recutita*) tincture
Add tinctures together and mix well. Take 60-90 drops before bed, or upon awakening in the middle of the night. If not asleep within 20 minutes, take another dose.

Sleep Easy Tea
This calming tea is safe for both children and adults. You can also put the tea into an evening bath for babies, small children, or those that find it hard to drink tea.
•1 part Chamomile Flowers (*Matricaria recutita)*
•1 part Skullcap Herb (*Scutellaria spp.*)
•1 part Spearmint Leaves (*Mentha spicata)*
•1 part Lemon Balm Leaves (*Melissa officinalis)*
•1/2 part Lavender Flowers (*Lavandula spp.)*
Mix all herbs together and store in an airtight glass jar. For one lovely cup of tea, pour one cup of boiling over 1 tablespoon of Sleep Easy Tea and let it steep for 20–30 minutes. Strain and enjoy!
Additional Information:

Determining Dosages for Children:
•**Fried's Rule:** The dose of an herb for an infant less than 2 years old is obtained by multiplying the child's age in months by the adult dose and then dividing the result by 150. An example would be if an adult tincture dosage is 20 drops. For an 8 month old child you would take 20 x 8 to get 160. Then divide: 160/150 = which would be approximately 1 drop of tincture.
•**Clark's Rule:** for children aged 2-17. Take the child's weight in pounds and divide by 150 pounds. Multiply the fractional result by the adult dose to find the equivalent child dosage. For example, if an adult dose of tincture calls for 30 drops and the child weighs 30 pounds, divide the child's weight by 150 (30/150) to get 1/5. Multiply 1/5 times 30 drops to get 6 drops. This method can also be used for elders, dogs and cats.

Chelation therapy: is a very useful treatment for metal poisoning. In this treatment, chemicals bind to heavy metals in the body and prevent them from binding to other agents. They are then excreted from the body. It is worth checking into this therapy if you have a child with a neurological issue or learning disability.

Medical Tests to Run Both Prenatally and for Children:
There is significant research confirming that the health of the parents, their toxic load (if you will) before conception and the health of the mother throughout her pregnancy can dramatically influence the mental, physical and emotional health of a child. Below are some tests I recommend to help clarify compromised physiological pathways, and any hormones or nutrient deficiencies that may need to be addressed. It is best to do these before conception and rectify problems then, but these tests are also very helpful for children with special needs.

1. MTHFR stands for the methylenetetrahydrofolate reductase gene (methyl-ene-tetra-hydro-folate-reductase). If the MTHFR gene is slightly altered (mutated), the MTHFR enzyme will not function properly in processing amino acids, the building blocks of proteins. It is also essential for a chemical reaction involving forms of the B-vitamin folate (also called folic acid or vitamin B9), which is crucial to healthy nervous system function. ("MTHFR").
2. Thyroid: Hypothyroidism can cause birth defects, Down Syndrome, autism and developmental issues. Ask for Labs: TSH, T3, T4, Reverse T3 enzyme, Thyroid Antibodies: (autoimmune issue) TPO and thyroglobulin
3. Ferritin: iron levels - 50 or above is good.
4. Adrenals: a saliva test works great!
5. DHEA levels
6. Oxidative stress: oxidative stress on the DNS (urinary test)
7. Lipid panel (look for elevated cholesterol and high triglycerides) (Dr. Erica Peirson)

In Conclusion:
I have been continually amazed and humbled watching parents and caregivers support and nurture their special children. I have immense respect and empathy for the beautiful and often painful journeys of these families. I hope this information helps ease their road and increase other's understanding in some small way. Remember that as your child changes and grows, so will the herbs and remedies that work the best for them. I hope this article gives you some helpful tools for the journey.

References:

"Changeling." . Wikipedia, 22 July 2014. Web. 28 July 2014. <http://en.wikipedia.org/wiki/Changeling>.
"Children & Youth With Special Health Care Needs (CYSHCN)." National Center for Medical Home Implementation. N.p., n.d. Web. 28 July 2014. <http://www.medicalhomeinfo.org/how/care_delivery/cyshcn.aspx>.
"Clean Your Plate: Six Steps to Removing Harmful Chemicals From Your Diet | Autism Companion." Autism Companion. N.p., n.d. Web. 28 July 2014. <http://www.autismcompanion.com/clean-your-plate-six-steps-to-removing-harmful-chemicals-from-your-diet/>.

Digitale, Erin. "Non-genetic factors play surprisingly large role in determining autism, says study by group." *News Center*. Stanford Medicine, 4 July 2011. Web. 4 Aug. 2014. <http://med.stanford.edu/news/all-news/2011/07/non-genetic-factors-play-surprisingly-large-role-in-determining-autism-says-study-by-group.html>.

"Environmental Toxins Linked to Rise in Autism." Mercola.com. N.p., n.d. Web. 28 July 2014. <http://articles.mercola.com/sites/articles/archive/2014/04/02/environmental-toxin-exposure.aspx>.

Epel, Elissa S. , Elizabeth H. Blackburn, Jue Lin, Firdaus S. Dhabhar, Nancy E. Adler, Jason D. Morrow , and Richard M. Cawthon. "Accelerated telomere shortening in response to life stress." PNAS 101: 17312-17315. Web. 29 July 2014.

"Health Problems." KidsHealth - the Web's most visited site about children's health. The Nemours Foundation, n.d. Web. 28 July 2014. <http://kidshealth.org/kid/health_problems/>.

"How Does Our Sense Of Smell Work?." - *Intelihealth*. AETNA, 12 Feb. 2010. Web. 30 July 2014. <http://www.intelihealth.com/article/how-does-our-sense-of-smell-work>.

Kirkpatrick, Betty . "Horseshoes, herbs and urine: all useful for warding off fairies - The Caledonian Mercury." *The Caledonian Mercury*. Caledonian Mercury, n.d. Web. 30 July 2014. <http://caledonianmercury.com/2011/03/15/horseshoes-herbs-and-urine-all-useful-for-warding-off-fairies/0015522>.

"Minnesota Department of Health." Chemicals of Special Concern to Children's Health. N.p., n.d. Web. 28 July 2014. <http://www.health.state.mn.us/divs/eh/children/chemicals.html#voc>.

Morell, Virginia. "Why Do Animals Sometimes Kill Their Babies?." . National Geographic, 28 Mar. 2014. Web. 4 Aug. 2014. <http://news.nationalgeographic.com/news/2014/03/140328-sloth-bear-zoo-infanticide-chimps-bonobos-animals/>.

"MTHFR gene." *Genetics Home Reference*. Genetic Home Reference, 28 July

"Proprioception." *Medterms*. Medicinenet.com, 19 Mar. 2012. Web. 4 Aug. 2014. <http://www.medterms.com/script/main/art.asp?articlckcy=6393>.

Robbers, Sylvana, Meike Bartels, C. E. M. Toos van Beijsterveldt, Frank Verhulst, Anja Huizink, and Dorret Boomsma. "Abstract." National Center for Biotechnology Information. U.S. National Library of Medicine, 7 Mar. 2010. Web. 29 July 2014. <http://www.ncbi.nlm.nih.gov/pmc/articles/PMC3056000/?report=classic#CR21>.

"Special Needs Digest." : Autism and Toxic Chemicals: Are Pollutants Fueling Rising Prevalence?. N.p., n.d. Web. 28 July 2014. <http://www.specialneedsdigest.com/2014/03/autism-and-toxic-chemicals-are.html>.

"Survey Results." CSHCN 2009/10: Use of alternative health care or treatment, Nationwide. N.p., n.d. Web. 28 July 2014. <http://www.childhealthdata.org/browse/survey/results?q=1815&r=1>.

"The Changeling." : *The Changeling*. Faerydae's Tales, Hedge Witchery Books, 23 June 2010. Web. 4 Aug. 2014. <http://faerydaestales.blogspot.com/2010/06/changeling.html>.

U.S. Department of Health and Human Services, Health Resources and Services Administration, Maternal and Child Health Bureau. The National Survey of Children with Special Health Care Needs Chartbook 2005–2006. Rockville, Maryland: U.S. Department of Health and Human Services, 2007.

"Women and Caregiving: Facts and Figures." *Family Caregiver Alliance*. Family Caregiving Alliance, National Center on Caregiving, 31 Dec. 2003. Web. 4 Aug. 2014. <https://www.caregiver.org/women-and-caregiving-facts-and-figures>.

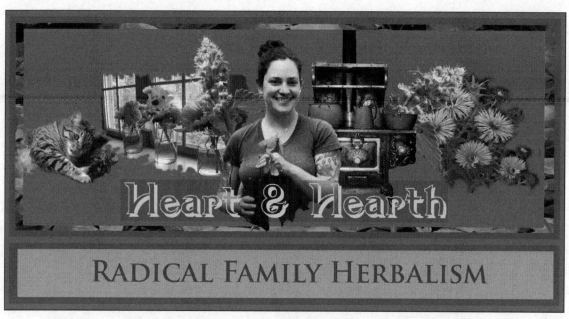

Heart & Hearth

RADICAL FAMILY HERBALISM

TREATMENTS FOR TODDLERS & CHILDREN

by Juliette Abigail Carr

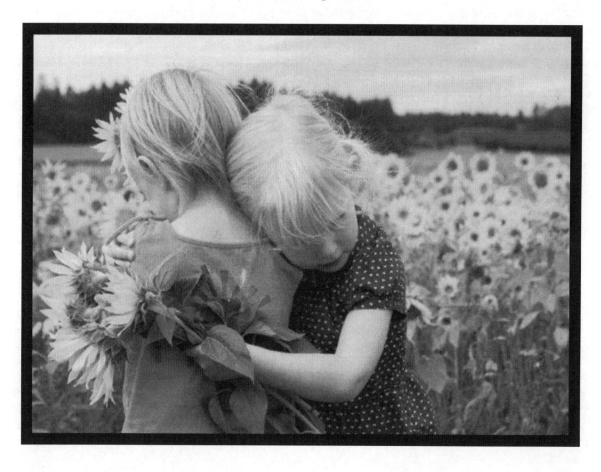

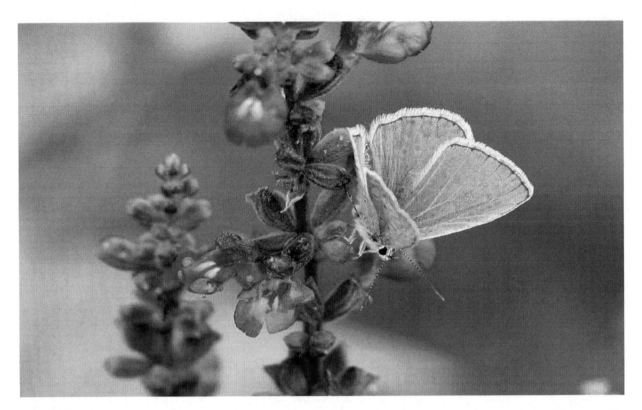

Home herbalism is who we are and how our families work, healing practiced around the kitchen table around the world and across the centuries. Thank the Good Green Earth that home herbalism happens as a reflex, intuition built on a foundation of herbal fluency that allows us to live as herbalists in every moment. Caring for our own children is the entry point into herbalism for many of us, inspired by the awe of a new life to look for safe, natural, inexpensive means of nurture.

However, many herbal references either start with older children, glossing over the unique needs of the preschool and younger crowd entirely, or try to cover all children as a monolith. This ignores the incredible spiritual and transformative power of littles' lives, both in their daily personal growth and change, and in their powerful role within a family and community. Children this age often need our support as they explore the world and how their body relates to it, engage with other beings, and discover their own perceptions. Families of young children likewise need community support to flourish during a time that is simultaneously joyful and challenging, infuriating and enlightening, frustrating and transformative.

Herb Choice: Look Ye To The Olde Wyves

In any given moment of using herbs, we consider Materia Medica, that lovely organizational system of the vast repository of herbal knowledge. What herbs are useful for a dry, hacking cough, or a stuck, wet cough, or a cough with back pain or a sinus headache or postnasal drip? Of the many herbs for cough, which is the perfect herb or combination for this unique cough?

When we work with toddlers and young children, there are extra considerations, given that they are fierce but tiny, and in a more-or-less constant state of anabolism and mental and physical development.

The first question to consider when choosing an herb or creating a formula for the daycare and preschool set is this: *Is this herb traditionally used in young children?*

358

It may sound obvious, but we live in a culture where the new thing is often confused with the best thing. It can be easy to forget amid the hullabaloo of the next incredible panacea from across the globe featured in glossy magazines and the nightly news, but the Olde Wyves knew what they were about. We do not want to be experimenting on our littles, we want to reach for the right herb the first time.

When searching for the right herb for a child, the best place to look is tradition: what have people always used for this issue in a person this age? What did our ancestors use, in our current region or elsewhere? What do the native people in our area traditionally use? In using traditional remedies we turn to thousands of years of healing tradition for guidance, and stand together with those who came before in practicing the healing arts. There is power, honor, and love in upholding good traditions (and in revamping bad ones: I'm looking at you, system of Eurocentric heteronormative racist misogynistic oppression). There is also safety: allow those who have come before to teach you their accomplishments, instead of reinventing the wheel at your kitchen table.

The second question to consider for herb choice is: *How welcoming is this herb?*

Some herbs are so safe to consume that they're food ingredients or spices, like Burdock, Nettles, Peppermint, and Fennel. Other herbs are not food but still extremely benign, like Catnip, Lavender, and Anise-Hyssop. Then there are herbs that are benign but definitively medicinal, like Skullcap, Passionflower, and Bee Balm. Beyond that there is a whole range of herbs, up to dose-dependent medicinals that make you sick (or worse) in doses beyond a few drops of tincture.

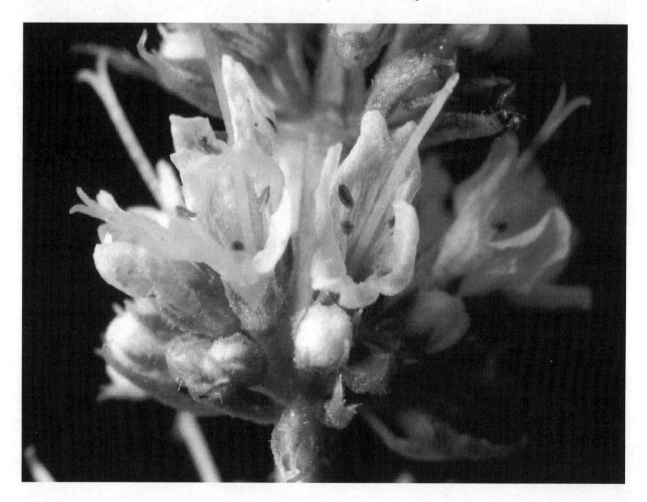

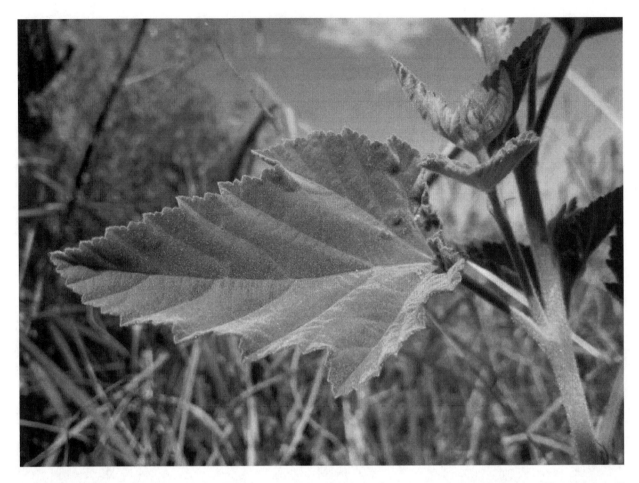

I think of this as how welcoming an herb is, as to a disorderly houseguest: peppermint and burdock will let me stumble around in muddy boots and leave dishes in the sink without reprimand, but the lovely lobelia demands a hostess gift and a deep bow to get through the door. For young children, the best herbs are food herbs, herbs that are not food but almost food (you could make an argument for lavender cookies), and benign medicinals, which to be very safe and gentle.

The third question to consider for herb choice is: *Is this the gentlest herb you can think of?*

Young children tend to be very sensitive: to medicines, to energetics, to spiritual awareness, to interpersonal dynamics, unhealthy relationships, unspoken nuance, and the vast mysteries of the universe. We always start with a small amount of the gentlest herbs we can find in the hopes of bolstering their innate vitality and helping maintain balance in their little bodies, not overbalancing them or spinning them way out on an energetic limb.

The last question to consider for herb choice is: *How safe is this herb?*

We have brushed up against this already, but part of critical thinking is a formal check-back: you think you have your herb, now check back intentionally to be sure that you couldn't possibly harm anyone. What other actions does the herb have? Are there any known contraindications? If the child in questions is on pharmaceuticals, extreme caution is required to avoid any potential interactions; depending on the situation, a professional clinical herbalist with pediatric experience may be your best bet for medically fragile children (who are usually tough as nails, "fragile" is a hell of a misnomer). Avoid dose dependent herbs, and anything potentially dangerous or toxic.

So, does the Materia Medica reflect an appropriate herb choice? Is this herb traditionally used in young children? Is it a food herb, completely benign, or very benign medicinally? Is this the gentlest herb you can find for this issue in this person? Is it undoubtedly safe? A series of resounding *yes's* means you're on the track of the right herb/formula for toddlers and young children.

Formula Construction: Stay Centered

Often, toddlers and young children do very well when given a simple (just one herb). Since they're so sensitive to both nuance and intervention, we can often do a lot with a very small dose of the one right herb delivered in just the right way.

That said, sometimes they benefit from formulas. In these cases, it is essential to remember that this age group is both very receptive and in a constant state of growth and change, physically, mentally, and spiritually.

Balance

Balance is at the heart of all schools of holistic medicine. As we have discussed throughout this column, it is a focus on nurturing our existing strengths and restoring areas that have eroded. We use herbs to maintain balance, or to return a system to balance when things get wonky, without overcompensating in the other direction.

Toddlers and young children are more sensitive and receptive than older children, teens, and adults, so it is extremely important to keep the principle of balance at the center of your mind when formulating for this age group. Choose gentle herbs with balanced or gentle energetics (more about this in a minute), and formulate with balance as a central focus.

Synergy

The principle of synergy states that the whole is greater than the sum of its parts. This is pivotal in formulation, when we combine plants and ask them to work together for greater healing. For toddlers and young children, looking at traditional formulas for enlightenment as to ideal combinations is a good place to start. Trust your intuition about which herbs seem to magnify each other: Hawthorn and Rose, Hyssop and Bee Balm, Witch Hazel and Marshmallow—which combinations do you find the most powerful?

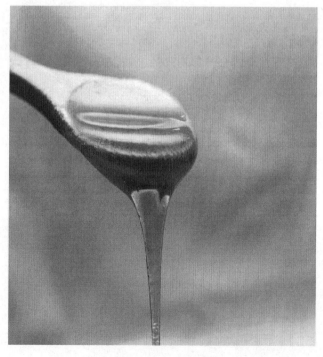

Remember that synergy can be enhanced by the route of administration, so consider how you will deliver your remedy. Will this be most powerful as a syrup, the soothing slide of honey accentuating the magic of elecampane? Or maybe a steam, taking advantage of thyme's volatile oils as they evaporate into the ether? Not all things must be tea.

"Gathering Wild Roses" -
from the book for kids
I'm a Medicine Woman Too!
by Jesse Wolf Hardin
(Hops Press)

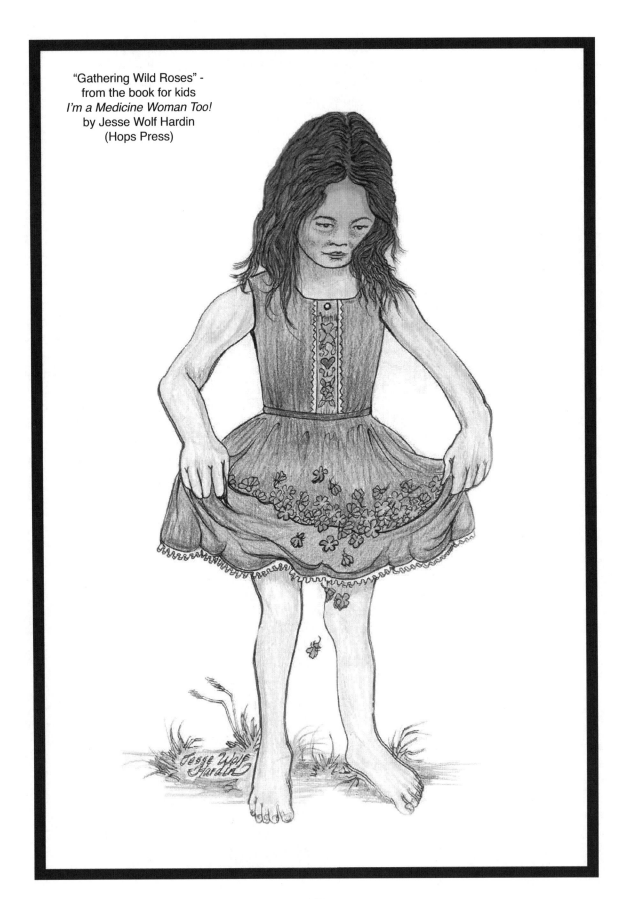

Electuaries are herbs that make a formula taste good, such as Lavender, Rose, Licorice, Elderberry, Peppermint, etc. They drastically increase the efficacy of formulas for toddlers and young children, as demon-possessed orangutans thankfully haven't lost their sweet tooth (and if your child is perfectly well-behaved when they don't feel good, just keep that to yourself, thank you). Obviously, if the remedy tastes good, they're more likely to take it.

Consider synergy: what flavors enhance each other? Is that a sign that perhaps the herbs are boosting each other in other ways too?

A sweet taste is very appropriate for young children, as it appeals to their active anabolic nature, providing grounding nourishment to send medicine deep, along with a replenishing energy boost. They crave it for a reason, after all; all that growth and change requires a lot of input, and the brain lives on glucose.

Energetics

Young children's energetics are noticeably different from their older counterparts. They are more delicate and sensitive as a baseline. How they manifest illness and imbalance varies by the individual of course, but the incredible anabolism and transformation of this age tends itself toward a balanced state that is more toward the warm and moist part of the circle, with plenty of movement and little stagnation or constriction (we grow into that, lucky things). Regardless of which philosophy of energetics you're using, remember to focus on gently restoring balance. Children this age are extremely sensitive and it is very easy to overbalance them in the other direction if we intervene too significantly. Nudging them gently in the right direction is usually enough. Many of the herbs we use have stronger and milder parts; for instance, I find marshmallow leaves to be more than sufficient in this age group, and see no need to use the far more intense root.

When making a formula in advance, I often make it relatively neutral energetically, and then add to it in the moment based on what is actually going on, by adding infused ice cubes, tinctures, honeys, etc. This has the advantage of being versatile enough to meet the needs of numerous people at once, important in my busy family and my life ruled by the seasons—I make cough syrup in September when the garden gives, not in January when everyone around me is at various stages of hack-hack-hacking.

Autonomy

Discussing a very rudimentary version of energetics with a child can aid in choosing the right herb, as well as assisting in the child's sense of self and autonomy, which are major developmental tasks for this age group. As a radical community we strive to raise our children with a deeply rooted sense of self-empowerment and consent, and that starts young. Asking if a tummy ache is stuck or moving invites the child to consider their body autonomously, especially if we then reflect back their feelings to reinforce the idea that they are in charge of their own body and we are here to assist. It seems like a silly little thing, but remember that they are actively constructing how they fit in the world ("no! mine!"), so treating that journey with respect teaches them that they deserve respect. As they get older, deferring to their assessment of their bodies can help teach self-empowerment and increase engagement, but in order to self-empower they must first develop a self (and honestly, my 2-year-old's idea of self-empowerment involves climbing the bookshelf, so less of that, please). The same is true when remedies taste good: if they like taking them, they consent and we can honor their consent instead of forcing them to take some disgusting mess we've concocted—and they learn lessons about bodily autonomy and mutual respect.

For a more in-depth discussion of balance, synergy, electuaries, and energetics, please see previous issues of Heart & Hearth #1 *in* Plant Healer Magazine.

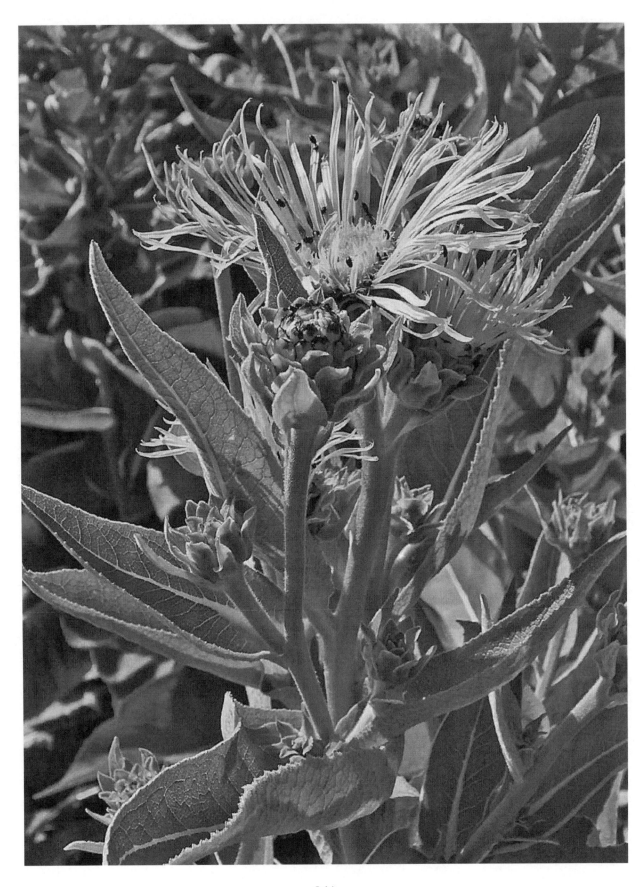

And Finally...

Pinpointing which herb is the most appropriate in a given situation is one of the main hurdles we must leap as we develop our skills as home herbalists. These decisions are especially fraught when we're working with limited supplies, limited experience, and a furious toddler, perhaps on limited sleep. As you tailor your home apothecary to your family's unique needs, I hope these tips are helpful for choosing appropriate herbs.

But if you only take two pieces of advice from me today, let them be these:

1. **Make it in advance:** unless it is truly impossible, spare yourself the misery of infusing honey with a child screaming "uppy uppy uppy" amid bouts of coughing.

2. **Treat the parents and siblings too:** if Baby gets a nervine, so does Mama! We need all the patience and grace we can muster to support littles when they're not at their best. You are also a person, if no one has reminded you of that today.

Next, Heart & Hearth *will explore useful methods of preparation and dosage for toddlers and young children.*

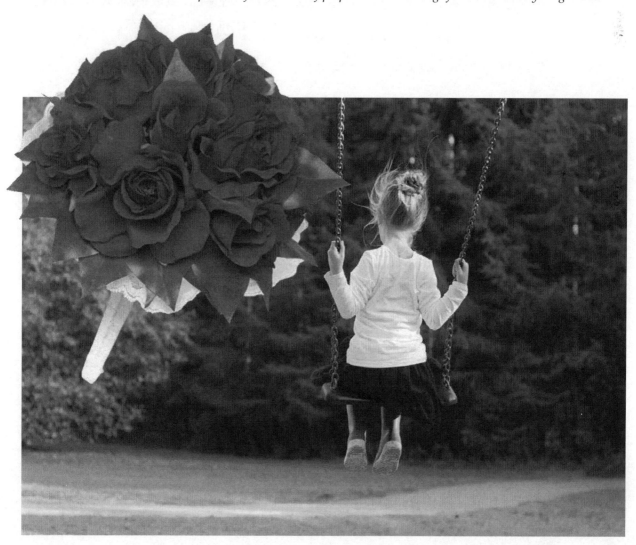

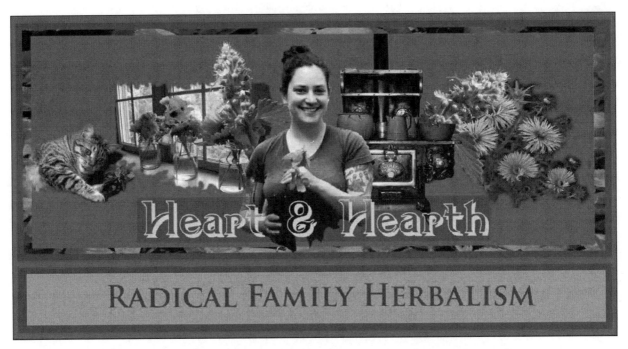

RADICAL FAMILY HERBALISM

THE BEST REMEDY FORMS
FOR TODDLERS & YOUNG CHILDREN

by Juliette Abigail Carr

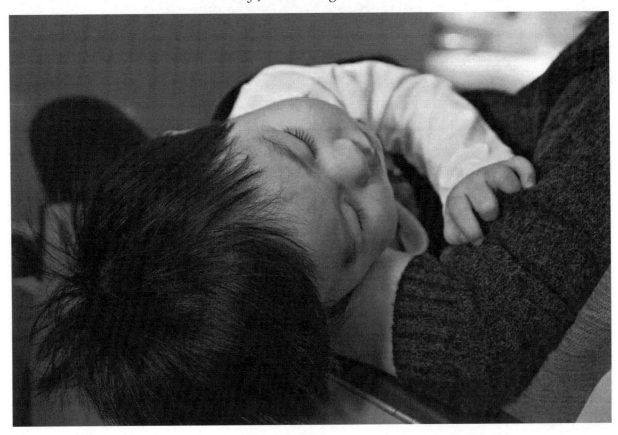

Home herbalism is who we are and how our families work, healing practiced around the kitchen table around the world and across the centuries. Thank the Good Green Earth that home herbalism happens as a reflex, intuition built on a foundation of herbal fluency that allows us to live as herbalists in every moment. Caring for our own children is the entry point into herbalism for many of us, inspired by the awe of a new life to look for safe, natural, inexpensive means of nurture.

As discussed in the previous issue, this year my Heart & Hearth column in Plant Healer Quarterly is focusing on the safe, effective, and useful application of herbal remedies for toddlers and young children. Last time we explored choosing herbs and safety; still to come is a discussion of useful methods of preparation, dosage, and essential materia medica for this glorious era of transformation, for the child and family. Join me at the 2020 Lands of Enchantment Faire to explore these topics in real life.

Not All Things Must Be Tea: Choosing a Method of Preparation

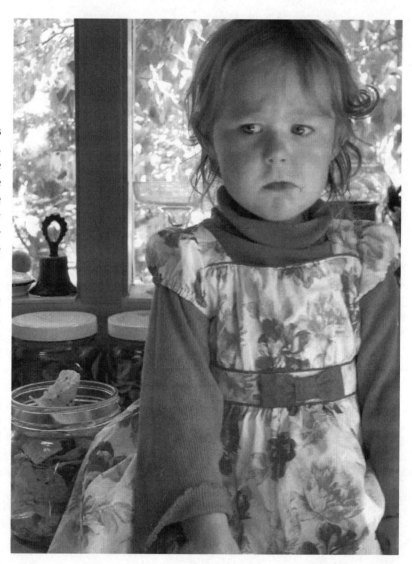

Ticking Time Bomb of a Miserable Toddler

Often when we prepare medicines for toddlers and young children, we are focused most on what the easiest, fastest method is, while our child is busily climbing the cabinets or screaming bloody murder or some other behavior that requires the bulk of our attention.

Many preparations appropriate for this age group can be made well in advance and stored, which is ideal; others can be thrown together quickly as needed.

Anything that doesn't fall into one of those two categories should be closely examined for usefulness, and most likely discarded until they're older if you can't find a way to prepare it that allows you to do it *not* during a crisis, when they need your focused attention.

Synergy

In the previous issue we discussed how the principle of synergy guides formulation, in that we look for herbs that magnify and expand upon each other's effects. This can also be true of remedy forms: there is tangible love in an infused honey, and honey's own medicinal effects can magnify a formula for sore throats or wounds or inflammation. The water that boils to make a steam is stimulating and invigorating, as is the thyme or eucalyptus we add. A digestive preparation in vinegar has additional digestive stimulation and live cultures, as well as superior mineral content to a tea.

Electuaries

Another important consideration is what can we actually get into them? An unwell toddler or preschooler can be a very stubborn adversary indeed: perhaps reconsider that slurry. We discussed electuary herbs, or herbs that make a formula taste good, in the previous issue. Electuaries increase the efficacy of formulas: they actually take it, so it actually works. The discussion of electuary herbs in the previous article applies to methods of preparation as well. Infused honey, syrup, oxymel, vinegar, yogurt, bath, and ice cubes can be delicious and/or fun, which makes it far easier to administer medicine and helps the young child consent to what needs to happen.

Solubility

Solubility is absolutely essential when choosing a remedy form. Does the medicine you're trying to make dissolve in the route of administration? Choosing the most effective extraction method goes a long way toward having a useful apothecary for the young child, as you will probably not be able to get vast quantities into them.

Energetics

What are the energetic properties of the method of preparation? Is it warming, cooling, stimulating, dispersing, constricting, drying, moistening? Can you choose a method of preparation that magnifies the energetic properties of the herbs?

Please refer to the previous Heart & Hearth articles for a fuller discussion of energetics, solubility, and synergy.

Autonomy

As we discussed last time, developing a sense of self and autonomy is an essential developmental task for this age group, so everything we as a community can do to support their sense of bodily autonomy and consent is wonderful. In terms of remedies, offering them medicines that are delicious or fun to take allows them to consent and be treated with respect; if we offer them a valerian slurry (ick, don't) we will have a battle on our hands that does not reinforce any positive messages about their personhood.

Indispensable Remedy Forms for Toddlers and Young Children

See my blog for easy instructions on making most of these remedy forms, www.oldwaysherbal.com

Tea: Infusions and decoctions are easy and fast to make, and if you make it tasty, often easy enough to get in to a thirsty child. If they're used to drinking tea it's especially comforting; my family loves tea through a bombilla (mate straw), so this usually works unless they're so sick they won't drink.

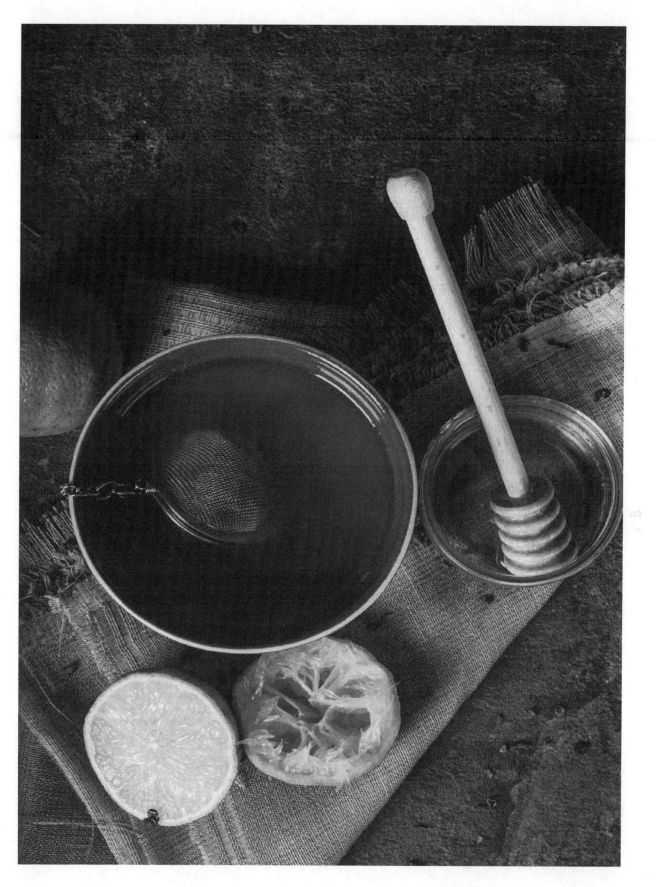

Tincture/Glycerite: Tinctures are extremely easy to give in that the dose is usually several drops, but mostly they don't taste good. A few drops added to honey or yogurt is an easy way to give it. Many people add tinctures to tea to evaporate off the bulk of the alcohol, but then the child needs to get all the water down to get the dose. Some people are concerned about the alcohol content; however, the actual alcohol in 5-10 drops of tincture is minuscule, certainly far less than children in Europe are getting in their watered wine, and certainly nothing a liver can't handle. Glycerine tinctures are a nice alternative, but they extract less medicinal constituents and only have a shelf life of about a year (compared to up to 8 years for alcohol tinctures).

Honey/Syrup/Elixir: Honey medicines are the gold standard for toddlers and young children. They are delicious and synergistic, medicinal in their own right. They can be made in advance and stored for a long time, and can include both water- and alcohol-soluble constituents if you include tincture in your syrup.

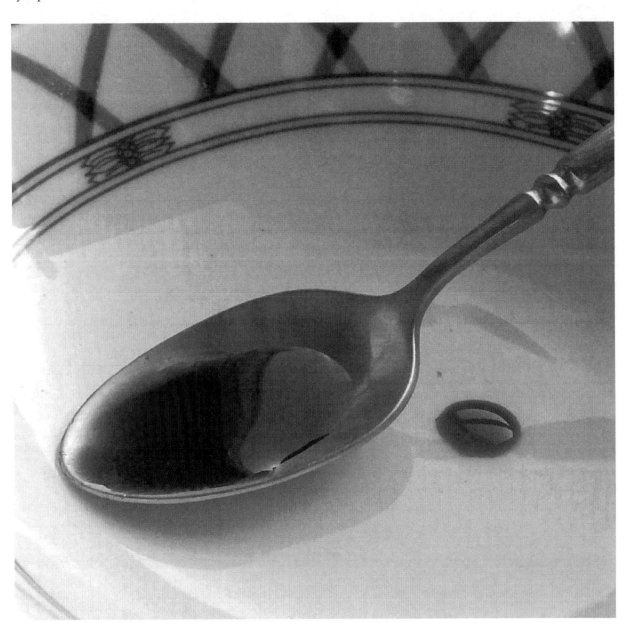

Oxymel/Vinegar: Vinegar medicines are one of the best methods for water-soluble constituents, especially minerals, which extract phenomenally in vinegar. These medicines are delicious and synergistic, and can be made far in advance.

Ice Pop/Ice Cube/Yogurt: Turn infusions and decoctions into delicious, fun remedies that go down easy, just by freezing them into popsicle or ice cube trays (pop them into bags for easier storage). If dehydration is a concern, combine an infusion with honey sweetened lemonade before freezing for a tasty, electrolyte-rich remedy. Infusions can also be blended with yogurt for flavored frozen yogurts, especially nice for kids prone to tummy trouble, and those who stop eating when things go awry.

Oil: Infused oils can be gently warmed and used for massage, added to bath water, or several drops added to humidifier. Consider an oil rub on the chest for bad chest colds. Oils only last about a year in a cool place, less if they are heated during the infusion process. Note: I'm talking about infused oils, not essential oils. I no longer use essential oils due to their negative environmental impact.

Steam: Add fresh or dried herbs or tincture to a bowl of boiling water, and cuddle your child in an enclosed space as close to the bowl as is safe. A fort under the kitchen table, a closet, or a shower stall all work. Strained infusions can be added to humidifiers, just be sure to clean it after. Older children and adults can breath steam through a paper bag or with a towel over their head, but this is not safe for this age group.

Bath: Add a very strong infusion or decoction to the bath, or use an infused oil. The added benefit of the steam helps them bring the medicine in through the lungs and sinuses, as well as soaking through the skin. A recognizable routine like bath time is helpful in soothing fraught moments.

Wash: A wash can be great if it needs to be done throughout the day, or an issue only affects a specific area (i.e. poison ivy). Strong infusions/decoctions or tinctures diluted in warm water are useful.

Compress: soak thick washcloths (or cloth prefold diapers) in a strong wash, or make a slurry of herbs with a little water or oil, then apply and cover with a dry cloth. If possible, wrap with an ace bandage or similar. If applying to the chest of a congested child, leave off the dry cloth so the steam and volatile oils rise. Compresses are genuinely hard to keep on a young child, so plan to only use it for a few minutes; often a bath is more effective.

Nursing: If a toddler is still nursing, a safe and effective means of delivering herbs is by taking them yourself and letting your milk filter out most potentially harmful things. Caveat: fat-soluble molecules tend to concentrate in breast milk, so some compounds are actually stronger in breastmilk than they would otherwise be (for instance, THC) so have an awareness of that.

Therapeutic Touch Remedies

The skin is like a sponge, but we often don't think of applying topical remedies with the same frequency as internal ones. Toddlers and young children love to snuggle, especially if they don't feel well, and therapeutic touch can be used to deliver comfort and love as well as an herbal remedy. An all-over massage can be nice, but also consider targeting areas that strongly affect other parts of the body. In particular, the temples, ears, neck, chest, hands, and feet are extremely effective. Use an infused oil or a strong wash as you massage. If you can do it in close proximity to a steam bowl, even better. A quiet room and your undivided attention add to the remedy.

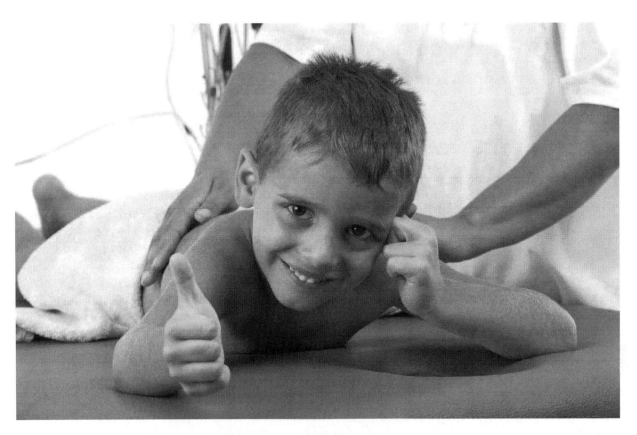

Alternative Alternative Medicine

Some of our most interesting home remedies come to us from the old wives' tales of kitchen witching, and should not be ignored. Half a burnt onion on an ear to draw out an ear infection really does equalize the pressure; grated raw potato is amazing for mastitis; a cabbage leaf in a bra decreases milk supply; warm garlic oil on the soles of the feet helps break a fever. Let us not discard our less sciency preparations simply on the basis of weirdness, as they really can work. Rosemary Gladstar's collection of works are rich in these types of remedies, as she has spent much of her illustrious career reclaiming disappearing kitchen healing traditions.

Dose

Dosing internal medicines for littles can be challenging, as they are so sensitive and responsive to intervention, and as they lack the vocabulary to fully describe their symptoms. The good news is that since you're working exclusively with very benign herbs, you have wiggle room to start low and increase until you see a change.

7Song talks about using drop dosing as an energetic test of a remedy, giving just a drop and watching the person's subconscious, nonverbal body language to assess if it's the right herb: if they sigh, relax, drop their shoulders for a split second etc. then he knows it's a good match. I love this idea and try to apply it when appropriate, and with very young children you're usually working on body language and behavior so it can be a nice idea to keep in mind as you decide if another dose is warranted. They might still be uncomfortable or upset, but do they seem more comfortable or relaxed in their body? Often we continue to feel bad for a while even after a remedy has started to work, and children this age may lack the vocabulary to describe feeling "a little better but still lousy." Sometimes, the earache feels better, but now their throat hurts from all the screaming; in this case, it's not another dose that's needed, but a different remedy entirely.

Mary Bove has some nice starting places for dosing in The Encyclopedia of Natural Healing for Children and Infants. You will need to tweak it based on the child's constitution and weight since dosing is not one-size-fits-all, but it's a good starting place if you're feeling totally at sea. The dose will vary based on the herbs, the preparation, and the child's weight. As a general guideline, stick with drop dosing (i.e. 5 drops, instead of mls or dropperfuls). Start low and increase every 20-30 minutes if needed. Tinctures, glycerites, and vinegars will require the lowest dose, followed by infused honeys, then syrups, and teas require a larger dose.

In the end, remember that dosing isn't an exact science: use safe herbs, have patience with your patient and with yourself, and trust your intuition.

Next time, Heart & Hearth will explore essential Materia Medica for toddlers and young children.

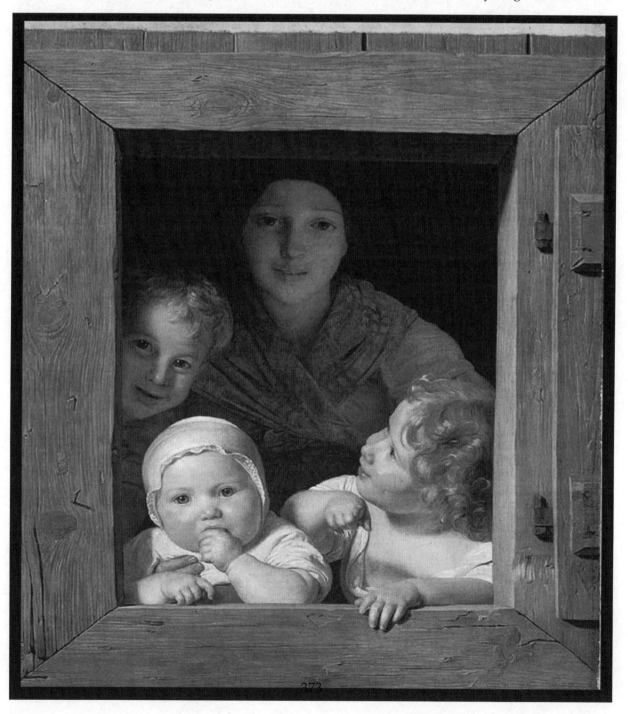

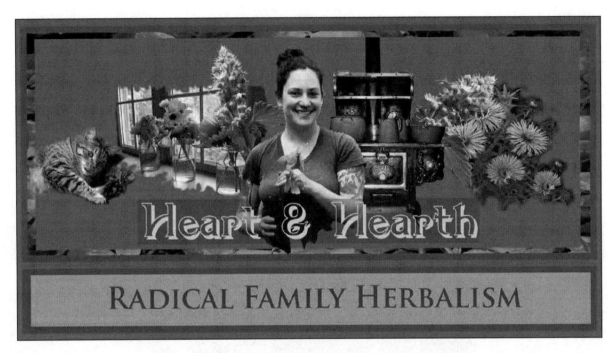

Radical Family Herbalism

Essential Materia Medica
for Toddlers & Young Children

by Juliette Abigail Carr

Home herbalism is who we are and how our families work, healing practiced around the kitchen table around the world and across the centuries. Thank the Good Green Earth that home herbalism happens as a reflex, intuition built on a foundation of herbal fluency that allows us to live as herbalists in every moment. Caring for our own children is the entry point into herbalism for many of us, inspired by the awe of a new life to look for safe, natural, inexpensive means of nurture.

This year *Heart & Hearth* is focusing on the safe, effective, and useful application of herbal remedies for toddlers and young children. We have explored choosing herbs, safety, useful methods of preparation, and dosage; in this issue, we will discuss essential materia medica for this glorious era of transformation.

The era of toddlers and young children is a uniquely transformative time for both the child and family as a whole. It is important to support the incredible growth of their physical, emotional, and spiritual lives as they constantly build and adapt to the world around them.

Supporting the family constellation is key. The sleepless teething baby's parents need nervines just as the baby does, and limbic resonance and a calm, patient presence go a long way toward soothing both! Immune support, nervines, aches and pains: do not forget the rest of the constellation when working with the most demanding star.

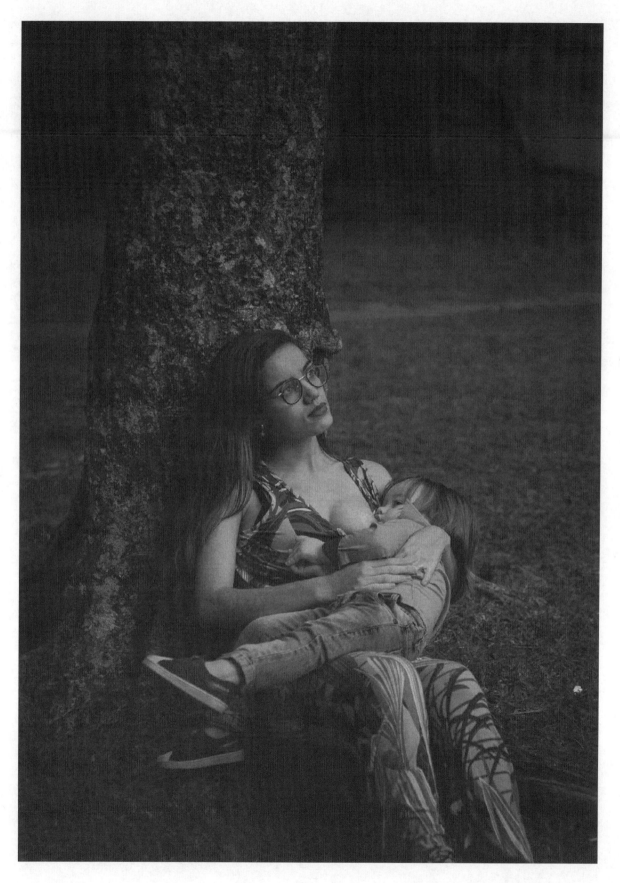

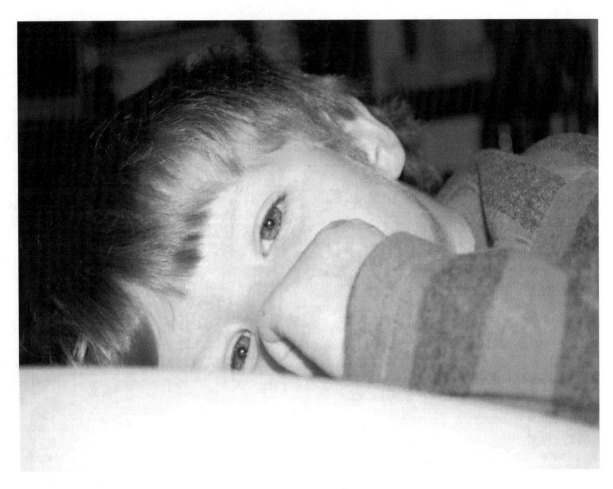

Little Bodies, Big Differences

When working with toddlers and young children, we are well-served to pay close attention to the confluence of physical and emotional states, as that is where they live. Because young children's normal state is one of constant growth and change, things that we see in adults as disparate symptoms, or related by stress or inflammation or whatever, are often directly or causally linked in this age group as their complex systems develop. Illness, trouble sleeping, digestive upset and more can be manifestations of emotional or spiritual disruption. Temper tantrums might signal a headache or ear infection, as well as obvious stress or exhaustion. Stress in the overall environment, disruptions to routine, the overall family emotional state: these can tie closely with a bout of constipation or headache or trouble sleeping.

Additionally, physical systems function differently as they develop from how they will at maturity, so the common assumption that young children can be treated like tiny adults is inappropriate. As young children progressively develop their active immunity by encountering the world, their digestive tracts play an essential role in their immune system. The developing immune system relies on gut acidity and the microbiome to help defend a child from infection, so ensuring a healthy flora is essential to preventing sickness and developing allergies. It is also absolutely key to understand that the digestive tract is where we often see the first signs of illness, stress, anxiety, or other types of distress manifested, so looking solely at digestive herbs for digestive issues in toddlers is not enough: consider what else is at play.

Some Favorite Herbs

There is an incredible plethora of safe, effective herbs for common problems with this age group. The following are a few of the herbs that I turn to over and over again, filtered specifically for broadest use and ease of growing: these grow easily across the country and are freely or cheaply accessible to most families.

Catnip, *Nepeta cataria*

I use the cool, dry above ground parts of catnip as a nervine, antispasmodic, carminative, analgesic and febrifuge. One of the most useful things about catnip is the broadness of its use with this age group, when seemingly disparate symptoms occur together as manifestations of the same issue (i.e. tummy ache and nightmares from interrupted-routine stress).

For stress, anxiety, trouble sleeping (especially with nightmares), and pain, catnip is useful internally, or as a massage, bath, or pillow stuffing, alone or combined with lavender or chamomile.

For tummy aches or gas, catnip is especially useful internally or as a belly massage with fennel, chamomile, or ginger (depending if the balance point is cooler or warmer). It is doubly, especially, particularly indicated when indigestion or gas is accompanied by stress or pain.

Catnip helps break a fever by inducing sweating without increasing hypothalamic-regulated body temperature, which is key in the toddler set, as they are prone to runaway fevers. It is especially useful when fevers are accompanied by headache or other pain. It is ideally used internally and externally at the same time, as a bath and tea. For this application it combines well with chamomile and thyme, plus immune herbs like elderberry and echinacea internally if an infection or sickness is at work.

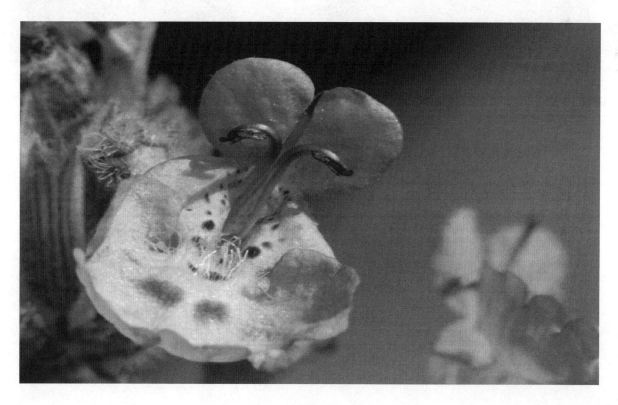

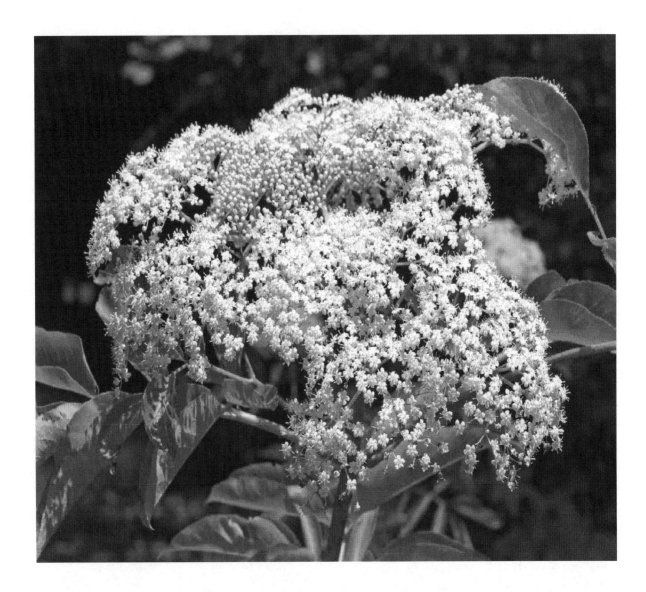

Elderberry, *Sambucus canadensis*

The fruit of this safe, effective, versatile immune stimulant and febrifuge is absolutely indispensable in the home apothecary. Older toddlers and young children can help harvest berries and make honey or syrup once they get into pouring as a hobby, which engenders a sense of pride and self-efficacy. Elderberry is used in small doses on a daily basis to help prevent seasonal illness. It is wonderful as a syrup with cinnamon, ginger, and garlic (what my daughter wants when she asks for "medicine"), or just on its own as a simple infused honey.

Elderberry is used in slightly larger doses when a child is actually sick, internally with other safe immune stimulants and herbs for specific symptoms. I make a very strong infusion of thyme, hyssop, and bee balm in late summer, sweeten it with elderberry honey, and add some echinacea tincture, then freeze the whole thing into mini-popsicles for when a child is sick: they think they're getting a treat, you think they're getting hydration and medicine, so everybody wins. For my clinical practice, I often just do a syrup with these or similar herbs, depending on what is called for, as popsicles don't travel well, but I can't speak highly enough of them in the home setting.

378

Fennel, *Foeniculum vulgare*

Fennel seed is already in many parents' home apothecary, as it is one of our favorite herbs for increasing breast milk supply, and especially useful when nursing colicy babies. As our children grow it continues to be a favorite, as it is perennially useful as a warming, stimulating carminative and aromatic bitter, dispersing upper GI grumpiness and getting the lower GI motor started for bloating and mild constipation. When parents bring me infant clients after being encouraged to start pharmaceutical reflux medication, fennel is often a central herb, as it can help disperse that hot digestive irritability, especially with catnip.

Fennel is a versatile digestive herb that works for many different kinds of digestive upset. It eases tummy aches that rumble and shudder without going anywhere, with chamomile to soothe and cool. It also works just as well for stuck, bloated balloon bellies with thyme and catnip. It is extremely helpful for stress constipation with catnip or chamomile. Fennel is wonderful as a tea or honey, and also very useful as a wash or gentle tummy and lower back massage for tummy aches and constipation.

Fennel's astringency makes it useful in formulas as a child's astringent in general, perhaps with marshmallow leaf, violet, or mullein for dry, irritated mucous membranes, to help hold the moisture in parched tissues.

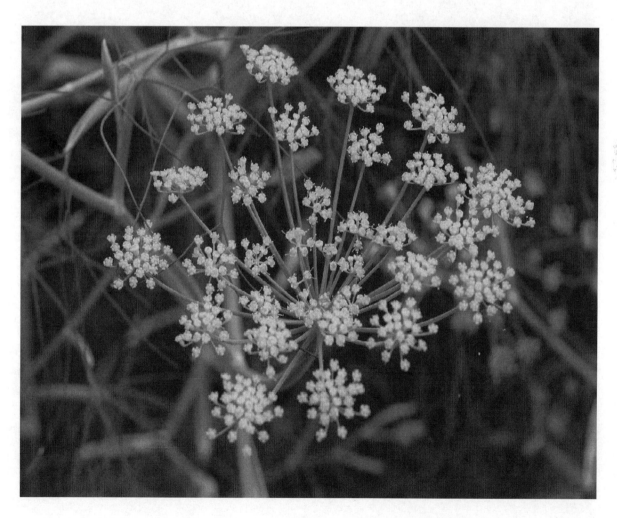

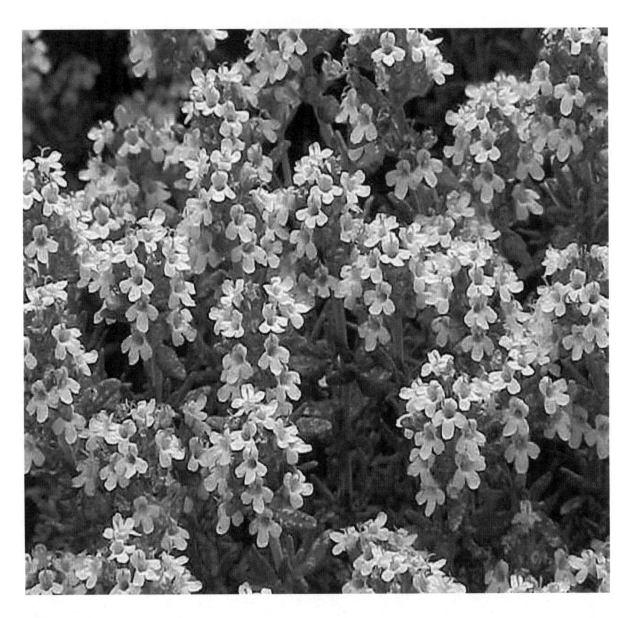

Thyme, *Thymus vulgaris*

The enticingly aromatic above ground parts of thyme are useful as a warming, antimicrobial, decongestant and immune stimulant, as well as a warming, stimulating digestive aid. I use it internally and externally for respiratory infections, ear infections, sinus congestion, and any infection that is causing congestion. It is wonderful as a steam, chest rub, or in the bath with other aromatic herbs like eucalyptus and hyssop. Thyme is truly glorious fresh in honey or syrup with other immune herbs, like echinacea and bee balm. If it is too warming, or there is an irritated cough along with the congestion, mullein leaf tea can provide a nice soothing balance, or marshmallow leaf and flower honey.

Thyme is extremely useful as a digestive aid for stuck, cold tummy aches, bloating, and mild constipation, which makes a honey preparation double useful for the probiotic content. It is nice in this context with fennel, or catnip if there is a stress component.

380

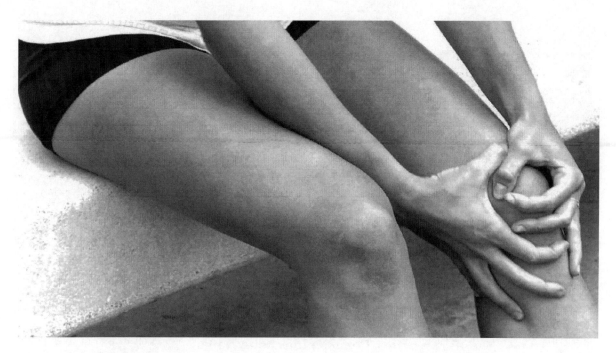

Bumps and Boo-boos

Having a nice salve or cream on hand for bumps and boo-boos is key. As toddlers learn about their bodies and the world through direct experience, they tend to hurl themselves into the path of danger on a moment-to-moment basis, heedless of the heart attack they're giving you, and minor wounds are the result, as are gross motor skills, self-efficacy, and problem-solving abilities.

A perfect salve for bumps and boo-boos is balanced between moistening and drying herbs, as you cannot predict what fresh hell is around the next bend and should be prepared for bee stings as well as scrapes. Combining an astringent like witch hazel with a demulcent like violet or marshmallow leaf provides balance and helps the skin retain moisture, they work better together to decrease inflammation and provide a soothing, moist healing environment.

Several vulnerary herbs are usually a good idea, as they bring different benefits in addition to their wound-healing properties. I like calendula and yarrow for their extra antimicrobial and anti-inflammatory awesomeness, plus plantain for how it draws things out of wounds (dirt, thorns, bee stingers), and chamomile for soothing pain relief. There are many other fantastic vulnerary herbs, simply choose 2 or 3 that grow near you, and make sure you've got an astringent and a demulcent involved (either one of the vulneraries, or in addition), and make a salve in advance so you have it on hand. Often the ritual of a kiss and a little boo-boo cream takes away most of the emotional crisis.

Families with young children are well-served to identify 5 to 10 herbs that they find particularly helpful for a wide variety of conditions, and keep them on hand in useful preparations. Toddlers and young children cherish routines and rituals, looking to stability in times of disruption. Young families benefit from working normal routines into a hard day, as well as creating their own healing rituals for times of need. Holding a calm, focused presence, maintaining quiet space, and giving a young child your undivided attention are all essential remedies in their own right—although this can feel impossible with limited sleep and plenty of stress, which is why it is so important to support the family as a whole. Preparing remedies in advance and treating the family as a constellation really help maintain harmony on difficult days.

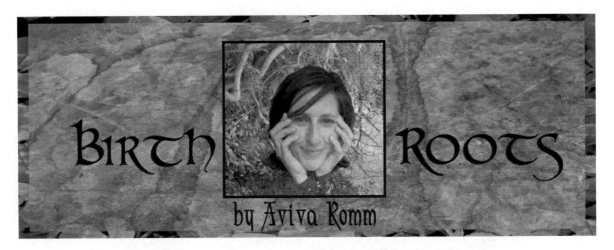

BIRTH ROOTS

by Aviva Romm

September 1, 2011, the Centers for Disease Control (CDC) released a report on the problem of unnecessary antibiotic prescribing for kids. They found that doctors are unnecessarily prescribing antibiotics for kids more than 50% of the time, most often for upper respiratory infections (colds, coughs, ear infections, sinusitis, and sore throats).

Inappropriate antibiotic prescribing is the primary cause of antibiotic resistance, which is a major global public health problem. Further, medical science is waking up to the fact that pediatric antibiotic exposure is not benign for the individual, and may lead to asthma, eczema, and the development of inflammatory bowel diseases such as ulcerative colitis and Crohn's disease later in life. Finally, antibiotics that may their way into the environment whether through industrial manufacturing, use in animal husbandry, or human excretion, also have an impact.

Other commonly prescribed adjunct therapies for common kids' infections, for example, Tylenol and ibuprofen also carry the potential for serious side

Kids, Common Infections, Herbs & Antibiotics

by Aviva Romm

effects, including the development of asthma and gastrointestinal bleeding, respectively. Tylenol overuse is one of the most common causes of liver failure in the United States. While antibiotics can be are lifesaving when necessary, when overprescribed and misused, the consequences can be deadly!

Antibiotics are often given unnecessarily for common pediatric infections because doctors think that parents want or expect them. Indeed, I've had to talk dozens of parents out of an antibiotics prescription---they are accustomed to doctors giving meds, and they are afraid and don't want their kids to suffer. Doctors also prescribe antibiotics because they are worried about missing a serious diagnosis --- and then there is also fear of litigation for the rare missed or under-treated infection.

If you haven't caught my subtext by now, I'm a big advocate of avoiding unnecessary antibiotic use, and the fact is, for common pediatric infections, they're unnecessary. And herbs can play a huge role in supporting health and comfort while avoiding unnecessary medications.

It's amazing, though, how many herbalists and naturally inclined folks are confident using herbs until it comes to their young'uns getting sick. The fever of 103 degrees, the cough that lasts for 2, 3, or 4 weeks, or the middle-ear infection can bring even the bravest hearts to their knees at the pediatrician's office. You find yourself tentatively taking that antibiotic prescription that is handed out as freely as candy on Halloween. And then there is the ensuing dilemma when you get home-- do you give the antibiotic or do you stick with the herbs just a little longer? Too often fear trumps evidence and intuition.

Sometimes we're comfortable making the decision to forego antibiotics for our own kids, but lack confidence as clinical herbalists when it comes to advising an anxious mom about whether her kiddo can be treated botanically or really does need an antibiotic. After all, we're not entirely immune to the fear of litigation, as herbalists and we don't want to hurt anybody!

This article is intended to provide you with clear, simple guidelines that you can use to help parents—or yourself-- make intelligent choices about herbs versus antibiotic use, and some of my favorite recipes for fever, cough, and ear infections in kids.

Herbal Care or Medical Attention?

Here's the meat in a nutshell:

Here are symptoms to *worry* about. If you see any of these, a doctor's appointment is appropriate and medications are likely warranted:

• Any baby less than 1 month old with a fever *requires* immediate medical attention!
• High (> 103.5 F) or persistent fever in any aged child
• A child is having to work extra hard to breathe or if her breathing is as fast, labored, or accompanied by stridor, whooping sounds, or wheezing
• Persistent pain (nothing relieves it) such as an earache, sore throat, severe headache or stomach ache
• Frequent vomiting or diarrhea if a child us unable to keep down enough liquids to urinate at least once

every six to eight hours-- this could be a sign of dehydration
• Thick eye discharge that doesn't get better during the day
• A stiff neck, extreme lack of energy or the illness seems to be getting worse rather than staying the same for more than five days
• Blood in the vomit or diarrhea
• If the child has been exposed to a contagious disease such as mono, pertussis, measles, the flu, or has travelled out of the country recently
• If your treatment for a mild condition is not helping, and the condition persists or worsens

Reassuring signs that you can, in good confidence, continue to treat an illness botanically include:

• The child, in spite of not feeling well, continues to play and act generally normally, and is able to be awake, and alert even though he or she may be more sleepy than usual
• The child's appetite may be decreased from normal, but he or she continues to take fluids and perhaps a small amount of food
• The child is peeing a normal amount compared to usual
• The symptoms slowly improve over the course of several days

Fever

You do not have to treat fever. Comfort measures and hydration are the most important treatments unless the child has a serious bacterial infection. Most kids who become seriously ill during a fever do so because of dehydration. Water (you can add lemon and honey or maple syrup), tea, broth, and even ice pops if all else fails, are optimal fluids. Fever may continue for a number of days or even ebb and flow for a week—particularly in the afternoon and evening. This is usually not a problem if the child is taking plenty of fluids and seems otherwise well.

Botanicals

Botanicals can be used to help ease the *symptoms* associated with a fever —aches, headache, tummy discomforts, and chills. Following are some of my favorite remedies.

Kudzu *(Pueraria lobata)* **Apple Juice:** Kudzu is known in TCM for relieving chills, aches, indigestion, and other symptoms of colds. To prepare, heat 3/4 cup unfiltered apple juice in a saucepan until it begins to simmer. Dissolve 1-teaspoon kudzu root into 1/4-cup cold apple juice. Stir this into the saucepan, and continue to stir until it comes to a boil. Reduce the temperature to low, and stir continuously for two to three minutes more. Cool until drinkable and then enjoy. The juice can be used as the child's main nourishment for a day. You can use pear juice in place of apple juice. A pinch of cinnamon can be added to either if the child has severe chills, diarrhea, or stomach upset.

Catnip *(Nepeta cataria)*, **lemon balm** *(Melissa officinalis)*, **and elder blossom** *(Sambucus nigra)* **Infusion:** Steep 1/3 oz. of each herb in a covered quart jar of boiling water for 20 minutes. Strain and sweeten lightly (no honey for kids under 2 years old; maple syrup is a good alternative). Give as warm as the child will take it, and often (up to 2 cups), until a sweat results. Eases headache, nausea, and aches, and promotes sleep.

Fever is not an illness. It is the body's innate, beneficial response to infection! Fevers are not inherently dangerous. A temperature over 100.4 degrees F is considered a fever. Anything less than that is not! Most fevers are in the range of 101-103.5 degrees. A high fever is over 103.5!

When to Consult with a Doctor

•A doctor should see all babies under 1 month old with fever immediately! This can be a medical emergency!
•Babies under 3 months old with a *high* fever (see above) should be seen by a doctor
•Any kids who are not taking fluids, not urinating a normal amount compared to usual, or are just not "acting right" should be seen by the doctor
•Any kids with fever along with stiff neck or neck, persistent vomiting, or severe headache should be seen by the doctor
•If the child has severe ear pain or severe belly pain
•If the child is lethargic—that is, he just isn't really waking up fully, seems weak, or just seems sort of limp, is just lying there, and doesn't really make eye contact
•Fevers that stay high for more than 3-5 days
•If you or the parents feel worried that child has a serious illness, take the child is best seen by a doctor: Remember, trust momma's (and your own) intuition! (and better safe than sorry)

Cough

A cough is a reaction to airway irritation or inflammation, usually caused by viral upper respiratory infection (also called a cold) or something in the environment (i.e., dust). Asthma and gastroesophageal reflux can also cause cough. This is a discussion of cough due to viral infection. Coughs can last from days to even weeks. In fact, you might have noticed that sometimes after a cold, a child can have a lingering cough for even 6 weeks. This can actually be completely normal, is called post-viral airway reactivity, and is due to persistent irritation in the upper airway.

Antibiotics do not treat coughs due to viral infections and are almost never indicated for coughs due to colds.

Botanicals

Aunty Aviva's Cough Syrup Blend

This remedy is effective and pleasant for use with children.
•½ ounce dried mullein leaves *(Verbascum thapsus)*
•½ ounce marshmallow root *(Althea officinalis)*
• ½ ounce licorice root *(Glycyrrhiza glabra)*
• ½ ounce thyme *(Thymus vulgaris)*
• ½ ounce anise seeds *(Pimpinella anisum)*
• ½ ounce wild cherry bark *(Prunus serotina)*
•½ ounce slippery elm bark *(Ulmus rubra)*
•1 quart of boiling water

Combine all the herbs. Put 1 ounce of the mixture in a glass jar, add the boiling water, cover, and steep for 2 hours. Strain the liquid into a pot and simmer gently until it is reduced to 1 cup (discard the plant material). Sweeten with H cup of honey (for children under one year, omit the honey and replace with maple syrup or sugar to taste). After the syrup cools to room temperature, store it in a jar in the fridge. It will keep for up to 2 months.

Dose: 1-2 teaspoons as needed for children one to three years old, 1 tablespoon as needed for older children.

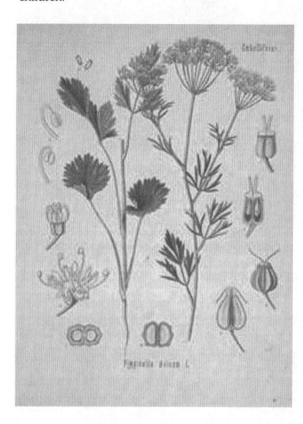

Quiet Cough Formula

This sweet-tasting, glycerin-based tincture is relaxing, expectorant, and antimicrobial for the respiratory passages.

•½ ounce anise seed tincture (*Pimpinella anisum*)
•½ ounce cramp bark tincture (*Viburnum opulus*)
•½ ounce thyme tincture (*Thymus vulgaris*)
•½ ounce elecampane tincture (*Inula helenium*)
•½ ounce red clover blossom tincture (*Trifolium pretense*)
•½ ounce black cohosh tincture (*Actea racemosa* syn. *Cimicifuga racemosa*)
•1-ounce vegetable glycerin

Mix all the ingredients in a 4-ounce dark amber bottle. Shake well before each use. It will store indefinitely. Refrigeration is not necessary.

Dose: Give 1/2 to 1 teaspoon up to every 30 minutes for 2 hours for acute coughing bouts, or two to four times daily for milder or chronic coughs.

When to Consult with a Doctor

•All babies under 1 month old with persistent cough should be evaluate by a doctor
•If the child is wheezing and has no history of asthma
•If the child has asthma and wheezing that is causing him significant difficulty breathing, with no relief from prescribed medications.
•The child's breathing is rapid *and* labored (fever by itself can cause breathing to be faster than usual, but it should not make a child work harder to breathe)
•The child's lips or mouth are turning blue due to labored breathing or shortness of breath.

Ear Infections (Otitis media)

Ear infection is the most common reason for a pediatric office visit, and one of the most common conditions leading to antibiotic over-prescription. Antibiotics treatment is considered appropriate (though not always necessary) for babies under 6 months old with known or suspected ear infections, and sometimes for children ages 6 months to 2 years with severe infection.

The American Academy of Pediatrics recommends giving parents the option of waiting 48-72 hours to see if symptoms resolve on their own before using an antibiotic. Approximately 80% of kids with acute otitis media get better without antibiotics!

Botanicals

•**Garlic-Mullein Oil:** (*Allium sativum* and *Verbascum Thapsus*) The classic herbal remedy for ear infections is garlic-mullein oil. In 30 years of herbal practice, I've rarely had to turn to anything else. Garlic is a natural antimicrobial, addressing infections of both

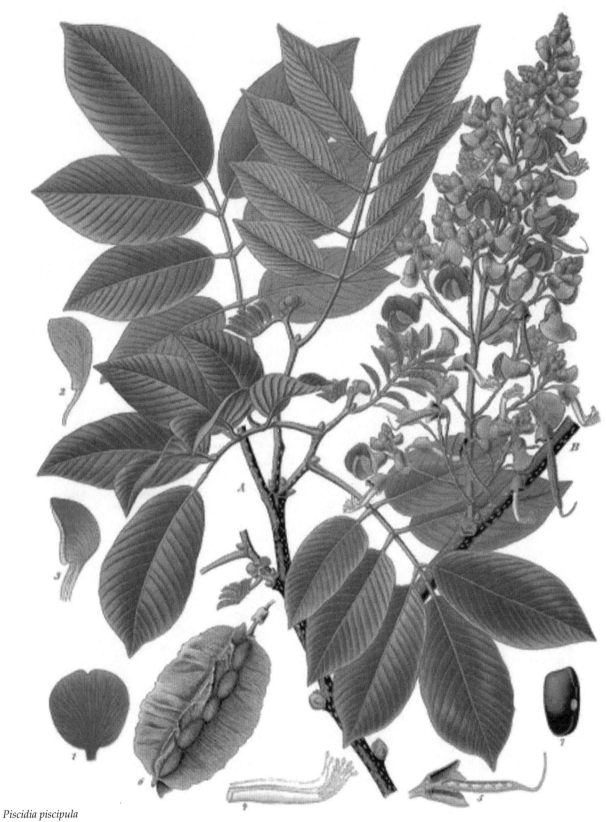

Piscidia piscipula

a bacterial and viral nature. Mullein is an analgesic, relieving the pain associated with earaches. *Never put anything in the ear if you suspect eardrum rupture or if there is drainage from the ear.*

•

•**St John's Wort** (*Hypericum perforatum*) Oil is a natural antiviral and analgesic, and can be used as an alternative to garlic-mullein oil, though I prefer the latter.

•

•**Jamaican Dogwood** (*Piscidia piscipula*) – Cramp Bark (*Viburnum opulus*) tincture (a 50/50 combination) is a reliable alternative to ibuprofen or Tylenol for pain relief. Give 5-10 drops to children under 5; 10-20 drops to children 5-12, and 2-3 mL to older children. Repeat the dose in 15- 20 minutes, then every 2-4 hours as needed. Jamaican dogwood is said to cause respiratory paralysis in excessive doses; do not exceed the above doses and keep out of reach of children.

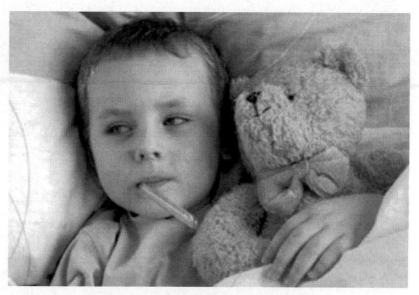

Here are additional helpful measures:

•Let the child sleep on a slightly filled hot water bottle—if it is overly full it will be too firm to rest on comfortable (do NOT use a heating pad)
•Use firm but gentle massage all around the jaw and head in the area adjacent to the ear. Massage in a downward direction behind the ear on the neck and apply gentle inward pressure in front of the ear toward the cheek (about where sideburns would be).
•Kids who drink a lot of juice and dairy products may get more earaches. Cut back on juice and milk during the infection and for at least three days after the earache symptoms have resolved.

When to Consult with a Doctor

•Pain that won't resolve
•High fever and persistent ear pain
•Drainage from the ear
•Neck pain or stiffness

Herbal pediatrics is an important but under utilized art because so many folks are afraid to treat kids, especially young children. It is critically important to know when medications are necessary, and also equally important to know when they are not. The health of the individual and the balance of the planet are at stake when medications are inappropriately and over used. Paying close attention to healthy kids, and spending time around kids when they are sick will help you to learn the difference. A family physician or pediatrician in your community can be an ally for you and your family or patients, and you an asset for him or her as many physicians treating kids want to know how to use alternatives but don't know where to learn or who/what to trust.

For those of you interested in learning more about botanical pediatrics, and for those of you seriously interested in specializing in this field, please sign up on my website at www.avivaromm.com. I also welcome your questions.

387

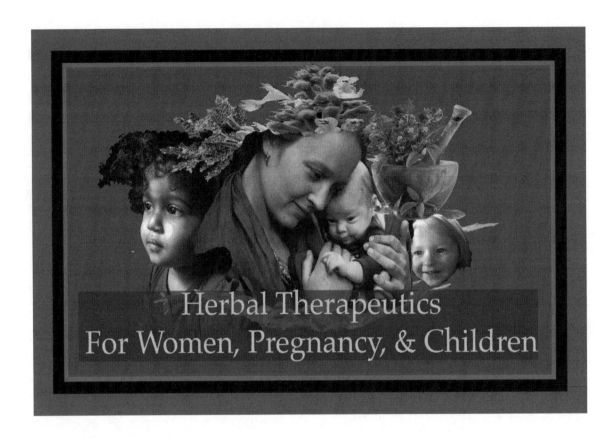

STRATEGIES FOR ACUTE ILLNESS IN CHILDREN

PART I: AVOIDING PHARMACEUTICALS

by Kenneth Proefrock

Expanding the herbalist's tool box with nebulizers, eye drops, nasal sprays, mouthwash/gargles and enemas for the most common acute pediatric conditions. This presentation includes fundamental strategies for addressing the most pressing needs of the patient and their families, natural courses for the resolution of those conditions and ways to assist the child's body in that resolution. Included are specific botanical medicine strategies, using tinctures, powders, topical agents and hydrotherapy techniques. Conditions that will be addressed will include EENT/Respiratory infections, digestive upsets, and skin infections.

There are two inevitably controversial subjects that come up whenever we discuss acute illness in children, antibiotic resistance and immunization. Antibiotic resistance is definitely one of the most urgent emerging threats to the public's health and the subject of immunization has become so socially politicized that it is nearly impossible to have a reasonable conversation about the actual pros and cons.

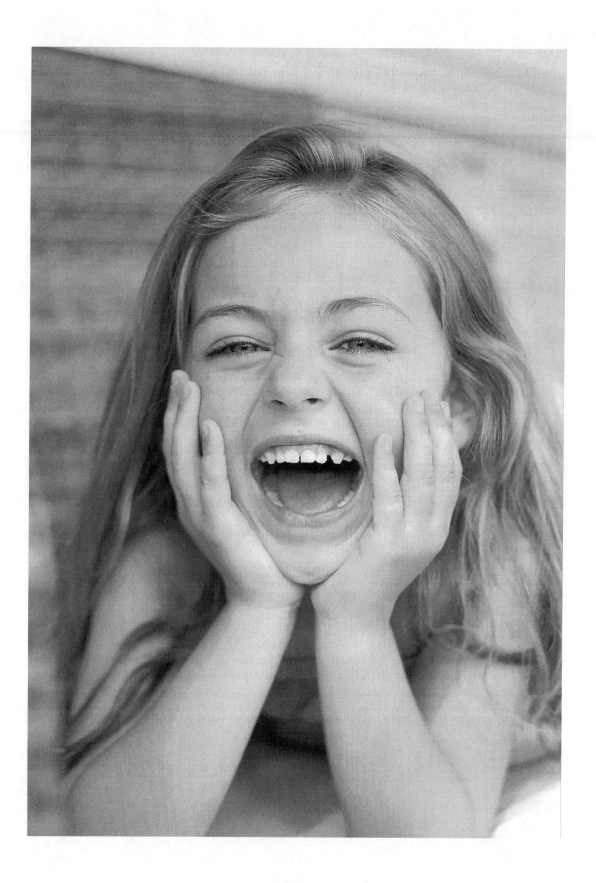

Antibiotic resistance has, by contrast, a much less political and more logical backstory. Every time a person takes an antibiotic, bacteria sensitive to that agent are killed while resistant ones may be left to grow and multiply. Very straightforwardly, overuse of antibiotics is a major cause of increases in drug-resistant bacteria, and antibiotic resistance in children and older adults is of particular concern because these age groups have the highest rates of antibiotic use. Decreasing inappropriate antibiotic use is a key strategy to control antibiotic resistance.

Immunization, on the other hand, is a much less straightforward topic of discussion and I won't dwell on it very long here. As in every other controversial subject, those opinions that are held from the extremes of both sides of the conversation are usually wrong. As a people, as educated citizens of a democracy that espouses the virtues of personal liberty and freedom, we are sadly led to our extremes by rhetoric, it is hard to find common ground when we are constantly defending extreme perspectives.

"Reality must take precedence over public relations as nature can't be fooled"
- Prof R. P. Feynman

Antibiotic Prescribing: Attitudes, Behaviors, Trends & Cost

According to a study published in the Journal of the American Medical Association, at least 30% of antibiotic courses prescribed in the outpatient setting are unnecessary, meaning no antibiotic was needed at all. Most of this unnecessary use is for acute respiratory conditions, such as colds, bronchitis, sore throats caused by viruses, and even some sinus and ear infections[1]. According to a survey conducted by the Centers for Disease Control in 2011, total inappropriate antibiotic use (which includes unnecessary antibiotic use plus inappropriate antibiotic selection, dosing, and duration) may approach 50% of all outpatient antibiotic use[2,3,4].

Antibiotics cause 1 out of 5 emergency department visits for adverse drug events (ADEs)[7, 8] and antibiotics are the most frequent cause of ADEs leading to emergency department visits in children. 7 of the top 10 drugs involved in ADEs leading to emergency room visits are antibiotics[9]. We spent $10.7 billion on antibiotics in the United States in 2009, including $6.5 billion among patients who visit physician offices and $3.5 billion among hospitalized patients[10].

Unfortunately, we have spent much of the past 60 years in pediatric medicine over-focused on antibiotic interventions to such a degree that many of the simpler, home remedy-type interventions, previously considered 'common sense', have been relegated to our social margins. Quite simply, most physicians end up writing a prescription because they don't know what else to do and there is a cultural expectation from the parents or guardians of the child that that is what it means to have their concerns taken seriously. The cultural double-bind is that parents expect a prescription and the physician often has no better recourse, it is a situation that is exacerbated by the companies that make the prescription items spending more money on advertising than they do on the development of the drugs and creating a cultural expectation that this is 'real' and effective medicine.

As a Naturopathic Physician, I have certain philosophical biases in my practice of medicine, so, for the purpose of this discussion, I have taken the organizing schema and the information regarding antibiotic use and overuse straight off of the website of the Centers for Disease Control (CDC.gov). All of the statistics regarding inappropriate antibiotic use, although consistent with my bias, come from that very public and government funded webpage. I have, and still do, prescribe antibiotics on occasion for certain manifestations of acute illness in pediatric patients. Through this discussion, I am hopeful that we can discuss how, when and what might be the most appropriate prescription for an acute presentation. As such, there will be a discussion of technical antibiotic prescribing that is consistent with current standards of care in pediatric medicine. The vast majority of the time, such prescribing is unnecessary as botanical medicine, hydrotherapy, nutrition and, gasp, homeopathy, are usually more than adequate interventions for most presentations of acute illness in children.

Acute Otitis Media

AOM is the most common childhood bacterial infection for which antibiotics are prescribed worldwide. The most common pathogens causing AOM in children are Streptococcus pneumoniae, non-typeable Haemophilus influenzae, Moraxella catarrhalis and Group A streptococcus. Antibiotic resistance is increasing among the bacterial pathogens causing AOM, with percentages of penicillin- and macrolide-resistant S. pneumoniae strains estimated to be between 30 and 70%, and of beta-lactamase-producing H. influenzae ranging between 20 and 40%[11].

4-10% of children with AOM treated with antibiotics experience adverse effects.[4]

Definitive diagnosis requires either:

• Moderate or severe bulging of tympanic membrane (TM)/Otorrhea not due to otitis externa.

• Mild bulging of the TM AND recent (<48h) onset of otalgia (holding, tugging, rubbing of the ear in a nonverbal child)/intense erythema of the TM.

• AOM should not be diagnosed in children without middle ear effusion (based on pneumatic otoscopy and/or tympanometry).

• Mild cases with unilateral symptoms in children 6-23 months of age or unilateral or bilateral symptoms in children >2 years may be appropriate for watchful waiting based on shared decision-making.

• Amoxicillin remains first line therapy for children who have not received amoxicillin within the past 30 days.

• Amoxicillin/clavulanate is recommended if amoxicillin has been taken within the past 30 days, if concurrent purulent conjunctivitis is present, or if the child has a history of recurrent AOM unresponsive to amoxicillin.

•For children with a non-type I hypersensitivity to penicillin: cefdinir, cefuroxime, cefpodoxime, or ceftriaxone may be appropriate choices.

•Prophylactic antibiotics are often prescribed, but NOT recommended to reduce the frequency of recurrent AOM.[3]

The central issue with Otitis media is really the inability of the eustachian tube to stay patent and communicative with its pharyngeal opening; somewhere along its path, it becomes blocked and establishes an anaerobic environment in the middle ear. Common culprits include mucus plugs from thick and chunky mucus that simply can't flow through such a tiny tube, colonization of microorganisms due to bottles and sippy cups being used while the child is laying down on their backs, excess sugar in liquids administered through bottles and sippy cups, and overuse of dietary wheat, dairy and eggs, that contribute to thicker, more tenacious mucus.

The anaerobic environment of the inner ear allows a micro-organismal overgrowth that produces pressure within the inner ear that pushes against the eardrum and hurts like crazy. It is self-limiting in that once the membrane ruptures, the bacterial overgrowth resolves in the now aerobic environment. If the environment remains susceptible, as soon as that tympanic membrane knits and recreates an anaerobic environment, pressure will build again and re-rupture the freshly knitted and not quite cured membrane and the ensuing scar tissue can compromise the ability of the eardrum to properly transmit sound and hearing loss can occur. This is a great source of consternation for parents of small children and a major reason why parents visit emergency rooms at all times of the day and night. It is one of the most common reasons why children are given antibiotic prescriptions that then disrupt the intestinal microbiome, facilitate fungal overgrowths and start cycles of ecological and immune dysfunction. We have better answers!! Avoiding sugar and dairy helps a majority of children with this issue...as does limiting wheat, soy and eggs (these are all 'globular' proteins that impart a thick, globular consistency to mucus)[12]. Lean proteins and fresh fruits and vegetables are practically foreign to families that start their days with cold cereal and milk, toast and eggs, engage in fast food burger/chicken nugget lunches, with macaroni and cheese or cheese crisp snacks and pizza for dinner. Judicious application of normal sleep cycles, lots of loving touch, soothing language, Apples, Pears, Plums, Blueberries, Blackberries, Avocados, lean meats and nuts and seeds through the days of small children's lives is practically miraculous. Herbal teas with a small amount of agave syrup through crazy straws are fun and therapeutic. Hydrotherapy techniques like alternating hot and cold, wet sheet packs, and wet socks are amazingly effective in resolving the inevitable upper respiratory infections of childhood. The classic herbs, Echinacea, Thyme, Anemopsis, Baptisia, Licorice, Ginger, even Datura and Lobelia can be extremely helpful in stimulating immune responses, opening up Eustachian tubes and sinus passageways and resolving infectious conditions. N-Acetyl-Cysteine as a powder smells like a fart but tastes a little sour and can be mixed in applesauce at 300 mg 2-3 times a day and works well for thinning the mucus secretion and resolving otitis media. Swollen lymph nodes in the head and neck respond to small amounts of Iris and Phytolacca. Swollen, indurated tonsils and sore throats respond to throat sprays of Spilanthes, Zanthoxylum and Echinacea, with tinctures of Baptisia, Sambucus, Elecampane and Salvia apania.

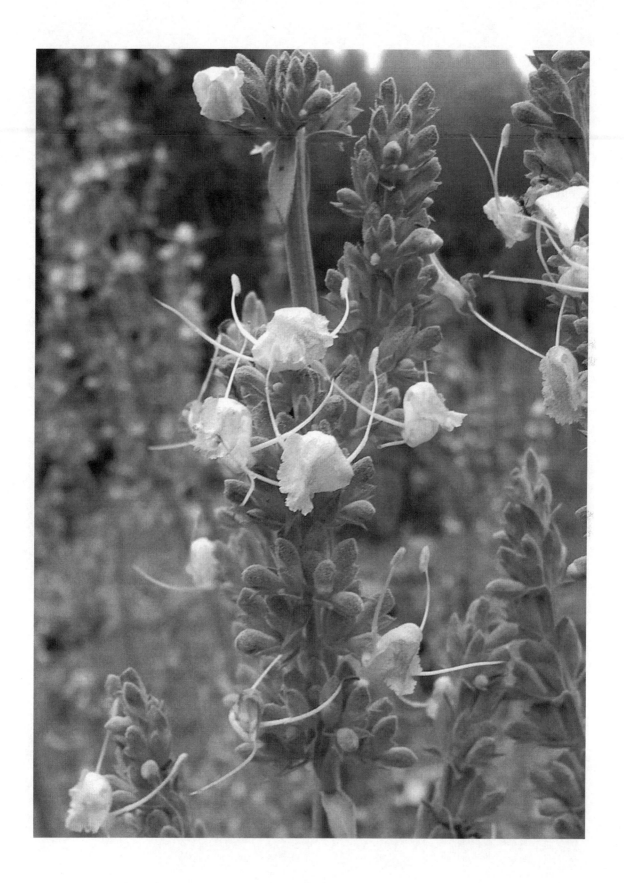

More specifically, I will include small amounts of Lobelia and/or Datura to a tincture for a patient with otitis media...typically on the order of 5 ml of either one or both in a 60 ml tincture that I am dosing 30 drops 4-6 times a day. The tropane alkaloids have a relaxing and dilating effect on the eustachian tube and impart a drying effect to the inner ear. Application of alternating hot/cold, four minutes hot, one minute cold, to the area of the ear down into the neck is helpful to get more exuberant blood flow into and out of the areas that are affected, with 8-9 hot/cold applications often being very helpful before laying down for bed. The pain is the hardest part of the process for the patient and their parents to deal with and often results in a very hard to console child. A warming light bulb placed at the opening of the ear can help, one should place their hand between the light bulb and the child's skin to ensure it is not hot enough to burn them...if you are using an LED bulb...forget about it, it is not likely to ever get warm enough to be effective. A blow dryer on a low speed that allows for the introduction of warming air into the ear canal can also be helpful. I will often use a few drops of 2% procaine with 2 drops of Aconitum tincture into the ear canal just to numb the area to provide a measure of relief...Caution! if you see enough pressure in the ear such that the TM is bulging and looks likely to rupture...the good news is that if it ruptures, the patient will be out of pain. but they won't be able to hear for a while after...however, if material has been placed into the ear canal, it will now be able to freely move into the compartment of the inner ear and cause no end of problems. I have seen this be the case more often than I could count with things like Garlic and Mullein ear drops...using sterile, water soluble materials is going to cause fewer issues than an oil based substance. In 24 years of practice, I have had to rely on antibiotic interventions for Acute Otitis Media only a handful of times and every time because of a rupture after administration of an OTC ear drop that secondarily contaminated the inner ear.

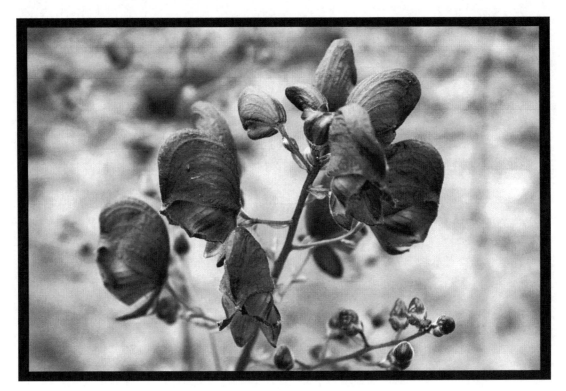

Acute Sinusitis

Acute sinusitis is most often caused by viral or bacterial organisms, and antibiotics are not guaranteed to help even if the causative agent is bacterial. The most common presenting symptoms include halitosis, fatigue, headache, decreased appetite, but most physical exam findings are non-specific and do not distinguish bacterial from viral causes. Environmental allergy can be a common predisposing factor and many cases of subacute, chronic sinusitis involve a secondary fungal presence that has to be dealt with in order to completely resolve the chronicity.

According to the CDC, a bacterial diagnosis may be established based on the presence of one of the following criteria:

• **Persistent symptoms without improvement**: nasal discharge or daytime cough >10 days.

• **Worsening symptoms**: worsening or new onset fever, daytime cough, or nasal discharge after initial improvement of a viral URI.

• **Severe symptoms:** fever ≥101°F, purulent nasal discharge for at least 3 consecutive days.

Imaging tests are no longer recommended for uncomplicated cases.

If a bacterial infection is established:

• Watchful waiting for up to 3 days may be offered for children with acute bacterial sinusitis with persistent symptoms.

• Antibiotic therapy is suggested for children with acute bacterial sinusitis with severe or worsening disease.

• Amoxicillin or amoxicillin/clavulanate (Augmentin) remain first-line therapy.

Recommendations for treatment of children with a history of type I hypersensitivity to penicillin: cefdinir, cefuroxime, cefpodoxime, or ceftriaxone may be appropriate choices.
In children who are vomiting or who cannot tolerate oral medication, a single injection dose of ceftriaxone can be used and then can be switched to oral antibiotics if improving.[1,2]

Sinusitis is one of the most common complaints in North American medical visits, and one of the main reasons for antibiotic prescriptions. About 135 in 1,000 persons – 31 million people - are affected yearly in the US. The general classification of rhinosinusitis is according to the length of the condition, acute cases last less than 12 weeks and chronic cases are those lasting over 12 weeks. Chronic rhinosinusitis sufferers may present with nasal polyps, associated with neutrophilic presence and a likely fungal infection where those without polyps are largely associated with allergic eosinophilic infiltration. Biofilm expression in rhinosinusitis cases has been studied since 2001 when scanning electron microscopy (SEM) was initially used to identify biofilms in Eustachian tubes, sinus passageways, ventilation tubes, and also associated with chronic otitis media. Biofilms have also been demonstrated in cholesteatomas, chronic tonsillitis, adenoids of patients with chronic sinusitis, and infections associated with biomaterials such as voice prostheses and myringotomy tubes. In children, it is important to recognize that it is common for them to have some level of predisposing allergic response and that acute sinusitis becomes chronic when the underlying allergy is not appropriately addressed.

Topical application to the sinus passageways of therapeutic materials through nasal sprays and nasal washes can be a very effective way to treat sinusitis and there are several agents that I have used quite extensively in this way. The first of these agents is reduced L-Glutathione, made as a saline solution of 100 mg/ml or 200 mg/ml in sterile saline. Gutathione is a tripeptide of the amino acids glycine, glutamine and N-acetyl-cysteine; it is heavily involved in tissue detoxification reactions and requires selenium as a cofactor. Glutathione is one of the most versatile and important antioxidants produced by our bodies. It has a specific affinity for liver and mucus membrane tissues where it has been shown to inhibit angiogenesis, facilitate the repair of DNA, scavenge free radicals, have anti-tumor activity and is required for optimal activation of T-lymphocytes. It is generally well tolerated in eyedrops, nasal sprays, nebulizers and is dosed 4 times a day. I generally augment it with NAC, in half the concentration of the glutathione, as an agent that helps keep the glutathione in a reduced form and as a mucolytic agent, helping to make mucus have a less globular and more planar structure, making it more protective and less likely to get stuck in the smaller vessels of the sinuses. NAC is also a very strong free radical scavenger, inhibits angiogenesis, facilitates the repair of DNA, inhibits further bacterial growth as well as being a major component of glutathione. Other systemic considerations that are often helpful include 1/8-1/2 tsp of local bee pollen consumed daily (start small and work up to the higher doses) to create an oral desensitization to commonly occurring pollens in your area. An amino acid powder consisting of half L-Threonine and half N-Acetyl-Glutamine, orally dosed at 5-10 grams per day is often very helpful in repairing damaged membranes as well as creating newer membranes that are more durable and for stimulating a more effective immune response.

L-Threonine is an essential amino acid that has several important functions in the body and is a precursor to the other amino acids, serine and glycine. All three of these amino acids are necessary for muscle tissue production, proper immune function and muscle coordination and control. L-Threonine helps to produce the mucus gel layer that covers and protects the mucus membranes of the body. This mucus layer is a protective barrier from the outside world and is supportive to the bacteria that make up the microbiome, it is also a major component of the secreted immune proteins of the mucosal tissues. L-threonine is specifically involved in the production of antibodies within the immune system. The thymus gland, which resides in the middle of our chest, is especially active in childhood, is responsible for making and maturing T lymphocytes (T- cells), L-threonine is a critical component of this process.

L-Glutamine is the most abundant amino acid in the body and accounts for 60% of the intracellular amino acid pool, it is considered to be conditionally essential as a deficiency can occur rapidly after infection or injury. Glutamine is the primary fuel source for rapidly dividing cells like epithelial cells of the mucus membranes during healing. Like NAC, it is a potent antioxidant and a component of the intracellular glutathione system. It also has direct immunological function by stimulating lymphocyte proliferation and is the rate-limiting agent for new protein synthesis.

Herbal teas can be quite effective when applied as nasal washes, sprays, eyewashes/drops. I generally make the tea, then try to get it to an iso-osmolar concentration by creating a 0.9% solution of sodium chloride and potassium bicarbonate (1 measured teaspoon of finely ground sea salt is approximately 7.5 grams and ¼ teaspoon of potassium bicarbonate or sodium bicarbonate (baking soda)=1.5 grams added to a quart of water or tea).

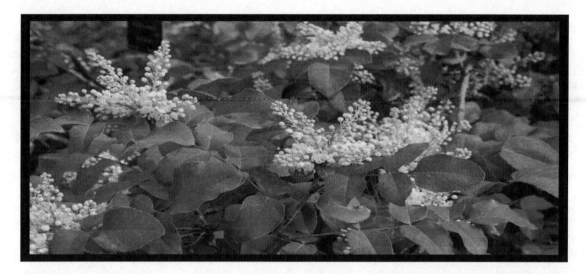

The best course of action in initiating this type of therapy is to start with dilute, weak teas and then make them stronger as the need might present. Green and black teas exert an astringent effect in the nasal passageway, which is helpful in boggy, swollen, polypoid conditions, 2 tbsps colloidal silver in a quart of nasal wash can be nicely anti-microbial, Licorice tea is nicely demulcent, soothing and anti-inflammatory in a nasal wash. Berberis, Mahonia, Hydrastis, and Achalypha have been shown to be helpful in breaking down biofilms. Twice a day application of 30-50 ml of nasal wash through a neti-pot can be wildly effective, but a hard sell in smaller children who are quite sure that you are drowning them. In smaller children, judiciously (4-6 times a day) applied nasal sprays can be very effective.

Mucus chemistry is a very fascinating aspect of membrane health that can be dramatically affected by shifting both osmolarity and pH. Mucus is a conglomeration of the secreted protein mucin and the numerous saccharides that glycosylate it. Some of the most critical of these saccharides are the family of sialic acids, and within this family, the compound neuraminic acid. Sialic acids contribute greatly to the viscosity of mucus, the more acidic the internal environment, the higher the viscosity or thickness of the mucus; alternately, the more alkaline the internal environment, the thinner the mucus. The acidic nature of the infectious process creates a thickening of the mucoid secretions, making them significantly more "sticky", a measure which impedes further progression of the infection. Moreover, the acidic environment of the mucus membranes is conducive to tissue constriction through the neural reflex (acidity creates 'tension' in the tissues), inhibition of histamine breakdown, and is a contributor to tissue irritation. One of the reasons why the Influenza family of viruses is so virulent is that it has evolved a neuraminidase enzyme that allows the viral particles to cleave through the thickening and protective neuraminic acid component of the mucus and infect adjacent tissues to the primary site of infection. Neutralizing the acidity of mucus makes it a looser, thinner mucus, facilitating liquefaction of the harder secretions, promoting relaxation and improvement of blood flow into and out of affected tissues while inactivating histamines. Applying relatively alkaline solutions to the affected tissues represents a decided advantage in the treatment of patients with many congestive conditions of the mucus membranes. I find that using potassium bicarbonate, where reasonable (baking soda, sodium bicarbonate, is far more readily available), as a buffer to bring the pH of a topical solution into a slightly alkaline realm adds even more greatly to the therapeutic potential.

Closely related to the idea of mucus chemistry is the concept of biofilm. According to JW Costerton at the Center for Biofilm Engineering in Montana, a bacterial biofilm as "a structured community of bacterial cells enclosed in a self-produced polymeric matrix and adherent to an inert or living surface"[13]. In other words, bacteria can join together on essentially any surface and start to form a protective matrix around their colony. This matrix, or syncytium, has many of the same physical properties that mucus does and is made of similar polymers composed of molecules with repeating structural units that are connected by chemical bonds. These biofilms form when bacteria adhere to surfaces in aqueous environments and begin to excrete their slimy, glue-like polymeric substances that anchor them to some substrate material, which could be metals, plastics, soil particles, medical implant materials and, most significantly, human or animal tissue. The first bacterial colonists to adhere to a surface initially do so by inducing weak, reversible bonds called van der Waals forces. If the colonists are not immediately separated from the surface, they can anchor themselves more permanently using cell adhesion molecules. These bacteria facilitate and support the presence of other pathogens by providing more diverse adhesion sites. They also continue to build the matrix that holds the biofilm together, allowing an environment conducive to the presence of more and more micro-organisms, many that would not be able to survive in the host on their own. Several studies have shown that while a biofilm is being created, the pathogens inside it can communicate with each other via a phenomenon called quorum sensing which allows them to communicate their presence by emitting chemical messages that their fellow infectious agents are able to recognize. Although the mechanisms behind quorum sensing are not fully understood, the phenomenon allows a single-celled bacterium to perceive how many other bacteria are in close proximity. When a bacterium senses the presence of other microbes, it is more inclined to join them and contribute to the formation of a biofilm. When the messages grow strong enough, the bacteria respond en masse, behaving as a group. Quorum sensing can occur within a single bacterial species as well as between diverse species, and can regulate a host of different processes, essentially serving as a simple communication network that allows the biofilm community of organisms to act as a single organism.

As the biofilm grows through a combination of cell division and recruitment it allows the cells inside to become more resistant to antibiotics administered in a standard fashion. In fact, depending on the organism and type of antimicrobial, biofilm bacteria can be up to a thousand times more resistant to antimicrobial stress than free-swimming bacteria of the same species. Biofilms tend to grow slowly, in diverse locations, and biofilm infections are often slow to produce overt symptoms. However, biofilm bacteria can move in ways that allow them to insidiously expand and infect new tissues. Biofilms move collectively, by rippling or rolling across the surface, or by detaching in clumps. Sometimes, in a dispersal strategy referred to as "swarming/seeding", a biofilm colony differentiates to form an outer "wall" of stationary bacteria, while the inner region of the biofilm "liquefies", allowing planktonic cells to "swim" out of the biofilm and leave behind a hollow mound. Research on the molecular and genetic basis of biofilm development has made it clear that when cells switch from independent, planktonic to community mode, they also undergo a shift in behavior that involves alterations in the activity of numerous genes. There is evidence that specific genes must be transcribed during the attachment phase of biofilm development. In many cases, the activation of these genes is required for synthesis of the extracellular matrix that protects the pathogens inside. This represents an epigenetic phenomenon within the microorganisms themselves and speaks to how single organisms may have been able to consolidate and evolve into multi-cellular organisms.

According to Costerton, the genes that allow a biofilm to develop are activated after some critical mass number of cells attach to a solid surface. "Thus, it appears that attachment itself is what stimulates synthesis of the extracellular matrix in which the sessile bacteria are embedded," states the molecular biologist. "This notion that bacteria have a sense of touch that enables detection of a surface and the expression of specific genes, is, in itself, an exciting area of research." Biofilms can be broken down by topical application of hyperosmolar saline solutions, radical shifts of pH, and the judicious use of chelating agents like EDTA, DMSA and DMPS, sulfur products like Glutathione and N-Acetyl-Cysteine, mineral products like bismuth subnitrate and subgallate, proteolytic enzymes like lysozymes, hyaluronidases and serratiopeptidases as well as botanical agents like *Achalypha mexicana, Achillea, Allium sativa, Althaea, Anemopsis, Arctostaphylos* Uva Ursi, *Baptisia, Boswellia, Bursera, Calendula, Commiphora myrrha, Echinacea, Hydrastis, Hypericum, Larrea, Myrica, Plantago*, Propolis, and *Thuja*, among others. Most modern antibiotics are not effective against these biofilm communities; in fact, it is these types of communities that are direct contributors to the formation of antibiotic resistant strains of bacteria. It requires some physical as well as physiological/biochemical methods to break down and eradicate a biofilm community.

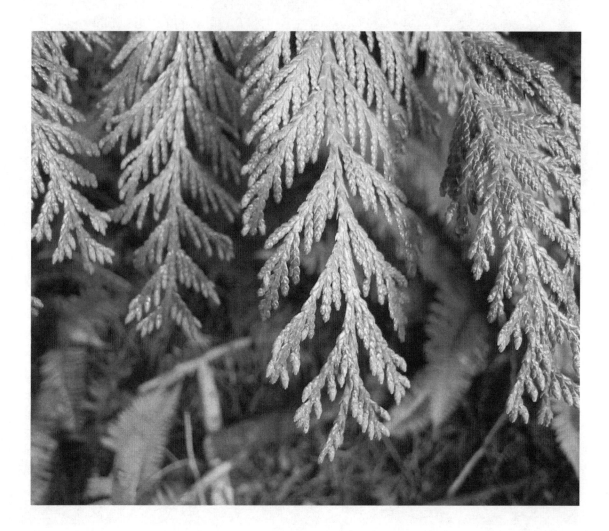

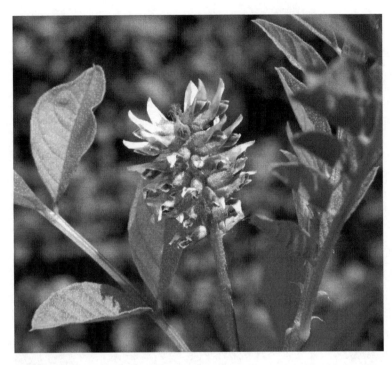

The components of a nasal spray can vary tremendously but, in my practice, usually consist of a base of L-Glutathione (100 mg/ml), N-Acetyl-Cysteine (50 mg/ml, and the licorice saponin, Glycyrrhizinate, 5 mg/ml. Glycyrrhizic acid is a glycosylated saponin (a soap-like molecule) that is directly anti-microbial, inhibiting of biofilm formation, and anti-inflammatory.

The practicality of making this kind of preparation at home or in one's office setting requires the ability to weigh the ingredients. All three of these components are acidic and need to be made neutral in their pH or they will be highly irritating to the mucus membrane tissues. Fortunately, they are all reactive with bicarbonate and at a 2:1 ratio by weight. Specifically, if one was to make a liter/quart of such a solution, they would start with a large vessel--2-3 times larger, by volume than what they think because this is a chemical reaction that is going to create a very foamy product that will smell like sulfur and get everywhere if it is not contained. For every 100 grams of L-Glutathione, one needs 50 grams of sodium bicarbonate to neutralize the pH, for every 50 grams of NAC, one will need 25 grams of sodium bicarbonate, and for every 5 grams of glycyrrhizic acid, one will need 2.5 grams of bicarbonate, this would be enough material to make a liter of finished product. So, 155 gms of material is going to require 77.5 gms of sodium bicarbonate/baking soda to appropriately neutralize the pH. 80 gms of bicarbonate will ensure that the final product has an alkaline pH and will have a better effect on mucus viscosity. A reasonable strategy for mixing is to place the mixed powders in the bottom of a vessel and slowly add distilled water, controlling the rate at which the materials react with the water by controlling how quickly it is added, until a final volume of 1 liter is reached. Such a nasal spray/wash can be administered 6 times a day, one spray into each nostril with really good effect. Often, I will also add 1 mg/ml Lysozyme to the nasal spray to improve penetration into the tissues and provide better immune 'clean-up'.

Lysozymes are enzymes that damage bacteria by catalyzing hydrolysis of 1,4-beta-linkages in the cell wall. They are naturally abundant in human secretions, such as tears, saliva, human milk, and mucus. They are also present in cytoplasmic granules of the macrophages and the neutrophils and play a significant role in non-specific immune response. Lysozymes are commercially prepared from egg whites, we purchase 100 gms at a time and mix them into eyedrops, nasal sprays, nebulizer solutions, and for wound healing poultices and compresses at a 1mg/ml.

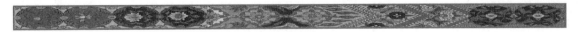

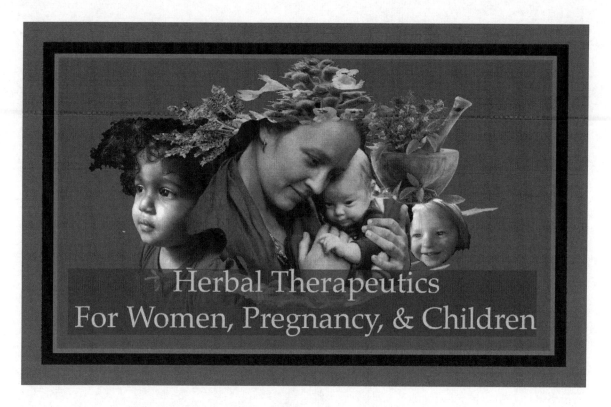

STRATEGIES FOR ACUTE ILLNESS
IN CHILDREN
PART II

by Kenneth Proefrock

Pharyngitis

Pharyngitis is the universal manifestation of the 'sore throat', and often equated to "Strep Throat" in the minds of parents everywhere. Recent pediatric guidelines aim to minimize unnecessary antibiotic exposure by emphasizing appropriate use of rapid antigen detection test (RADT) testing and subsequent treatment. During the Winter and Spring, up to 20% of asymptomatic children can be colonized with group A beta-hemolytic streptococci (GAS), leading to more false positives from RADT-testing and increases in unnecessary antibiotic exposure.

• Streptococcal pharyngitis is primarily a disease of children 5-15 years old and is rare in children < 3 years.
• Clinical features alone do not distinguish between streptococcal and viral pharyngitis.
• Children with sore throat plus 2 or more of the following features should be considered candidates for a rapid strep test:
  •absence of cough
  •presence of tonsillar exudates or swelling
  •history of fever
  •presence of swollen and tender anterior cervical lymph nodes

Testing should generally not be performed in children < 3 years in whom GAS rarely causes pharyngitis and rheumatic fever is uncommon.

In children and adolescents, the standard of care is that negative rapid strep tests should be backed up by a throat culture; positive tests do not require a back-up culture.

Amoxicillin and penicillin V remain first-line therapy. Recommended treatment course for all oral beta lactams is 10 days.

For children with a non-type I hypersensitivity to penicillin: cephalexin, cefadroxil, clindamycin, clarithromycin, or azithromycin are recommended.

For children with an immediate type I hypersensitivity to penicillin: clindamycin, clarithromycin, or azithromycin are recommended.

By far, the majority of pharyngitis cases seen in my practice are viral in origin, if I suspect a bacterial presence, usually indicated by a higher than 102^0 F fever and purulent white patches on the tonsils, I will usually start with a topical spray to reduce the pain and inflammation locally as well as to initiate a different immune response.

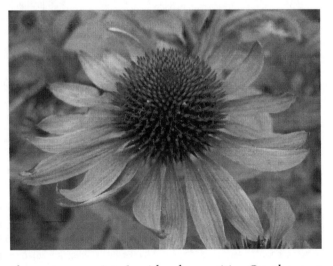

My usual throat spray preparations include *Echinacea angustifolia & purpurea*, propolis, *Hyssopus officinalis*, *Zanthoxylum clava-herculis*, *Monarda fistulosa*, *Ligusticum porteri*, bitter and sweet orange essential oils. In some cases, I will exchange the Echinacea for *Rudbeckia laciniata*, a yellow cone flower endemic to the Southwest US and Mexico that is also nicely immuno-stimulating, adding 1-2 ml of Iris to a 1 oz preparation can initiate a nice lymph moving effect for patients with unusually large tonsils, *Spilanthes acmella* is complimentary to the *Zanthoxylum* and *Echinacea* in reducing the pain associated with pharyngitis. On the rare occasion, I will add colloidal silver to the spray in order to generate a stronger anti-microbial effect, sometimes it seems to work and seldom makes the situation worse.

Throat poultices, which consist of grated Potatoes, Carrots, Jicama, or other bulky plant material encased in cheesecloth or linen and wrapped around the neck with a scarf, can be helpful in improving blood flow into and out of the tonsillar area...essentially we are making a warming poultice, which is cool when applied and stimulates increased blood flow through the region while the body tries to warm it up. The grated plant material adds biomass that requires more effort, i.e. blood flow, to properly warm up and makes the poultice effect more dramatic. Once the poultice is warmed to body temperature, it is removed, rinsed with cold water and reapplied.

Common Cold or Non-Specific Upper Respiratory Tract Infection (URI)

This is, as the name suggests, very common. There are at least 200 known viruses that are able to cause the common cold and the course of most uncomplicated viral URIs is 5 – 10 days.

- Viral URIs are often characterized by nasal discharge and congestion or cough. Usually nasal discharge begins as clear and changes throughout the course of the illness.

- Fever, if present, is typically low-grade ($<102^0$) and occurs early in the illness.

- According to the CDC, management of the common cold, nonspecific URI, and acute cough illness should focus on symptomatic relief. They suggest that antibiotics should not be prescribed for these conditions.

There is potential for harm and no proven benefit from over-the-counter cough and cold medications in children < 6 years. These substances are among the top 20 substances leading to death in children <5 years. Low-dose inhaled corticosteroids and oral prednisolone do not improve outcomes in children without asthma (and are seldom more than temporarily helpful in those with asthma).

This is an arena where botanical medicine and hydrotherapy really shine. Something as simple as wet socks or a wet sheet pack can be wildly helpful. Wet socks consists of applying a pair of damp cotton socks and then dry wool socks to the feet of the patient before bed. The rationale is that the body will increase peripheral blood flow in order to resolve the dampness of the socks, the wool socks keep the feet from getting cold and allow the moisture to evaporate. As blood flow is improved peripherally, lymph flow is also improved and the endogenous immune response becomes more effective. Administering this treatment at the beginning of a URI and persisting nightly will, typically, allow for a deeper, more restful sleep and faster resolution of the condition. A wet sheet pack consists of placing the child in a warm to hot bath with a warm to hot tea to drink (Ginger with honey and lemon works well for children, but, really, any diaphoretic tea that they will drink will work). When the child is removed from the bath, they are immediately, without drying them off, wrapped in a flannel or linen sheet and then wrapped in a wool blanket. Smaller children can be held, older children are put to bed and allowed to generate a fever. I have seen a 103^0 from this treatment within an hour of being bundled. This therapy can be quite profound, even in the most hardcore URI.

Fever is an important subject to address here as it is a very important part of how an immune system operates, however, it is also one of the manifestations of illness that contribute to parental anxiety[14]. Mostly, a fever is a very beneficial process that is generated by the cytokine interleukin 1 (IL-1) which participates in the regulation of immune response, inflammatory reactions and hematopoesis, it is produced by macrophages, endothelial cells, B-cells, and fibroblast cells. IL-1 has direct central nervous system effects that include producing fever and shivering while augmenting corticosteroid release. As a whole body process, fever is beneficial by enhancing the effects of immune regulating interferons, inhibiting the growth of many organisms and enhancing the performance of phagocytes and the specific immune response while accelerating tissue remodeling and repair. The ideal temperature for a fever to accomplish these objectives is 102-103^0 F. A fever that goes too high and or lasts too long can begin to have adverse effects that outweigh the positive effects as a fever also contributes to the denaturing of biological proteins, inhibits nerve impulses, and contributes to dehydration.

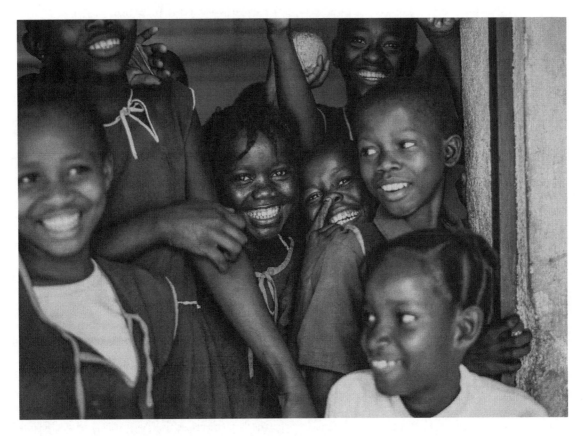

Many parents have false beliefs about fever, they think fever will hurt their child so they worry and lose sleep when their child is feverish. My approach is to reassure them and encourage them to stimulate a fever through a wet sheet pack.

About 80% of children who act sick and feel warm do have a fever. If you want to be sure, take the temperature. These are the cutoffs for fever using different types of thermometers:

•Rectal, ear or forehead temperature: 100.4° F (38.0° C) or higher

•Oral (mouth) temperature: 100° F (37.8° C) or higher

•Under the arm (Armpit) temperature: 99° F (37.2° C) or higher

We have to emphasize that a fever turns on the body's immune system and helps the body fight off the infection. Normal fevers between 100° and 104° F (37.8° - 40° C) are generally good. Fevers with infections don't cause brain damage. Only temperatures above 108° F (42° C) can cause brain damage and it's very rare for the body temperature to climb this high. It only happens if the air temperature is very high, like summers in Arizona or if one is left in a closed car during hot weather.

Fevers only need to be treated if they cause discomfort and most fevers don't cause discomfort until they go above 102° or 103° F (39° or 39.5° C). Most fevers from infection don't go above 103° or 104° F (39.5°- 40° C), and very rarely go up to 105° or 106° F (40.6° or 41.1° C). While these are "high" fevers, they are generally harmless.

Only 4% of children have seizures associated with fever, they are generally related to dehydration and electrolyte imbalances. These seizures are scary to watch, but they stop within 5 minutes. They don't cause any permanent harm. They don't increase the risk for speech delays, learning problems, or seizures without fever[14].

With pharmacologic treatment, most fevers only come down 2° or 3° F (1° or 1.5° C).

Fevers that don't come down to normal can be caused by viruses or bacteria. The response to fever medicines tells us nothing about the cause of the infection. It's normal for fevers with most viral infections to last for 2 or 3 days. When the fever suppressant wears off, the fever will come back. The fever will go away and not return once the body overpowers the virus. Most often, this is day 3 or 4.

If the fever is high, the cause may or may not be serious. If the patient looks very sick, the cause is more likely to be serious. The child who is playing with the toys in the waiting area of your office is less concerning than the child who is lethargic and slow. How a person presents is what's important. The exact temperature number is not necessarily so important.

Viral infections are a serious threat to the health of people in all parts of the world. For most bacterial diseases, several antibiotic drugs are available, viral diseases are often more difficult to treat because viruses spread and mutate very rapidly. The control and treatment of a viral infection in the conventional medical model depends mainly on the availability of antiviral drugs, which are few and usually are not virucidal but simply prevent replication in the host. It has become imperative to develop effective medical strategies for the management of common viral diseases like influenza, which can assume pandemic proportions and become a major threat to humanity. Complementary and alternative medicines have been used effectively by humans over several centuries for treating various diseases and can be effectively employed to target the host response during influenza outbreaks.

True anti-viral agents are few and far between in the world of pharmaceutical agents as well as in botanical medicine, however, botanical medicine offers a rich variety of options for modifying the immune response and engaging more and less anti-viral host defense mechanisms. The agents that I employ for such conditions is very dependent on the presentation of the patient.

Oseltamivir (Tamiflu), a neuraminidase inhibitor, was approved for the treatment of influenza by the US Food and Drug Administration in 1999. It is a sialic acid analog, ultimately made from star anise, Illicium vera, that restrains viral population to one generation, decreases viral load, and so, theoretically, contains the infection and its outcomes. Oseltamivir is taken orally and is potentiated in the liver by the action of carboxyl esterase. Its half-life is 6–10 h with good oral bioavailability. The side effects include nausea, diarrhea, insomnia, abdominal pain, and headache[15].

A number of randomized controlled trials, systematic reviews, and meta-analysis originally suggested that the drug was safe and efficacious, unfortunately, the majority of those studies were funded by Roche, which also first marketed and promoted this drug. In 2005 and 2009, the looming fear of pandemic flu led to recommendation by prominent regulatory bodies such as the World Health Organization (WHO), Centers for Disease Control and Prevention, European Medicines Agency and others for its use in treatment and prophylaxis of influenza, and it's stockpiling as a measure to tide over the crisis. As the drug became more widely used, some reports of serious adverse events began to surface, especially notable were neuropsychiatric events in children.

There had been no mention of adverse effects associated with the use of this drug in the published trials. Post-marketing surveillance had uncovered adverse effects like raised liver enzymes, hepatitis, neuropsychiatric events, cardiac arrhythmia, skin hypersensitivity reactions including toxic epidermal necrolysis, Stevens-Johnson syndrome and erythema multiforme, metabolic side effects and renal events[16]. In some cases, increased QTc prolongation was seen in ECG in the treatment group compared with placebo during on-treatment periods. The most important serious adverse events which raised concerns were neuropsychiatric events such as depressed mood, behavior disturbance, panic attack, suicidal ideation, delusion, delirium, convulsion, and encephalitis. These were reported more frequently in children than in adults and generally occurred within 48 h of drug intake[17].

A recent Cochrane review (2014) and related articles have questioned the risk-benefit ratio of the drug, besides raising doubts about the regulatory decision of approving it. The recommendations for stockpiling the said drug as given by various international organizations like the WHO and CDC have also been put to scrutiny. It would appear that a climate of pandemic panic, publicity propaganda, and scientific misconduct turned a new medicine with only modest efficacy into a blockbuster. It appears that the multiple regulatory checks and balances gave way as science lost its primacy and pharmaceutical enterprise lost no time in making the most of it. Another neuraminidase inhibitor has been brought to market more recently, Relenza (Zanamivir), but, overuse of Tamiflu seems to have encouraged resistance to both drugs.

There is no shortage of botanical agents that share a myriad of host immune stimulating effects as well as antimicrobial influences. Nearly every system of traditional medicine from every culture on the planet have their favorites, from *Glycyrrhiza*, *Sambucus*, *Ocimum*, *Eupatorium*, *Mentha*, *Melissa*, *Hypericum* and *Azadirachta*. It goes beyond the scope of our discussion to go into depth on these agents. It may suffice to say that frequent consumption of warm herbal beverages is sensorially pleasing and impactful of immune systems while helping to mitigate some of the presenting symptoms of a viral infection. Inasmuch as they contribute to hydration, manage nausea, encourage expectoration and occupy the mind, they are immeasurably helpful. A little honey and a crazy straw will entice even the most reluctant toddler to consume some *Melissa*, *Sambucus* or *Zingiber* tea.

Bronchiolitis

This is the most common lower respiratory tract infection in infants. It is most often caused by respiratory syncytial virus but can be caused by many other respiratory viruses. Bronchiolitis occurs in children<24 months and is characterized by rhinorrhea, cough, wheezing, tachypnea, and/ or increased respiratory effort.

• Routine laboratory tests and radiologic studies are not recommended, but a chest x-ray may be warranted in atypical disease (absence of viral symptoms, severe distress, frequent recurrences, lack of improvement).

• Usually patients worsen between 3-5 days, followed by improvement.

• Antibiotics are not helpful and should not be used.

• Nasal suctioning is mainstay of therapy.

• Neither albuterol nor nebulized racemic epinephrine should be administered to infants and children with bronchiolitis who are not hospitalized.

• There is no evidence to support routine suctioning of the lower pharynx or larynx (deep suctioning).

• There is no role for corticosteroids, ribavirin, or chest physiotherapy in the management of bronchiolitis[18].

Nasal sprays and nebulizer solutions of slightly alkaline saline solutions are the mainstays of treatment for infants with bronchiolitis in my practice. A pulse oxymeter is a very useful, even essential, tool in the treatment of infants with pulmonary conditions, they can be purchased online and fit on baby toes to register their oxygen saturation levels. Supplemental oxygen can be administered with the nebulizer treatment and the infant's response can be monitored by the changing O_2 levels.

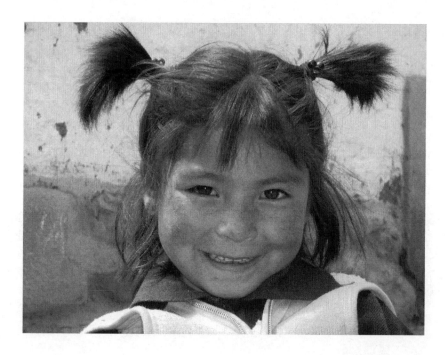

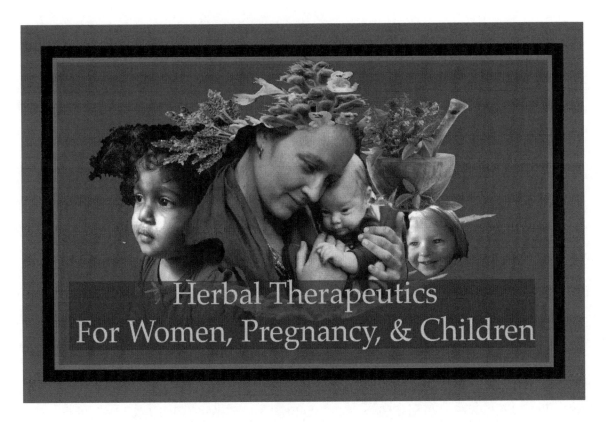

Herbal Therapeutics
For Women, Pregnancy, & Children

STRATEGIES FOR ACUTE ILLNESS IN CHILDREN
PART III

by Kenneth Proefrock

Urinary Tract Infections

Urinary tract infections (UTIs) are common in children, affecting 8% of girls and 2% of boys by age 7. The most common causative pathogen is E. coli, accounting for approximately 85% of cases. In infants, fever and or strong-smelling urine are common. In school-aged children, dysuria, frequency, or urgency are common. A definitive diagnosis requires both a urinalysis suggestive of infection and at least 50,000 CFUs/mL of a single uropathogen from urine obtained through catheterization or suprapubic aspiration (NOT urine collected in a bag) for children 2–24 months...I do not recommend this approach...catheterizing a child who is suspected of having a bladder infection is most certainly going to spread that infection further into the urinary tract. It may take some effort, time and patience, but most of the time a urine sample can be procured from a child without traumatizing them.

• Urinalysis is suggestive of infection with the presence of pyuria (leukocyte esterase or ≥5 WBCs per high powered field), bacteriuria, or nitrites.

• Nitrites are not a sensitive measure for UTI in children and cannot be used to rule out UTIs.

• The decision to assess for UTI by urine testing for all children 2--24 months with unexplained fever is no longer recommended and should be based on the child's likelihood of UTI[9].

• Initial antibiotic treatment should be based on local antimicrobial susceptibility patterns. • Suggested agents include TMP/SMX, amoxicillin/clavulanate, cefixime, cefpodoxime, cefprozil, or cephalexin in children 2-24 months.

• Duration of therapy should be 7-14 days in children 2-24 months.

• Antibiotic treatment of asymptomatic bacteriuria in children is not recommended.

• Febrile infants with UTIs should undergo renal and bladder ultrasonography during or following their first UTI. Abnormal imaging results require further testing.

Causation of UTI's in children can become a tricky arena, bubble bath can be a culprit as can other bath soaps as they can compromise and diminish the protective mucus lining in the urethra, girls are more susceptible than boys but it can happen to both. Personal hygiene practices are important to consider, infants and toddlers left too long in dirty diapers become susceptible to UTI's, teaching children to wipe themselves from front to back after using the bathroom is likewise important. Recurrent UTI's can be associated with foreign objects and dirty fingers, the patient's own or someone else's and that is a conversation that should be had more frequently than it does.

The prevalence of child sexual abuse is difficult to determine because it is often under-reported; experts agree that the incidence is far greater than what is reported to authorities. CSA is also not uniformly defined, so statistics may vary. Statistics below represent some of the research done on child sexual abuse[19].

The U.S. Department of Health and Human Services' Children's Bureau report Child Maltreatment 2010 found that 9.2% of victimized children admitted to being sexually assaulted. Studies by David Finkelhor, Director of the Crimes Against Children Research Center, show that:

•1 in 5 girls and 1 in 20 boys is a reported victim of child sexual abuse (actual cases are estimated by the FBI to be closer to 3 out of 5 girls experiencing inappropriate sexual contact and 1 in 5 boys);

•Self-report studies show that at least 20% of adult females and 5-10% of adult males recall a childhood sexual assault or sexual abuse incident;

•During a one-year period in the U.S., 16% of youth ages 14 to 17 had been sexually victimized;

•Over the course of their lifetime, 28% of U.S. youth ages 14 to 17 had been sexually victimized;

•Children are most vulnerable to CSA between the ages of 7 and 13.

•According to a 2003 National Institute of Justice report, 3 out of 4 adolescents who have been sexually assaulted were victimized by someone they knew well.

•A study conducted in 1986 found that 63% of women who had suffered sexual abuse by a family member also reported a rape or attempted rape after the age of 14. Recent studies in 2000, 2002, and 2005 have all concluded similar results.

•A child who is the victim of prolonged sexual abuse usually develops low self-esteem, a feeling of worthlessness and an abnormal or distorted view of sex. The child may become withdrawn and mistrustful of adults, and often become suicidal.

•Children who do not live with both parents as well as children living in homes marked by parental discord, divorce, or domestic violence, have a higher risk of being sexually abused.

•In the vast majority of cases where there is credible evidence that a child has been violated, only between 5 and 15% of those children will have genital injuries consistent with sexual abuse.

This can be a difficult conversation to have with families, and the awkwardness makes a lot of practitioners shy away from the uncomfortable subject. It is an unfortunate reality and we don't serve these children if we don't provide the opportunity to shed light on these dark places.

Regardless of the cause of UTI's, there are a number of effective botanical and nutritional interventions that are very helpful. It should go without saying that the first step needs to be consuming enough water, about an ounce of water per kilo (2 lbs) of body weight for pediatric patients.

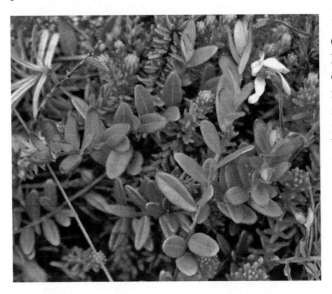

Vaccinium macrocarpon - American Cranberry has a long historical use in North American botanical medicine, especially in the treatment of urinary tract infections. The name of the berry comes from a contraction of "crane berry" which is a nickname of another Vaccinium, the bilberry, which is also somewhat effective in the prevention of UTI's. In fact, most of the Vaccinium family of plants have shown some measure of effectiveness in preventing and treating urinary tract infections. The constituents that are believed to play at least some role in the therapeutic effects include a family of anthocyanidins, proanthocyanidins and tannins that function as an antimicrobial defense system for the plants. The proanthocyandins appear to be specifically inhibitory to the adhesion process of E. coli to the urethral and bladder walls. The tannins have an astringent and antiseptic effect on the tissue walls, and D-mannose, a sugar found in all of the Vaccinia family of plants, also prevents bacterial adherence to the tissue walls. Unsweetened cranberry is sour and most kids won't care for it...I find that sweetening the cranberry juice with some blueberry juice and D-Mannose, and occasionally L-Threonine improves compliance. Such a recipe would look like a 50/50 mix (4 ozs) of unsweetened blueberry/cranberry juices with 1/2 tsp each of D-mannose and L-Threonine, dosed 4-6 times per day.

Arctostaphylos Uva-Ursi and *glauca*- Bearberry and Manzanita leaves, as well as the leaves of the Madrone tree, *Arbutus menziesii*, contain up to 10% of the glycoside, arbutin. Arbutin, under alkaline conditions in the kidney, is cleaved into glucose and hydroquinone. Hydroquinone is specifically antiseptic to the bladder and urethra and impedes adhesion and migration of bacterial cells. These plants also contain very astringent tannins that are also anti-microbial and serve to improve the tone in swollen boggy tissues. These are not very flavorful botanicals as teas, but I can often persuade children to take a tincture if I add Melissa, Schisandra or Albizia as a glycerite. Echinacea glycerite is also a useful agent to add to such a preparation. Dosage of a tincture that is arbutin rich of 1-5 ml 4-6 times a day is often effective.

Sometimes a urinary tract infection can be painful, both from the rawness of one's urethra as well as from cramping in the bladder. *Piscidia erythrina*, now *piscipula*, Jamaican dogwood, inner bark is very effective for bladder cramping, it is palatable as a glycerite and doses as low as 5 drops or as high as 15 drops can be very effective in reducing pain. Piper methysticum, Kava Kava is also very helpful in reducing the pain of irritated urethras, alongside *Zea mays*, cornsilk and demulcents like Althaea, Calendula, and *Asparagus racemosa*, Shatavari.

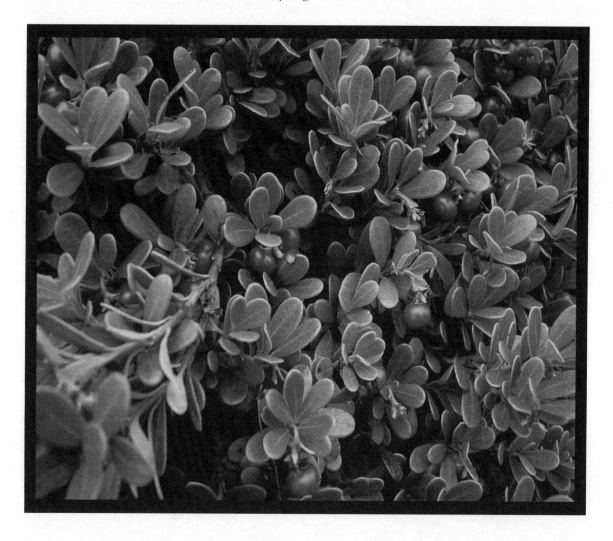

Diarrhea

Diarrhea remains one of the most common illnesses of children, and it is associated with 9% of all hospitalizations of children less than 5 years of age. One hundred years ago, diarrheal diseases were among the principal causes of death of children in the United States, with seasonal epidemics occurring during summer. Today, this pattern of illness is replicated on a wider scale in many developing countries, where 1.5 billion episodes of diarrhea and 4 million associated deaths occur among children each year[20,21].

These statistics translate to an average of 3.3 episodes of diarrhea per year for a child less than 5 years of age and greater than 10,000 childhood deaths worldwide per day. In the United States children less than 5 years of age still experience 20-35 million episodes of diarrhea per year, which result in 2-3.5 million doctor visits, greater than 200,000 hospitalizations, and 325-425 deaths[22-25].

Rotavirus is the most common cause of acute diarrhea among children, accounting for one-fourth of all cases[26], but many other viruses can cause childhood diarrhea as well, including Norwalk-like viruses, enteric adenoviruses, astroviruses, and caliciviruses. Important bacterial pathogens include Salmonella, Shigella, Yersinia, Campylobacter, and certain strains of Escherichia coli. Common parasitic causes of diarrhea include Giardia, Cryptosporidium, and Entamoeba histolytica. Despite the wide range of organisms associated with gastrointestinal infections, the mainstay of the treatment of a person with acute watery diarrhea is appropriate fluid and electrolyte therapy and nutritional management.

Oral rehydration therapy (ORT) is the preferred treatment of mild to moderate dehydration caused by diarrhea in children. Appropriate oral rehydration therapy can be as effective as intravenous fluid in managing fluid and electrolyte losses and has several advantages. Goals of oral rehydration therapy are restoration of circulating blood volume, restoration of interstitial fluid volume, and then maintenance of rehydration. Here we discuss different ORT solutions and discuss pros and cons of each preparation.

The perfect solution will meet the particular needs of the individual in that moment...no one product will cover everyone's needs. The general idea is that we will need some carbohydrate content, electrolytes like sodium, chloride, potassium and bicarbonate in clean water. During the past 25 years, WHO and UNICEF have recommended a single formulation of glucose-based oral rehydration salts to prevent or treat dehydration from diarrhea regardless of the cause or age group affected. This product, which provides a solution containing 90 mEq/l of sodium with a total osmolarity of 311 mOsm/l, has proven clinically effective the world over and has contributed substantially to the dramatic global reduction in mortality from diarrheal disease.

The general guidelines for an appropriate ORT as established by the World Health Organization:

The total substance concentration, osmolarity, (including that contributed by glucose) should be within the range of **200-310 mmol/l**.

The individual substance concentration:

Glucose	should at least equal that of sodium but **should not exceed 111 mmol/l**
Sodium	should be within the range of **60-90 mEq/l**
Potassium	should be within the range of **15-25 mEq/l**
Citrate	should be within the range of **8-12 mmol/l**
Chloride	should be within the range of **50-80 mEq/l**

For the past 20 years, numerous studies have been undertaken to develop an "improved" ORS. The goal was a product that would be at least as safe and effective as standard ORS for preventing or treating dehydration from all types of diarrhea but which, in addition, would reduce stool output or have other important clinical benefits. Normal blood osmolarity rests somewhere between 280 and 310 mOsm/l. Several worldwide studies over the past two decades have concluded that a hypo-osmolar solution between 210-268 mOsm/l, with 75-90 mEq/l sodium, and 75 mmol/l glucose reduces the need for supplemental IV therapy in children by 33%. In addition, stool output was reduced by about 20% and the incidence of vomiting by about 30%. Currently, the most universally effective formulation consists of the following solids per liter of water:

NaCl-2.6 gms
KCl-1.5 gms
Trisodium citrate dihydrate-2.9 gms
Glucose-anhydrous-13.5 gms
This produces a solution that is 75 mmol/l of sodium, 65 mmol/l chloride, 75 mmol/l glucose, 20 mEq/l potassium, 10 mEq/l Citrate with a total osmolarity of 245 mOsm/l.

Not everyone has potassium chloride and trisodium citrate in their cupboard...Perhaps the simplest, therapeutically effective solution that is easily prepared from items found in most kitchens, but not appropriate for long-term use as it has no potassium:

• 6 level teaspoons of sugar or honey
• 1/2 teaspoon sea salt
• 1 liter of clean water
• Although this solution is far from complete, it will work for short term rehydration with materials that are often easier to gather.

A better, slightly more difficult preparation requiring some forethought:

- 1/2 teaspoon salt
- 2 tablespoons plus 3/4 teaspoon sugar
- 1/2 teaspoon salt substitute (Morton's)
- 1 1/4 teaspoons trisodium citrate dihydrate*
- Water (to make 1 liter)

To a one liter container, add about 1/2 the needed water. Add the dry ingredients, stir well, then add the remaining water to make a final volume of one liter.

- Total sodium = 70 mEq
- Total potassium = 20 mEq
- Total carbohydrate = 27 g
- Osmolarity: 245 mOsm/L
  Available from Amazon or 'Prescribed For Life' at $12.95 a pound.

A widely available, inexpensive option:

- TRIORAL Oral Rehydration Salts packet is a sealed, pre-measured and pre-formulated powder that contains: Glucose anhydrous 13.5g, Trisodium Citrate Dehydrate 2.9g, Sodium •
- Chloride 2.6g and Potassium Chloride 1.5g.
- Total sodium = 75 mEq
- Total potassium = 20 mEq
- Total carbohydrate = 13.5 g
- Osmolarity: 245 mOsm/L

Another not great but ok solution:

- 1 quart of ready to drink Gatorade® G2 Low Calorie
- 1/2 teaspoon salt

Add salt to ready to drink Gatorade G2 and shake well.

Total sodium = 68 mEq

Total potassium = 3.2 mEq

Total carbohydrate = 18.6 g

Osmolarity: 256 mOsm/L

Note: potassium levels in this Gatorade® G2 recipe are well below the recommended amount for an ORS.

Another proprietary product, a rice based electrolyte:

- 1 packet of CeraLyte 70®
- 1 liter (L) of water

Briskly mix 1 cup of warm water with CeraLyte® and shake until dissolved.

Add additional cold water to make a one liter volume.

- Total sodium = 70 mEq
- Total potassium = 20 mEq
- Total carbohydrate = 41 g
- Osmolarity: 235 mOsm/L

A preparation that I have found useful in hydration and slowing diarrhea, and what we make in our office:

- NaCl-1/2 tsp (2.6 gms)
- $KHCO_3$-1/4 tsp (1 gm)
- Zinc gluconate 75 mg (providing 10 mg Zn)
- 2 1/2 tablespoons turbinado sugar
- 1 1/4 teaspoons trisodium citrate dihydrate in 1 liter of water.
- Total sodium = 70 mEq
- Total potassium = 20 mEq
- Total carbohydrate = 27 g
- Osmolarity: 245 mOsm/L

The added zinc helps resolve the diarrhea more rapidly, international studies show that children have shorter courses of infectious diarrhea after taking zinc supplements[29]. The children in these studies received 4–40 mg of zinc a day in the form of zinc acetate, zinc gluconate, or zinc sulfate[29,30]. Similar findings were reported in a meta-analysis published in 2008 and a 2007 review of zinc supplementation for preventing and treating diarrhea[31,32]. The effects of zinc supplementation on diarrhea in children with adequate zinc status is not clear, even so, the World Health Organization and UNICEF now recommend short-term zinc supplementation (20 mg of zinc per day, or 10 mg for infants under 6 months, for 10–14 days) to treat acute childhood diarrhea[28].

The most widely used ORS's in the United States are Pedialyte and Ricelyte, which contain 45 and 50mEq/L of sodium, respectively. These fluids are intended for maintenance of hydration and prevention of dehydration in clinical practice. Ricelyte has been used successfully for rehydration and maintenance therapy in one study; however, the effectiveness of Pedialyte for rehydration has not been studied. Although solutions with higher sodium concentrations (75-90 mEq/L) are preferable, Pedialyte, Ricelyte, and other similar low-sodium solutions can be used for rehydration when the alternative is physiologically inappropriate liquids or IV fluids. When the rate of purging is very high (e.g., greater than 10 ML/kg/hour), solutions with 75-90 mEq/L are recommended for rehydration.

For the mildly dehydrated patient (3%-5% fluid deficit), oral rehydration should begin with a fluid containing 50-90 mEq/L of sodium. The amount of fluid administered should be 50 mL/kg over a period of 2-4 hours. Using a teaspoon, syringe, or medicine dropper, the caregiver should initially provide small volumes of fluid and then gradually increase the amount, as tolerated. After 2-4 hours, hydration status should be reassessed. If the patient is rehydrated, treatment should progress to a maintenance phase. If the patient is still dehydrated, the fluid deficit should be re-estimated and rehydration therapy should begin again.

For the moderately dehydrated patient (6%-9% fluid deficit), ORS should be administered by the same procedures as used for the mildly dehydrated patient. The initial amount of fluid administered for rehydration should be increased to 100 mL/kg, administered over 2 hours.

Severe dehydration (greater than or equal to 10% fluid deficit, shock or near shock) constitutes a medical emergency. IV rehydration should begin immediately. Boluses (20 mL/kg) of Ringer's lactate solution, normal saline, or a similar solution should be administered until pulse, perfusion, and mental status return to normal. This treatment may require two IV lines or even alternate access sites (e.g., venous cutdown, femoral vein, intraosseous infusion). When the patient's level of consciousness returns to normal, he or she can take the remaining estimated deficit by mouth. As with less severely ill patients, hydration status should be assessed frequently to monitor the adequacy of replacement therapy.

Antimicrobial therapy of acute diarrhea varies depending on the etiologic agent, viral agents are the predominant cause of acute diarrhea and are not responsive to antimicrobial therapy. Bloody diarrhea or the presence of white blood cells on methylene blue stain of the stool specimen suggests a bacterial agent causing invasive mucosal damage and indicates that stool cultures should be performed to identify the organism. Other clinical clues suggesting a cause of infectious diarrhea amenable to antimicrobial therapy include a history of recent antibiotic use (in which case Clostridium difficile should be suspected), exposure to children in day care centers where Giardia or Shigella is prevalent, recent foreign travel, and immunodeficiency, in which infectious causes of diarrhea should be diligently evaluated. Conversely, watery diarrhea and vomiting in a child less than 2 years of age most likely represent viral gastroenteritis and therefore do not require antimicrobial therapy.

The use of nonspecific antidiarrheal agents such as adsorbents (e.g., kaolin-pectin), antimotility agents (e.g., loperamide), antisecretory drugs, or toxin binders (e.g., cholestyramine) is a common practice in conventional medical arenas. Despite the theoretical benefits from their use, available data do not demonstrate their effectiveness in reducing diarrhea volume or duration. For example, although stool consistency can be improved by binding agents, stool water losses are unchanged and electrolyte losses may increase. Indeed, side effects of these drugs are well known, including medication-induced ileus, drowsiness and nausea due to medication side-effects, and binding of nutrients and other drugs. Charcoal, bentonite clay and oat bran fiber are as effective in most cases as the medications. Reliance on antidiarrheal agents shifts the therapeutic focus away from appropriate fluid, electrolyte, and nutritional therapy; can interfere with oral therapy; and can unnecessarily add to the economic cost of the illness. Little evidence exists to support the use of nonspecific drug therapy in children.

Ideally, management of acute diarrhea should begin at home, since effective early interventions can reduce complications, such as dehydration and poor nutrition. Families with infants and small children should be encouraged to keep a supply of ORS at home at all times and use the solution when diarrhea first occurs in the child. Early home management will result in fewer office or emergency room visits, hospitalizations, and deaths. This type of management is best realized through support and education of mothers by health-care personnel at centers that use oral therapy. All families, particularly those in rural areas or poor urban neighborhoods where access to health care may be delayed, should be encouraged to have a supply of ORS in the home at all times. Our clinic maintains the components for ORS, they are very inexpensive, and we often give them to families to have on hand. Most of these solutions are more palatable if they are frozen in ice cube trays and the child is able to eat them like a mini-popsicle.

Humans are amazingly adaptable creatures, young humans are very resilient, very often it is easier for well-meaning parents and medical providers to do to too much. Often, there is a socio-cultural expectation on the part of parents to want some kind of intervention, there is also an idea that agents that require a prescription are 'stronger' and more effective medicines. This is not usually true, however, the anxious parent's an often be pacified with a prescription and the admonition to not get it filled for a day or two, first seeing how the child does with the other recommended measures. Most of the time, they never need the prescription, but there is something reassuring about having it available for them.

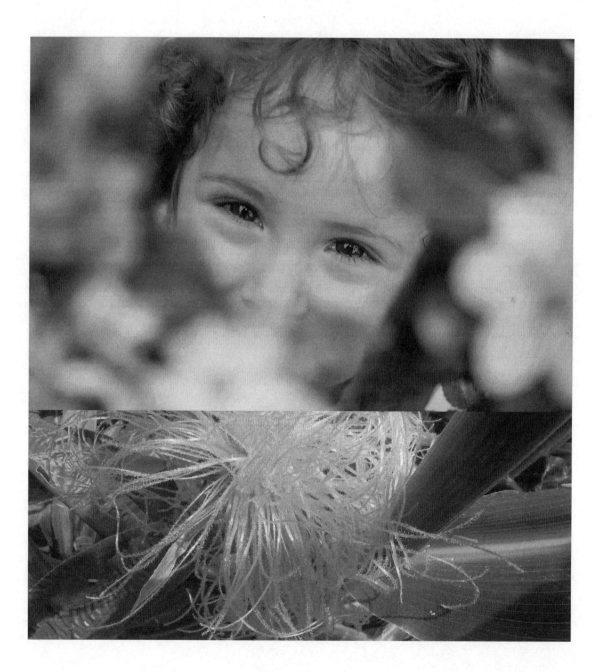

1. Fleming-Dutra, K., et al. (2016). "Prevalence of Inappropriate Antibiotic Prescriptions Among US Ambulatory Care Visits, 2010-2011 External." JAMA: The Journal of the American Medical Association 315(17): 1864-1873.

2. Centers for Disease Control and Prevention (CDC). Office-related antibiotic prescribing for persons aged ≤14 years — United States, 1993—1994 to 2007—2008. MMWR Morb Mortal Wkly Rep. 2011;60(34):1153-6.

3. Pichichero ME. Dynamics of antibiotic prescribing for children-External. JAMA. June 19, 2002;287(23): 3133-5.

4. Shapiro DJ, Hicks LA, Pavia AT, Hersh AL. Antibiotic prescribing for adults in ambulatory care in the USA, 2007-09 External. J Antimicrob Chemother. 2014;69(1):234-40.

5. Vaz LE, Kleinman KP, Raebel MA, Nordin JD, Lakoma MD, Dutta-Linn MM, Finkelstein JA. Recent trends in outpatient antibiotic use in children. Pediatrics. 2014;133(3):375-85.

6. CDC. Antibiotic Resistance Patient Safety Atlas.

7. Bourgeois FT, Mandl KD, Valim C, Shannon MW. Pediatric adverse drug events in the outpatient setting: An 11-year national analysis. Pediatrics. 2009;124(4):e744-50.

8. Budnitz DS, Pollock DA, Weidenbach KN, Mendelsohn AB, Schroeder TJ, Annest JL. National surveillance of emergency department visits for outpatient adverse drug events. JAMA. 2006;296(15): 1858-66.

9. Shehab, N., et al. (2016). "US emergency department visits for outpatient adverse drug events, 2013-2014." JAMA 316(20): 2115-2125.

10. Suda KJ, Hicks LA, Roberts RM, Hunkler RJ, Danziger LH. A national evaluation of antibiotic expenditures by healthcare setting in the United States, 2009. J Antimicrob Chemother. 2013;68(3):715-18.

11. Leibovitz E, Broides A, Greenberg D, Newman N. Current management of pediatric acute otitis media. Expert Rev Anti Infect Ther. 2010 Feb;8(2):151-61.

12. Pinnock CB, Graham NM, Mylvaganam A, Douglas RM. Relationship between milk intake and mucus production in adult volunteers challenged with rhinovirus-2. Am Rev Respir Dis. 1990 Feb;141(2):352-6.

13. Costerton JW1, Lewandowski Z, Caldwell DE, Korber DR, Lappin-Scott HM. Microbial biofilms. Annu Rev Microbiol. 1995;49:711-45.

14. Schmitt BD. Fever phobia: misconceptions of parents about fevers. Am J Dis Child. 1980 Feb;134(2): 176-81.

15. Moscona A. Neuraminidase inhibitors for influenza. N Engl J Med. 2005;353:1363–73.

16. Jefferson T, Jones M, Doshi P, Spencer EA, Onakpoya I, Heneghan CJ. Oseltamivir for influenza in adults and children: Systematic review of clinical study reports and summary of regulatory comments. BMJ. 2014;348:g2545.

17. Simon RJ. Oseltamivir and neuropsychiatric disturbance in adolescents. The case is not proved but caution is advisable. Br Med J. 2007;334:1232–3.

18. Øymar K, Ove H, I Skjerven, M Bruun. Acute bronchiolitis in infants, a review. Scand J Trauma Resusc Emerg Med. 2014; 22: 23.

19. "Child Sexual Abuse". Facts for Families, No. 9. American Academy of Child and Adolescent Psychiatry. May 2008.

20. Claeson M, Merson MH. Global progress in the control of diarrheal diseases. Pediatr Infect Dis J 1990;9:345-5.

21. Bern C, Martines J, de Zoysa I, Glass RI. The magnitude of the global problem of diarrheal disease: a ten year update. Bull WHO 1992; 70(6).

22. Ho MS, Glass RI, Pinsky PF, Anderson LJ. Rotavirus as a cause of diarrheal morbidity and mortality in the United States. J Infect Dis 1988;158:1112-6.

23. Glass RI, Lew JF, Gangarosa RE, LeBaron CW, Ho MS. Estimates of morbidity and mortality rates for diarrheal diseases in American children. J Pediatr 1991;118:S27-33.

24. Ho MS, Glass RI, Pinsky PF, et al. Diarrheal deaths in American children -- are they preventable? JAMA 1988;260:3281-5.

25. Gangarosa RE, Glass RI, Lew JF, Boring JR. Hospitalizations involving gastroenteritis in the United States, 1985: the special burden of the disease among the elderly. Am J Epidemiol 1992;135:281-90.

26. Cohen MB. Etiology and mechanisms of acute infectious diarrhea in infants in the United States. J Pediatr 1991;118:S34-9.

27. Nalin DR. Nutritional benefits related to oral therapy: an overview. In: Bellanti JA, ed. Acute diarrhea: its nutritional consequences in children. Nestle Nutrition Workshop Series, Vol. 2. New York, NY: Raven Press, 1983:185

28. World Health Organization and United Nations Children Fund. Clinical management of acute diarrhea. WHO/UNICEF Joint Statement, August, 2004.

29. Black RE. Therapeutic and preventive effects of zinc on serious childhood infectious diseases in developing countries. Am J Clin Nutr 1998;68:476S-9S.

30. Bhutta ZA, Bird SM, Black RE, Brown KH, Gardner JM, Hidayat A, et al. Therapeutic effects of oral zinc in acute and persistent diarrhea in children in developing countries: pooled analysis of randomized controlled trials. Am J Clin Nutr 2000;72:1516-22.

31. Lukacik M, Thomas RL, Aranda JV. A meta-analysis of the effects of oral zinc in the treatment of acute and persistent diarrhea. Pediatrics 2008;121:326-36.

32. Fischer Walker CL, Black RE. Micronutrients and diarrheal disease. Clin Infect Dis 2007;45 (1 Suppl):S73-7.

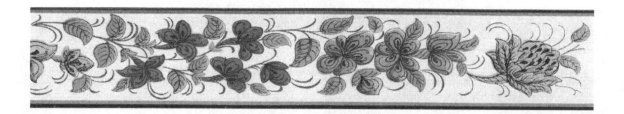

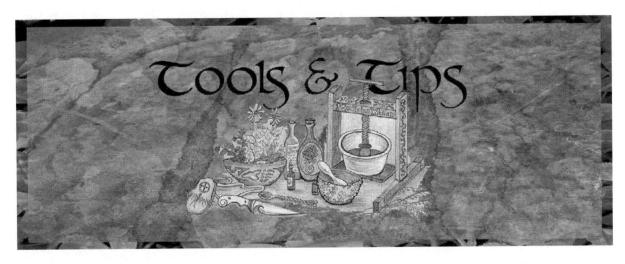

Puberty, most of us would agree, ia not very fun. Pimples, mood swings, body changes – all at a time when everyone is discovering alienating things like "popularity" and appearances are starting to matter more than whether or not someone is nice. As we watch our children entering this stage, we might feel at a loss, wondering how to help them. Some of it is just a rite of passage, but a great deal of it can be supported with herbs, simple lifestyle modifications, diet, and movement.

The most important thing you need to know about puberty is that it's a great deal of work! The conversion of a child body into an adult body is a huge task. Anyone who has ever renovated a kitchen, for example, knows that the process always takes longer than you think and is terribly inconvenient. Imagine trying to renovate your entire house – every room simultaneously - while you're still living in

Supporting Your Child Through Puberty

Part I: It's All About Hormones
by Katja Swift

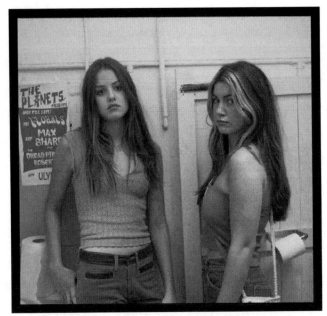

it! That's what puberty is. Another way to say that is, puberty is productivity.

We live in a productivity-driven, achievement-driven society, where many children are pushed from a young age to be involved in as many extra-curricular activities as possible, hoping to beef up their young resumes to get them into the right college. Even kids who aren't on that track are often over-scheduled, just with afterschool activities that they enjoy or that occupy them while their parents work, plus their personal pile of homework. These kids are already very busy, and adding the giant transitional work of puberty to the pile is precarious. To look at this not just from the privileged point of view, many kids lack even basic nutrition, a safe place to live or even sleep, or a family or community that can support their needs through this transition – making the job even more difficult.

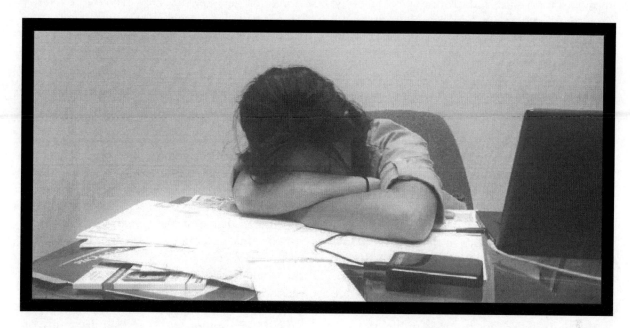

So a major focus of our work for our kids in puberty is to reduce the amount of "stuff" on their to-do lists, and give them some breathing room to make this change smoothly. We want to increase their nutrition during this time so that they have the tools they need to renovate their bodies, increase their sleep, and make sure they stay active – but wait: you're probably already thinking, this might mean some big changes for your kids! Change is hard, no matter who you are, so it's important to have some compassion around these suggestions. First, educate your child(ren) about why the changes are necessary, and what the kids will get out of it. Let them read this article, or read it together as a family. Make a plan together about how to tackle the changes, and most importantly, make those changes as a family as much as possible. It will benefit every member of the family to sleep a little more, to eat a little better. Showing solidarity as a family for the transitions your teen is going through is a beautiful gift – it's tangible proof that you're really there for your kid.

None of the following suggestions are exactly easy, and we live in busy times. Here's some motivation for you: not only is the transition of puberty a lot of work, but that work needs to be done well in order to create a healthy adult. A woman who has her first period before the age of 12 is 50% more likely to get breast cancer than a woman whose first period comes in her teens. I haven't yet found any such statistics for boys, though I'm sure they're out there, but if we can track that kind of influence over one factor, there must be others. For me, looking at my daughter, that statistic alone is pretty motivating.

One more thing before we dig in: although the focus of this article is on puberty, it's important to note that it's never too early to start. If your children aren't to puberty yet, start now with these suggestions! Even if they're just babies, go ahead and get started – you'll be giving them a strong foundation for success!

It's All About Hormones

The word "hormone" in our culture is synonymous with sex hormones – estrogen/progesterone and testosterone, because that's what we identify with. The simplified story we learn is that those hormones make us who we are – men or women – so we think they must be very important! While it's true that especially in puberty, these hormones are not irrelevant, we have to recognize that these hormones are dead last on a very long list of hormones that are critical to our daily survival. Many of our

421

hormones play a life-and-death role in the body every day, and unless we have those in good working order, there's no way we can hope to have our estrogen and testosterone where they need to be. Here are some of the most important hormones:

Insulin

Insulin is a hormone, and if insulin is in a state of dysregulation, we absolutely will die. Whenever we work with anyone with hormone problems, we always start with insulin – even if the problem doesn't seem to have anything to do with insulin – because it's at the very top. How can we resolve issues with hormones further down the line if the one at the top is out of whack? Insulin has several functions that are relevant to puberty. First, insulin signals the cells in the body to accept glucose – which is fuel. Without fuel, there's no energy to get the work done! Of course, the body has a backup system, and that's fat: if you skip a meal, for example, your body will just break down your fat stores and burn that as energy. However, insulin also shuts down the ability of your body to burn fat – because if there's insulin around, that means you already have a bunch of glucose to burn. You don't need to burn fat when there's glucose available, and your body would rather conserve your fat for a time when you don't have any glucose.

Every time you eat something, your body releases insulin – more if that food was high in sugar/carbs, less if it was protein and less (or none) if it was fat. A snack of pretzels and a soda would require a lot of insulin to process; a snack of macadamia nuts and beef jerky would require less.

There are other hormones that are shut off in the presence of insulin – for example, growth hormone, which we'll get to next. Another very important one is thyroid hormone. Your body produces thyroid hormone and stores it in a deactivated form, because of course if you store it in the active form, it would be stimulating your thyroid to overwork. When you need more thyroid hormone, your body just activates those stores and gets to work. However, that activation cannot take place concurrently with insulin. Just with these two examples, we're starting to get a picture here – the body doesn't want to have insulin running all the time. You may have heard that "4-6 or 6-8 small meals a day is healthy, because it keeps your metabolism/insulin levels steady throughout the day" – but when we look at the body functions, we see that insulin should not be steady throughout the day. Much like your house – if you're always putting things away, you have no time to make a nice dinner or relax with a good book. At some point, you want the things that must be put away to stay put away so that you can go on to other things.

So what does this all mean for your kid? For starters, it's time to reign in the snacking. In other countries, people don't really snack. A very young child might snack, but adults rarely do, and at some point it's not appropriate for older children to either. Perhaps you remember being told by your own mom, "you'll spoil your supper". Snacking constantly means insulin constantly, which means there's not enough time to be doing the work of all that body renovation, because you're too busy putting all the snacks away!

But mom, I'm hungry! That's ok. It's good to be hungry sometimes. Come to mealtimes good and hungry, and really enjoy every bite of delicious dinner. Curbing snacking doesn't in any way mean calorie restriction – in fact, at this age, kids will probably need more calories. But let's encourage kids to get those calories during breakfast, lunch, and dinner, instead of by grazing through their day. A side benefit is more opportunity for family meals!

Also, if kids are hungry, we need to make sure we're feeding them nutrient dense foods, as opposed to empty snacks. My family didn't snack so much when I was a kid, but I remember my much younger brother had a steady stream of hot pockets and chips and salsa. His band would practice in the basement and my mom stocked them up with industrial sized boxes of Mountain Dew and unlimited microwavable snacks. Your son might think that's the idyllic

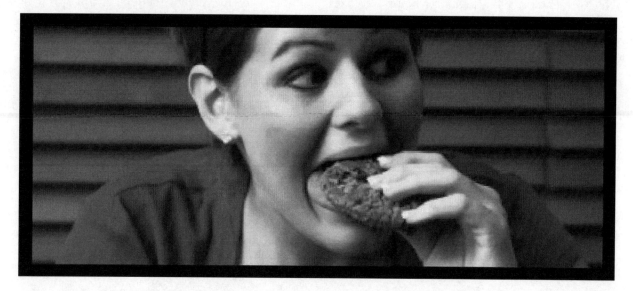

setup, but asking him to wait till dinner, and then stuffing him with beef roast, sweet potatoes, and kale will yield better insulin levels.

What if they really do need a snack, and what about younger kids? Try to stick to proteins and fats, and whole carbs such as fruit – all of which require less insulin than "snack foods". That may be less convenient, because these are things that don't readily come in packages, but there are many snack foods you can make up on the weekend and have ready for the whole week. Some examples would be berry muffins made from nut meal and lots of eggs (I usually use at least one egg per muffin), and just a bit of honey for sweetener. I like to make sure there's a generous amount of cinnamon in the mix, as cinnamon is very helpful for controlling blood sugar levels. There is some very interesting modern research going on in this area, but you don't have to tell your kid that – they'll just think it tastes great!

Another make-ahead idea is eggs-and-meat in a muffin tin: just crack an egg into each muffin section, add crumbled sausage or bacon, and maybe some chopped peppers and scallions. Bake it up and you have a breakfast sandwich without the sandwich. If you beat the eggs, it's an omelet you can eat with your hands! Even easier, nuts, hard boiled eggs, carrots, and jerky are grab-and-go snacks. Ryn loves sardines, straight out of the tin, and Wild Planet makes a

BPA-free tin. Of course, kids might not think that's delicious, but if they could, it's an amazingly healthful snack.

At this age, a lot of kids decide that breakfast isn't "cool". Maybe they need that time to fix their hair or to get to school early to hang out with friends. It's true though, breakfast is the most important meal of the day! A hearty breakfast that features plenty of protein and fat sets up ideal hormone production through the whole day – not just insulin levels, but also leptin, ghrelin, and other hormones that have to do with hunger, satiety, and circadian rhythms.

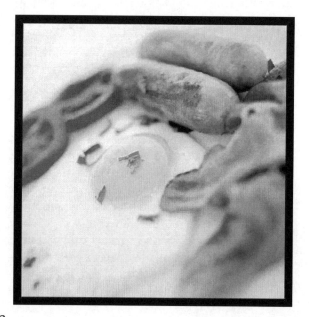

423

Not to mention, a big breakfast helps stabilize mood through the day (reason enough right there!), and wards off the desire to snack – not just for teens! Make a big protein breakfast a new family tradition and everyone will feel better for it!

Growth Hormone

Growth hormone is exactly what you think it is – it grows stuff! It's not just for children and teens, even adults need growth hormone to heal wounds, etc. It also increases the mineralization of bones (and teeth) – which makes them stronger, stimulates the immune system, and helps repair and maintain the pancreas. Growing kids and kids in puberty obviously need the highest levels of growth hormone,

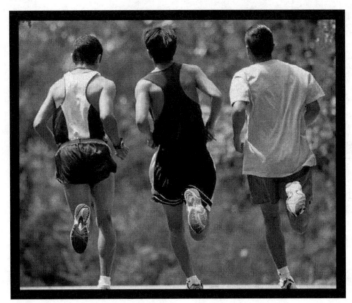

but there are some significant inhibitors – the most important being insulin. Insulin and growth hormone are like yin and yang – both are important, but they're not in the same space at the same time. The way to make sure you have enough growth hormone is the same as how you make sure you don't have too much insulin: less snacking, more nutrient-dense foods.

Removing the impediments to growth hormone production is one approach – another is to seek out ways to stimulate its release. This is where movement comes in. You could say that exercising (especially resistance training and sprinting) stimulates the release of high amounts of growth hormone – or you could say that a sedentary lifestyle removes an ancestral stimulus that results in ordinary levels of growth hormone.

Either way, movement matters! A full sprint or resistance workout three times a week will make a huge difference in growth hormone levels, both during and after the exercise itself, but also on rest days due to the accumulation of trained muscle. This isn't about going for a jog – jogging is a kind of exercise that is stuck in the middle. Instead, think about going for a walk with some sprints added in, or playing games like ultimate Frisbee, soccer and basketball – these are games with short bursts of high energy mixed with some rest times.

Active movement habits are useful in another way, in that they help kids get good-quality sleep. And in fact, another inhibitor of growth hormone is sleep deprivation! The body expects the highest concentration of growth hormone to occur overnight – and here is the beginning of the concept that sleep is productive. When you go to sleep, your body is literally taking many of your systems "off line", so that other systems can go to work. Very much like a janitorial and repair staff at the local school who does their work once the students and teachers have gone home and the buildings are empty, your body stops certain activities in order to perform cleanup and repair tasks. Kids in puberty require more sleep – at least 10-12 hours per night, and more in a time of stress! – but most of them are getting much less than that. Which brings us to melatonin:

Melatonin

Melatonin is the hormone that gets us to sleep. Its production is stimulated by decreasing light – that's all you need! (Well, that and sufficient nutrients in your diet to give you the raw materials, of course.) But don't sell melatonin short – it has many other functions in the body, and we haven't even discovered them all yet. Melatonin is a powerful anti-oxidant – studies have shown it to be twice as powerful as vitamin E (which was previously thought to be the most powerful antioxidant. Of course, now we're learning that the story is quite a bit more complicated, but melatonin is still up at the top of the pack).

But wait – there's more: melatonin plays a very important role in the immune system as well – it stimulates the activity of NK cells, which fight off viruses and cancerous cells. And, melatonin levels are also implicated in the onset of puberty – lowered levels of melatonin mean earlier puberty. (Lower levels of melatonin are also associated with autism and diabetes in recent studies.)

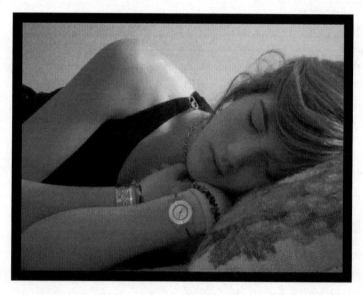

None of that means you should go out and get a melatonin supplement – in fact, that's really not a good idea on multiple levels! You have probably experienced the phenomenon, perhaps during a time of stress or overwork, of caffeine dependence. First you drink one cup of coffee to get you up-and-at'em in the morning, but after a while, one cup doesn't cut it anymore, so you drink two. And not only does one cup not do the job anymore, but if you don't have it, you experience withdrawal. That's because caffeine stimulates adrenaline – another hormone – and it's the adrenaline that you're really responding to. This phenomenon of dependence and resistance is true for all the hormones. When we supplement melatonin, we are increasing the body's dependence on that supplement, decreasing the ability to produce it independently, and becoming resistant to normal levels of melatonin, requiring the higher levels found in the supplements. Besides that, it's clear that melatonin is a hormone with lots of effects, many of which we haven't discovered yet. Supplementing could cause significant dysregulation with unknown consequences.

What's the alternative? Turn out the lights! Get some candles. Light in the blue spectrum inhibits melatonin production – so make sure to get outside during the day in the bright light (when the body is not supposed to be making melatonin). As the sun goes down, try not to turn on lights, so that your body will make melatonin. Let the lights you do use be candles or low-wattage, yellow-spectrum light bulbs (incandescents), which do not inhibit melatonin production as strongly. Limit screen time – a good idea in general – to daytime hours, so that your child is not exposed to the blue light spectrum after dark. Make sure that your kids' bedroom is really dark (and yours too!) – using light block curtains and getting away from nightlights, even for younger children – night should be dark.

But what if your kids are afraid of the dark? First, have compassion – after all, no one really likes to sleep alone. Have some relaxing music playing so that despite the darkness, there is comforting noise in the room. Lay down with your child for a while and talk quietly about the day – in the dark, they may find it easier to talk about emotional events than they do in the harsh light of after-school time. This can be a good relaxing way for you to help a child give their day some closure and move into sleep.

The time before bedtime is also important! Right after dinner, start dimming lights – and screen time! Especially screen time, because screens (both the old ones and LCD ones, as well as iPads and iPhones) operate in the blue spectrum: your after dinner movie is telling your body the sun is still shining! If you have bright lights on right up until bedtime, like as not you'll just lay there waiting for sleep and being frustrated, because your body hasn't started making any melatonin yet. It takes a while to get up to a fall-asleep level, so start early – as soon as dinner is done, switch to candles or low lamps with incandescent bulbs. You can listen to recorded herbal lectures (sure to put your kids to sleep!) as a family, or audio books, or read out loud to each other. You can listen to relaxing music and do simple handwork that doesn't require too much light. When the whole family gets into this, everyone will start sleeping better!

If sleep is still difficult, there are plenty of herbs to help! You may already have your favorites, but here are some my family loves: Amber particularly enjoys Linden tea, and lately her favorite is Linden and Peppermint. I thought the Mint would be too strong to taste the Linden, but I was really wrong – it's delightful! Sometimes I slip some Chamomile in there for her too. My favorite before bed tea is Chamomile and Ginger, though often other herbs get put in the mix, especially Wood Betony, and Linden if it's been a rough day. Ryn usually likes whatever we're drinking, more on the ginger side, but if he really needs to sleep, Hops knocks him out every time – even just in a foot bath! A nice cup of tea during the after-dinner time, or a foot bath, are wonderfully relaxing ways to help you calm right down as you transition from your day towards bed.

If it's too close to bedtime for tea, I like Wild Lettuce tincture myself – often with Skullcap and Passionflower added, and Amber likes an elixir of Linden and Chamomile.

To be clear: none of us have owl eyes. Human adults require a minimum of 9 hours of sleep a night. In puberty, sleep requirements are at least 10 – 12 hours. Your kids might not love that, but remember, they're doing a huge amount of work in puberty, and a majority of that work gets done while they're asleep!

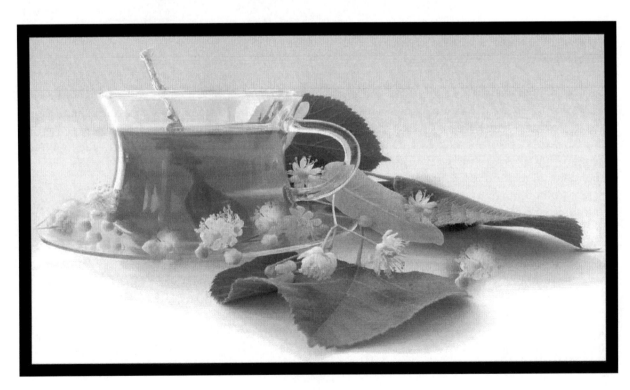

Adrenaline

Adrenaline is the opposite of sleep: adrenaline is zing! – and our culture is addicted to it. Not just with coffee: check out the media lineup. Action and adventure gives you a big adrenaline boost, because your subconscious brain doesn't really understand that what you're watching isn't real. But it's not just shoot'em-up movies that amp you up: thrillers, suspense, intense drama, even agitating documentaries and political news will get your adrenaline levels up, not to mention video games. Any kind of stressful event is responded to with adrenaline, along with its friend cortisol. School is a fairly stressful place these days too: bullies are finding new and more novel ways to be cruel, children live with emergency drills to learn how they would handle a school shooting, and there's ever more pressure to get good grades.

As puberty sets in, many kids start drinking coffee, either to be cool or to stay awake after long nights of studying (or procrastinating). Many will also start smoking – both of these stimulate adrenaline. Here in Boston, and I suspect it's true in other areas, kids at the "good" high schools report that many of their high achieving friends are taking Ritalin – not for ADD, but because it is speed. They do it so that they can overachieve.

How can we help our kids keep their stress levels down? As much as I'd love for television to broadcast nothing but David Attenborough nature documentaries, the reality is, kids like media. But we as parents can limit media to appropriate times, saving the adrenaline movies for the weekend, perhaps, when they can watch them during the day and still have time to come down again before bed. Helping them to handle their stresses is important too – even though their dramatic crises might seem silly to us as adults, each one they go through is an opportunity to help them practice managing their emotions.

And here's where the herbs really shine! Tulsi is my very favorite for unmanageable emotions. Tulsi is a great pick-me-up, especially when

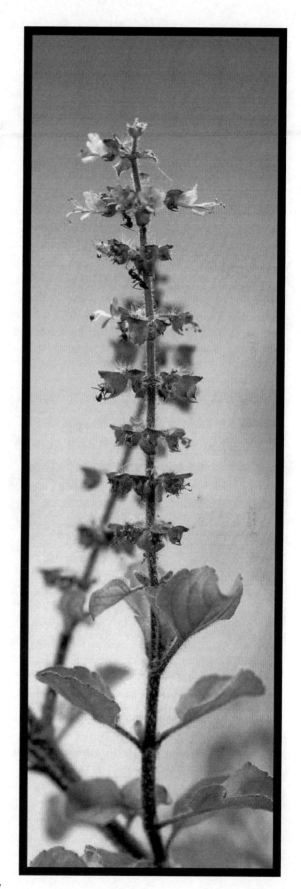

everything is all wrong and you just can't possibly show your face in public ever again! On top of that, Tulsi has beneficial impact on lots of hormones, as well as the hippocampus – the center in your brain where you process your short term memory into long term memory. In other words, your hippocampus is where you "get over it" – every time you wish you could just say those words to your teen, hand them a cup of Tulsi tea instead!

And what about coffee? It's true, it's trendy! You can hear the wailing already – but ma-aaaaaaaahhm, everyone drinks coffee! So give your kid a designer brew instead! Lately my favorite "un-coffee" is a long decoction of Burdock, Dandelion, Codonopsis, Chaga, Ashwagandha, a bit of Solomon's Seal and Black Seed, and just a spoonful of decaf fair trade coffee. That spoonful is enough to give the blend "authentic" coffee flavor, without the caffeine.

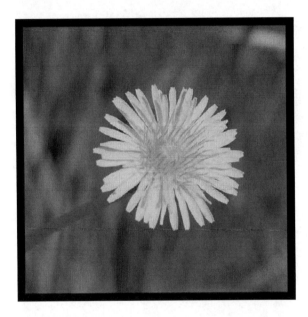

Mix in some almond milk, and it's absolutely delicious. Don't try to pull a fast one on your kid though – once they've had a sip and declared it passable, stuff them full of information about why this is so much better for them. You know your kid, so present the information in the way that's right for them - which might simply be leaving your own "homework" out on the table with some bullet points about the benefits of each plant in the mix! The information isn't

useful if your kid tunes it out, but if you can get it in there, you're not just affecting your own kid – wait and see, I predict that she'll be asking you to make a larger quantity for her to share with her friends at school. Kids are really pressuring each other at this age, and if you can fortify your kid with knowledge, she'll not only be able to stand up to the pressure, but even to help other kids learn as well!

Xenoestrogens

Unfortunately, there are hormones at work in the environment that we have less control over. With names such as BPA and phthalates, these come from plastics and chemicals primarily, and they're such a danger because of the way our bodies used to work. If you go back far enough in evolution, the human body didn't produce sufficient estrogen for itself, instead absorbing it from the environment (much like we absorb vitmamin C from our environment – by eating it - instead of producing it ourselves, like cats can). Historically, this absorption would have been mostly from plant sources, and interestingly, plant estrogens, such as those in Red Clover, are generally beta-estrogens. Beta-estrogens are responsible for checking growth and shutting down the activity of alpha-estrogens; alpha-estrogens are responsible for growth, and things that are associated with the words "estrogen dominant...". As we evolved, we developed the ability to produce estrogen on our own, but we never lost the ability to absorb it from the environment. This absorption capability is tremendously efficient, which is extra problematic at this point in history. Unlike plant estrogens, xenoestrogens (modern environmental estrogens) are alpha-estrogens. Much of this environmental absorption happens in breast tissue, but not all of it. (There's much more detailed information about this in Breasts: a Natural and Unnatural History, by Florence Williams – a fantastic read!)

Major sources of xenoestrogens are plastics and things treated with certain chemicals, such as flame retardants. Since so many children are surrounded with large quantities of these two items from birth (and since their mothers were as

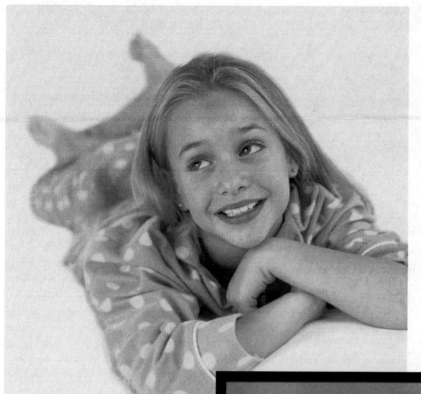

the participants consumed nothing that had ever touched plastic, and within the timeframe of the study they were able to significantly reduce their xenoestrogen load – so all is not lost! Additionally, get your kids hooked on Red Clover! Add mint or any other flavor your kids like – and why not add some Nettle as well, to keep mineral levels up! Red Clover's beta-estrogens will help combat the alpha-estrogens in the environment, so while you're reducing the ones you can control, you can count on Red Clover to be reducing the ones you can't control.

well, and these chemicals are transmitted to the growing fetus), our children may be entering puberty very differently than we and our mothers did. Xenoestrogens play a major role (not the only role – all those other hormones we've already mentioned also contribute) in the trend towards entering puberty earlier, and exposure to xenoestrogens before and during puberty tracks with increased risk of breast cancers later in life.

How do we avoid environmental estrogens? Rid your house of plastics, don't buy flame retardant clothing and bedding, try not to purchase foods in plastics. A great study was done in Newton, MA recently wherein

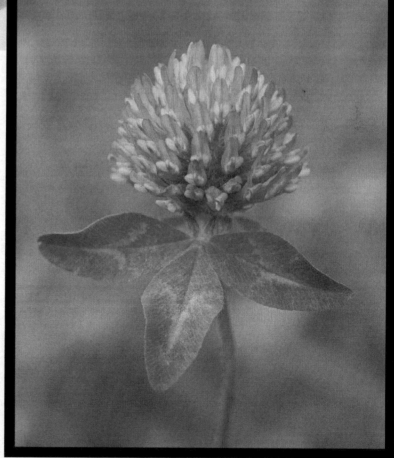

Love that Liver

The liver plays so many important roles in the body, we could talk about it for days. But just at the moment, one particular function we're quite interested in has to do with – hormones!

Hormones are communicators – they send messages around the body. When their job is finished, they end up in the liver to be broken down, and recycled or excreted. When the liver isn't up to snuff, the hormones hang around too long, and that disrupts the balance. This is why when clients come in with severe PMS complaints, a major way to resolve this is through the liver – the PMS is so bad because hormones are not being broken down in a timely manner, which means that there's too much of various hormones at any given time, which means PMS is worse.

In puberty, it's not just that the hormones are in overdrive – the liver needs

Supporting Your Child Through Puberty

Part II:
It's Not Just About Hormones

by Katja Swift

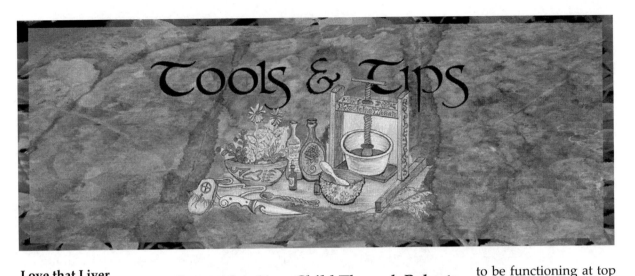

Pituitary gland

Growth hormone

Muscle growth

Bone growth

Liver

IGF-1

to be functioning at top speed as well, in order to keep up! But kids' livers are facing a big challenge today – our carbohydrate and sugar driven society means more insulin to break down, and since insulin is the most critical hormone in terms of life support, it takes priority over the rest of the hormones, both in manufacture and in breakdown. More stress – stress at school, but also the adrenaline rush from movies and video games, as well as the adrenaline required to fuel a body not getting enough sleep – means more stress hormones to break down. More xenoestrogens from the environment means more work for the liver too – but it's not just hormones! The liver is responsible for breaking down all the toxins in the body, like the chemical dyes in snack foods and soda. Of course this is the time when kids want to have more of all of these things: exciting movies, sugary treats with coloring and preservatives, late nights – but it's all taking a huge toll on the liver.

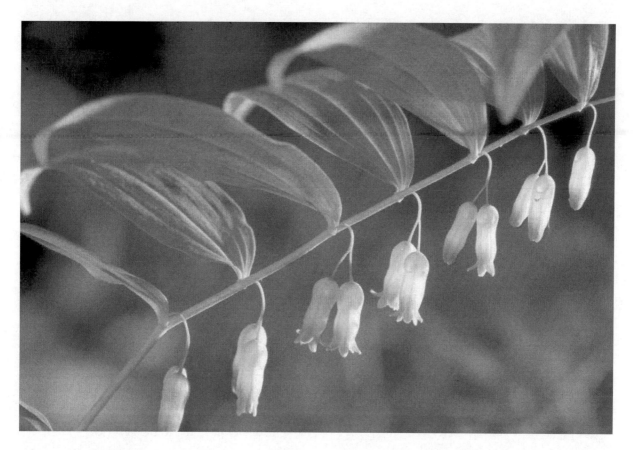

What to do? Well, this is a job for our "un-coffee" recipe from earlier! All that Burdock and Dandelion root is just what the liver ordered, and with the way kids go through coffee, you can be sure they'll get plenty of it this way. Not to mention the adaptogenic effects of Codonopsis, Ashwagandha, and Chaga. We'll talk about emotional support in later sections but here's a preview: in this formula, it's the Solomon's Seal.

Solomon's seal has been a vital part of our practice for quite some time, not just for folks with twisted ankles and stressed wrists, but also those who need a little help being flexible and graceful when our expectations and our realities don't quite match up. As plans change underneath us, Solomon's Seal gives us a feeling of firm footing, and that feeling of security can be just the thing to ward off a temper tantrum (they're not just for toddlers anymore!). Digging even deeper, Karyn Sanders has spoken about Solomon's Seal as medicine for people who can't be true to themselves: sounds like medicine made for puberty! Being true to yourself at that

age is so difficult: your Self is in the middle of drastic change, with peer pressure and achievement pressure on top of it. Solomon's Seal has been such an ally for me in uncertain situations, when I was expected to respond before I even quite knew how I felt. If only I had known this dear plant friend as a teenager!

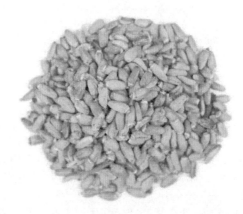

Maybe your kid doesn't love coffee? Milk Thistle is a liver aid anyone can handle. It's gentle but effective, and if you need to, a good quality capsule will be just fine. Just make sure that the only ingredients are ground organic Milk Thistle seeds, and you'll be all set. Bitters are great here too – and if you haven't introduced bitters to your family yet, this is definitely a great time to start! Have a selection of different bitters: we have a row of them in our kitchen, including Calamus, Yellow Dock, lovely Lavender and Sage bitters and Juniper and Pinon Pine bitters from King's Road Apothecary, Maple bitters from Urban Moonshine, and a variety of bitter teas as well. Before meals, everyone gets to choose which bitters they want to have – maybe Calamus when you're feeling cold and sluggish, or Pinon when you're just missing the desert (as Amber often is!) – and we all take them together. If your kids don't like the flavor, don't censor them! Let them make the biggest yuck face they can conjure – in fact, have yuck face contests! Bitters are supposed to be bitter. It's ok if you make funny faces, and besides that, it's fun to make funny faces! Your kids won't really mind the flavor so much if everyone, even mom and dad, are joining in a little pre-dinner silliness.

Kidneys

When I look at pictures of my childhood self, the first things that jump out at me are dark rings under each eye. They're even in my elementary school photographs, as early as first grade! Of course, back then school was nothing like as stressful as today, and we still got plenty of recess – a luxury kids don't have today (40% of American schools have banished recess altogether!). When I see children today, in the grocery store, at the library, or even the children of our friends, there are those dark rings under each eye – what's going on?

Something's happening with the kidneys: the center of emotion and hormonal activity, regulators of minerals and water in the bloodstream, and the soil that our adrenal glands thrive in – or don't. We're all aware that dark rings under the eyes come with sleep deprivation, but there's more to the story than that. They are an indication of depletion on a much deeper level: late nights, stressful situations, and lots of hormones mean a lot of extra strain on the kidneys. Even if you can't get

your kids into bed earlier, there are things you can do to help.

Nettle and Friends – a blend of Nettle, Dandelion, Red Clover, and a bit of Licorice, with Mint or Ginger for flavor if you like - is one of our favorite teas for teens. It incorporates the Red Clover – for combating xenoestrogens, among other exciting actions – along with Nettle and Dandelion, which are kidney powerhouses. The Licorice supports adrenal health, and also makes it tasty! It's important to steep this brew overnight so that you get the full concentration of minerals – in particular calcium, which is poorly absorbed from supplements, and magnesium, which is direly lacking in modern diets.

Some other great herbs here are Tulsi – not only an adaptogen but also an herb to help with emotions – and Ashwagandha, which we love for helping to balance circadian cycles. You might put the Ashwagandha into your kid's designer "un-coffee", or let them have it as a tincture along with some Licorice – both are great!

Finally, of all things for depletion, bone broth might be king! Toss in whatever bones you have – meat, poultry, fish – they're all good! Add in some good grounding roots like Burdock, Dandelion, and Codonopsis – and don't forget some Seaweeds – and you've got an extremely nourishing concoction. You can even give it to your kid in a thermos for breakfast on the go!

Feed Your Kid!

Hormones – not to mention muscles, and even cell walls – are made of fats and proteins, which means your kids have to eat fats and proteins. It's very important that protein sources include fish, meat, and eggs from healthy animals, and in particular organ meats whenever possible. Meat from animals that were raised in confinement operations (most grocery store meat in this country) and fish that are farm-raised come along with their own puberty disruption toxins and xenoestrogens, so it is very important to make sure that you find good sources for meat and eggs. If you're willing and able to drive a little way, or have a farmer's market in your area, you can buy meat direct from a farmer, which means better quality meat at much better prices.

Organ meats are not always popular with kids, but I've found that grinding them and mixing them into some flavorful recipe like chili or curry hides both the flavor and texture so effectively that no one even knows they are there. Also important are all the other parts – skin, bones, cartilage. These are parts of animals that were historically always in the human diet, but are not commonly found today. We need to bring them back though, as they contain critical nutrients for growth and for health. Here's another way to look at it: as herbalists, most of us tend to prefer tea over isolated constituents removed from herbs and put into tablets. Consider muscle meat an isolated constituent of animal protein! In order to get the full health benefits from animal protein, we need the whole package – the whole egg, including the yolk; the whole animal, including the organs and cartilage and bone.

Vegetables are also super important! In every study everywhere, people who eat more vegetables win. Protein and fat are super important for making hormones, but vegetables are just as critical to good health. Teach your kids to choose vegetables with dark and bright colors – the pigments themselves are bioflavonoids, anthocyanins, and other phytonutrient compounds! Maybe your kids didn't love vegetables in the past, but let them know that palates change at this time in life, and sometimes things that we didn't like as children become favorite new foods as our tastes mature with our bodies. And if you're having trouble with vegetables, you can always get creative: make vegetables into fancy hors d'oeuvres, give them a tasty sauce or seasoning, and if all else fails, serve them with bacon (from happy pigs, of course!).

Above all, this is a time to limit, as much as possible, refined carbohydrates, sugary foods, and any food allergens you may or may not have discovered. Many people have serious issues with gluten and dairy that they don't discover until much later in life – trying an elimination diet now can save your kid years of discomfort

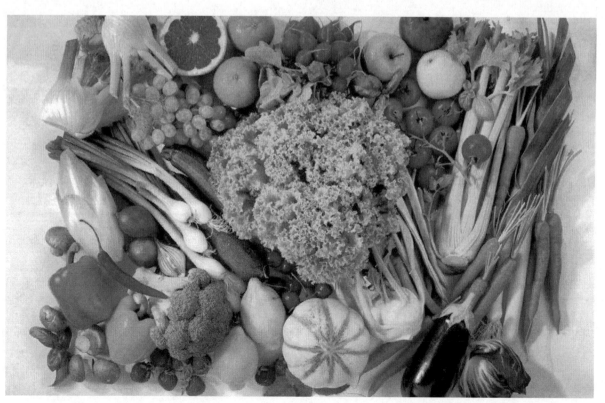

433

and make the puberty process much less frustrating. In our clinic and among our students, we have found that eliminating just gluten or just dairy isn't enough, since the two have such similar and overlapping effects. These days we suggest The Whole 30 (www.whole30.com) as an elimination diet, and we've seen drastically more success with this method than single eliminations. An added benefit is that it's only 30 days, which isn't too intimidating. In 30 days you'll get some good solid data that you can use to make choices about what foods are best for your body in the long term, instead of making a lifetime commitment on a hunch.

Of course kids like to have delicious things – I keep a lot of tasty recipes on our website for everything from party hor d'oeuvres to delectable vegetables to paleo cakes (2 cups of almonds, 13 eggs, coconut oil and honey...), and you'll find lots of other recipes all around the internet. Googling "paleo cookies", for example, will definitely get you started with low-sugar treats free of refined carbs. CommonWealthHerbs.com is our website, and NomNomPaleo.com is a good place to start for paleo recipes.

Beauty Products

It happens almost overnight: one day your kid couldn't care less about the dirt all over her face, the next suddenly she's crying at the mirror over a tiny speck of a potential pimple that you can't see at all. Face cleansers, makeup, deodorant – suddenly these things become super important. Fortunately these days it's not so difficult to find products that are trustworthy, but you do need to be vigilant: beauty products contain all kinds of problem ingredients, from gluten in lipstick, to parabens in lotion and shampoos, to neurotoxins and carcinogens in perfumes. Ingredients in deodorant show up in the lymphatic fluids of breast cancer patients, and even menstrual pads and tampons are full of chlorine and other chemicals. What to do? Here's a list:

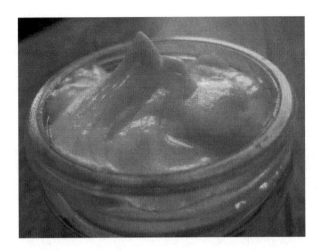

Making your own products is both cost effective and quality controlled! My favorite anti-acne preparation is very simple – just half apple cider vinegar and half rose water. Use it on the face as a wash daily, and you can use it as a spot treatment for individual pimples as well. If you have a particularly troublesome spot, you can use apple cider vinegar straight instead, but I generally recommend this only for nighttime since you'll smell like a salad for a while!

My favorite lotion is just as simple: although I love Rosemary's Famous Face Cream, I generally only have time for "just-in-time" lotion. First I take a spraybottle with rose water and spray it all over my face. Then I massage a little olive or rosehip oil 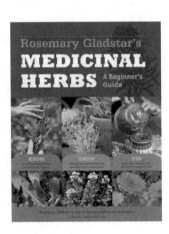 into my face, and voila! The best lotion ever, and you didn't even have to clean the blender!

Pure powdered mineral make up can be found online and at many health food stores, even including mascara and eye liner that are paraben and petroleum free. I particularly like the HopScotch, Piggy Paint, Go Natural, and PeaceKeeper nail polishes, and they each have their own lines of non-toxic polish remover as well.

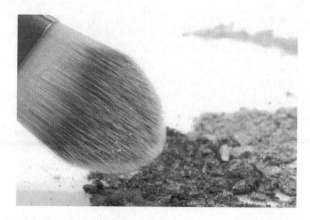

Lotion and hair care is best made at home too, but that's a bigger undertaking. There are great recipes all around the internet, but if you find you just don't have the time, don't despair – there are some trustworthy brands out there. You could make an order from your favorite herbal apothecary, and we also like Desert Essence coconut based shampoo and conditioner, and Shea Yeleen body butter, which is not just free of icky stuff, it's also fair trade.

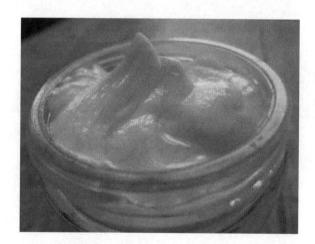

Why does it matter? Because parabens are endocrine disruptors and accumulate in breast cancer tissue, among other problems. They've been shown to be highly absorbable through the skin, and over the years research is showing that they are more harmful than we first thought.

Menstrual products are a quandary. I can remember hating tampons when I was young, and then loving them so much I even used them overnight, for a while. Over the years though, I've broken my tampon dependence and switched just to cloths – and I'll never go back.

Besides all the research about how tampons are harmful to the body, and how products with chlorine and added fragrances can cause problems, for me the biggest factor is this: with cloths I get less cramping, and they never leak. I just cut an old towel into the exact right length for me (I'm tall, so commercial products are usually too short), and zig-zag stitch the edges. I have some sturdy cotton panties that hold the folded-over cloths in place even without a safety pin – and I walk five miles a day back and forth to work! If you cut the cloth to the right size, it really doesn't show under clothes, but you can always wear an extra layer during your cycle if you're worried. And in 11 years of using my cloth pads? Not one single leak. That's pretty fantastic!

If girls feel they really want to use a tampon to participate in sports, make very sure to use organic cotton tampons, and to remove it right away after the activity – the less time you have a tampon in, the better! The Diva Cup is another option, and works well for lots of women.

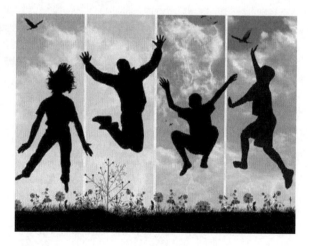

Move Around!

Writing about the lack of physical movement in kids' lives today is a topic that could fill a book. In teaching, what we find is that over and over again, young adults are saying that their younger siblings or their nieces and nephews don't play outside, but spend most of their leisure time indoors on video games. My own daughter, while she doesn't have any video

435

games at my house, does at her father's. One day she said in a conversation: "I was in a bad mood so I killed a bunch of stuff in my [video game] and then I felt better". Those are intense words. It seemed perfectly reasonable to her, and I've heard the same kinds of things said by adults and children in other contexts as well – but she wouldn't have gone outside and killed a bunch of squirrels. So here's the first aspect of moving around: Movement is better therapy for a bad mood than killing video game zombies. Now, any one of my students can tell you I hate video games, so let's not trust my opinion: in medical studies, 30 minutes of "exercise" was more effective at combating depression than prescription Zoloft.

But getting your body moving doesn't just improve your mood – though that's reason enough! The effect of movement on organ systems – in particular the lymphatic and circulatory systems – is critical for daily health, no matter what your age. The lymphatic system doesn't have a pump or any

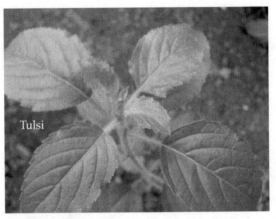
Tulsi

musculature, and depends necessarily on the movement of skeletal muscles to do its work: taking out the trash! Movement is also a big part of prevention of osteoporosis and arthritis – there are many studies showing that girls who jump regularly as children, such as jumping rope, greatly decrease their risk of osteoporosis in adulthood. Why? Because impact and traction are the ways to increase bone density: they're mechanical signals which stimulate the activity of osteoblasts. This means that a child who is jumping and hanging is going to build strong effective bone and connective tissue – all the more important during puberty, when children are growing and solidifying their adult bodies!

Kids don't have to be gymnasts or athletes – it's enough to go for a walk every day, and to go to the playground. Make it a family habit: walk to the playground together, swing from the monkey bars, sprint around the ball field, throw things and catch them. Video games are said to be good for hand-eye coordination, but so is tossing a ball, and when you toss a ball, you get to move your whole body! Do you have an artsy kid? Consider some really creative things like circus arts, juggling, or spinning poi. Do you have an athlete? Consider rock climbing, hiking, or parkour. A team player? Go for ultimate Frisbee. These are all fun activities that also have a strong component of self-teaching and community teaching, as well as community support over competitiveness, and it is not at all abnormal to find young people teaching older people these skills. Now you have an environment where your kid is active and being respected for their accomplishments as an equal in community, which is fantastic!

Emotional Support

Kids – and parents! – need a lot of emotional support during puberty. I'm not really sure which is worse: the crippling drama of the moment to moment crises of being a tween and a teen, or the exhausting endurance sport of trying to be patient from one to the next as a parent. How can we help them, and help ourselves? First, kids need time to process. They need plenty of sleep, and they need some quiet time alone sometimes. It's most ideal if they can get time away from electricity. Think about it: everyone feels a little skittish about those big metal electrical boxes on the city streets. They hum and have scary danger stickers and they're imposing enough that we believe the danger is real. We believe it because on some innate level, we feel it, and we feel it because humans are electrically wired. That hum, the buzz that is so apparent next to one of those big transformer boxes is all around us – modern houses have that same buzz, albeit quieter, running constantly in the background. Now imagine if your five year old was pretending he's a bee, and buzzing everywhere: for a while it's cute, and then it's really, really annoying. You start to feel your stress level rising, and suddenly you're yelling at your sweet little bumblebee.

That same process happens with electricity – and it's not just kids. So get outside, get away from any wifi, electric lights, buzzing boxes. Get away from power lines. Even if you can only do it on the weekends, pack up your kids and go to the beach, to the woods, to the anywhere that is free of electricity. Walk around as a family some, and then give them some freedom to be independent. Start a family tradition of drawing, of journaling; make a game out of it. Everyone could draw a picture of something, and then you could all trade pictures and try to find the thing in the drawing you have. Or you could have a big family game of capture the flag – anything it takes to get kids out of stressville, into nature, and moving around. It will make a huge difference in their moods, and yours! Besides, if you can see your children as people outside of their repetitive dramas, you'll be seeing your kids' real selves, and the same is true in reverse!

Need something a little more immediate? On our back porch we have a hammock, and Amber loves time there. She goes out even in the winter; she'll just take a bunch of blankets and sit herself in the hammock. She takes a book, but I think she doesn't really read it most of the time. I think she's really just laying there letting her head get good and empty: she always comes back in a better mood.

There are so many herbs that can help here too – Tulsi just keeps coming up, again and again. But Linden – a hug in a mug! – is a great helper when you're feeling battered by drama, no matter what your age. Hawthorn and Rose are two particular favorites, especially when personal growth is on the line. Growing, maturing, it's tricky business, for kids and adults. It's scary to be someone new, to react in new ways – but it can be so much easier if you have a little cover. Hawthorn and rose are two plants with fabulous thorns: Wild Rose is a favorite hiding place for bunnies when there are hawks and foxes about, so when you feel like prey, Rose can be your protection. Hawthorn

thorns, spread so far apart, aren't there to protect the tree from dainty eaters like deer, but are an evolution left over from the time of prehistoric giant ground sloths. If your problems seem bigger than hawks and foxes, more likely to gobble you up whole, Hawthorn's got you covered.

Remember that you don't have to have an answer to everything your kids say. Simple little things that convey empathy are sufficient much of the time! Just "oh man, that's rough" is enough to make them feel heard, and saves you having to get so involved in their drama that suddenly you're feeling it with them. Leaving them to figure out their own approach to their problems, even if it doesn't match yours, also gives them the opportunity to learn what works and what doesn't for themselves. It can be really hard to turn off the steady stream of advice that seems to flow so easily from the parental mouth (even if you promised yourself you'd never be that parent!), but time and time again it pays off. And, it saves you from having to relive all the drama yourself. A good hug, a cup of tea, and a nice walk with the dog can be much more powerful – and empowering! - than even good advice.

Well, there you have it. The idea of implementing this much change might seem as daunting as puberty itself – or maybe it's not so different from where your family already is. Wherever you fall, take one step at a time. Make one change, see if it sticks. If not, try again or move on to something else for a while. If it does, great - time for another change!

It can seem extreme, compared to what's "normal" these days, or like a lot of effort compared to what you remember – we didn't have to go through this much when we were kids! Well, when we were kids we didn't have so much media to stand up to, and we went outside to play more readily. There was less junk food available, and we still had recess at school. We didn't carry the internet around in our pockets, and video games were just barely invented. And even at that, we weren't balanced. Even at that, we didn't all grow up healthy: our generation is the one that moved the chronic elder diseases – Parkinsons, MS, diabetes, etc – into middle age, and even younger. When we recognize that, we can realize, in order to find some balance, in order to give our children a chance to be healthier than we are, we might need to take a stand that looks extreme by today's standards. Today's standards aren't necessarily right just because we've come this far, and they aren't necessarily good. But they are common, and standing against them isn't easy.

In order to have success, be honest with your kids. Tell them your goals, give them the whole story. Let them understand what's at risk. It might take them a little while, but I've watched kids become educated and slowly make their own choices about caring for their health. They don't need to be coerced: they need to see family members choosing to take care of themselves, choosing to get educated about their bodies and how to keep them healthy, choosing to share and support one another. It's ok if your family does things differently than their friends' families do. As long as your child understands why, you might be quite pleased to see that they can be willing to make changes that surprise you!

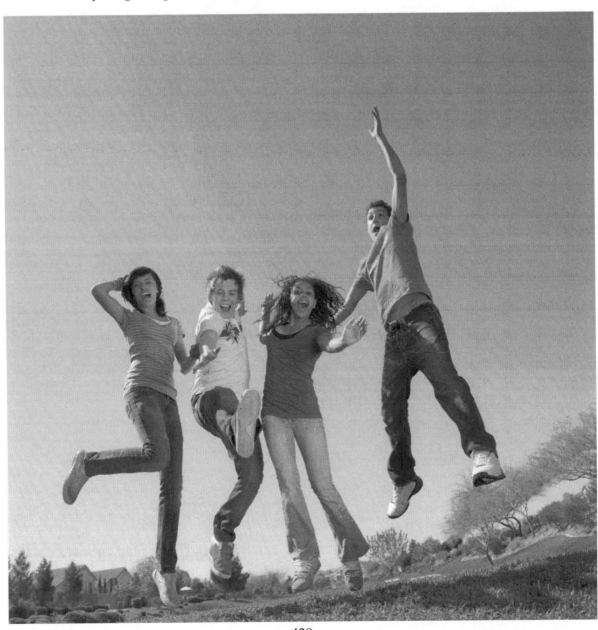

438

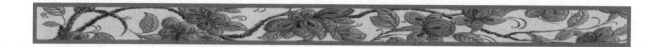

CONTRIBUTORS

In Alphabetical Order

Juliet Blankespoor is the director and primary instructor at the Chestnut School of Herbal Medicine, and hosts some of the most beautiful and comprehensive online herbal courses, featuring botany, plant identification, human anatomy and physiology, cultivation and food preparation, and bioregional roots herbalism. Enraptured by the diversity and intricacies of the green world, Juliet received her B.S. in Botany and furthered her studies by completing over 1200 hours of herbal education. Being obsessed with plants, she has spent much of her adult life botanizing and wildcrafting in diverse settings throughout North America. She is also an avid edible and medicinal mushroom hunter. Her previous herbal business endeavors include an herbal tincture line, natural body care products and prepared wild foods. Her love of plants is also expressed through writing herbal articles and botanical photography. Juliet lives with her family outside of Asheville, NC, where they nurture a small herb farm and the Chestnut Herb Nursery, a medicinal herb and native plant nursery. In addition, she maintains a varied herbal apothecary, primarily from herbs grown on the farm or wildcrafted in the surrounding area. She believes that growing and gathering food and medicine is empowering, revolutionary, and highly entertaining. www.ChestnutHerbs.com

Juliette Abigail Carr, RH (AHG), RNC, is a clinical practitioner and proprietor of Old Ways Herbal School of Plant Medicine (Newfane, VT), which offers hands-on learning in her Botanical Sanctuary forest classroom. Multiple levels of learning include beginner and intermediate courses, and a rigorous apprenticeship tailored to student interest in cultivation, medicine-making, and more. Clinical consultations specializing in the health of women, babies, and children are available, including fertility, pregnancy, and postpartum concerns. She writes a regular column for Plant Healer Quarterly entitled "Heart & Hearth: Radical Home Herbalism," as well as for other magazines and her popular blog. She also works as an RNC at her local birthing center, and raises pastured heritage meats with her family in the grand tradition of multi-tasking Vermont farmers.

Rosalee de la Forêt is a clinical herbalist and Structural Medicine Specialist living in Washington State. She contributes regularly to Herb Mentor where she enjoys answering questions in the community forums and providing herbal education through ebooks, articles, videos and photography. Rosalee's roots in herbal medicine began by studying stone age living and she and her husband cYou can visit her website at www.Rosalee.info

Astrid Grove is a midwife, herbalist and ceremonialist. Her passion for herbs began as a teenager in Vermont and has since wandered through Massachusetts, New York, Maine, Florida, Washington, California and now Colorado. She has gathered much knowledge the last 20 years from her teachers, mainly the plants, and also wise herbalists (mainly Susun Weed) and her clients. She works mostly with women, with the core belief that a culture where women are tended to and cared for will be healthy and strong. She is the co-founder of Red Earth Herbal Gathering, learn more at: www.redearthherbalgathering.com.

Jesse Wolf Hardin is an impactful author, ecosopher, ecological and societal activist, personal counsel, graphic artist, musician, and historian – a champion of both human and bio diversity, as well as of nature's medicines. Wolf has been a featured presenter at hundreds of conferences and universities, and was the creator of cross cultural ecospiritual collaborations appropriately called "Medicine Shows," melding his powerful spoken word with live music, indigenous presenters, and focused activism. With his wife Kiva Rose, he founded Plant Healer's international Good Medicine Confluence gathering in 2008. He is the author of over 800 published articles in over 200 different publications, as well as of over 25 books, his work earning the praises of luminaries such as Gary Snyder, Joanna Macy, Ralph Metzner, Starhawk, and Rosemary Gladstar. He has appeared in *The Encyclopedia of Nature & Religion* (Continuum 2005) and many other compilations. His published works include early titles *Full Circle* , *Kindred Spirit* and *Gaia Eros*, along with *The Practice of Herbalism* and *The Plant Healer's Path* covering the core whys and hows of an herbal practice, *The Healing Terrain* on sense of place, cultivation, and the healing power of nature... as well as an inspiring historical novel *The Medicine Bear*, a book of herbs and empowerment for kids *I'm a Medicine Woman Too!* (Hops Press 2009), and *The Traveling Medicine Show: Pitchmen & Plant Healers of Early America*. His inspiring book *The Enchanted Healer* also comes in a version for an audience beyond herbalists titled *Wonderments*, with both being focused on heightened awareness, the senses, plant spirit and the spiritual heart of healing, A number of his books are available on the Bookstore page of their website, and the remainder can usually be located on Amazon. Wolf's work is also featured in the lauded *Plant Healer Quarterly* as well as the free *Herbaria Monthly* which you can subscribe to on the Plant Healer website. His most recent project is creating courses, writings, audio and visual content for a wide audience of seekers and practitioners under the umbrella The Alder Mysteries Hedge Guild. His latest writings and art in progress are featured sharings on his Patreon pages: patreon.com/HedgeGuild, which you are personally invited to join. As Terry Tempest Williams opined, *"Wolf's voice inspires our passion to take us further —seeing the world whole — even holy."* For more information and opportunities, go to: PlantHealer.org

Kiva Rose Hardin is a botanist, editor, botanical perfumer, and author whose work is rooted in her relationship with plants, fungi, and the more than human world. She lectures and writes on the subjects of plant medicine, mythology, animism, ecology, and depth psychology with an emphasis on fairy tale motifs, embodied enchantment, and the forest as archetype With sixteen years experience as a clinical herbalist and counselor, Kiva now focuses on the formulation of aromatic potions, exploring the delights of woodland terroir, forging a deeper understanding of forest ecology, and writing both fiction and non-fiction. She lives off grid in a remote riparian canyon deep in the Gila Forest of southwest New Mexico with her beloved husband, Jesse Wolf Hardin, and their two children, Inga and Thorn. She spends her days chasing her feral toddler son, gathering wild plants, cooking up woodland foods made with forest-harvested ingredients in her cottage kitchen, and writing whenever she can. Kiva's first book, *The Weedwife's Remedy: Folk Herbalism For The Hedgewise* was published in December of 2019 and her next book, *The Folkloric Forest: Healing Trees For The Hedgewise* is forthcoming from Plant Healer Press in Spring of 2020, and more of her writing, as well as her handcrafted Hedgefumes can be found at The Enchanter's Green http://enchantersgreen.com - She also co-directs the annual Plant Healer's HerbalConfluence in Durango, Colorado, each May and is co-editor of Plant Healer Quarterly with Jesse which you can find at http://planthealer.org

Wendy Hounsel lives in Eugene, OR, where she is an herbalist and RN with the Occupy Medical health clinic, a cardiac nurse at Sacred Heart Medical Center, and a teacher of affordable herbal and holistic health classes in the community. Born and raised in the South, she moved to Eugene in 2013 from New Orleans, where she co-created the herbal medicine program at Common Ground Health Clinic and co-founded Maypop Community Herb Shop. Her work is reflective of her belief in health care as a human right. Common Ground was a free, anti-racist, primary care and herbal clinic until 2013. Occupy Medical offers free primary care, herbal medicine, social work, and wound care to the Eugene community, and is the recipient of the 2015 AHG Community Service Award. Wendy is currently pursuing a graduate degree as a family nurse practitioner in order to facilitate increased access to truly holistic and integrative health care.

Julie James is an herbalist, and director of Green Wisdom Herbal Studies, an herb school based in Long Beach, CA. With over 30 years of experience and training, she focuses on expanding understanding of traditional Western herbalism, deep plant love, medicine-making, wellness and holistic nutrition. She has taught for numerous organizations and events throughout the United States, and has created a large body of herbal education curricula for adults and children. Teaching about plant medicines is her passion and her joy. Check out the calendar of upcoming classes and events at www.greenwisdomherbalstudies.com

Angela Justis is passionate about inspiring children's first curiosity with plants. With an education in biology and herbal medicine, Angela has worked as a science teacher in a hands-on preschool environment for over 10 years. Enjoying this unique opportunity, she shares her passion for plants through the creation of innovative, fun activities for children to learn about herbalism, science and the world around them. Her projects are designed to engage all of a child's senses incorporating an element of crafting that brings out the creative herbalist in kids encouraging facilitate self-expression, learning, and increasing confidence. Angela has developed several educational offerings including a free Introduction to Herbs for Kids mini-course, a six week Kids Summer Camp, and an empowering parent-focused Family Herbs series. She is also has an extensive and ever growing Herbs for Kids section on Mama Rosemary devoted to sharing herbal crafts to inspire children along with of resources for the whole family! Follow Angela's adventures at mamarosemary.com.

Adrie Lester writes and works with plants and people in western MA. She is trained as a clinical herbalist in the traditions of western herbalism, wise women, and Ayurvedic medicine. She is also a practitioner of Shambhala Buddhism, training as a compassionate warrior. She is also a mother, a poet, and a dreamer. You can find her on Instagram @gladheartherbals or at www.gladheartherbals.weebly.com

Phyllis D. Light is a practicing herbalist and health educator with over 30 years of herbal experience. She is traditionally trained in Southern and Appalachian Folk Medicine and began her studies with her Creek/Cherokee grandmother in the deep woods of North Alabama. Phyllis continued her studies with her father and other Appalachian elders, such as Tommie Bass, as well as studies in conventional Western bio-medicine. She holds a Master's of Health Studies degree from the University of Alabama. Phyllis is Director of the Appalachian Center for Natural Health, offering herbal and natural health classes in north Alabama as well as an online program. Phyllis travels and teaches classes in integrative medicine and herbalism at universities, hospitals, and symposia across the country. She is currently secretary of the AHG, president of the American Naturopathic Certification Board, and board member of Old Spirits, New Lives, a non-profit organization dedicated to preserving Indigenous knowledge. Above all, Phyllis devotes herself to building a bridge between traditional knowledge and modern-day science; to help hold sacred the traditional herbal and healing knowledge that has been handed down from generation to generation while embracing the relevant scientific knowledge of today. Please see: www.phyllisdlight.com

Sabrina Lutes has been part of the herbal and healing community since 2001 when she began studying midwifery and doula work. During this time she received her license in massage therapy and opened a busy practice in Gainesville Florida, serving women and families by offering massage, doula services, and blessing ways. Herbs have been a part of her life for nearly 12 years and they infuse her healing and work. Since giving birth to her son in 2008, her focus has narrowed and she has immersed herself in healing her family with herbal medicines as well as helping friends. The richness that is the plant world now encompasses much of her time. She spends her days wild crafting, teaching her son the healing plants as well as cooking and creating with them and being a part of beautiful and gentle mountains of North Carolina she now calls home. She is currently enrolled in Aviva Romm's distance course, has completed Rosemary Gladstar's distance course, studied with Gail Faith Edwards and Pam England as well as attended a myriad of herbal and healing conferences. She is a mother, midwife assistant , retired massage therapist, writer, artist, and lover of the natural world. http://www.heartwoodbirth.com/

Juanita Nelson has been a practicing midwife for 38 years in the Four Corners region of the Southwest, as well as a mother and a grandmother, artist, gardener, and a being of spirit. Included in her practice is ongoing clinical herbal care for moms, babies, and families. She has a particular passion for working with this population, and has always been interested in the ways that herbs can be used safely and effectively to support and assist them. Juanita is licensed as a midwife in both New Mexico and Colorado, and nationally certified as a Certified Professional Midwife, requiring ongoing educational and clinical development on a yearly basis. She works with women and their families in all stages of their lives providing preconception, prenatal, birth, postpartum, newborn, and well-women care, as well as providing breastfeeding and herbal consultations. She worked as the Director of the National College of Midwifery's Mexico Midwifery Immersion Program for many years, giving her the opportunity to work with traditional midwives and herbalists, and to train midwifery students with a goal of providing the cultural sensitivity lacking in so many other programs. Juanita is dedicated to teaching and sharing information with women and families that empowers them to birth naturally and fully present, trusting themselves and their bodies. For more information, check out her website at: FourCornersHomeBirth.com

Erin Piorier is a Traditional Western Herbalist who has been offering consultations, herbal education, and plant-based medicine to the Twin Cities community for over eight years. Erin is available for private consultation and provides her clients with handmade wildcrafted herbal products gathered from the fields and forest of the upper Midwest or grown in her organic garden. She is committed to safe, collaborative, respectful natural health care that treats the whole person. Erin is also a traditional midwife who offer homebirth services as well as classes and consultations focusing on women and family health. Erin is a mother of two children and lives with her family in St. Paul. Find her on the web at www.minnesotaherbalist.wordpress.com

Dr. Kenneth Proefrock graduated from Southwest College of Naturopathic Medicine in 1996. He and his family live deep in the desert of Arizona with numerous reptiles, amphibians, ducks, chickens, horses and goats. Prior to naturopathic medical school, he received degrees in Chemistry and Zoology from Northern Arizona University and worked as a Research and Development/Quality Assurance Chemist for Procter & Gamble. For the past 20 years, he has conducted a very busy Naturopathic medical practice in Surprise, Arizona. He is also sole owner and formulator for Vital Force Naturopathic Compounding, which provides consulting services and a wide variety of unique and effective compounds for other Naturopathic Physicians and their patients. He speaks at conferences across the country sharing his perspective on the modern practice of Naturopathic Medicine. Kenneth is also the Vice-President for the North American Board of Naturopathic Examiners, the chairperson for the biochemistry portion of the Naturopathic Physician's Licensing Exam, and co-founder and current President of the Naturopathic Oncology Research Institute (NORI). In his spare time, when such a thing really exists, he can be found in the desert with his kids, honing his skills in primitive archery, gardening, home-brewing, wildcrafting, reading and writing poetry and studying obscure and old texts on spiritual matters, healing, and philosophy. For more information please see the Vital Force Naturopathic Compounding & Total Wellness Medical Center website.

Anja Robinson is founder of Mana Medicinals, a small holistic health company focused around women's health, nutrition and empowerment. She is a Clinical Herbalist, Ayurvedic Health Counselor, Holistic Nutrition Consultant, Woman's Health Educator and Birth Doula. Anja is passionate about women's health and believes that it is every woman's birthright to have access to a healthy lifestyle in sync with the body's natural rhythms. She believes in the body's innate capacity for healing and a woman's own intuition around her well-being. She helps empower women to take back their health through body literacy, syncing with their natural cycles, hormone and blood sugar regulation as well as holistic nutrition education and body-mind-spirit medicine techniques. She believes that healing is elemental, and through exploring the ways in which the elements are expressed in each woman's individual constitution, insight is gained into the pathways towards optimal health. She is passionate about whole foods nutrition, botanical medicine and sustainability; for bodies and lifestyles, as well as for the Earth. Anja's organic apothecary, whole health consultations and classes represent a compassionate system of healing that bridges traditional western herbalism, holistic nutrition, functional medicine and the wisdom of Ayurveda to help women, families and communities lead healthy, vibrant lives in harmony with our sacred ecosystems. Click here to check out her Mana Medicinals, website.

Aviva Romm is highly respected for her work in botanical medicine, childbirth, women's and pediatric children's health, who practiced as a homebirth midwife and herbalist for over 20 years, before becoming a physician (Yale 2009). Her books include *The Natural Pregnancy Book, Naturally Healthy Babies and Children, Natural Health After Birth, Vaccinations: A Thoughtful Parent's Guide, ADHD Alternatives* (with her husband Tracy Romm, EdD), *A Pocket Guide to Midwifery*, and the textbook *Botanical Medicine for Women's Health* (Elsevier), and are regarded as standards for women's and children's health. Aviva is the Director of *Herbal Medicine for Women*, a distance learning program, and *Pediatrics for Parents*, an innovative and intensive seminar empowering parents. Aviva combines skills as a physician, midwife, and herbalist to offer comprehensive, insightful clinical care, education, writing, and consulting on general health, pregnancy and birth, women's health, women's and pediatric botanical medicine, health and ecology, and natural living. . www.AvivaRomm.com

Elaine Sheff has been studying medicinal plants since 1987. A Clinical Herbalist, she is a graduate of both the Rocky Mountain Center for Botanical Studies and the Southwest School of Botanical Medicine. Elaine is a certified instructor of Fertility Awareness and Natural Family Planning, a safe, effective birth control method used to avoid or achieve pregnancy. She has a long-standing clinical practice providing herbal consultations for individuals with health concerns. Elaine is a bestselling author and teaches herb classes throughout the United States. She was the co-founder of Meadowsweet Herbs and is the co-director of Green Path Herb School in Missoula, Montana. She is the proud mama of two boys, one of whom has special needs. You can often find Elaine in her garden, or cooking gluten free. www.GreenPathHerbSchool.com

Jennie Isbell Shinn is a multi-modality practitioner who in another era might have been the crazy-haired woman living at the edge of town. As it is, she offers massage and bodywork, yoga therapy, spiritual direction, and herbal consultations from her in-home office on an island off the coast of Massachusetts. At the local library and in pop-up spaces, she leads dreamwork circles, beginner- and home-herbalism classes, and free clinics. Jennie is oriented toward vitalism and the wise woman tradition, because of their shared focus on nourishment of whole persons—body, mind and spirit. Her formal training includes masters degrees in the humanities and Christian spirituality, training as a spiritual director, yoga therapist, doula, Reiki practitioner, and two years of herbal apprenticeship and a year of clinical herbal study. Jennie is a 47-year-old mother of a preschooler, who lived a very different—and not nearly as exciting— life prior to her initiation into motherhood. www.jennieisbell.com

Jen Stovall grew up in the North Georgia piedmont and spent her summers in the Southern Appalachians surrounded by the verdant abundance of medicinal plants. Driven and inspired by her thirst for autodidactic education, she left Georgia at seventeen and traveled extensively throughout the US and internationally. As the wind blew her hither and thither, she became entranced by the beauty and mysteries of plant medicine and sought more formal training with many amazing teachers including 7song, Michael Moore, Phyllis D. Light, Patricia Kyritsi Howell, and DeAnna Batdorff. In 2004, Jen moved to New Orleans, a city permeated by the fragrances of Jasmine and Sweet Olive, and where the plants grow in wild abandon, taking over anything in their path. She has spent the years since then learning to love the swamp and getting to know the sub-tropical plants that grow in it. In 2011, Jen opened the collectively run Maypop Community Herb Shop, which many people in the community rely on as their primary source of healthcare. She also graduated with a BSN-RN from Louisiana State University School of Nursing and obtained her NADA Ear Acupuncture Detox Specialist & Trainer license, both of which continue to inform her herbal practice. At present, Jen works as a Community Herbalist & Health Educator, using a blend of Southern Folk Medicine, Western Herbalism, and harm reduction in her classes and with her clients. She has found herbalism to be both a potent tool for pursuing social justice in the world, and a powerful manifestation of the ethical and ideological path she walks in her personal life. She believes that health care should be accessible to everyone and that the most powerful strategy for this is educating and empowering people to choose their own path to health. She is constantly renewed and inspired by witnessing the magic spark that occurs when people are introduced to plant allies through consultations, herb walks, medicine making, & health education. You can catch up with her at jenstovall.com

Debra Swanson is the founder and owner of Dancing Willow Herbs in Durango, Colorado. Dancing Willow was opened in late 1991 and has been a pioneer for herbalism in the four corners. The store has been the heart of community herbalism serving and educating many of thousands of people for a variety of health concerns. Dancing Willow has had a strong commitment to local sustainability, as well as furthering education and opportunities for aspiring Herbalists. Debra has had over 30 years of clinical experience.

Katja Swift is a clinical herbalist and teacher, practicing currently in Boston. Although most people thought she was crazy for moving away from a farm in Vermont (that herbal oasis!), Katja thinks that city people need plants too. In the clinic and in teaching, Katja works with adults, children, and families rebuild their relationships with their bodies and with their own ability to heal. She sees the strength of the grassroots herbal movement coming from the tight web of support and connection those roots weave between people, plants, and the land, and how this counteracts the distancing, anonymizing influences of modern culture. She is also the director of the CommonWealth School of Herbal Medicine www.commonwealthherbs.com

Briana Wiles is author of "Mountain States Foraging" and owner of Rooted Apothecary in Crested Butte, Colorado, where she offers her skills as town herbalist, and practitioner of a form of bodywork called Structural Integration. A Michigan native, she has studied with herbal teachers from across the country with a focus on plants that enrich our lives. After 10 years in the Colorado Rockies she has found a love to talk about plants, while collaborating and learning with others. As an educator she encourages others to listen to the path that is calling to them with excitement for the plant allies that surround us. She is deeply concerned with passing on plant knowledge to the next generation and takes her young son foraging often. She can be found spending her days creating herbal remedies, foraging, writing, teaching, seeing clients, and finding excuses to escape to the woods. rooted-apothecary.com

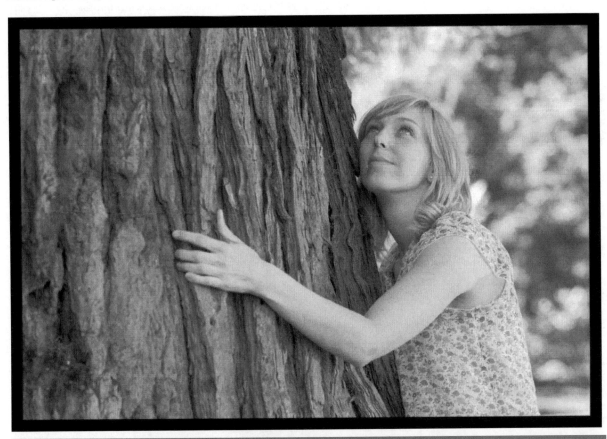

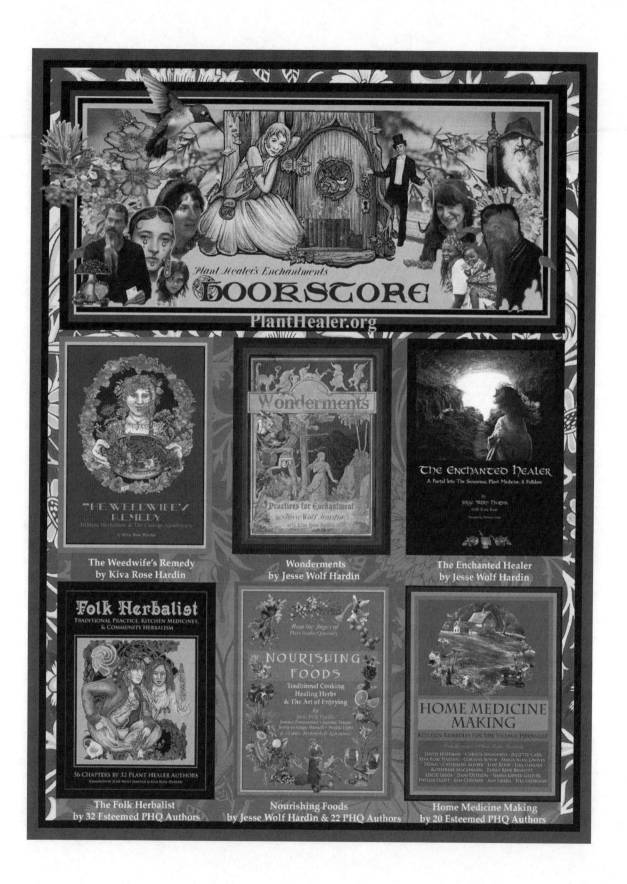

Plant Healer's Enchantments
DOORSTORE

PlantHealer.org

The Weedwife's Remedy
by Kiva Rose Hardin

Wonderments
by Jesse Wolf Hardin

The Enchanted Healer
by Jesse Wolf Hardin

The Folk Herbalist
by 32 Esteemed PHQ Authors

Nourishing Foods
by Jesse Wolf Hardin & 22 PHQ Authors

Home Medicine Making
by 20 Esteemed PHQ Authors

445

Softbound & Color Ebooks – Order from the Bookstore Page at PlantHealer.org

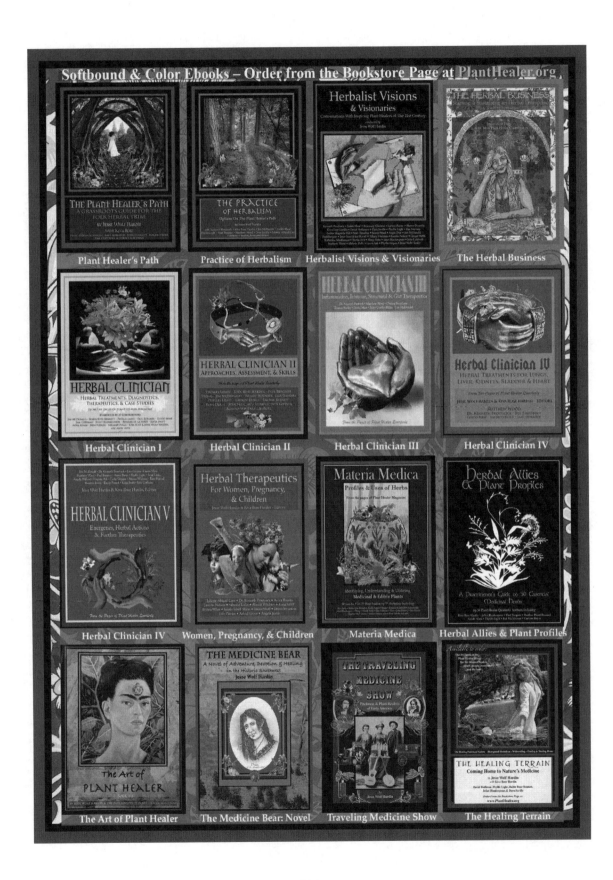

Plant Healer's Path	Practice of Herbalism	Herbalist Visions & Visionaries	The Herbal Business
Herbal Clinician I	Herbal Clinician II	Herbal Clinician III	Herbal Clinician IV
Herbal Clinician IV	Women, Pregnancy, & Children	Materia Medica	Herbal Allies & Plant Profiles
The Art of Plant Healer	The Medicine Bear: Novel	Traveling Medicine Show	The Healing Terrain

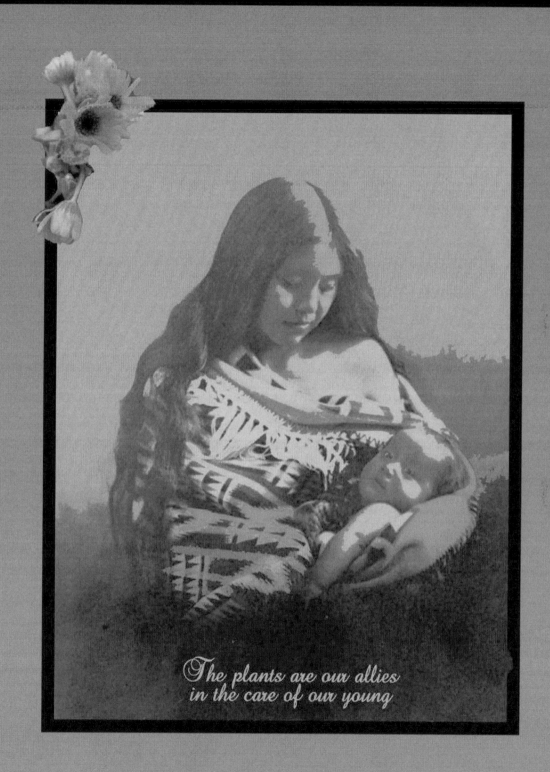

The plants are our allies
in the care of our young

Made in the USA
Middletown, DE
09 September 2024

60645962R00247